Nutrition Science: Challenges and Concerns

Nutrition Science: Challenges and Concerns

Edited by Dorothy Green

SYRAWOOD
PUBLISHING HOUSE
New York

Published by Syrawood Publishing House,
750 Third Avenue, 9th Floor,
New York, NY 10017, USA
www.syrawoodpublishinghouse.com

Nutrition Science: Challenges and Concerns
Edited by Dorothy Green

International Standard Book Number: 978-1-68286-548-4 (Hardback)

Cataloging-in-Publication Data

Nutrition science : challenges and concerns / edited by Dorothy Green.
p. cm.
Includes bibliographical references and index.
ISBN 978-1-68286-548-4
1. Nutrition. 2. Diet. 3. Food. 4. Health. I. Green, Dorothy.
QP141 .N88 2018
613.2--dc23

Printed in China.

TABLE OF CONTENTS

PREFACE

Nutrition is the science that studies nutrients present in the food and the effects of food components on the metabolism, growth and health of humans and animals. It also focuses on how diseases and certain medical conditions can be prevented or limited with a healthy diet. The aim of this book is to present researches that have transformed this discipline and aided its advancement. In this book, using case studies and examples, constant effort has been made to make the understanding of the subject of nutrition science as easy and informative as possible, for the readers.

This book is a result of research of several months to collate the most relevant data in the field.

When I was approached with the idea of this book and the proposal to edit it, I was overwhelmed. It gave me an opportunity to reach out to all those who share a common interest with me in this field. I had 3 main parameters for editing this text:

1. Accuracy - The data and information provided in this book should be up-to-date and valuable to the readers.
2. Structure - The data must be presented in a structured format for easy understanding and better grasping of the readers.
3. Universal Approach - This book not only targets students but also experts and innovators in the field, thus my aim was to present topics which are of use to all.

Thus, it took me a couple of months to finish the editing of this book.

I would like to make a special mention of my publisher who considered me worthy of this opportunity and also supported me throughout the editing process. I would also like to thank the editing team at the back-end who extended their help whenever required.

Editor

Maternal Serum and Breast Milk Vitamin D Levels: Findings from the Universiti Sains Malaysia Pregnancy Cohort Study

Hamid Jan Jan Mohamed[1]*, Angela Rowan[2], Bertram Fong[3], See-Ling Loy[1]

1 Nutrition Program, School of Health Sciences, Universiti Sains Malaysia, Kubang Kerian, Kelantan, Malaysia, **2** Fonterra Co-operative Group Ltd, Palmerston North, New Zealand, **3** Fonterra Research and Development Centre, Palmerston North, New Zealand

Abstract

Background: Vitamin D deficiency has become a global health issue in pregnant women. This study aimed to assess the adequacy of maternal vitamin D status by measuring maternal serum and breast milk 25-hydroxyvitamin D [25(OH)D] levels and to determine the association between maternal serum and milk 25(OH)D levels.

Methods: Data was obtained from the Universiti Sains Malaysia Pregnancy Cohort Study. This study was conducted from April 2010 to December 2012 in the state of Kelantan, Malaysia. Blood samples from pregnant women aged 19 to 40 years were drawn in the second and third trimesters of pregnancy, while breast milk samples at delivery, 2, 6 and 12 months postpartum were collected to analyze for 25(OH)D levels. A total of 102 pregnant women were included in the analysis.

Results: Vitamin D deficiency [25(OH)D $<$50 nmol/L] was detected in 60% and 37% of women in the second and third trimesters of pregnancy, respectively. There were 6% and 23% of women who reached normal level of vitamin D status in the second trimester and the third trimester, respectively. Multivitamin intakes during pregnancy were significantly associated with higher serum 25(OH)D levels in the second trimester ($\beta = 9.16$, $p = 0.005$) and the third trimester ($\beta = 13.65$, $p = 0.003$). 25(OH)D levels in breast milk during the first year of lactation ranged from 1.01 to 1.26 nmol/L. Higher maternal serum 25(OH)D level in the second trimester of pregnancy was associated with an elevated level of 25(OH)D in breast milk at delivery ($\beta = 0.002$, $p = 0.026$).

Conclusions: This study shows that high proportions of Malay pregnant women are at risk of vitamin D deficiency. Maternal vitamin D status in the second trimester of pregnancy was found to influence vitamin D level in breast milk at delivery.

Editor: Kenji Hashimoto, Chiba University Center for Forensic Mental Health, Japan

Funding: This work was supported by Universiti Sains Malaysia Research University Grant Scheme (1001/PPSK/811087). See-Ling Loy was funded by Universiti Sains Malaysia Fellowship Scheme. Financial support for the analytical work was provided through the New Zealand Primary Growth Partnerships post-farmgate dairy programme, funded by Fonterra Co-operative group and the NZ Ministry for Primary Industries (MPI). The funders had no role in study design, data collection and analysis, decision to publish, or preparation of the manuscript.

Competing Interests: Hamid Jan Jan Mohamed has read the journal's policy and has the following conflicts. Angela Rowan and Bertram Fong are employees of Fonterra Co-operative Group Ltd, New Zealand. This funder provided support in the form of analytical materials and expertise, but did not have any additional role in the study design, data collection and analysis, decision to publish, or preparation of the manuscript. The specific roles of these authors are articulated in the 'author contributions' section.

* Email: hamidjan@usm.my

Introduction

The role of vitamin D in health outcomes related to pregnancy, the perinatal period and young children has received considerable interest recently. Although evidence is inconsistent, numerous studies have reported that low maternal vitamin D status is associated with multiple adverse obstetric outcomes and thereby, is increasingly recognized as a global health problem [1]. Vitamin D deficiency during pregnancy has been linked with maternal osteomalacia, gestational diabetes, preeclampsia, small birth size, respiratory diseases, impaired fetal growth and bone development later in childhood [1–4], and more recently adequate vitamin D status has been linked to fetal neurodevelopment [5,6].

The major circulating form of vitamin D in blood is 25-hydroxyvitamin D [25(OH)D]. Serum 25(OH)D is currently accepted as the best biochemical indicator of vitamin D status [7]. However, the level of circulating 25(OH)D required for optimal health is uncertain, and the normal range of 25(OH)D concentration in pregnancy and lactation is unknown [3,8]. Few guidelines have been established in defining the cut-off point for vitamin D status [9–12]. Overall, most researchers agree that serum 25(OH)D levels below 50 nmol/L are defined as deficiency [13–15]. It has been reported that both maternal and infant complications associated with low vitamin D occur more often with a serum vitamin D level below 50 nmol/L [2]. The cut-off that defines vitamin D insufficiency is based on a threshold for serum 25(OH)D above which there is no further suppression of parathyroid hormone (PTH) to reduce bone loss [16,17]. It is suggested that poor calcium intakes require higher 25(OH)D levels to exert maximal suppression of PTH [17].

Breast milk is considered the optimal source of nutrition during early infancy. There are, however, increasing reports that exclusively breastfed infants with inadequate sunlight exposure and without vitamin D supplementation have an increased risk of rickets [18,19]. Although human milk is generally thought to be a poor source of vitamin D [7], there is a need to reassess breast milk vitamin D levels and factors that may affect this in order to investigate a strategy to optimize levels of vitamin D in breast milk and thus improve the vitamin D status of the breastfed infant [19]. This study therefore aimed (i) to examine maternal serum and breast milk 25(OH)D levels; and (ii) to associate 25(OH)D levels in breast milk during the first year postpartum with maternal values during pregnancy.

Materials and Methods

Ethics statement

The present data was obtained from the Universiti Sains Malaysia (USM) Pregnancy Cohort Study which was conducted between April 2010 and December 2012 in Kelantan, Malaysia [20]. The study protocol was approved by the Human Research Ethics Committee of USM and Medical Research Ethics Committee of Ministry of Health, Malaysia.

Study design and participants

A subsample of pregnant women (n = 102) from the cohort with complete data on 25(OH)D analysis were used in this study. Pregnant women were recruited from the Obstetrics and Gynecology (O & G) Clinic of Hospital Universiti Sains Malaysia (HUSM) and Kubang Kerian Health Clinic, Kota Bharu. Convenience sampling technique was adopted for sample selection. The inclusion criteria were defined as i) Malaysian and Malay ethnicity, ii) aged 19 to 40 years, iii) singleton pregnancy, iv) gestational age 24 weeks and less based on the last menstrual period or early ultrasound examination, v) plan to give birth in HUSM, and vi) live within a distance of 50 km from HUSM. Exclusion criteria included i) diagnosed with pre-existing chronic diseases or pregnancy complications and ii) preterm delivery before 37 weeks of gestation. The study objective and procedure were explained to the eligible women and the written informed consent documents were signed. These recruited women were followed from the second trimester (14–24 gestational weeks) to the third trimester of pregnancy (≥32 gestational weeks), 1 to 14 days after giving birth, 2, 6 and 12 months postpartum. Data on sociodemographic characteristics, obstetrics history, smoking status, physical activity, dietary intake, multivitamin intake that included vitamin B complex, vitamin C, folic acid, iron and vitamin D supplements during pregnancy were collected using questionnaires via interview.

Anthropometry

Maternal height was measured with a microtoise tape (Seca 206, Hamburg, Germany) while pre-pregnancy weight was based on the maternal recall. Body mass index (BMI) was computed from maternal weight (kg)/height (m^2).

Dietary assessment

Maternal dietary calcium intake was assessed using 24-hour diet recalls in the second and third trimesters of pregnancy. A four stage, multiple-pass interviewing technique was used to conduct the diet recalls [21]. Atlas of Food Exchanged & Portion Sizes was used to aid in quantifying food portion sizes [22]. Dietary calcium intake was derived using the Nutritionist Pro Diet Analysis software (Axxya Systems LLC., USA) based on Nutrient Composition of Malaysian Foods database and U.S. Department of Agriculture (USDA) Foods database.

Physical activity

A short form of the International Physical Activity Questionnaire (IPAQ) was used to assess maternal physical activity in the second and third trimesters of pregnancy. Three specific types of activity were included in the questionnaire, which were walking, moderate-intensity activities and vigorous-intensity activities. Total activity score was computed from the summation of the duration (in minutes) and frequency (days) of these three types of activity. The score was expressed in metabolic equivalents (Mets-minutes/week) and categorized as low, moderate and high levels of physical activity [23].

25(OH)D analysis

A fasting venous blood sample was collected from each woman in the second and third trimesters of pregnancy. These blood samples were centrifuged at 3500 rpm for 10 min at 4°C (Eppendorf Centrifuge 5810R, Hamburg, Germany). Breast milk samples were collected using a mini electric breast pump (Medela, Illinous, USA) within 1–14 days after delivery, at 2, 6 and 12 months postpartum. Both serum and breast milk samples were stored in −80°C freezer (Thermo Fisher Scientific 702, USA) until analysis. The 25(OH)D analysis was performed by High Performance Liquid Chromatography (HPLC) with a C8 column coupled to an API 3200 Q-trap mass spectrometer (MS, AB SCIEX Framingham, MA, USA), as described by Lewis and Elder [24]. The limit of quantification was at ~2 nmol/L. The serum and breast milk 25(OH)D results were expressed in nmol/L. Breast milk 25(OH)D levels were also shown in IU/L (40 IU/L = 1 ug/L, MW = 404 g/mol) for the purpose of comparison with other studies [19]. Depending on maternal serum 25(OH)D levels, the women were categorized as severe vitamin D deficiency (<25 nmol/L), mild vitamin D deficiency (25–<50 nmol/L), vitamin D insufficiency (50–<75 nmol/L) and vitamin D sufficiency (≥75 nmol/L).

Statistical Analysis

Data was analyzed using IBM SPSS statistics, Version 19.0 (USA). Difference in serum 25(OH)D levels between second and third trimesters of pregnancy was compared using paired t-test. Differences in serum 25(OH)D levels according to maternal factors were compared using One-Way ANOVA. Differences in breast milk 25(OH)D levels during the first year lactation were compared using repeated measures ANOVA. Multiple linear regression analysis with confounders forcibly entered was used to examine the association between maternal factor (independent variable) and serum 25(OH)D level (dependent variables), and the association between maternal serum (independent variable) and breast milk 25(OH)D levels (dependent variable). Skewed data were log-transformed to reduce the influence of outliers. Finding at $p<0.05$ for a two-sided test was considered statistically significant.

Results

Table 1 shows the distributions of pregnant women by characteristics. The mean age of the women was 29.11 years (SD 4.50). Most women were multiparous (42.2%), employed (78.4%) and within normal BMI status (57.8%). Less than 30% of them were supplemented with multivitamin during pregnancy. By comparing to the RNI for pregnant women [25], median percentage of RNI for calcium was below 50%. Generally, the

Table 1. Characteristics of the pregnant women (n = 102).

Variables	Second trimester	Third trimester
Gestational age, weeks [mean (SD)]	18.41 (3.71)	34.56 (1.84)
Age, years [n(%)]		
19–29	62 (60.8)	58 (56.9)
30–40	40 (39.2)	44 (43.1)
Parity [n(%)]		
0	25 (24.5)	
1	34 (33.3)	
≥2	43 (42.2)	
Employment [n(%)]		
Unemployed	22 (21.6)	
Working	80 (78.4)	
Pre-pregnancy BMI, kgm^{-2} [mean (SD)]	22.35 (4.27)	
Pre-pregnancy BMI categories [n(%)]		
<18.5	17 (16.7)	
18.5–24.99	59 (57.8)	
≥25.0	26 (25.5)	
Maternal BMI, kgm^{-2} [mean (SD)]	23.63 (4.19)	26.45 (4.03)
Maternal BMI categories [n(%)]		
<18.5	8 (7.8)	0
18.5–24.99	57 (55.9)	42 (41.2)
≥25.0	37 (36.3)	60 (58.8)
Multivitamin intake [n(%)]		
No	75 (73.5)	77 (75.5)
Yes	27 (26.5)	25 (24.5)
Dietary calcium, mg/day [median (IQR)]	486.81 (318.81–708.41)	485.31 (315.59–788.54)
Activity score, Mets [median (IQR)]	405.00 (120.00–1188.00)	480.75 (198.00–1253.63)
Activity status [n(%)]		
Low	64 (62.7)	59 (57.8)
Moderate	25 (24.5)	39 (38.2)
High	13 (12.7)	4 (3.9)

SD = standard deviation, IQR = interquartile range, BMI = body mass index, Mets = metabolic equivalents.

women had low activity level based on the medium Mets scores [23]. History of smoking or alcohol consumption was not reported among the women.

Maternal serum 25(OH)D levels during pregnancy are indicated in Table 2. In the second trimester, vitamin D deficiency [25(OH)D <50 nmol/L] was detected in 59.8% women. Of

Table 2. Maternal vitamin D levels during pregnancy (n = 102).

Serum 25(OH)D levels	Second trimester	Third trimester	p*
mean (SD)	48.45 (15.27)	58.99 (20.43)	<0.001
Vitamin D status, n (%)			
Severe deficiency (< 25 nmol/L)	4 (3.9)	0	
Mild deficiency (25–<50 nmol/L)	57 (55.9)	38 (37.3)	
Insufficiency (50–<75 nmol/L)	35 (34.3)	41 (40.2)	
Sufficiency (≥75 nmol/L)	6 (5.9)	23 (22.5)	
Total	102 (100.0)	102 (100.0)	

SD = standard deviation.
*p value obtained from paired t-test.

Table 3. Comparisons of maternal serum 25(OH)D levels according to maternal factors during pregnancy (n = 102).

		Serum 25(OH)D, nmol/L			
		Second trimester		Third trimester	
		Mean (SD)	p*	Mean (SD)	p*
Pre-pregnancy BMI, kgm^{-2}	<18.5	52.41 (17.34)	0.166	61.59 (18.16)	0.807
	18.5–24.99	46.02 (15.11)		58.95 (21.53)	
	≥25	51.38 (13.67)		57.38 (19.79)	
Maternal BMI, kgm^{-2}	<18.5	44.00 (17.05)	0.436	-	0.187
	18.5–24.99	47.60 (15.41)		62.19 (19.60)	
	≥25	50.73 (14.75)		56.75 (20.68)	
Multivitamin intake	No	45.31 (12.75)	**0.004**	55.51 (18.10)	**0.002**
	Yes	57.19 (18.32)		69.72 (23.66)	
Dietary calcium, mg/day	T1	45.21 (11.98)	0.318	60.59 (21.55)	0.719
	T2	49.91 (14.68)		59.68 (23.29)	
	T3	50.24 (18.40)		56.71 (16.18)	
Physical activity, Mets	Low	47.66 (15.97)	0.498	58.42 (22.69)	0.745
	Moderate/High	49.79 (14.11)		59.77 (17.06)	

BMI = body mass index, SD = standard deviation, T = tertile, Mets = metabolic equivalents.
*p values obtained from F tests using ANOVA. Bold print shows significant p<0.05.
Dietary calcium in the second trimester: T1 = <378 mg/day; T2 = 378–592 mg/day; T3 = >592 mg/day; Dietary calcium in the third trimester: T1 = <348 mg/day; T2 = 348–657 mg/day; T3 = >657 mg/day.

these, 3.9% women had severe vitamin D deficiency [25(OH)D < 25 nmol/L] and 55.9% women had mild vitamin D deficiency [25(OH)D 25–<50 nmol/L]. The proportion of women having vitamin D deficiency decreased to 37.3% in the third trimester. More than one third of women had vitamin D insufficiency [25(OH)D 50–<75 nmol/L in the second trimester (34.3%) and third trimester (40.2%). Vitamin D sufficiency was found in 5.9% women in the second trimester and 22.5% women in the third trimester. Overall, mean levels of maternal serum 25(OH)D increased significantly from 48.45 nmol/L (SD 15.27) in the second trimester to 58.99 nmol/L (SD 20.43) in the third trimester of pregnancy (p<0.001).

Table 3 presents the comparisons of maternal serum 25(OH)D levels during pregnancy based on several maternal factors. Levels of maternal 25(OH)D were not different according to pre-pregnancy BMI, maternal BMI, calcium intake and physical activity (p>0.05). On the other hand, women with multivitamin intake had significantly higher serum 25(OH)D than those without multivitamin intake in the second (p = 0.004) and third trimesters of pregnancy (p = 0.002). After adjusting for confounders, multivitamin intakes remained significantly associated with serum 25(OH)D levels during pregnancy (Table 4).

Table 5 shows that mean levels of 25(OH)D in breast milk were 1.26 nmol/L, 1.18 nmol/L, 1.01 nmol/L and 1.16 nmol/L at delivery, 2, 6 and 12 months postpartum, respectively. As indicated in Table 6, there were no significant differences in two comparisons of each lactation stage (p>0.05).

The associations between maternal serum and breast milk 25(OH)D levels are shown in Table 7. There was a positive association between serum 25(OH)D level in the second trimester and breast milk 25(OH)D level at delivery (β = 0.002, p = 0.026); whereas breast milk 25(OH)D levels at 2, 6 and 12 months postpartum were not associated with maternal values in the second trimester. Similarly, no association was observed between levels of 25(OH)D in maternal serum in the third trimester and breast milk.

Table 4. Associations between maternal factors during pregnancy and serum 25(OH)D levels after adjusting for confounders[a] (n = 102).

Maternal factors	Serum 25(OH)D in the second trimester, nmol/L[a]		Serum 25(OH)D in the third trimester, nmol/L[a]	
	β (95% CI)	p	β (95% CI)	p
Prepregnancy BMI, kgm^{-2}	−0.06 (−0.74,0.62)	0.855	−0.40 (−1.37,0.57)	0.413
Maternal BMI, kgm^{-2}	−0.20 (−0.90,0.49)	0.562	−0.68 (−1.69,0.33)	0.186
Multivitamin intake	9.16 (2.79,15.53)	**0.005**	13.65 (4.73,22.57)	**0.003**
Dietary calcium, mg/day	0.002 (−0.01,0.01)	0.706	−0.01 (−0.02,0.01)	0.281
Activity score, Mets (log unit)	−1.95 (−4.60,0.71)	0.148	2.18 (−2.20,6.55)	0.326

BMI = body mass index, Mets = metabolic equivalents. Bold print shows significant p<0.05.
[a]Adjusted for maternal age and gestational age.

Table 5. The 25(OH)D levels of breast milk.

Postnatal age	n	25(OH)D levels of breast milk, mean (95% CI)	
		nmol/L	IU/L
At delivery[a]	101	1.26 (1.09, 1.42)	20.16 (17.51, 22.81)
2 months	90	1.18 (1.09, 1.27)	19.21 (17.70, 20.73)
6 months	69	1.01 (0.99, 1.04)	16.39 (15.93, 16.86)
12 months	49	1.16 (1.02, 1.31)	18.80 (16.41, 21.19)

[a]Between 1 and 14 days postpartum.

Discussion

This study provides the first data on vitamin D status in Malaysian pregnant women. Less than 4% of women were shown to have severe vitamin D deficiency (<25 nmol/L) during pregnancy, suggesting that this population may have a low risk of developing maternal osteomalacia [19]. However, 40% to 60% of women were found to have vitamin D deficiency (<50 nmol/L), which may impose negative effects on immune health, bone health, neural development and increase the risk of fracture in the offspring during childhood [26]. Compared to other studies in the Asian region, a relatively lower proportion of maternal vitamin D deficiency was observed in our study. Recent studies in India [27] and China [28] revealed that 74% and 97% of pregnant women had serum 25(OH)D below 50 nmol/L. Although optimal concentrations of maternal 25(OH)D at different gestational periods are not known, there is emerging evidence showing that low vitamin D status (<50 nmol/L) is currently common in pregnant women [8,29].

Despite living in a country with an abundance of sunshine, the majority of women in Malaysia had inadequate levels of vitamin D (<75 nmol/L). This phenomenon could be attributable to the combined influences of darker skin, cultural avoidance of sun exposure and clothing style that cover most of the body while outdoors [29,30]. Green et al. [17] and Moy and Bulgiba [30] found that the means of serum 25(OH)D in Malay women of childbearing age were 43 nmol/L and 36 nmol/L, respectively. Rahman et al. [31] indicated that Malay postmenopausal women had serum 25(OH)D at the mean level of 44 nmol/L. A recent study which was conducted among urban and rural women in Malaysia showed that 25(OH)D concentration was at the mean of 65 nmol/L [32]. Our results which showed maternal serum 25(OH)D levels at 48 nmol/L and 59 nmol/L were comparable to these reported values.

In general, the circulating 25(OH)D levels during gestation do not change [33], although one report from Spain noted a significant decline in 25(OH)D levels by the third trimester of pregnancy [13]. However, the opposite effect was observed in our study. The maternal 25(OH)D levels significantly increased from the second to the third trimesters of pregnancy. This result is in agreement with a Thai study which showed significant increment of maternal serum 25(OH)D levels during the course of pregnancy [14]. Even after removing women who were using vitamin supplementation throughout gestation, the current findings remained similar (data not shown). It is suggested that such enhanced levels of serum 25(OH)D are unlikely to be caused by altered vitamin D metabolism during pregnancy. As reported previously, 25(OH)D levels are relatively unaffected by pregnancy despite there is an increase of calcitriol level during pregnancy and passage of 25(OH)D across the placenta to the fetus [10]. Instead, it could be due to the changes in lifestyle factors towards the end of pregnancy, such as higher vitamin-fortified milk consumption [14] or more sunlight exposure [10] which represents the key factor on influencing vitamin D status. Otherwise, genetic factors and changes in adipose tissue deposition during pregnancy may also effect maternal serum 25(OH)D levels [10,14]. Further investigations are required in this area.

Instead of vitamin D supplementation alone, pregnant women in Malaysia are commonly supplemented with multivitamins which contain 400 IU of vitamin D. These multivitamin intakes were consistently associated with higher maternal serum 25(OH)D levels in the second and third trimesters of pregnancy, which is in line with previous reviews that indicated the positive effect of vitamin D supplementation on increasing serum vitamin D status [7,34]. On the other hand, maternal BMI, pre-pregnancy BMI, dietary calcium intake and physical activity were not significantly associated with serum 25(OH)D during pregnancy. It may be that most women in this study had normal BMI status, did not meet the RNI for calcium intake and were not physically active enough to

Table 6. Comparison of breast milk 25(OH)D levels at different stages during the first year of lactation.

Comparison	25(OH)D levels of breast milk (nmol/L), mean difference (95% CI)	p
At delivery - 2 months	0.17 (−0.29, 0.63)	>0.95
At delivery - 6 months	0.31 (−0.09, 0.72)	0.228
At delivery - 12 months	0.19 (−0.27, 0.64)	>0.95
2 months - 6 months	0.15 (−0.06, 0.35)	0.307
2 months - 12 months	0.02 (−0.27, 0.31)	>0.95
6 months - 12 months	−0.13 (−0.34, 0.09)	0.657

Repeated measures ANOVA within group analysis was applied followed by pairwise comparison with confidence interval adjustment.

Table 7. Associations between maternal serum and breast milk 25(OH)D levels after adjusting for confounders.[a]

Maternal serum 25(OH)D levels, nmol/L	25(OH)D levels of human milk, nmol/L (log)							
	At delivery		2 months		6 months		12 months	
	β	p	β	p	β	p	β	p
Second trimester	0.002 (0,0.003)	**0.026**	0 (−0.001,0.001)	0.591	0 (−0.001,0.001)	0.639	−0.001 (−0.002,0.001)	0.389
Third trimester	0.001 (0,0.002)	0.098	0 (−0.001,0.001)	0.622	0 (−0.001,0.001	0.241	0.001 (−0.001,0.002)	0.424

Bold print shows significant $p<0.05$.
[a]Adjusted for maternal age and prenatal multivitamin intake.

exert an effect on the levels of maternal serum 25(OH)D during pregnancy. Supportive evidence has been reported in a few studies. Nurbazlin et al. [32] showed that body fat percentage did not appear as a significant contributor to 25(OH)D level. Rahman et al. [31] reported a non-significant association between physical activity and 25(OH)D level. Green et al. [17] found that the relationship between 25(OH)D and parathyroid hormone (PTH) concentrations did not differ between women with low, medium or high calcium intake.

As reviewed by Dawodu and Tsang [19], most studies of breast milk vitamin D levels were reported more than two decades ago from North America and Europe. Assessment of vitamin D in breast milk among Asians has not previously been reported. In general, the mean of breast milk total vitamin D activity in healthy lactating women ranged from 10 to 80 IU/L [19]. The 25(OH)D has been shown to contribute to about 33 IU/L of vitamin D activity in breast milk [35], which is relatively higher than our findings that ranged from 16 to 20 IU/L. These levels of breast milk 25(OH)D did not appear to change significantly during the first year of lactation. Since vitamin D levels in breast milk are dependent on maternal vitamin D status [36], the current result is therefore reflecting that maternal serum vitamin D levels remained similar during lactation. A recent study in Malawi indicated that vitamin D was undetectable in breast milk at delivery and 2 months postpartum [37]. Earlier reports have shown that milk of healthy lactating women contains relatively small amount of vitamin D and is a poor source of vitamin D for the infants [10,19].

The 25(OH)D levels in the milk from mothers in our study are closer to that observed in dark skinned than white skinned women [38], which may be attributable to increased skin pigmentation that reduces the skin's ability to produce vitamin D from sunlight. Otherwise, it may reflect low intake of vitamin D or sunlight exposure among the women. Such low levels of vitamin D in breast milk might result in low intake of vitamin D among breastfed infants as compared to the recommended intake of 400 IU/d of vitamin D [10]. It is therefore expected that a significant proportion of exclusively breastfed infants are at risk of vitamin D deficiency. According to Balasubramanian and Ganesh [18], there is rising recognition of vitamin D deficiency during infancy and this has become a public health and pediatric problem in many countries.

It has been reported that cord blood 25(OH)D level was correlated positively with maternal value [27,39], indicating infant vitamin D stores at birth rely on maternal vitamin D status during pregnancy. An early study by Hollis et al. [40] showed that all vitamin D compounds in breast milk were associated with maternal levels during lactation. Our finding provides additional evidence that breast milk 25(OH)D level at delivery was associated with maternal serum 25(OH)D in the second trimester of pregnancy instead of third trimester of pregnancy. This situation may be explained by the mechanism of breast milk vitamin D production. It is possible that there could be some lag between elevated levels of vitamin D in the blood and breast milk whereby times are required to enable vitamin D from the adipose tissue to be made available for milk production. This suggests that maternal vitamin D status during mid gestation is potentially affecting vitamin D level in breast milk at delivery and thereby, influencing vitamin D status of the breastfed infants in their early life. This situation should be of concern, especially if the mother plans to exclusively breastfeed. Currently, there are ongoing research activities which focus on high-dose maternal vitamin D supplementation alone during lactation to increase vitamin D level in breast milk [19].

The present results may not be generalizable to all pregnant women in Malaysia as convenience sampling technique was adopted. Only Malay women within a particular region with specific local ethnic practice were recruited. Also, other factors associated with vitamin D status were not measured, such as PTH and sunlight exposure, as well as influencing factors during lactation which might affect human milk vitamin D levels. Therefore, the findings that indicated a positive association between maternal serum and breast milk vitamin D levels shall be cautiously interpreted as there was limited adjustment for confounders. Nevertheless, this study represents the first study in Malaysia to investigate vitamin D status in pregnant women and breast milk. The present study adds to the small number of studies that have reported vitamin D changes during pregnancy and lactation. These data are important for future intervention studies which aim to increase vitamin D status in pregnant women, lactating women or breastfed infants. Furthermore, application of a longitudinal approach reduces inter-individual variation in studying vitamin D changes during pregnancy and lactation. Also, vitamin D levels in this study were measured using gold standard HPLC-MS method which has greater specificity and increased results precision compared with immunoassays and HPLC-UV methods [41].

In conclusion, vitamin D insufficiency was common in Malay pregnant women. Maternal serum 25(OH)D in the second trimester of pregnancy was potentially associated with 25(OH)D level in breast milk at delivery, which is expected to affect the vitamin D status of the breastfed infant in early life. This result suggests that intervention to optimize vitamin D in breast milk should be started early in pregnancy, rather than during the lactation period.

Acknowledgments

We thank the hospital staff and pregnant women for their cooperation and support throughout the study. We thank Kevin Ma, Fonterra Research and Development Centre for assistance in the laboratory, and Dr Linda Schollum of Fonterra Co-operative Group Ltd for editorial assistance. Vitamin D analysis was conducted by Canterbury Health Laboratories, Christchurch, New Zealand.

Author Contributions

Conceived and designed the experiments: HJJM. Performed the experiments: SLL. Analyzed the data: HJJM SLL. Contributed reagents/materials/analysis tools: AR BF. Wrote the paper: HJJM SLL. Provided analytical and technical support and interpreted the data: AR BF. Final approval of the version to be published: HJJM AR BF SLL.

References

1. Aghajafari F, Nagulesapillai T, Ronksley PE, Tough SC, O'Beirne M, et al. (2013) Association between maternal serum 25-hydroxyvitamin D level and pregnancy and neonatal outcomes: systematic review and meta-analysis of observational studies. BMJ 346: f1169. doi: http://dx.doi.org/10.1136/bmj.f1169
2. Barrett H, McElduff A (2010) Vitamin D and pregnancy: An old problem revisited. Best Pract Res Clin Endocrinol Metab 24(4): 527–539. doi: 10.1016/j.beem.2010.05.010
3. Principi N, Bianchini S, Baggi E, Esposito S (2013) Implications of maternal vitamin D deficiency for the fetus, the neonate and the young infant. Eur J Nutr 52(3): 859–867. doi: 10.1007/s00394-012-0476-4
4. Specker BL (2012) Does vitamin D during pregnancy impact offspring growth and bone? Proceedings of the Nutrition Society 71(01): 38-45. doi: 10.1017/S0029665111003053
5. Whitehouse AJO, Holt BJ, Serralha M, Holt PG, Kusel MMH, et al. (2012) Maternal Serum Vitamin D Levels During Pregnancy and Offspring Neurocognitive Development. Pediatrics 129(3): 485–493. doi: 10.1542/peds.2011-2644
6. Morales E, Guxens M, Llop S, Rodriguez-Bernal CL, Tardon A, et al. (2012) Circulating 25-hydroxyvitamin D3 in pregnancy and infant neuropsychological development. Pediatrics 130(4): e913–e920. doi: 10.1542/peds.2011-3289
7. Thorne-Lyman A, Fawzi WW (2012) Vitamin D during pregnancy and maternal, neonatal and infant health outcomes: a systematic review and meta-analysis. Paediatr Perinat Epidemiol 26 Suppl 1: 75–90. doi: 10.1111/j.1365-3016.2012.01283.x
8. Nassar N, Halligan GH, Roberts CL, Morris JM, Ashton AW (2011) Systematic review of first-trimester vitamin D normative levels and outcomes of pregnancy. Am J Obstet Gynecol 205(3): 208 e1–7. doi: 10.1016/j.ajog.2011.03.058
9. Holick MF, Binkley NC, Bischoff-Ferrari HA, Gordon CM, Hanley DA, et al. (2011) Evaluation, treatment, and prevention of vitamin D deficiency: an Endocrine Society clinical practice guideline. J Clin Endocrinol Metab 96(7): 1911–1930. doi: 10.1210/jc.2011-0385
10. Institute of Medicine (2011) Dietary reference intakes for calcium and vitamin D. Washington, DC: The National Academies Press.
11. Ross AC, Manson JE, Abrams SA, Aloia JF, Brannon PM, et al. (2011) The 2011 report on dietary reference intakes for calcium and vitamin D from the Institute of Medicine: what clinicians need to know. J Clin Endocrinol Metab 96(1): 53–58. doi: 10.1210/jc.2010-2704
12. DSM (2012) DSM Nutritional Products. Global vitamin D map launched – DSM calls for urgent action to address major public health issue. Kaiseraugst, Switzerland: Press Release.
13. Fernandez-Alonso AM, Dionis-Sanchez EC, Chedraui P, Gonzalez-Salmeron MD, Perez-Lopez FR, et al. (2012) First-trimester maternal serum 25-hydroxyvitamin D(3) status and pregnancy outcome. Int J Gynaecol Obstet 116(1): 6–9. doi: 10.1016/j.ijgo.2011.07.029
14. Charatcharoenwitthaya N, Nanthakomon T, Somprasit C, Chanthasenanont A, Chailurkit L, et al. (2013) Maternal vitamin D status, its associated factors and the course of pregnancy in Thai women. Clin Endocrinol 78: 126–133. doi: 10.1111/j.1365-2265.2012.04470.x
15. Song SJ, Zhou L, Si S, Liu J, Zhou J, et al. (2013) The high prevalence of vitamin D deficiency and its related maternal factors in pregnant women in Beijing. PLoS One 8(12):e85081. doi: 10.1371/journal.pone.0085081
16. Aloia JF, Talwar SA, Pollack S, Feuerman M, Yeh JK (2006) Optimal vitamin D status and serum parathyroid hormone concentrations in African American women. Am J Clin Nutr 84(3): 602–609.
17. Green TJ, Skeaff CM, Rockell JE, Venn BJ, Lambert A, et al. (2008) Vitamin D status and its association with parathyroid hormone concentrations in women of child-bearing age living in Jakarta and Kuala Lumpur. Eur J Clin Nutr 62(3): 373–378. doi:10.1038/sj.ejcn.1602696
18. Balasubramanian S, Ganesh R (2008) Vitamin D deficiency in exclusively breast-fed infants. Indian J Med Res 127(3): 250–255.
19. Dawodu A, Tsang RC (2012) Maternal vitamin D status: effect on milk vitamin D content and vitamin D status of breastfeeding infants. Adv Nutr 3(3): 353–361. doi: 10.3945/an.111.000950
20. Loy SL, Hamid Jan JM (2014) The Universiti Sains Malaysia Pregnancy Cohort Study: Maternal-infant adiposity development until the first year of life. Health Environ J 5(1): 50–64.
21. Fahmida U, Dillon DHS (2011) Nutritional assessment 2nd edition. Jakarta: South East Asian Ministers of Education Organization, Regional Centre for Food and Nutrition (SEAMEO RECFON), University of Indonesia.
22. Suzana S, Noor Aini MY, Nik Shanita S, Rafidah G, Roslina A (2009) Atlas of food exchanges & portion sizes. 2nd ed. Kuala Lumpur: MDC Publishers Sdn Bhd (91168-A).
23. IPAQ (2005) Guidelines for Data Processing and Analysis of the International Physical Activity Questionnaire (IPAQ) – Short and Long Forms, revised on November 2005. Available: http://www.ipaq.ki.se/scoring.pdf Accessed 15 March 2010.
24. Lewis JG, Elder PA (2008) Serum 25-OH vitamin D2 and D3 are stable under exaggerated conditions. Clin Chem 54(11): 1931–1932. doi: 10.1373/clinchem.2008.111526
25. NCCFN (2005) Recommended nutrient intakes for Malaysia. A report of the Technical Working Group on Nutritional Guidelines. Putrajaya: National Coordinating Committee on Food and Nutrition, Ministry of Health Malaysia.
26. Javaid MK, Crozier SR, Harvey NC, Gale CR, Dennison EM, et al. (2006) Maternal vitamin D status during pregnancy and childhood bone mass at age 9 years: a longitudinal study. Lancet 367(9504): 36–43.
27. Sahu M, Bhatia V, Aggarwal A, Rawat V, Saxena P, et al. (2009) Vitamin D deficiency in rural girls and pregnant women despite abundant sunshine in northern India. Clin Endocrinol (Oxf) 70(5): 680–684. doi:10.1111/j.1365-2265.2008.03360.x
28. Song SJ, Zhou L, Si S, Liu J, Zhou J, et al. (2013) The high prevalence of vitamin D deficiency and its related maternal factors in pregnant women in Beijing. PLoS One: 8(12):e85081. doi: 10.1371/journal.pone.0085081
29. Lucas R, Xiang F, Ponsonby AL (2013) Vitamin D sufficiency in pregnancy. BMJ 346: f1675. doi: 10.1136/bmj.f1675
30. Moy FM, Bulgiba A (2011) High prevalence of vitamin D insufficiency and its association with obesity and metabolic syndrome among Malay adults in Kuala Lumpur, Malaysia. BMC Public Health 11: 735. doi:10.1186/1471-2458-11-735

31. Rahman SA, Chee WS, Yassin Z, Chan SP (2004) Vitamin D status among postmenopausal Malaysian women. Asia Pac J Clin Nutr 13(3): 255–260.
32. Nurbazlin M, Chee WS, Rokiah P, Tan AT, Chew YY, et al. (2013) Effects of sun exposure on 25(OH) vitamin D concentration in urban and rural women in Malaysia. Asia Pac J Clin Nutr 22(3): 391–399. doi: 10.6133/apjcn.2013.22.3.15
33. Perez-Lopez FR (2007) Vitamin D: the secosteroid hormone and human reproduction. Gynecol Endocrinol 23(1): 13–24.
34. De-Regil LM, Palacios C, Ansary A, Kulier R, Pena-Rosas JP (2012) Vitamin D supplementation for women during pregnancy. Cochrane Database Syst Rev 2: CD008873. doi: 10.1002/14651858.CD008873.pub2
35. Reeve LE, Chesney RW, DeLuca HF (1982) Vitamin D of human milk: identification of biologically active forms. Am J Clin Nutr 36(1): 122–126.
36. Hollis BW, Wagner CL (2004) Vitamin D requirements during lactation: high-dose maternal supplementation as therapy to prevent hypovitaminosis D for both the mother and the nursing infant. Am J Clin Nutr 80(6 suppl):1752S–1758S.
37. Amukele TK, Soko D, Katundu P, Kamanga M, Sun J, et al. (2013) Vitamin D levels in Malawian infants from birth to 24 months. Arch Dis Child 98(3): 180–183. doi: 10.1136/archdischild-2012-302377
38. Specker BL, Tsang RC, Hollis BW (1985) Effect of race and diet on human-milk vitamin D and 25-hydroxyvitamin D. Am J Dis Child 139(11): 1134–1137.
39. Maghbooli Z, Hossein-Nezhad A, Shafaei AR, Karimi F, Madani FS, et al. (2007) Vitamin D status in mothers and their newborns in Iran. BMC Pregnancy Childbirth 7: 1. doi: 10.1186/1471-2393-7-1
40. Hollis BW, Pittard WB 3rd, Reinhardt TA (1986) Relationships among vitamin D, 25-hydroxyvitamin D, and vitamin D-binding protein concentrations in the plasma and milk of human subjects. J Clin Endocrinol Metab 62(1): 41–44.
41. Roth HJ, Schmidt-Gayk H, Weber H, Niederau C (2008) Accuracy and clinical implications of seven 25-hydroxyvitamin D methods compared with liquid chromatography-tandem mass spectrometry as a reference. Ann Clin Biochem 45(Pt 2): 153–159. doi: 10.1258/acb.2007.007091

2

Pyrophosphate-Mediated Iron Acquisition from Transferrin in *Neisseria meningitidis* Does Not Require TonB Activity

Francis Biville*, Christophe Brézillon, Dario Giorgini, Muhamed-Kheir Taha

Unité des Infections Bactériennes invasives, Département Infection et Epidémiologie, Institut Pasteur, Paris, France

Abstract

The ability to acquire iron from various sources has been demonstrated to be a major determinant in the pathogenesis of *Neisseria meningitidis*. Outside the cells, iron is bound to transferrin in serum, or to lactoferrin in mucosal secretions. Meningococci can extract iron from iron-loaded human transferrin by the TbpA/TbpB outer membrane complex. Moreover, *N. meningitidis* expresses the LbpA/LbpB outer membrane complex, which can extract iron from iron-loaded human lactoferrin. Iron transport through the outer membrane requires energy provided by the ExbB-ExbD-TonB complex. After transportation through the outer membrane, iron is bound by periplasmic protein FbpA and is addressed to the FbpBC inner membrane transporter. Iron-complexing compounds like citrate and pyrophosphate have been shown to support meningococcal growth *ex vivo*. The use of iron pyrophosphate as an iron source by *N. meningitidis* was previously described, but has not been investigated. Pyrophosphate was shown to participate in iron transfer from transferrin to ferritin. In this report, we investigated the use of ferric pyrophosphate as an iron source by *N. meningitidis* both *ex vivo* and in a mouse model. We showed that pyrophosphate was able to sustain *N. meningitidis* growth when desferal was used as an iron chelator. Addition of a pyrophosphate analogue to bacterial suspension at millimolar concentrations supported *N. meningitidis* survival in the mouse model. Finally, we show that pyrophosphate enabled TonB-independent *ex vivo* use of iron-loaded human or bovine transferrin as an iron source by *N. meningitidis*. Our data suggest that, in addition to acquiring iron through sophisticated systems, *N. meningitidis* is able to use simple strategies to acquire iron from a wide range of sources so as to sustain bacterial survival.

Editor: Eric Cascales, Centre National de la Recherche Scientifique, Aix-Marseille Université, France

Funding: This work was supported by Pasteur Institute and the Institut de veille sanitaire. The funders had no role in study design, data collection and analysis, decision to publish, or preparation of the manuscript.

Competing Interests: The authors have declared that no competing interests exist.

* Email: fbiville@pasteur.fr

Introduction

Neisseria meningitidis (*Nm*) is found exclusively in humans, and although it is frequently present in the nasopharynx of asymptomatic carriers, it may be the causative agent of life-threatening invasive infections such as septicemia and meningitis [1]. Ability to acquire iron from various sources has been demonstrated to be a major determinant in the pathogenesis of *Nm* [2]. In mammals, iron sequestration is the main form of nutritional immunity [3], [4]. Obtaining iron required for bacterial growth is a challenge, since 99.9% of total body iron is sequestered inside the cells [5]. Outside the cells, iron is bound to transferrin in the serum or to lactoferrin in mucosal secretions [2]. Another iron source in mammals is heme, mainly contained in hemoproteins like hemoglobin. When freed after erythrocyte lysis, most hemoglobin is bound by haptoglobin. Hemoglobin degradation allows the release of heme that is sequestered by hemopexin to prevent its toxicity [5]. Bacterial acquisition of iron in mammals requires the activity of transport systems allowing uptake of iron and/or heme bound to proteins. In *Nm*, the HmbR [6] and HpuAB outer membrane transport systems [7] allow the bacteria to use heme-loaded proteins as a heme source. HmbR and HpuAB systems differ according to their substrate specificity. HmbR can obtain heme from hemoglobin with better efficiency for human hemoglobin [6]. In contrast, HpuAB not does not exhibit specificity toward the human forms of its two substrates, characterized as hemoglobin and haptoglobin-hemoglobin complexes [8]. *Nm* strains express HmbR, HpuAB or both systems [9]. Most invasive strains express HmbR alone or both heme uptake systems, as reported in isolates of the hyperinvasive genotype ST-11 [9]. Strains expressing only the HpuAB heme transport system were mostly described as carriage strains [9]. The periplasmic heme binding protein and the inner membrane heme transporter are not yet identified. Inside the cytoplasm, heme is degraded by HemO, a bacterial heme oxygenase, thus allowing the release of iron [10].

The main source of iron in blood is iron-loaded transferrin. Iron is extracted from iron-loaded human transferrin by the TbpA/TbpB outer membrane complex [11]. Also, *Nm* expresses the LbpA/LbpB outer membrane complex, which can extract iron from iron-loaded human lactoferrin [12]. After transportation through the outer membrane, iron is bound by the periplasmic protein FbpA and directed to the FbpBC inner membrane transporter [13]. Most of heme and iron outer membrane transport systems require energy provided by the ExbB-ExbD-TonB system [14]. TonB independent iron transport processes were also reported. [15], [16]. Alongside the two systems allowing the obtaining of iron contained in human protein, *Neisseriae* genomes encode systems enabling uptake of free iron. The transport of iron-loaded xenosiderophores has been investigated in *Neisseria gonorrhoeae* [17]. Iron-loaded xenosiderophores are transported by the TonB-dependent outer membrane transporter FetA [18], sent by FbpA to the inner membrane FbpBC transporter and degraded inside the cytoplasm to allow iron release [15]. TonB-independent transport of xenosiderophores through the outer membrane has been described in *N. gonorrhoeae*, but the mechanism remains hypothetical [17]. In contrast, the role of the FbpABC inner membrane ABC transporter in TonB-independent use of enterobactin, salmochelin and other xenosiderophores has been clearly demonstrated [15]. The absence of siderophore biosynthesis was reported for *Nm* [19]. Only the use of a ferrated form of three dihydroxamate siderophores (schizokinen, arthrobactin, aerobactin) can stimulate growth of *Nm* [20]. Recently, the binding of Ferric enterobactin by the factor H binding protein was described [21].

Iron-complexing compounds like citrate and pyrophosphate have been shown to support *Nm* growth *ex vivo* [19]. The use of iron pyrophosphate as an iron source by *N. meningitis* was described, but not investigated. Pyrophosphate-dependent use of iron was investigated in *Escherichia coli* [22], [23]. In that bacterium, pyrophosphate facilitates the enterobactin-dependent iron uptake process [24]. In the absence of enterobactin, pyrophosphate acts as an iron chelator and strongly inhibits *E. coli* growth [25]. Also, pyrophosphate was shown to participate in iron transfer from transferrin to ferritin [26]. This report aimed to investigate the mechanism that allows use of ferric pyrophosphate as an iron source and its impact on meningococcal virulence.

Materials and Methods

Ethics statement

This study was carried out in strict accordance with the European Union Directive 2010/63/EU (and its revision 86/609/EEC) on the protection of animals used for scientific purposes. Our laboratory has the administrative authorization for animal experimentation (Permit Number 75–1554) and the protocol was approved by the Institut Pasteur Review Board that is part of in the Regional Committee of Ethics of Animal Experiments of the Paris region (CETEA 2013-0190).

Bacterial strains and plasmids

Bacterial strains and plasmids used in this study are listed in Table 1.

Media and growth conditions

Human (Sigma; ref: T4132) and bovine (Sigma; ref: T1283) transferrin were prepared in water at 0.25 mM final concentration, filter-sterilized and stored at −20°C. Bovine hemoglobin (Sigma; ref: H2500) was dissolved in 100 mM NaCl, filter-sterilized and stored at −20°C. The hemoglobin concentration was calculated on the basis of the heme monomer. Tetrasodium pyrophosphate (Sigma; ref: P8010) was prepared at a 200 mM final concentration in water, buffered at pH 7 with HCl, filter-sterilized and stored at room temperature. Imdidodiphosphate (Sigma; ref: 10631) and methylenediphosphonic acid (Sigma; ref: M9508) were prepared according to the same protocol and stored at −20°C. Iron pyrophosphate (Sigma; ref: P6526) was prepared in water at a 10 mM final concentration, filter-sterilized and stored at room temperature. Desferal (Sigma; ref: D9533) was prepared in water at 15 mM, filter-sterilized and stored at −20°C. All solutions were filter-sterilized using 0.20 μm Millipore filters. *Nm* strains were grown on GCB agar plates supplemented with Kellogg supplement solution [27]. To create iron depletion, supplement S2 was substituted for desferal (30 μM final concentration). When required, kanamycin (Kan) and erythromycin (Ery) were added at 50 μg/ml, and 2 μg/ml respectively. *Nm* strains were grown at 37°C under a 5% CO_2 atmosphere. *E. coli* strains were grown on LB medium [28] at 37°C. Solid media agar contained 1.5% agar.

Use of iron source assays

To evaluate the effect of mutation of the *Nm* capacity to use various iron sources, strains were first isolated on GCB plates supplemented with S1 and S2 complements and grown for 18 h at 37°C in the presence of 5% CO_2. Bacteria were isolated on the test plates and incubated for 18 h at 37°C in the presence of 5% CO_2. Iron-depleted GCB plates (see above) were supplemented with the tested iron sources.

Invasion assays in mice

Nm tested strains were grown on GCB plates for 18 h at 37°C under a 5% CO_2 atmosphere. Bacteria collected from one plate were suspended in physiological serum and the density of the cell suspension was adjusted to 2.5×10^6 bacteria/ml. Four-hundred μl of the bacterial suspension were supplemented with 100-μl of the tested iron source, and the mixture was inoculated intraperitoneally into 7-week-old BalbC mice (Janvier). The number of viable bacteria before inoculation was then determined by plating serial dilutions on GCB plates. At t = 6 h, blood and intraperitoneal samples were collected, diluted in physiological serum and serial dilutions were plated on GCB plates supplemented with S1 and S2 and kanamycin (50 μg/ml). After 18 h incubation at 37°C under a 5% CO_2 atmosphere, colonies were counted.

Imaging of bioluminescence from animals

Mice were then anesthetized with a constant flow of 2.5% isoflurane mixed with oxygen, using an XGI-8 anesthesia induction chamber (Xenogen Corp.). The mice were maintained for at least 5 min. Bacterial infection images were acquired using an IVIS spectrum system (Xenogen Corp., Alameda, CA) according to instructions from the manufacturer. Analysis and acquisition were performed using Living Image 3.1 software (Xenogen Corp.). Images were acquired using a 1 min integration time with a binning of 16. All other parameters were held constant. Quantifying was performed using the photons per second emitted by each mouse.

Genetic techniques

Nm was transformed using linear 3-partner PCR fragments obtained as described below. *Nm* strains were grown on GCB plates for 18 h at 37°C under a 5% CO_2 atmosphere. Bacteria collected from one plate were suspended in GCB medium completed with S1 and S2 supplements and MgCl2 at a 5 mM final concentration (GCBMg medium). Bacterial density was adjusted at OD_{600}:1. Three hundred microliters of the bacterial suspension were placed inside a well of a 24-well multiwell plate (Falcon), supplemented with a PCR fragment (100 to 500 ng) and incubated for 30 min at 37°C under a 5% CO_2 atmosphere. The mixture was supplemented with 700 μl of GCBMg medium and incubated for 5 h at 37°C under a 5% CO_2 atmosphere. One-

Table 1. Strains and plasmids used in this study.

Escherichia coli strain	**Genotype**	**Origin**
Xl1 blue	F^- *supE44 hdsR17 recA1 endA1 gyrA46 thi relA1 lac*$^-$ *F' proAB*$^-$ *lacI*^{q} *lacZΔM15 Tn10* (Tet^R)	Laboratory collection
***Nm* strains**	**Genotype**	**Origin**
2C4.3	wild-type strain	[59]
2C4.3::*lux*	2C4.3::*lux*, Km^R	This work
2C4.3 *ΔtonB::Ery*	2C4.3 *ΔtonB::Ery*, Ery^R	This work
2C4.3 *ΔfbpABCD::Ery*	2C4.3 *ΔfbpABCD::Ery*, Ery^R	This work
2C4.3 *ΔporA::Ery*	2C4.3 *ΔporA::Ery*, Ery^R	This work
2C4.3 *ΔporB::Ery*	2C4.3 *ΔporB::Ery*, Ery^R	This work
2C4.3::*lux ΔtonB::Ery*	2C4.3::*lux ΔtonB::Ery*, Km^R, Ery^R	This work
Plasmids	**Antibiotic resistance**	**Origin**
pXen-13	Amp^R	Xenogen
pTE-KM	Amp^R, Km^R	[29]
pDG33	Amp^R	This work
pDG34	Amp^R, Km^R	This work

hundred and 500 µl samples of the mixture were plated on GCB complete medium supplemented with selective antibiotic and incubated for 18 h at 37°C under a 5% CO_2 atmosphere. Six clones were isolated on selective medium, screened using PCR and positive clones were stored at −80°C in complete GCB medium supplemented with glycerol (20% final concentration). For *fbpABC* mutants, GCB supplemented with S1 Kellogg supplement solution [27], bovine hemoglobin (10^{-6} M) and erythromycin was used as selective medium.

DNA manipulations

DNA fragments were amplified from chromosomal *Nm* strain 2C4.3 in a Hybaid PCR thermocycler using Phusion DNA polymerase (Finnzymes). Restriction, modification and ligation were carried out according to the manufacturer's recommendations. Purification of DNA fragments from the PCR reaction, the restriction reaction and agarose gels was performed using the Macherey-Nagel NucleoSpin Extract II kit.

Construction of the 2C4.3::*lux* strain

Plasmid pXen-13 (Xenogen Corp., Alameda, CA) containing the *Photorhabdus luminescens luxCDABE* operon was modified by insertion of an *Nm*-specific promoter sequence. To express the *luxCDABE* operon under the PproB meningococcal promoter *Nm*, a 600 bp promoter sequence of the *porB* gene (PporB) from strain 2C4.3 was amplified using primers PorB3 and PorB4 (Table 2) and cloned into a *Bam*HI site upstream of the *luxCDABE* operon after Kleenow filling. The generated plasmid was named pDG33. The fragment encompassing the *luxCDABE* cassette and the *porB* promoter was extracted by digesting pDG33 with KpnI and SacI restriction enzymes and inserted into the *Bam*HI site of plasmid pTE-KM [29], upstream from the kanamycin resistance cassette *aph3'*. In the resulting vector, named pDG34, the PporB-*luxCDABE-aph3'* was flanked by the meningococcal *pilE* gene and, 120 bp downstream, by the *pilE* gene to facilitate chromosomal integration upon transformation.

Construction of knockout mutants in *Nm*

Non-polar mutations that delete entire genes were created by allelic exchange with the non-polar Ery gene cassette. For knockout genes in *Nm*, the methods already described require the use of *E. coli* to clone, in plasmids, *Nm* DNA fragments containing a gene of interest, disrupted by insertion of a cartridge expressing antibiotic resistance [30]. These methods require cloning steps and are subordinated to the stability of the recombinant plasmids and their absence of toxicity when introduced into *E. coli*. To avoid the use of cloning steps, we directly introduced into *Nm* the disrupted genes contained in the DNA fragment obtained using a two-step PCR procedure. The two-step PCR procedure was used to produce a PCR product in which the Ery gene cassette is flanked by arms of about 500 to 1,000 bp, corresponding to sequences upstream from the start codon and downstream from the stop codon of the gene of interest. The erythromycin cartridge was amplified from plasmid pMGC20 [31] using Eram1 and Eram3 as primers (Table 2). The primers used for *tonB* were TonBAmtAmt and TonBAmtAvlEry for the upstream region and TonBAvlAmtEry and TonBAvlAvl for the downstream region (Table 2). For *porA*, the primers used were PorAAmtAmt and PorAAmtAvlEry for the upstream region and PorAAvlAmtEry and PorAAvlAvl for the downstream region (Table 2). For *porB*, the primers used were PorBAmtAmt and PorBAmtAvlEry for the upstream region and PorBAvlAmtEry and PorBAvlAvl for the downstream region (Table 2). To delete *fbpABC*, the primers used were FbpABCAmtAmt and FbpABCAmtAvlEry for the upstream region and FbpABCAvlAmtEry and FbpABCAvlAvl for the downstream region (Table 2). For each gene of interest, the sequence of the 5′ end of the reverse primer used to amplify the upstream region was anti-parallel to the 5′end of Eram1 primer and the sequence of the 5′ end of the forward primer used to amplify the downstream region was anti-parallel to the 5′ Eram3 primer. For each gene of interest, a 1 µl sample of upstream and downstream regions was mixed with 1 µl of the erythromycin cartridge and the mixture was amplified using primers TonBAmtAmt and TonBAvlAvl for *tonB*, PorAAmtAmt

Table 2. Primers used in this study.

Name	Sequence 5′-3′
Eram 1	**GCAAACTTAAGAGTGTGTTGA**
Eram 3	**AAGCTTGCCGTCTGAATGGGACCTCTTTAGCTTCTTGG**
PorB3	**GGTGCTGAAGCACCAAGTGA**
PorB4	**GGCAATCAGGGATTTTTTCA**
TonBAmtAmt	**ACAGAATCGCATTGATCAGAATACCG**
TonBAmtAvlEry	**TCAACACACTCTTAAGTTTGCTAAAATTCGTTCTTTATCCATAATTC**
TonBAvlAmtEry	**CCAAGAAGCTAAAGAGGTCCCATTCAGACGGCAAGCTTAGTCCCCGTCAAGTTTGAATTGAATTAG**
TonBAvlAvl	**TCAGCTATCCTTTTGATTAAGCAGGC**
FbpABCAmtAmt	**GACGCATTGAGAAAAGAAATCCGCCACCTCCAAT**
FbpABCAmtAvlEry	**TCAACACACTCTTAAGTTTGCTCAGGGCTGCGGCAAGCAGTGCGTATCGGATAG**
FbpABCAvlAmtEry	**CCAAGAAGCTAAAGAGGTCCCATTCAGACGGCAAGCTTACGGTCCCGCCCTGTTCTTCCCCGGAAATACC**
FbpABCAvlAvl	**ATGGCGGCGGCTTGGACGGTGCGGGGTTCTG**
PorAAmtAmt	**TGTAGATGCCCGACGGTCTTTATAGCGG**
PorAAmtAvlEry	**TCAACACACTCTTAAGTTTGCTGTAAATTTGATAAAAACCTAAAAACATCG**
PorAAvlAmtEry	**CCAAGAAGCTAAAGAGGTCCCATTCAGACGGCAAGCTTGAAGCGGATAGCTTTGTTTTTGACGGCTCG**
PorAAvlAvl	**TATATTCCGCCATCTCTAAGATTTACAGCG**
PorBAmtAmt	**ATCGGTTCCGTACTATTTGTACTGTCTGCG**
PorBAmtAvlEry	**TCAACACACTCTTAAGTTTGCTCGTAGTTAAGAAATTTAAGCAGACCTAAC**
PorBAvlAmtEry	**CCAAGAAGCTAAAGAGGTCCCATTCAGACGGCAAGCTTTCTGAAAAGATTGGTATCAACAAAAAGCCTG**
PorBAvlAvl	**ACAGATAGTAGGGAACCGATTCACTTGGTG**

and PorAAvlAvl for *porA*, PorBAmtAmt and PorBAvlAvl for *porB* and FbpABCAmtAmt and FbpABCAmtAvl for *fbpABC*. Various amounts of the three partners PCR fragments were introduced into *Nm* using the transformation method described above. Correct localization of the chromosomal insertion was checked by PCR amplification using cat primers Eram1 and Eram3, in combination with primers TonBAvlAvl and TonBAmtAmt for *tonB* disruption, PorAAvlAvl and PorAAmtAmt for *porA* deletion, PorBAvlAvl and PorBAmtAmt for *porB* deletion or FbpABCAvl-tAvl and FbpABCAmtAmt for *fbpABC* deletion.

Iron binding assay

The ability of desferal, pyrophosphate and its structural analogues to bind iron Fe^{3+} was visualized with a classical assay used to quantify siderophores in solution [32].

Statistical analysis

Data are expressed as the mean ± SD of 5 samples, and the reproducibility was confirmed at least in three separate experiments. Statistical analysis were performed using two-way unpaired Student's *t*-test and considered significant if $P<0.05$.

Results

Ex vivo use of ferric pyrophosphate as an iron source

In a first set of experiments, we investigated the *ex vivo* use of ferric pyrophosphate as an iron source by *Nm* strain 2C4.3. The tested strain was cultured on GCB medium supplemented with S1 complement and desferal 15 μM or 30 μM to create iron depletion. On this medium, no growth of the *Nm* 2C4.3 strain was observed. The addition of iron pyrophosphate led to growth restoration (Table 3). The minimal concentration of iron pyrophosphate required for growth on GCB iron-depleted medium was 15 μM (Table 3). In iron pyrophosphate, the iron content was about one-tenth of the iron pyrophosphate compound in weight. In spite of the presence of desferal used as a chelator, *Nm* was able to use iron pyrophosphate as an iron source. This suggested that the affinity of pyrophosphate for iron was higher than that of desferal. This hypothesis was strengthened by comparing the ability of pyrophosphate and desferal to induce a color change in an iron dye complex used to detect and quantify siderophores [32]. This ability was related to the capacity to bind iron and release free dye [32]. As seen in Figure 1, pyrophosphate induced a strong color change at 630 nm, reflecting its ability to bind iron [24]. In contrast, with desferal, the free dye release occurred much more slowly (Figure 1).

The iron pyrophosphate transport pathway in *Nm*

In order to be used by the bacteria, the iron source must be transported through the outer membrane, the periplasm and the inner membrane. Outer membrane transport of iron and heme primarily involves transporters requiring the presence of the ExbB-ExbD-TonB complex as an energy provider [33]. We first checked for the effect of *tonB* disruption upon the ability of *Nm* to use iron pyrophosphate as an iron source. As shown in Figure 2, *tonB* disruption did not impair the use of iron pyrophosphate as an iron source. In contrast, the use of iron-loaded human transferrin and hemoglobin as an iron source was abolished in the *Nm tonB* mutant. Similarly, disruption of *porA* or *porB* structural genes encoding for the *Nm* major porins [34] had no effect on the use of iron pyrophosphate as an iron source (Figure 2). The inner membrane FbpABC transporter was shown to be required for the use of transferrin and xenosiderophores as iron sources [35], [15]. We thus tested the effect of *fbpABC* disruption of the capacity of *Nm* to use iron pyrophosphate as an iron source. As seen in

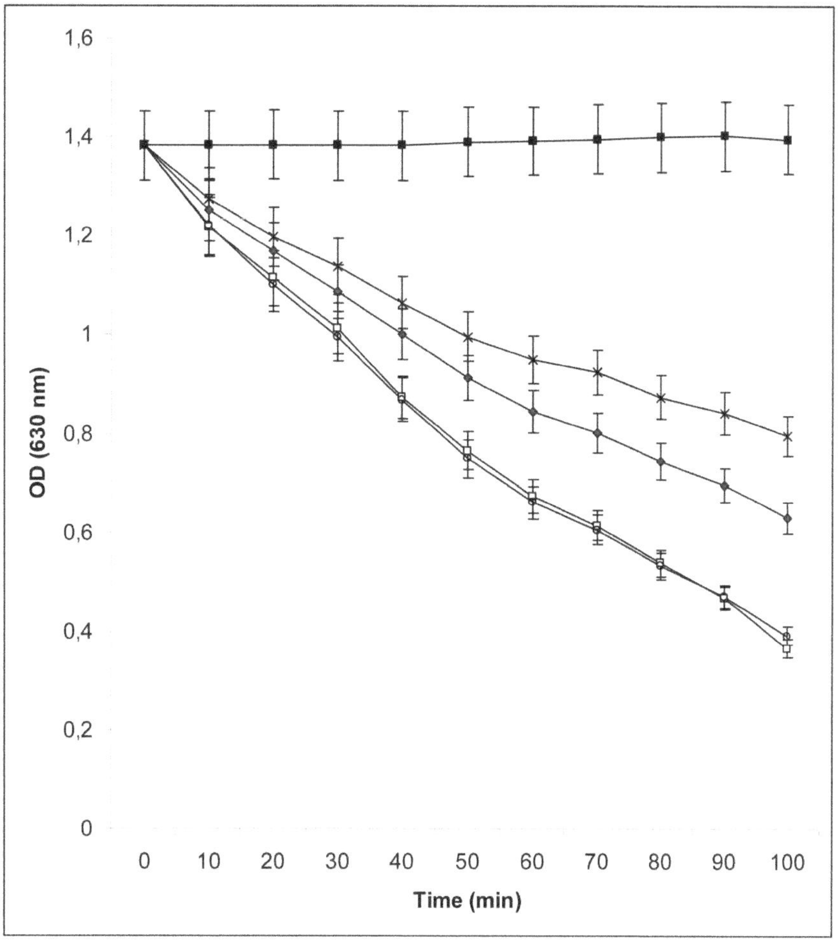

Figure 1. Assay of the ability of desferal, pyrophosphate (PPi), methylenediphosphonic acid (PcP) and imidodiphosphate (PnP) to bind iron. 150 nanomoles of desferal (♦), PPi (○), PcP (□), or PnP (X) were added to a 1 ml mix (1/4 V/3/4 V) of distilled water and CAS assay solution [32] at room temperature. Every 10 min for 60 min absorbance was measured at 630 nm. (■): No agent added. The experiment was repeated three times. A representative result is presented.

Figure 2, *fpbABC* disruption abolished the use of iron pyrophosphate as an iron source.

Exogenous pyrophosphate allows iron utilization in the presence of desferal

GCB medium can support *Nm* growth in the presence of supplement S1 and in the absence of supplement S2. Thus, iron traces present in the medium are sufficient for sustaining *Nm* growth. Addition of desferal at 15 μM or 30 μM abolished *Nm* growth on this medium. Addition of pyrophosphate, at 5 mM or higher, restored the growth of *Nm* on GCB S1 medium supplemented with desferal (Table 4). This result is in good agreement with the high affinity of pyrophosphate for iron [24]. The use of two structural analogues of pyrophosphate strengthened this conclusion. Imidodiphosphate and methylenediphosphonic acid were added to iron depleted GCB medium and growth of *Nm* was investigated. Our results demonstrated that methylenediphosphonic acid, similarly to pyrophosphate, allowed *Nm* growth on iron-depleted medium when added at a 5 mM final concentration (Table 4). In contrast, addition of imidodiphosphate did not support *Nm* growth on the same medium (Table 4). These results are in accordance with our results demonstrating that pyrophosphate and methylenediphosphonic acid, in contrast to imidodiphosphate, bind iron with higher affinity than desferal (Figure 1). Pyrophosphate and methylenediphosphonic-acid-dependent use of iron did not require TonB activity, but was abolished when *fbpABC* genes were disrupted (data not shown).

Pyrophosphate enables TonB-independent use of transferrin as an iron source

In *Nm*, the use of transferrin as an iron source is restricted to human transferrin [2]. Other transferrins are not used by *Nm* as an iron source. Transportation of iron from human transferrin requires the activity of the TonB-dependent outer membrane transporter TbpAB [2]. *In vitro* experiments demonstrated the role of pyrophosphate as a mediator of iron transfer from transferrin to ferritin [36]. According to these results, pyrophosphate can bind iron loaded on transferrin and deliver it to ferritin [26]. Other authors demonstrated transfer from iron-loaded transferrin to pyrophosphate [37], [38]. The results described in these reports prompted us to check for the effect of pyrophosphate on the use of iron-loaded transferrin as an iron source. In a first set of experiments, we investigated the effect of pyrophosphate on the use of human transferrin and bovine transferrin as an iron source. As shown in Figure 3, in the absence of pyrophosphate, *Nm* used only human transferrin as an iron source. In contrast, in the

Table 3. Use of iron pyrophosphate (FePPi), FeNo3 and FeCl3 as iron sources by *Nm*.

Desferal 15 µM					Desferal 30 µM			
µM	20	15	10	5	20	15	10	5
FePPi	+++	+++	−	−	+++	+++	−	−
FeNo3	+++	−	−	−	+	−	−	−
FeCl3	+++	−	−	−	−	−	−	−

Experiments were repeated three times. Representative results are presented. +++: large colonies (1 to 1.5 mm diameter); +: small colonies (<0.5 mm diameter); −: no growth.

presence of pyrophosphate, both bovine and human transferrins were iron sources for *Nm*. This cannot be explained by solubilization of contaminating iron, since the concentration of pyrophosphate used in this assay (1 mM) was not sufficient for supporting *Nm* growth in the presence of 30 µM desferal (Table 4). Since the TbpAB transport system exhibits absolute specificity for human transferrin, we hypothesized that the transport pathway used in the presence of pyrophosphate was independent of TbpAB activity. As a consequence, *tonB* disruption would not have an effect on the use of human or bovine transferrin in the presence of pyrophosphate. This was shown to be the case (Figure 3). Human and bovine transferrin as an iron source was also used in the presence of the two pyrophosphate analogues already tested in this report. As seen in Figure 3, imidodiphosphate addition did not alter the phenotype observed with wild type and *tonB* mutant strains. In contrast, similarly to pyrophosphate, methylenediphosphonic acid allowed TonB-independent use of human and bovine transferrin as iron sources (Figure 3).

Effect of methylenediphosphonic addition upon *Nm* survival in the mouse model

In the absence of a usable iron source, *Nm* is cleared from mice very rapidly after intraperitoneal injection [39]. Addition of human transferrin to the bacterial suspension allows *Nm* to survive in mice [39]. Since the above results demonstrated that addition of pyrophosphate and methylenediphosphonic acid enabled the use of non-human transferrin as an iron source, we hypothesized that the addition of pyrophosphate and its structural analog, methylenediphosphonic acid, could promote the use of mouse transferrin as an iron source and enhance the survival of *Nm* in the mouse model. The addition of iron pyrophosphate (50 µM final concentration), pyrophosphate (5 mM final concentration) or imidodiphosphate (5 mM final concentration) had no effect on survival of *Nm* in mice (data not shown). In contrast, addition of 5 mM methylenediphosphonic acid, which is not degraded by inorganic pyrophosphatase [24], [40], increased significantly the ability of wild-type *Nm* to survive in the mice compared to control untreated mice ($p = 0.026$) (Figure 4). However, this effect of methylenediphosphonic acid on *Nm* growth was less prominent than that obtained by the addition of human transferrin ($p = 0.0002$) compared to control untreated mice (Figure 4). As evidenced in *ex vivo* assays, the effects of methylenediphosphonic acid were not abolished by *tonB* disruption. We therefore tested, in the mouse model (*in vivo*), the impact of *tonB* disruption on bacterial survival. As shown in figure 4, dynamic imaging result showed that *tonB Nm* mutant still showed significant better survival in mice treated with PcP compared to untreated control ($p = 0.034$). At the opposite, no more difference of survival *tonB Nm* mutant in human transferrin-treated mice compared to untreated control ($p = 0.1$) (Figure 4). We further study the survival of the wild type and the *tonB* mutant during the experimental infection in mice by bacterial counting from the peritoneal cavity and from the blood. The bacterial counts in blood and peritoneal cavity corroborated the results of dynamic imaging obtained with the wild type strain (Figure 4). For the *tonB* mutant, the results of the bacterial count in blood and peritoneal cavity are in a good accordance with the results of dynamic imaging when human transferrin was added (Figure 4). When methylenediphosphonic acid was added, a non significant trend for higher bacterial counts in the blood was observed (Figure 4). These data suggest that methylenediphosphonic acid enables a wide range of iron acquisition during experimental infection.

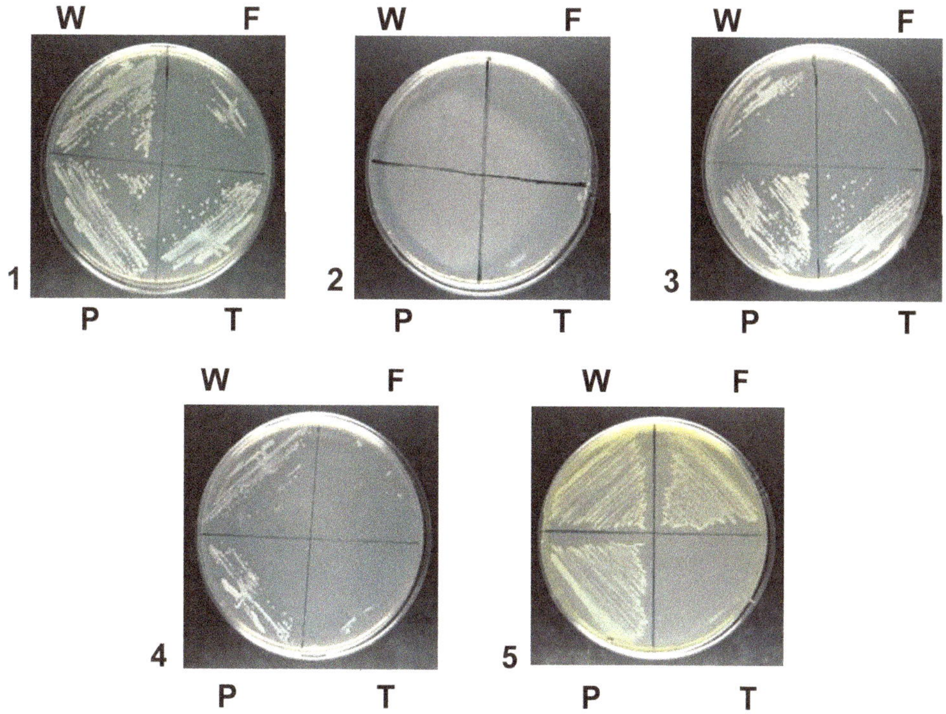

Figure 2. Mutations impairing iron pyrophosphate (FePPi) uptake in *Nm*. Strains 2C4.3 (W), 2C4.3 *ΔporA* or 2C4.3 *ΔporB* (P) and 2C4.3 *ΔtonB* (T) were isolated on a GCB plate supplemented with S1 and S2 complements and grown for 18 h at 37°C in the presence of 5% CO_2. For strain 2C4.3*ΔfbpABC* (F), GCB medium was supplemented with Kellogg supplement 1 solution [27] and human hemoglobin was added at a 5×10^{-6} M final concentration. All tested strains were then isolated on GCB medium (1), GCB medium with desferal (2), GCB medium with desferal and FePPi 15 μM (3), GCB medium with desferal and human transferrin 5×10^{-6} M (4), GCB medium with desferal and hemoglobin 5×10^{-6} M (5). Bacteria were isolated on the test plates and incubated for 18 h at 37°C in the presence of 5% CO_2. The experiment was repeated three times. Representative results are presented.

Discussion

Iron acquisition by pathogenic *Neisseria* within the host is a major virulence trait. Bacteria employ specific receptors to obtain this transition metal from iron-containing proteins (transferrin, lactoferrin) in a TonB-dependent manner. However, tonB-independent pathways have been described. The mechanisms and significance of these pathways are not yet understood. We describe here a TonB independent iron transport process in *Nm*. This TonB-independent process allows *ex vivo* transportation of the iron pyrophosphate complex through the outer membrane. *In vitro*, pyrophosphate and methylenediphosphonic acid (a structural analogue of pyrophosphate) bind iron with higher affinity than desferal, and rescue *Nm* growth on plates in the presence of desferal in a TonB-independent manner. Iron-complexing compounds like citrate and pyrophosphate have been shown to support *Nm* growth *ex vivo* on culture plates [19], but their transport pathways have not been investigated. Using a rapid method, we built various mutants that enabled demonstrating the TonB-independent mechanism responsible for transport of iron pyrophosphate. *porA* or *porB* inactivation did not abolish the ability to use iron pyrophosphate as an iron source. Iron-loaded pyrophosphate could pass the outer membrane through both PorA and PorB porins. This hypothesis is in good agreement with identification of phosphate and ATP as PorB ligands [41]. Also, iron pyrophosphate can pass the outer membrane through a porin hypothesized to be responsible for the TonB independent use of xenosiderophores [17]. Thus, the transport pathway of iron pyrophosphate through the *Nm* outer membrane remains to be elucidated. FbpABC was shown to be responsible for the transport of iron pyrophosphate through the inner membrane. This complex was already shown to be required for iron transport through the inner membrane in *Nm* [35] and *N. gonorrhoeae* [13].

Pyrophosphate was shown to have a siderophore-like activity when ferritin was used as an iron source [19]. Moreover, pyrophosphate was shown to transfer iron from transferrin to ferritin [26]. Accordingly, our data obtained on plates demonstrate that pyrophosphate permits TonB-independent use of iron that is loaded from both human and bovine transferrin. In contrast, the acquisition of iron from transferrin through the TbpAB transporter is highly specific to human transferrin [11]. Indeed, it was previously shown that transgenic mice expressing human transferrin, or injection of iron-loaded human transferrin mice, leads to meningococcal growth in these animal models [39], [42]. We therefore explored, in the mouse model (*in vivo*), the significance of our finding concerning the role of iron pyrophosphate, pyrophosphate and its analogues on plates (*ex vivo*). Addition of pyrophosphate did not increase survival capacity in the mice in the absence of added human transferrin. Pyrophosphate degradation by inorganic pyrophosphatase [43–45] can explain this result. Addition of methylenediphosphonic acid increases survival of *Nm* in mice (Figure 4). This effect, also observed on a *tonB* mutant, suggests that TonB-independent transport of iron bound to methylenediphosphonic acid can support the growth of *Nm* in mice. Bacterial CFU counting revealed that *tonB* disruption decreased the ability of *N. meningitidis* to survive in the mice model in the presence of both PcP and human transferrin (Figure 4). The effect may be due to a decreased use of murine hemoglobin as an iron source in a TonB-dependent manner [6].

Table 4. Effect of pyrophosphate (PPi), methylenediphosphonic acid (PcP) and imidodiphosphate (PnP) on *Nm* growth on iron-depleted medium.

	Desferal 15 µM				**Desferal 30 µM**			
mM	**10**	**5**	**2**	**1**	**10**	**5**	**2**	**1**
PPi	+++	+++	–	–	+++	+++	–	–
PcP	+++	+++	–	–	+++	+++	–	–
PnP	–	–	–	–	–	–	–	–

The experiment was repeated three times. Representative results are presented. +++: large colonies (1 to 1.5 mm diameter); –: no growth.

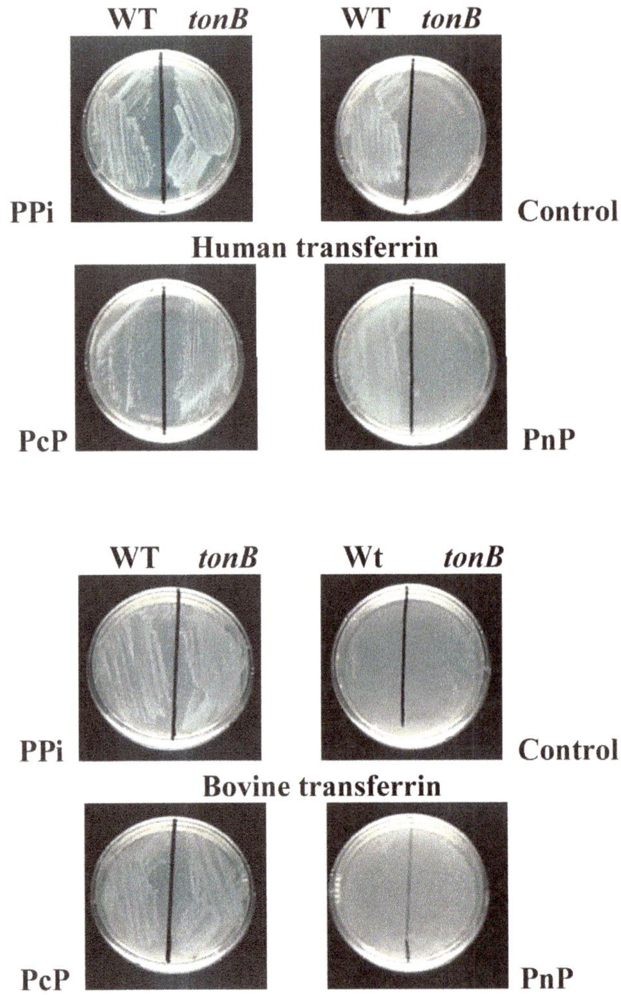

Figure 3. TonB-independent use of transferrin as an iron source. The tested strains were isolated on a GCB plate supplemented with S1 and S2 complements and grown for 18 h at 37°C in the presence of 5% CO_2. GCB plates depleted for iron by addition of desferal were supplemented with human or bovine transferrin added at a 5 µM final concentration. When specified, PPi, PcP and PnP were added at a 1 mM final concentration. Bacteria were isolated on test plates and incubated for 18 h at 37°C in the presence of 5% CO_2. The experiment was repeated three times. Representative results are presented.

However, the decrease was prominent in the presence of human transferrin. Since iron-loaded transferrin is the main iron source in mice, we propose that methylenediphosphonic acid is able to obtain iron from mouse transferrin, as from bovine and human transferrin, and to form a ferric complex that can be transported through the outer membrane. According to the results obtained with dynamic imaging method, the use of mouse transferrin in the presence of methylenediphosphonic acid not requires the TonB activity. The effect of methylenediphosphonic acid addition on *Nm tonB* mutant survival inside the mice cannot be related to *tonB* reversion, since bacteria recovered from the intraperitoneal cavity and from blood were unable to use human transferrin and hemoglobin on plates. Taken together, the data in this report demonstrate *ex vivo* and *in vivo* pyrophosphate-mediated use of iron-loaded transferrin as iron sources. *Ex vivo* data clearly demonstrate that the pyrophosphate-mediated use of iron-loaded transferrin as an iron source not requires the TonB activity.

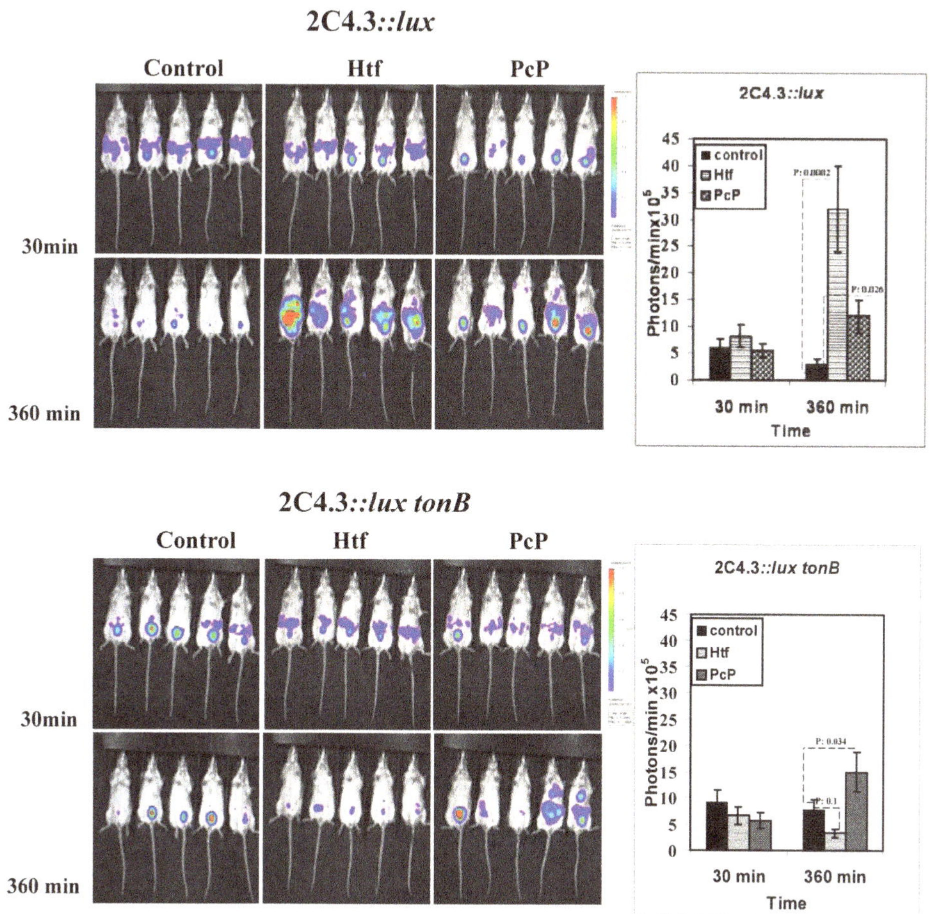

	Peritoneal fluid (UFC)	P* value	Blood (UFC)	P* value
2C4.3::*lux* control	8 ± 5	Ref	< 10	Ref
2C4.3::*lux* Htf	37000 ± 10000	0.002	374 ± 260	0.031
2C4.3::*lux* PcP	4800 ± 2000	0.003	224 ± 200	0.043
2C4.3::*lux tonB* control	< 10	Ref	< 10	Ref
2C4.3::*lux tonB* Htf	88 ± 40	0.139	< 10	1
2C4.3::*lux tonB* PcP	450 ± 674	0.196	45 ± 20	0.23

Figure 4. *Nm* growth in the mouse model in the presence of human transferrin (Htf) or methylenediphosphonic acid (PcP). The tested strains were isolated on a GCB plate supplemented with S1 and S2 complements and grown for 18 h at 37°C in the presence of 5% CO_2. Bacteria were suspended in sterile physiological serum to obtain a cell density of 2.5×10^6 bacteria/ml. When specified, 100 µl of the tested iron source were added to 400 µl of the bacterial suspension to obtain 0.05 mM for human transferrin and 5 mM for PcP. For the control experiment, 100 µl of physiological serum were added. For each experiment, the mixtures were injected intraperitoneally into five mice and bioluminescence was measured 30 min, and 360 min after injection, as described in Materials and methods. At t = 360 min, blood and peritoneal washes samples were taken, diluted in physiological serum and plated on GCB solid medium. After 18 h incubation at 37°C in the presence of 5% CO_2, the colonies were counted. Data represent the means ± SD from 3 independent experiments of groups of five mice per time point in each experiment. Student's *t*-test results were included in the figure and in the table. CFU: colony-forming unit.

Similarly to pyrophosphate-dependent iron uptake, other TonB-independent iron uptake processes have been described *ex vivo* in *Neisseria* [46], [15].

In *Escherichia coli*, pyrophosphate acts as an iron chelator in an *entF* strain that is unable to synthesize enterobactin, but is still able to produce dihydroxybenzoic acid [25]. This demonstrates that iron pyrophosphate cannot be used as an iron source in the absence of enterobactin in *E. coli*. In *Nm*, which was not demonstrated to produce siderophore, pyrophosphate addition counteracts the iron chelating of desferal, and iron pyrophosphate can be used as an iron source. The pore sizes of PorA (1.4 nm) [47] and PorB (1.6 nm) [48], [49] porins from *Nm* are close to those of OmpC (1,3 nm) and OmpF (1,4 nm) porins from *E. coli* [50], suggesting similar transport of iron pyrophosphate across the outer membrane. In *Neisseria*, the transport system responsible for transportation of iron pyrophosphate through the inner membrane was identified as FbpABC. This inner membrane transport system, was already demonstrated to be required for transport of iron from transferrin [35] and exogenous siderophores [15]. In FbpA, phosphate was identified as a synergistic anion allowing tight sequestration of iron [51]. Similarly to phosphate, pyrophosphate or methylenediphosphonic acid could play the role of a synergistic anion. This was suggested for pyrophosphate, and phosphatase activity was hypothesized for FbpA [51]. According to results obtained with methylenediphosphonic acid, this phosphatase activity is not required for the synergistic activity of pyrophosphate. In *E. coli*, that synthesizes siderophore, two periplasmic binding proteins and inner membrane transporters facilitate the transport of ferric-siderophore complexes. FhuD, the periplasmic protein responsible for directing ferric hydroxamate to the inner membrane $FhuBC_2$ ABC transporter, also facilitates the transport of ferrichrome, coprogen, ferrioxamine B and aerobactin [52]. FepB binds ferric enterobactin and enterobactin in the periplasm and directs it to the inner membrane ABC transporter $FepC_2D_2$ [53]. Moreover, *E. coli* synthesizes another ABC transporter, responsible for the transport of iron citrate through the inner membrane [54]. Similarly to FbpABCD from *Nm*, the FecBCDE inner membrane transport system transports iron Fe^{3+} but not the iron citrate complex [54]. In *E. coli*, FecBCDE can be hypothesized to also transport iron pyrophosphate. In *E. coli*, expression of the *fec* operon containing the structural genes of this inner membrane transport system is repressed by iron-loaded Fur and induced in the presence of iron-loaded citrate [55]. In the absence of iron-loaded citrate, basal expression of the *fecABCDE* operon would not be sufficient to promote a speculated FecBCDE-dependent transport of iron pyrophosphate through the inner membrane. Within the cytoplasm, intracellular pyrophosphatase can degrade pyrophosphate and facilitate iron release. In addition, reduction of iron by a ferric reductase [56], [57] could provoke its release from pyrophosphate and methylene diphosphonic acid. Iron reduction by a reductase was reported to be responsible for iron release from siderophores like coprogen and ferrioxamine [58].

Our work opens up new insights into iron acquisition in *Nm*. Indeed, *Nm* seems to preferentially use iron among the transition metals. Several systems have been selected to allow highly efficient iron acquisition in the natural habitat of *Nm*. Pyrophosphate could permit iron acquisition from a wide range of iron sources like lactoferrin at sites such as the nasopharynx, the natural habitat of *Nm*, and might support meningococcal growth when in competition with other microbial species that produce siderophores, exhibiting lower affinity for iron than enterobactin. Thus, the presence of pyrophosphate enables Nm to obtain iron using a simple, highly competitive pathway.

Acknowledgments

We thank Marie-Anne Nicola and Marek Szatanik for helpful discussion.

Author Contributions

Conceived and designed the experiments: FB MKT. Performed the experiments: FB CB DG MKT. Analyzed the data: FB MKT. Contributed reagents/materials/analysis tools: FB MKT. Contributed to the writing of the manuscript: FB MKT.

References

1. Rouphael NG, Stephens DS (2012) Neisseria meningitidis: biology, microbiology, and epidemiology. Methods Mol Biol 799: 1–20.
2. Perkins-Balding D, Ratliff-Griffin M, Stojiljkovic I (2004) Iron transport systems in Neisseria meningitidis. Microbiol Mol Biol Rev 68: 154–171.
3. Skaar EP (2010) The battle for iron between bacterial pathogens and their vertebrate hosts. PLoS Pathog 6: e1000949.
4. Cassat JE, Skaar EP (2013) Iron in infection and immunity. Cell Host Microbe 13: 509–519.
5. Wandersman C, Stojiljkovic I (2000) Bacterial heme sources: the role of heme, hemoprotein receptors and hemophores. Curr Opin Microbiol 3: 215–220.
6. Stojiljkovic I, Hwa V, de Saint Martin L, O'Gaora P, Nassif X, et al. (1995) The Neisseria meningitidis haemoglobin receptor: its role in iron utilization and virulence. Mol Microbiol 15: 531–541.
7. Lewis LA, Dyer DW (1995) Identification of an iron-regulated outer membrane protein of Neisseria meningitidis involved in the utilization of hemoglobin complexed to haptoglobin. J Bacteriol 177: 1299–1306.
8. Rohde KH, Gillaspy AF, Hatfield MD, Lewis LA, Dyer DW (2002) Interactions of haemoglobin with the Neisseria meningitidis receptor HpuAB: the role of TonB and an intact proton motive force. Mol Microbiol 43: 335–354.
9. Tauseef I, Harrison OB, Wooldridge KG, Feavers IM, Neal KR, et al. (2011) Influence of the combination and phase variation status of the haemoglobin receptors HmbR and HpuAB on meningococcal virulence. Microbiology 157: 1446–1456.
10. Zhu W, Wilks A, Stojiljkovic I (2000) Degradation of heme in gram-negative bacteria: the product of the hemO gene of Neisseriae is a heme oxygenase. J Bacteriol 182: 6783–6790.
11. Noinaj N, Buchanan SK, Cornelissen CN (2012) The transferrin-iron import system from pathogenic Neisseria species. Mol Microbiol 86: 246–257.
12. Schryvers AB, Morris LJ (1988) Identification and characterization of the human lactoferrin-binding protein from Neisseria meningitidis. Infect Immun 56: 1144–1149.
13. Adhikari P, Berish SA, Nowalk AJ, Veraldi KL, Morse SA, et al. (1996) The fbpABC locus of Neisseria gonorrhoeae functions in the periplasm-to-cytosol transport of iron. J Bacteriol 178: 2145–2149.
14. Stojiljkovic I, Srinivasan N (1997) Neisseria meningitidis tonB, exbB, and exbD genes: Ton-dependent utilization of protein-bound iron in Neisseriae. J Bacteriol 179: 805–812.
15. Strange HR, Zola TA, Cornelissen CN (2011) The fbpABC operon is required for Ton-independent utilization of xenosiderophores by Neisseria gonorrhoeae strain FA19. Infect Immun 79: 267–278.
16. Zola TA, Strange HR, Dominguez NM, Dillard JP, Cornelissen CN (2010) Type IV secretion machinery promotes ton-independent intracellular survival of Neisseria gonorrhoeae within cervical epithelial cells. Infect Immun 78: 2429–2437.
17. Cornelissen CN, Hollander A (2011) TonB-Dependent Transporters Expressed by Neisseria gonorrhoeae. Front Microbiol 2: 117.
18. Carson SD, Klebba PE, Newton SM, Sparling PF (1999) Ferric enterobactin binding and utilization by Neisseria gonorrhoeae. J Bacteriol 181: 2895–2901.
19. Archibald FS, DeVoe IW (1980) Iron acquisition by Neisseria meningitidis in vitro. Infect Immun 27: 322–334.
20. Yancey RJ, Finkelstein RA (1981) Assmilation of iron by pathogenic Neisseria spp. Infect Immun 32: 592–599.
21. Veggi D, Gentile MA, Cantini F, Lo Surdo P, Nardi-Dei V, et al. (2012) The factor H binding protein of Neisseria meningitidis interacts with xenosiderophores in vitro. Biochemistry 51: 9384–9393.
22. Biville F (1985) In vivo effects of pyrophosphate in *Escherichia coli*. FEMS Microbiol Lett 28: 73–76.
23. Biville F, Laurent-Winter C, Danchin A (1996) In vivo positive effects of exogenous pyrophosphate on Escherichia coli cell growth and stationary phase survival. Res Microbiol 147: 597–608.
24. Biville F, Oshima T, Mori H, Kawagoe Y, Bouvet O, et al. (2003) Escherichia coli response to exogenous pyrophosphate and analogs. J Mol Microbiol Biotechnol 5: 37–45.
25. Perrotte-Piquemal M, Danchin A, Biville F (1999) Pyrophosphate increases the efficiency of enterobactin-dependent iron uptake in Escherichia coli. Biochimie 81: 245–253.
26. Konopka K, Mareschal J, Crichton RR (1980) Iron transfer from transferrin to ferritin mediated by pyrophosphate. Biochemical & Biophysical Research Communications 96: 1408–1413.
27. Kellogg DS Jr, Peacock WL Jr, Deacon WE, Brown L, Pirkle DI (1963) Neisseria Gonorrhoeae. I. Virulence Genetically Linked to Clonal Variation. J Bacteriol 85: 1274–1279.
28. Miller JH (1972) Experiments in molecular genetics.: Cold Spring Harbor laboratory Press, Cold Spring Harbor, N.Y.
29. Taha MK, Morand PC, Pereira Y, Eugene E, Giorgini D, et al. (1998) Pilus-mediated adhesion of Neisseria meningitidis: the essential role of cell contact-dependent transcriptional upregulation of the PilC1 protein. Mol Microbiol 28: 1153–1163.

30. Taha MK, So M, Seifert HS, Billyard E, Marchal C (1988) Pilin expression in Neisseria gonorrhoeae is under both positive and negative transcriptional control. Embo J 7: 4367–4378.
31. Nassif X, Puaoi D, So M (1991) Transposition of Tn1545-delta 3 in the pathogenic Neisseriae: a genetic tool for mutagenesis. J Bacteriol 173: 2147–2154.
32. Schwyn B, Neilands JB (1987) Universal chemical assay for the detection and determination of siderophores. Anal Biochem 160: 47–56.
33. Krewulak KD, Vogel HJ (2011) TonB or not TonB: is that the question? Biochem Cell Biol 89: 87–97.
34. Tommassen J, Vermeij P, Struyve M, Benz R, Poolman JT (1990) Isolation of Neisseria meningitidis mutants deficient in class 1 (porA) and class 3 (porB) outer membrane proteins. Infect Immun 58: 1355–1359.
35. Khun HH, Kirby SD, Lee BC (1998) A Neisseria meningitidis fbpABC mutant is incapable of using nonheme iron for growth. Infect Immun 66: 2330–2336.
36. Konopka K, Romslo I (1980) Uptake of iron from transferrin by isolated rat-liver mitochondria mediated by phosphate compounds. Eur J Biochem 107: 433–439.
37. Harris WR, Brook CE, Spilling CD, Elleppan S, Peng W, et al. (2004) Release of iron from transferrin by phosphonocarboxylate and diphosphonate chelating agents. J Inorg Biochem 98: 1824–1836.
38. Brook CE, Harris WR, Spilling CD, Peng W, Harburn JJ, et al. (2005) Effect of ligand structure on the pathways for iron release from human serum transferrin. Inorg Chem 44: 5183–5191.
39. Szatanik M, Hong E, Ruckly C, Ledroit M, Giorgini D, et al. (2011) Experimental meningococcal sepsis in congenic transgenic mice expressing human transferrin. PLoS One 6: e22210.
40. Rodan GA (1998) Mechanisms of action of bisphosphonates. Annu Rev Pharmacol Toxicol 38: 375–388.
41. Zeth K, Kozjak-Pavlovic V, Faulstich M, Fraunholz M, Hurwitz R, et al. (2013) Structure and function of the PorB porin from disseminating Neisseria gonorrhoeae. Biochem J 454: 359.
42. Zarantonelli ML, Szatanik M, Giorgini D, Hong E, Huerre M, et al. (2007) Transgenic mice expressing human transferrin as a model for meningococcal infection. Infect Immun 75: 5609–5614.
43. Lahti R (1983) Microbial inorganic pyrophosphatases. Microbiol Rev 47: 169–178.
44. Pynes GD, Younathan ES (1967) Purification and some properties of inorganic pyrophosphatase from human erythrocytes. J Biol Chem 242: 2119–2123.
45. Kajander T, Kellosalo J, Goldman A (2013) Inorganic pyrophosphatases: one substrate, three mechanisms. FEBS Lett 587: 1863–1869.
46. Biswas GD, Anderson JE, Sparling PF (1997) Cloning and functional characterization of Neisseria gonorrhoeae tonB, exbB and exbD genes. Mol Microbiol 24: 169–179.
47. Song J, Minetti CA, Blake MS, Colombini M (1999) Meningococcal PorA/C1, a channel that combines high conductance and high selectivity. Biophys J 76: 804–813.
48. Jadhav SR, Rao KS, Zheng Y, Garavito RM, Worden RM (2013) Voltage dependent closure of PorB class II porin from Neisseria meningitidis investigated using impedance spectroscopy in a tethered bilayer lipid membrane interface. J Colloid Interface Sci 390: 211–216.
49. Rudel T, Schmid A, Benz R, Kolb HA, Lang F, et al. (1996) Modulation of Neisseria porin (PorB) by cytosolic ATP/GTP of target cells: parallels between pathogen accommodation and mitochondrial endosymbiosis. Cell 85: 391–402.
50. Mizuno T, Chou MY, Inouye M (1983) A comparative study on the genes for three porins of the Escherichia coli outer membrane. DNA sequence of the osmoregulated ompC gene. J Biol Chem 258: 6932–6940.
51. Parker Siburt CJ, Mietzner TA, Crumbliss AL (2012) FbpA–a bacterial transferrin with more to offer. Biochim Biophys Acta 1820: 379–392.
52. Braun V, Hantke K, Koster W (1998) Bacterial iron transport: mechanisms, genetics, and regulation. Met Ions Biol Syst 35: 67–145.
53. Sprencel C, Cao Z, Qi Z, Scott DC, Montague MA, et al. (2000) Binding of ferric enterobactin by the Escherichia coli periplasmic protein FepB. J Bacteriol 182: 5359–5364.
54. Braun V, Herrmann C (2007) Docking of the periplasmic FecB binding protein to the FecCD transmembrane proteins in the ferric citrate transport system of Escherichia coli. J Bacteriol 189: 6913–6918.
55. Braun V, Mahren S, Sauter A (2006) Gene regulation by transmembrane signaling. Biometals 19: 103–113.
56. Schroder I, Johnson E, de Vries S (2003) Microbial ferric iron reductases. FEMS Microbiol Rev 27: 427–447.
57. Le Faou AE, Morse SA (1991) Characterization of a soluble ferric reductase from Neisseria gonorrhoeae. Biol Met 4: 126–131.
58. Matzanke BF, Anemuller S, Schunemann V, Trautwein AX, Hantke K (2004) FhuF, part of a siderophore-reductase system. Biochemistry 43: 1386–1392.
59. Nassif X, Lowy J, Stenberg P, O'Gaora P, Ganji A, et al. (1993) Antigenic variation of pilin regulates adhesion of Neisseria meningitidis to human epithelial cells. Mol Microbiol 8: 719–725.

Impact of Vitamin D Supplementation during Lactation on Vitamin D Status and Body Composition of Mother-Infant Pairs: A MAVID Randomized Controlled Trial

Justyna Czech-Kowalska[1]*, Julita Latka-Grot[1], Dorota Bulsiewicz[1], Maciej Jaworski[2], Pawel Pludowski[2], Grazyna Wygledowska[3], Bogdan Chazan[4], Beata Pawlus[4], Anna Zochowska[5], Maria K. Borszewska-Kornacka[6], Elzbieta Karczmarewicz[2], Edyta Czekuc-Kryskiewicz[2], Anna Dobrzanska[1]

1 Department of Neonatology and Neonatal Intensive Care, The Children's Memorial Health Institute, Warsaw, Poland, **2** Department of Biochemistry, Radioimmunology, and Experimental Medicine, The Children's Memorial Health Institute, Warsaw, Poland, **3** Department of Neonatology, Miedzyleski Specialist Hospital, Warsaw, Poland, **4** Department of Neonatology, Holy Family Hospital, Warsaw, Poland, **5** Department of Neonatology, Public Hospital, Otwock, Poland, **6** Department of Neonatology, Warsaw Medical University Hospital, Warsaw, Poland

Abstract

Objective: The optimal vitamin D intake for nursing women is controversial. Deterioration, at least in bone mass, is reported during lactation. This study evaluated whether vitamin D supplementation during lactation enhances the maternal and infant's vitamin D status, bone mass and body composition.

Design and Methods: After term delivery, 174 healthy mothers were randomized to receive 1200 IU/d (800 IU/d+400 IU/d from multivitamins) or 400 IU/d (placebo+400 IU/d from multivitamins) of cholecalciferol for 6 months while breastfeeding. All infants received 400 IU/d of cholecalciferol. Serum 25-hydroxyvitamin D [25(OH)D], iPTH, calcium, urinary calcium, and densitometry were performed in mother-offspring pairs after delivery, and at 3 and 6 months later.

Results: A total of 137 (79%) (n = 70; 1200 IU/d, n = 67; 400 IU/d) completed the study. 25(OH)D was similar in both groups at baseline (13.7 ng/ml vs. 16.1 ng/ml; $P = 0.09$) and at 3 months (25.7 ng/ml vs. 24.5 ng/ml; $P = 0.09$), but appeared higher in the 1200 IU/d group at 6 months of supplementation (25.6 ng/ml vs. 23.1 ng/ml; $P = 0.009$). The prevalence of 25(OH)D < 20 ng/ml was comparable between groups at baseline (71% vs. 64%, $P = 0.36$) but lower in the 1200 IU/d group after 3 months (9% vs. 25%, $P = 0.009$) and 6 months (14% vs. 30%, $P = 0.03$). Maternal and infants' iPTH, calciuria, bone mass and body composition as well as infants' 25(OH)D levels were not significantly different between groups during the study. Significant negative correlations were noted between maternal 25(OH)D and fat mass ($R = -0.49$, $P = 0.00001$), android fat mass ($R = -0.53$, $P = 0.00001$), and gynoid fat mass ($R = -0.43$, $P = 0.00001$) after 6 months of supplementation.

Conclusions: Vitamin D supplementation at a dose of 400 IU/d was not sufficient to maintain 25(OH)D >20 ng/ml in nursing women, while 1200 IU/d appeared more effective, but had no effect on breastfed offspring vitamin D status, or changes in the bone mass and the body composition observed in both during breastfeeding.

Trial Registration: ClinicalTrials.gov NCT01506557

Editor: D. W. Cameron, University of Ottawa, Canada

Funding: The study was supported by research grant No. RG 3/2010 from Nutritia Fundation (www.fundacjanutricia.pl). The funder had no role in study design, data collection and analysis, the decision to publish, or preparation of the manuscript.

Competing Interests: The authors have declared that no competing interests exist.

* Email: j.kowalska@ipczd.pl

Introduction

Growing evidence suggests that vitamin D deficiency has a negative impact on the skeletal system and may be a potential risk factor for a wide range of diseases, including cancer, cardiovascular disease, hypertension, diabetes, autoimmune diseases, and allergies [1].

Previously, comparable serum 25-hydroxyvitamin D [25(OH)D] levels were reported in lactating and non-lactating women with stable 25(OH)D levels during lactation [2]. On the other hand, decreasing serum 25(OH)D level was observed during lactation in recent studies [3,4]. Postpartum deterioration of vitamin D status might be explained, at least in part, by less frequent multivitamin intake during lactation compared to pregnancy [5,6] and decreasing multivitamin intake in the course of lactation [2]. Vitamin D supplementation in lactating women may ensure appropriate maternal vitamin D status in cases of low vitamin D dietary consumption and restricted synthesis in the skin [7]. Most of the recently published RCT in lactating women have been focused on maternal supplementation as a method of achieving appropriate vitamin D status in both, mothers and their breastfed offspring [8–11]. It appeared that daily doses of 4000–6400 IU were needed to effectively increase and then to maintain 25(OH)D levels in the range considered by the authors as optimal, in both the infant and its mother. However, the optimal vitamin D intake as well as optimal 25(OH)D level for lactating women (based on estimated maternal needs) still remains not fully established, or at least not accepted worldwide. The recommended vitamin D intake varies from 400 IU/d to 2000 IU/d [7,12–16], but supplementation using less than 1000 IU/d may be inadequate for maintaining an "optimal" 25(OH)D level [17]. Breastfeeding is associated with increased bone turnover leading to release of calcium from the maternal skeleton that leads to bone mass loss during the first 6 months of lactation, with further recovery after weaning [18–21]. However, intervention limited to calcium supplementation only had a minimal effect on bone loss during lactation [21]. Increased bone turnover in lactating women may partly be explained by a decreased estradiol level and rise in prolactin, parathyroid hormone and parathyroid hormone-related protein concentrations during lactation [22,23]. Nevertheless, the precise mechanism of changes in bone metabolism during lactation is still not completely understood. Further, in addition to the body composition indices (fat and lean mass) vitamin D status seems an independent contributor to bone mineral density in girls and women [24,25]. A recently published RCT of vitamin D supplementation in breastfed infants showed no effect of different oral dosages of vitamin D (from 400 IU/d up to 1600 IU/d) on infants' bone mineral content [26].

To the best of our knowledge, bone mass and body composition have not been examined in lactating women and their offspring based on the level of maternal vitamin D intake in randomized control trials. We hypothesized that maternal vitamin D supplementation during lactation at a dose of 1200 IU/d, but not 400 IU/d, is more beneficial for both breastfeeding mothers and breastfed infants, when vitamin D status, bone mass and body composition are controlled for. Higher serum 25(OH)D levels, prevalence of vitamin D sufficiency, fat mass loss as well as a lower prevalence of vitamin D deficiency and decrease of bone mass are expected in lactating women.

Materials and Methods

Study design

The study was designed as a prospective, double-blinded, randomized, controlled trial of vitamin D supplementation during lactation. The trial was registered at ClinicalTrials.gov (NCT01506557) two months after the enrolment of the first participant by the principal investigator. There were no deviations from the study protocol between the first participant enrolment and the trial registration date. The protocol for this trial and supporting CONSORT checklist are available as supporting information; see Protocol S1, Protocol S2, and Checklist S1.

Study cohort and setting

Caucasian lactating mothers were recruited from four hospitals in Warsaw city, Poland (52°N) (Miedzyleski Specialist Hospital, Warsaw Medical University Hospital, Holy Family Hospital, Public Hospital in Otwock) between March 2011 and April 2012. Randomization, allocation, and follow-up (6 months) occurred at The Children's Memorial Health Institute in Warsaw. The follow–up visits took place between May 2011 and September 2012. Healthy women who delivered at term (gestational age 37–42 weeks) a single neonate with a birth weight appropriate for gestational age and declared breastfeeding for the next 6 months were eligible for the study. The exclusion criteria were: maternal and neonatal endocrine disorders (e.g., diabetes mellitus, thyroid disease, disturbed calcium-phosphorus homeostasis), renal and hepatic insufficiency, anticonvulsant treatment, and congenital malformations of the newborn infant.

Ethics statement

The study has been conducted according to the principles expressed in the Declaration of Helsinki and approved (46/KBE2009) by the Ethics Committee of The Children's Memorial Health Institute, Warsaw, Poland. The attached study protocol (Protocol S2) is the original version that was submitted to and approved by the Ethics Committee of The Children's Memorial Health Institute before the trial began. Written informed consent was obtained from each participant.

Intervention

Women were instructed to ingest two pills daily: one multivitamin tablet containing 400 IU of vitamin D3 and 200 mg of calcium (Prenatal Classic, Puritans Pride, Holbex, Poland) and one masked capsule containing 800 IU of cholecalciferol (VitaDerol forte, Sequoia, Poland) or placebo. The capsules were identical in appearance and prepared with a solution of medium-chain triglyceride oil, masked and certified by Sequoia (Poland). Multivitamin tablets as well as cholecalciferol capsules were produced according to Good Manufacturing Practice guidelines. Vitamin D intervention started approximately 3 weeks after delivery and continued up to 6 months after delivery. All infants received 400 IU/d of vitamin D3 from "twist-off" capsules throughout the study period. According to Polish recommendations, breastfed infants took an additional 25 μg/d of vitamin K1 (VitaDerol +K, Sequoia, Poland) up to 12 weeks of life, then only vitamin D3 (VitaDerol, Sequoia, Poland). Mothers received supplements at baseline and second visit with written instructions on how to use them and were asked to take all unused products for their next visit. Returned pills were recorded at each follow-up visit to calculate compliance and adherence to the intervention between study visits. Compliance was calculated separately for all study products (multivitamins and cholecalciferol) in mothers and infants at 3 and 6 months after delivery.

Randomization

Lactating mothers were randomly assigned (1:1) to 400 IU/d (placebo+400 IU/d from multivitamins) and 1200 IU/d (800 IU/d of cholecalciferol+400 IU/d from multivitamins) group using a computerized random number-generator (block size: 4) and stratified by season of delivery (winter: November–May; summer: June–October). A separate randomization list was generated for each season of delivery. The selected physician (not involved in the study in any other way) was responsible for the allocation procedure and provided the allocated study preparation and multivitamins. All investigators (including the principal), study subjects, health care providers, and laboratory staff remained blinded to the mother's intervention group throughout the study.

Data collection

A baseline visit occurred within 3 weeks after delivery (V0). A second visit occurred 3 months after delivery (V3) and the last visit 6 months after delivery (V6). At V0, the maternal socio-demographic and health data, prenatal vitamin intake, and neonatal status at birth were recorded using questionnaires. The infant's body weight, length, head circumference, and maternal weight and height, which were used to determine the maternal body mass index (BMI; kg/m^2) and the infant's Ponderal Index (PI; kg/m^3), were measured at all three visits.

Laboratory measurements

Blood samples were collected from the mother-infant pairs at every visit. The baseline neonatal biochemical status was analyzed using umbilical cord blood collected at delivery. Non-fasting spot urine samples to determine the urinary calcium/creatinine ratio (UCa/Cr) (normal range: adults <0.78 mmol/mmol, infants < 2.55 mmol/l) were obtained from mothers and infants at only V3 and V6. Serum calcium and UCa/Cr measurements were performed within 6 hours of collection, using a Cobas 6000 analyzer (Roche Diagnostics, Basel, Switzerland). Serum samples for total 25(OH)D and intact parathyroid hormone (iPTH) assays were stored at −80°C until assayed. Total serum 25(OH)D (25-hydroxyvitamin D_2 and 25-hydroxyvitamin D_3) level was determined using an immunochemiluminescent method (LIAISON, DiaSorin, Sallugia, Italy) at the laboratory, controlled and certified by the International Vitamin D Proficiency – Testing Program (DEQAS). The intra-assay and inter-assay precision for total serum 25(OH)D were <8% and <11%, respectively, both of which were assessed using a control 25(OH)D concentration of 25.1 ng/ml in our laboratory with infant serum samples. Antibody specificities were 100%, 104%, 40%, 17%, and 0% for 25(OH)D_2, 25(OH)D_3, 1,25$(OH)_2D_2$, 1,25$(OH)_2D_3$, and 3-epi-25-OHD_3, respectively. The cross-reactivity with other vitamin D metabolites and detection limit (4 ng/ml) was provided by the manufacturer (LIAISON, DiaSorin, Sallugia, Italy). Serum 25(OH)D <20 ng/ml defined the vitamin D deficiency state, whereas ≥30 ng/ml reflected vitamin D sufficiency [7]. Serum iPTH was determined by a fully automated electrochemiluminescence system (Elecsys 2010, Roche Diagnostics, Basel, Switzerland). The detection limit was 1.20 pg/ml; the manufacturer's normal range was 15–65 pg/ml and intra-assay and inter-assay coefficients of variation (CV) ≤ 2.7% and ≤6.5%, respectively.

Dual energy X-ray absorptiometry (DXA)

Bone mineral content (BMC), bone mineral density (BMD), total lean body mass (LBM), total fat mass (FM), gynoid FM, and android FM were measured by dual energy X-ray absorptiometry (Lunar Prodigy Advance, GE Healthcare, Madison, United States) at every visit. Measurements were made for the total body (BMC and BMD) and the L2–L4 lumbar spine (lumbar BMC and lumbar BMD) in mothers and the total body and total body less head (less head BMC and less head BMD) in infants. DXA acquisition times were less than 5 minutes for mothers and less than 3 minutes for infants. Optimal infant DXA scans without major artifacts were obtained during spontaneous sleep using special infant software provided by the manufacturer. To ensure the reproducibility of results, the infant's upper extremities were positioned away from the trunk, both the upper and lower extremities were gently bound using a cotton blanket to avoid movement artifacts, and the head was turned to the side. No sedation was used, only a soft silicon pacifier if acceptable by the baby. DXA scans were analyzed by an experienced Certified Clinical Densitometrist (M.J.) with special attention for region of interest (ROI) placing and for artifacts. Changes in body composition measurements were calculated as percentage differences between measurements obtained at the end of the study (6 months postpartum) and baseline values.

Dietary vitamin D intake

Infant dietary vitamin D intake was calculated at all visits using a questionnaire that assessed the type of feeding (exclusive breastfeeding, partial breastfeeding), daily volume of infant formula consumed, or complementary food ingested during the study period. The vitamin D concentration per 100 ml of infant formula or complementary food was obtained from the manufacturers. Mean daily dietary vitamin D intake was a product of the mean daily volume consumed during the study period and the vitamin D concentration of the formula. A precise calculation of vitamin D intake from breast milk was not possible. Because vitamin D concentration in human milk varies [27], a concentration of 4 IU/100 ml was arbitrarily chosen for further calculation. For statistical purposes, vitamin D intake from breast milk was estimated to be 20 IU/d (500 ml of breast milk) at baseline and 40 IU/d (1000 ml of breast milk) at follow-up visits. Mothers were questioned about average fish consumption (portions/month) during the last 3 months prior to each visit.

Sunlight exposure

Maternal UV exposure was assessed at every visit using a questionnaire. The duration of outdoor activity Monday–Friday and during weekends, use of sun-blockers, sunbathing, and holidays in sunny countries during last 3 months prior to each visit were recorded.

Sample size calculation

To detect a statistically significant difference in serum 25(OH)D level (primary outcome) by 4 ng/ml between the intervention groups after vitamin D supplementation at least 64 mother-infant pairs per group were required at 80% power using a two-sided t-test at $\alpha = 0.05$. It was based on an assumption that each 400 IU/d of vitamin D may increase 25(OHD) level by 2.8–4.8 ng/ml (mean ~4 ng/ml) and the standard deviation of 25(OH)D measurements was 8 [28,29]. Concerning the maternal secondary outcomes, the calculated highest group size was 67 participants per group for total body BMC (difference between groups 150 g, SD = 307; 80% power, $\alpha = 0.05$, a two-sided t-test), and 12 participants per group for total body BMD (difference between groups 0.06 g, SD = 0.05; 80% power, $\alpha = 0.05$, a two-sided t-test), and 64 participants per group for serum iPTH (difference between groups 5 pg/ml, SD = 10; 80% power, $\alpha = 0.05$, a two-sided t-test). To account for dropouts, we considered 75 pairs for each group (n = 150). Due to a higher dropout rate at the beginning of the study, the study population was increased to 174 (87 per intervention group).

Statistical analysis

The normality of the distribution of analyzed data was tested by the Shapiro-Wilk test. A two-factor repeated-measures ANOVA (with Box-Cox transformation for baseline maternal 25(OH)D level and infants' 25(OH)D levels at birth, and at 3 and 6 months of age) with time and vitamin D dose (group) as factors was used to analyze maternal and infants' serum 25(OH)D levels. The primary analysis of serum 25(OH)D levels (the separate models for mothers and infants) was modeled as a function of group, time and the interaction between group and time, while accounting for the repeated measurements across subjects. This was followed by analysis of difference between groups at each time point and within groups during time by the Fisher's LSD test with respect to repeated measurements and adjustment for multiple comparisons. For other analysis (comparison of an absolute value, increment, % change), we used the unpaired t-test for normally distributed variables, U Mann-Whitney for non- normally distributed variables, and chi -squared test/Fisher's exact test for categorical variables. Spearman correlations were used to assess the association between variables. Data were analyzed using Statistica PL, version 10.0. The results are presented as medians with the first and third quartile (Q1; Q3) unless otherwise indicated. *P*-values< 0.05 were considered significant.

The study was originally planned to conduct an intention-to-treat (ITT) analysis [30]. The ITT approach assesses the effectiveness of improving vitamin D status via different oral vitamin D supplementation, regardless of whether the subject adhered to the dosing regimen. However, under the circumstances only one case of administrative errors occurred (Fig. 1), that patient being analyzed according to the treatment actually received as recommended by Gillings and Koch [30]. Because the primary endpoint was maternal serum 25(OH)D during supplementation, primary analysis was restricted to women who provided a blood sample at baseline and V3 or V6. To support the ITT approach, we decided to impute missing values for V6 using the most recent previous value in 18 (13.1%) participants, as relatively constant biochemical values were noted for V3 and V6. In addition, taking into account adherence, the sub-analysis of primary outcome was performed only in subjects with compliance >80%.

Results

A total of 174 Caucasian lactating mothers were randomly assigned to the treatment group (Fig. 1); 137 (79%) provided data regarding primary outcome [25(OH)D] and were analyzed. The groups were similar in all baseline characteristics, including vitamin D status (Fig. 2, Fig. 3), but a higher maternal education level was found in the 1200 IU/d group (Table 1). The participants who exited the study had similar baseline characteristics as those in the analyzed population with the exception of a 2-fold higher rate of additional formula-feeding (Table 2).

Vitamin D status

Maternal 25(OH)D level was similar in both groups at baseline and after 3 months of vitamin D supplementation, however, at V6 significantly higher 25(OH)D levels were noted in the 1200 IU/d group (Fig. 3). The effect of group (vitamin D dose) x time interaction ($P = 0.0004$) and the effect of time ($P<0.0001$) on maternal serum 25(OH)D level were statistically significant, but the effect of group (vitamin D dose) was not ($P = 0.25$). The mean maternal 25(OH)D increment was 5.5±8.4 ng/ml in the 400 IU/d group and 10.8±9.4 ng/ml in the 1200 IU/d group ($P = 0.0009$) after 6 months of vitamin D supplementation. Baseline maternal 25(OH)D <20 ng/ml was noted in 67.9% of mothers postpartum and 64.2% of cord blood samples. The prevalence of maternal vitamin D deficiency was significantly higher in the 400 IU/d group at V3 (25.4% vs.8.6%; $P = 0.009$) and V6 (29.9% vs. 14.3%; $P = 0.028$) (Fig. 2). On the other hand, the prevalence of vitamin D sufficiency (≥30 ng/ml) was comparable across the intervention groups (400 IU/d vs. 1200 IU/d) during vitamin D supplementation, at V3 (22.4% vs. 22.8%; $P = 0.95$) and V6 (13.4% vs.24.9%; $P = 0.1$) (Fig. 2). As expected, a significant increase in 25(OH)D occurred in breastfed infants supplemented with 400 IU/d of vitamin D, and no differences were found between the study groups (Fig. 3). The effect of group (vitamin D dose) x time interaction ($P = 0.12$) and the effect of group ($P = 0.45$) on infants' serum 25(OH)D levels was not statistically significant, while the effect of time was statistically significant ($P<0.0001$) (Fig. 3). The prevalence of infants' vitamin D deficiency and sufficiency was also comparable across the study groups (Fig. 2). However, a higher percentage of vitamin D sufficient infants (up to 70%) than mothers was noted in both study groups (Fig. 2). There was a strong correlation between postpar-

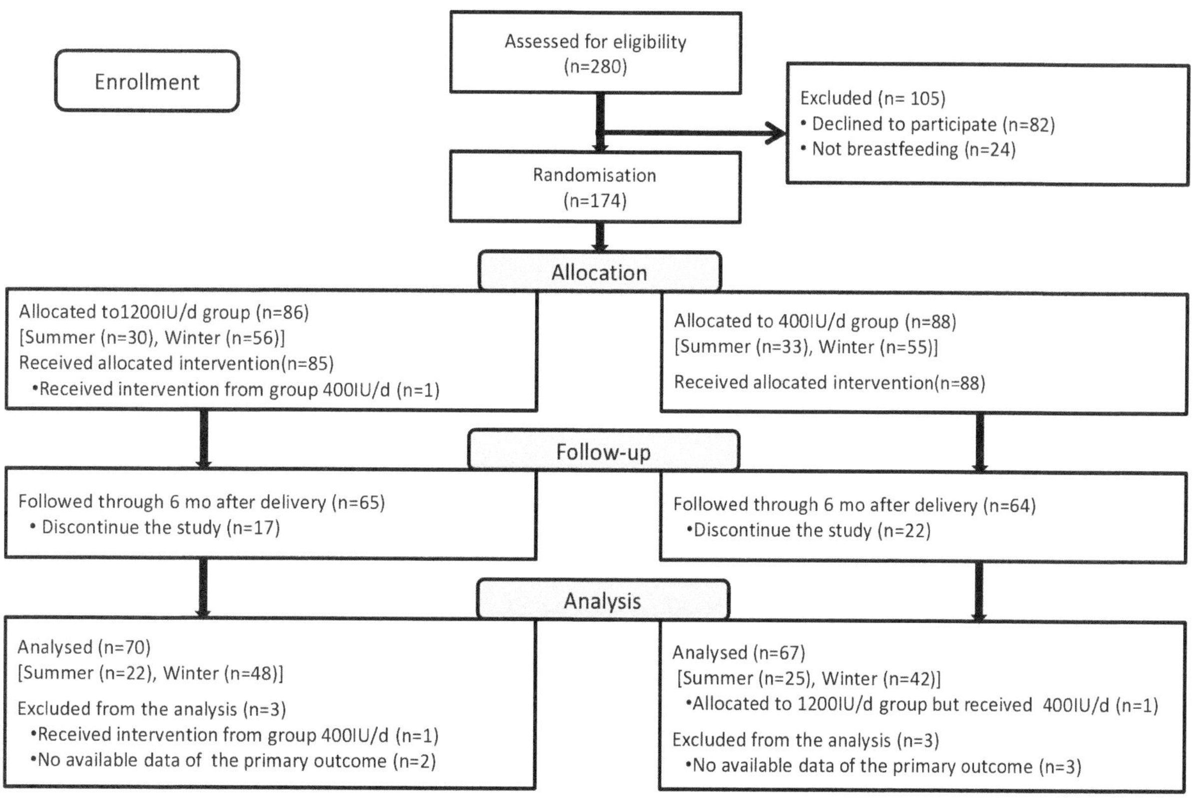

Figure 1. Flow chart of the subjects across the study.

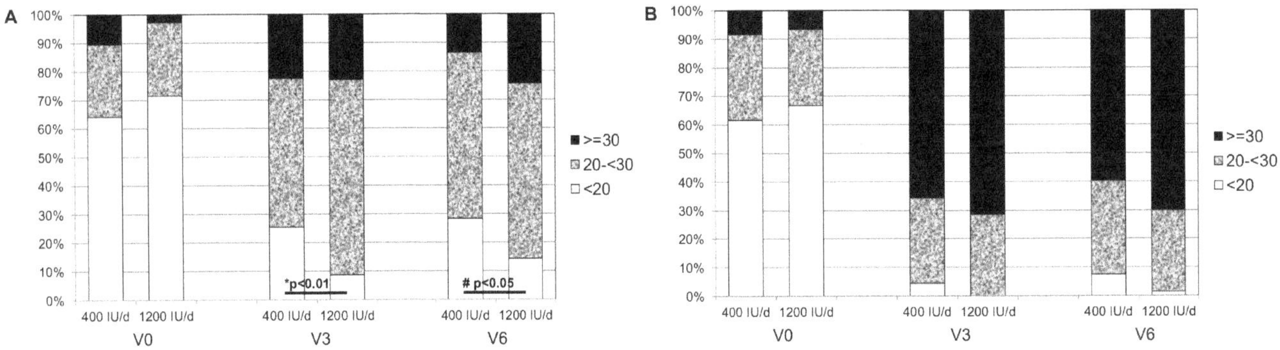

Figure 2. Maternal (A) and infants' (B) vitamin D status. Percentage of participants with serum 25(OH)D level <20 ng/ml, 20–29.9 ng/ml and >30 ng/ml in both study groups (maternal vitamin D intake 400 IU/d vs. 1200 IU/d). Significant (*P<0.05*) differences between the study groups are shown on the figures.

tum maternal and cord blood 25(OH)D levels in the 400 IU/d group (R = 0.86, *P*<0.0001) and in the 1200 IU/d group (R = 0.89, *P*<0.0001), respectively. A correlation between maternal and breastfed infants' 25(OH)D levels was still significant after 3 and 6 months of vitamin D supplementation but appeared weaker than the postpartum correlation: in the 400 IU/d group at V3 R = 0.35 (*P* = 0.003) and at V6 R = 0.4 (*P* = 0.0009), and in the 1200 IU/d group at V3 R = 0.3 (*P* = 0.01) and at V6 R = 0.39 (*P* = 0.0007), respectively.

Maternal and infant dietary vitamin D intake, sun exposure, and compliance are presented in Table 3. In a sub-analysis that included only participants with compliance >80%, maternal 25(OH)D appeared not significantly different between the study groups: 24.7 ng/ml (19.65–30.32 ng/ml) vs. 25.8 ng/ml (24–30.1 ng/ml) at V3 (*P* = 0.08) and 23.3 ng/ml (18.95–27.95 ng/ml) vs. 25.1 ng/ml (21.73–30.08 ng/ml) at V6 (*P* = 0.14) in the 400 IU/d and 1200 IU/d groups, respectively.

PTH levels

Maternal and infants' iPTH levels at baseline and increment (ΔiPTH) during the study period were comparable across intervention groups at every visit (*P*>0.05). However, different iPTH fluctuations at consecutive visits were observed (Table 4). A significant, negative correlation was noted between maternal iPTH and maternal 25(OH)D throughout the study (V0: R = −0.43, *P* = 0.00001; V3: R = −0.23, *P* = 0.008; V6: R = −0.24; *P* = 0.005). A similar weak correlation was found in infants at V3 (R = −0.23, *P* = 0.006) and V6 (R = −0.21, *P* = 0.01). However, when cord blood was controlled for, the correlation was not significant (R = 0.001, *P = 0.99*).

Calcemia and calciuria

No significant differences were found between intervention groups with regard to maternal calcemia and maternal and infants' calciuria (Table 4). No cases of hypercalcemia were found

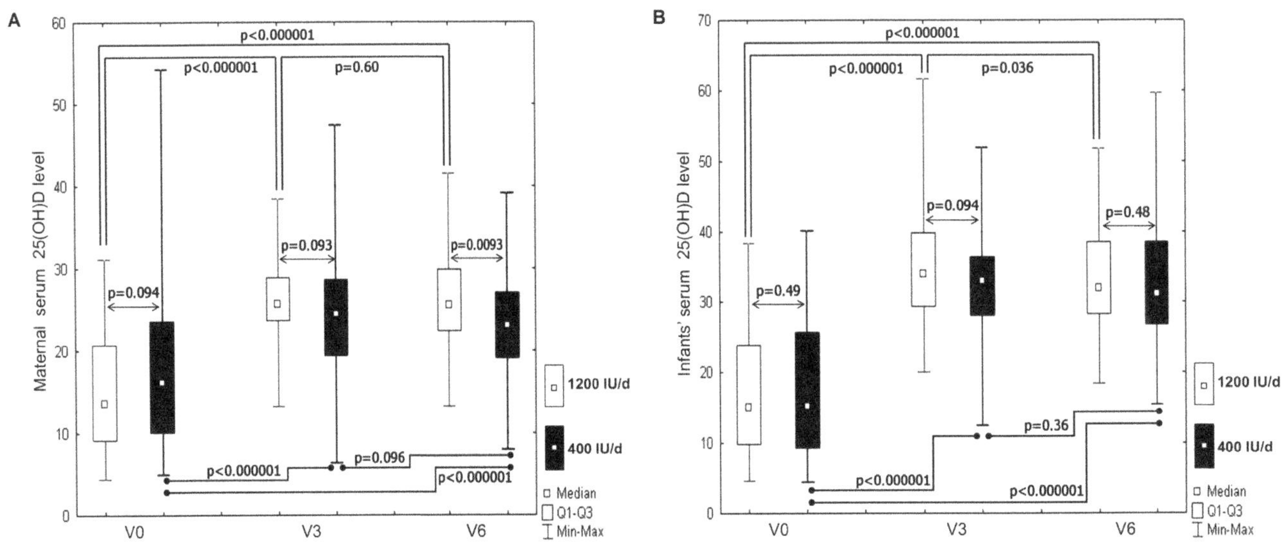

Figure 3. Maternal (A) and infants' (B) serum 25(OH)D concentrations at baseline and during vitamin D supplementation in the study groups (maternal vitamin D dose: 400 IU/d vs. 1200 IU/d). The effects of group (maternal vitamin D dose) × time interaction, group (maternal vitamin D dose) and time on maternal and infants' serum 25(OH)D levels were obtained from a two-factor repeated-measures ANOVA. *P*-values for these effects among mothers are 0.00042, <0.000001, 0.25, and among infants 0.12, <0.000001, 0.45, respectively. P-values presented on the figures (A, B) were obtained from post-test analysis (Fisher's LSD test) for differences in serum 25(OH) concentrations between the study groups and between the study visits. *P*-values<0.05 are significant. The study visits: V0- the baseline visit, V3, V6 – the visits after 3 and 6 months of vitamin D supplementation.

Table 1. Sociodemographic and clinical characteristics of the mothers and infants at study enrollment based on vitamin D supplementation group.

Parameter		400 IU/d group	1200 IU/d group	*P*-value between groups
Mathers		n = 67	n = 70	
Age, years		30 (27–33)	30 (26–34)	0.89
Baseline BMI, kg/m^2		24.4 (22.1–27.3)	23.8 (22.1–26.8)	0.49
BMI>30, n (%)		8 (12%)	5 (7%)	0.34
Weight before delivery, kg		77.4 (69–86)	74 (67–83)	0.26
Season at delivery, n (%)	June–October	25 (37%)	22 (31%)	0.47
	November–May	42 (63%)	48 (69%)	
Education, n (%)	>High school	5 (8%)	5 (7%)	0.04
	High school	27 (41%)	15 (21%)	
	College or more	34 (52%)	50 (71%)	
Monthly income, n (%)	<250 Euro/capita	16 (24%)	16 (23%)	0.59
	250–750 Euro/capita	32 (49%)	37 (54%)	
	>750 Euro/capita	18 (27%)	16 (23%)	
Vitamin D during pregnancy,	n (%)	46 (69%)	50 (71%)	0.73
	Daily dose, IU/d	400 (200–800)	400 (200–800)	0.70
	Duration, months	7 (6–9)	7 (5–9)	0.87
Infants		n = 67	n = 70	
Age at baseline visit, days		18 (14–22)	15 (13–20)	0.09
Boys, n (%)		29 (44%)	27 (38%)	0.48
Birth weight, g		3500 (3200–3815)	3480 (3280–3640)	0.80
Birth length, cm		55 (53–57)	55 (53–56)	0.25

Data are presented as median and interquartile range (Q1–Q3) or number and (%). *P-value*<0.05 are highlighted.

among participants. Hypercalciuria occurred in 3 mothers from the 400 IU/d group and 1 mother from the 1200 IU/d group at V3, and in 3 mothers from the 400 IU/d group at V6. Serum 25(OH)D concentrations were between 19 ng/ml and 28 ng/ml among the above-mentioned cases. Hypercalciuria was noted in 27 (20.44%) infants at V3 (13 infants of mothers receiving 400 IU/d, and 15 infants of mothers receiving 1200 IU/d; $P = 0.77$). At V6, hypercalciuria was observed in 10.95% of infants (5 from the 400 IU/d group, 10 from the 1200 IU/d group; $P = 0.20$).

Bone mass and body composition

No significant differences were found between the intervention groups with respect to maternal DXA measurements at any time point (Table 5). The mean maternal percent change in body composition parameters during the 6 months of breastfeeding was comparable between the intervention groups (Fig. 4). However, maternal total body fat mass was comparable between groups, significant negative correlations were noted between maternal 25(OH)D level and maternal fat mass ($R = -0.49$, $P = 0.00001$), android fat mass ($R = -0.53$, $P = 0.00001$), and gynoid fat mass ($R = -0.43$, $P = 0.00001$) after 6 months of vitamin D supplementation. The maternal 25(OH)D increment from V0 to V6 inversely correlated only with maternal android fat mass ($R = -0.18$, $P = 0.048$). Significant negative correlations were also noted between maternal 25(OH)D and maternal total body BMC ($R = -0.25$, $P = 0.006$) and lumbar BMC ($R = -0.18$, $P = 0.046$), but not total body BMD ($R = -0.13$, $P = 0.15$) and lumbar BMD ($R = -0.14$, $P = 0.13$). As expected, an increase in the infants' less-head total body BMC, BMD, LBM, and FM coincided with increasing infants' weight and length, with no significant differences between study groups (Fig. 4, Table 6).

Discussion

During this 6-month intervention study the dynamics of 25(OH)D levels and body composition parameters changes were examined among nursing mothers and their breastfed infants in relation to a vitamin D3 supplementation scheme. In our study maternal median 25(OH)D levels (~15 ng/ml) at the baseline visit, indicating vitamin D deficiency. More than 60% of mothers and newborns were vitamin D-deficient, and less than 10% of mothers and newborns had 25(OH)D >30 ng/ml. Fortunately, as early as 3 months after implementing vitamin D supplementation, 25(OH)D levels increased. Thereafter, maternal 25(OH)D levels tended to *plateau*, however a slight decline (by ~1.5 ng/ml) was noted in the 400 IU/d group. Hollis and Wagner [31] reported a much larger decline (by ~10 ng/ml) of maternal 25(OH)D3 level during the first 3 months of vitamin D supplementation at a dose of 400 IU/d. That difference can be explained, at least in part, by a higher baseline level (~25–30 ng/ml) and restricted sun exposure in the above-mentioned survey, compared to our population. In our study, women who took 1200 IU/d of vitamin D3 achieved a significantly higher 25(OH)D concentration compared to those supplemented using a dose of 400 IU/d only. However, a vitamin D daily dose of 1200 IU appeared too low to replenish vitamin D deficiency/insufficiency states in all breast-feeding mothers from the study group. It was shown that only 25% of women ingesting 1200 IU/d for 6 months achieved 25(OH) D levels higher than 30 ng/ml, the lowest value of optimal range

Table 2. Comparison of ITT population with participants lost to follow-up.

Parameter		ITT population	Patients not analyzed	*P*-value
Mothers		n = 137	n = 37	
Treatment group, n (%)	1200 IU/d	70 (51%)	16 (43%)	0.33
	400 IU/d	67 (49%)	21 (57%)	
Age, years		30 (27–33)	31 (27–35)	0.56
BMI, kg/m^2		24.2 (22.1–27.1)	25.3 (22.5–27.4)	0.36
BMI>30, n (%)		13 (10%)	2 (5%)	0.15
Season at delivery, n (%)	June–October	47 (34%)	16 (43%)	0.32
	November–May	90 (66%)	21 (57%)	
Education	>High school	10 (7%)	5 (14%)	0.32
	High school	42 (31%)	13 (36%)	
	College or more	84 (62%)	18 (50%)	
Monthly income, n (%)	<250 Euro/capita	32 (24%)	12 (33%)	0.38
	250–750 Euro/capita	69 (51%)	19 (53%)	
	>750 Euro/capita	34 (25%)	5 (14%)	
Vitamin D intake during pregnancy	Yes, n (%)	96 (70%)	27 (73%)	0.67
	Daily dose, IU/d	400 (200–800)	800 (400–800)	0.14
	Duration, months	7.0 (5.6–9.0)	6.0 (4.6–8.0)	0.17
Outdoor activity, hours	Mon-Fri	2.5 (2.0–4.0)	2.0 (1.9–4.6)	0.96
	Sat-Sun	3.5 (2.0–5.0)	4.0 (2.0–6.0)	0.34
Baseline 25(OH)D, ng/ml		15.2 (9.9–21.5)	15.8 (9.9–26.6)	0.28
25(OH)D >30 ng/ml, n (%)		9 (7%)	3 (8%)	0.72
25(OH)D <20 ng/ml, n (%)		93 (68%)	21 (57%)	0.63
Infants		n = 137	n = 37	
Boys, n (%)		56 (41%)	15 (41%)	0.97
Birth weight, g		3480 (3248–3756)	3450 (3180–3756)	0.79
Birth length, cm		55 (53–56)	54 (53–56)	0.22
Head circumference at birth, cm		34 (33–35)	34 (32–35)	0.29
Additional formula feeding, n (%)		21 (15%)	12 (32%)	0.02
Baseline 25(OH)D, ng/ml		15.2 (9.4–24.7) (n = 120)	12.7 (9.0–28.9) (n = 28)	0.84

Data are presented as median and interquartile range (Q1–Q3) or number and (%). *P-value*<0.05 are highlighted.

according to some authors [1,7,16], but not IOM experts (25(OH)D >20 ng/ml) [12]. In consequence, fundamental questions of: a) how much vitamin D is enough to reach and maintain optimal 25(OH)D level, and b) what is the optimal range for 25(OH)D levels, remain an issue of debate [32,33].

There is growing evidence showing serum 25(OH)D levels higher than 30 ng/ml, or even higher than 40 ng/ml as effective for expression of extra-skeletal effects related to proper vitamin D status [1,34,35]. On the other hand, the increased target level needs a much higher intake. The studies performed in healthy individuals indicate that vitamin D supplementation at a dose of 3000–7000 IU/d might be necessary to achieve a serum 25(OH)D level of at least 30 ng/ml in 97.5% of that population [17,35–37]. Our study was designed at the beginning of 2009, when recommended supplemental doses of vitamin D were around 400–600 IU/d. Keeping in mind recent literature, to address the question of the lowest effective and safe vitamin D dose needed to observe health benefits for both lactating mother and breastfed offspring, a higher vitamin D doses would be chosen and evaluated in our RCT (1500 IU/d vs. 2000 IU/d vs. 3000 IU/d).

Despite the aforementioned controversies, the improvement in vitamin D status in studied groups was achieved without any evidence of hypervitaminosis D, such as elevated 25(OH)D, hypercalcemia, or increased hypercalciuria. From a clinical point of view, the impact of 1200 IU/d vitamin D dose on the maternal 25(OH)D concentration was very subtle. The final intergroup difference in maternal 25(OH)D concentration was only 2.5 ng/ml. Unfortunately, the maternal compliance at V3 was significantly lower in the 400 IU/d group, which may have influenced the observed 25(OH)D level. When compliant mothers were compared, the difference in 25(OH)D levels between the 400 IU/d and 1200 IU/d groups was not any more significant. However, when the prevalence of vitamin D deficiency in intervention groups was considered, the clinical effect of the higher dose was much more distinct. Vitamin D deficiency affected women in the 400 IU/d group 2 to 3-times more frequently than those in the 1200 IU/d group. Undoubtedly, 400 IU/d of vitamin D appeared unsatisfactory for lactating women. Taking into account the maternal requirement, 1200 IU/d of vitamin D may protect against vitamin D deficiency, but seems too low to fully replenish vitamin D insufficiency (20 ng/ml<25(OH)D <30 ng/ml). Our

Table 3. Vitamin D intake, sun exposure, and compliance.

Parameter	Time	400 IU/d group	1200 IU/d group	*P*-value between groups
Mothers		n = 67	n = 70	
Fish consumption, portion/month	Baseline	2 (1–4)	2 (1–4)	0.62
	3 months	2 (1–4)	2 (1–4)	0.36
	6 months	2 (1–4)	2 (1–4)	0.86
Outdoor activity (Mon–Fri), hours	Baseline	2.5 (2.0–4.0)	2.0 (1.5–4.0)	0.21
	3 months	2.0 (1.0–3.0)	2.0 (1.8–3.5)	0.28
	6 months	2.0 (1.3–3.9)	2.0 (1.0–4.0)	0.68
Outdoor activity (Sat–Sun), hours	Baseline	3.5 (2.0–5.4)	3.0 (2.0–4.1)	0.27
	3 months	2.0 (1.3–3.4)	2.5 (1.8–4.5)	0.20
	6 months	3.0 (1.5–4)	2.5 (1.3–3.5)	0.77
Maternal sunblock usage, n (%)	Baseline	18 (27%)	17 (26%)	0.73
	3 months	6 (9%)	10 (14%)	0.34
	6 months	9 (13%)	7 (10%)	0.59
Maternal sunbathing, n (%)	Baseline	13(19%)	6(9%)	0.07
	3 months	8 (12%)	8 (11%)	0.93
	6 months	14 (21%)	14 (20%)	0.60
Holidays in sunny country, n (%)	Baseline	5 (8%)	7 (10%)	0.77
	3 months	0 (0%)	1 (1%)	0.49
	6 months	2 (3%)	3 (4%)	0.79
Mean compliance (Multivitamins), %	3 months	86%	92%	0.002
	6 months	86%	89%	0.03
Mean compliance (Cholecalciferol/placebo), %	3 months	89%	93%	0.02
	6 months	76%	88%	0.08
Infants		n = 67	n = 70	
Exclusive breastfeeding, n (%)	Baseline	57 (85%)	59 (84%)	0.90
	3 months	50 (75%)	53 (76%)	0.86
	6 months	2 (3%)	11 (16%)	0.03
Vitamin D intake from diet, IU/d	3 months	40 (40–40)	40 (40–40)	0.50
	6 months	40 (40–235)	40 (40–174)	0.36
Mean compliance, %	3 months	88%	89%	0.31
	6 months	85%	87%	0.73

Data are presented as median and interquartile range (Q1–Q3) or number and (%). *P-value*<0.05 are highlighted.

study findings are in contrast to the last IOM guideline defining the recommended dietary allowance (RDA) for lactating women as 600 IU/d [12]. Maternal supplementation at a dose twice lower than that of our study would likely not result in 25(OH)D >20 ng/ml, at least in a population living at a northern latitude. Though supplementation at a dose of 2000 IU/d was previously reported to increase maternal 25(OH)D to 30–39 ng/ml [35,38,39], it still might be insufficient for vitamin D-deficient women [40,41]. Even higher doses of vitamin D (4000–6400 IU/d) were tested in breastfeeding women as the combined maternal and breastfed infant supplementation [8–10,31,42]. Those high doses are not universally accepted, although not accompanied by any side effects. It is justified to recommend vitamin D supplementation in breastfeeding women based on their needs and separately in breastfed infants. Our results revealed that maternal vitamin D supplementation at a dose up to 1200 IU/d had no influence on the breastfed offspring's vitamin D status. Therefore, breastfeeding infants need additional vitamin D supplementation when maternal intake is 1200 IU/d.

Nevertheless, we should keep in mind that each 400 IU/d of vitamin D may increase serum 25(OH)D level by 2.8 ng/ml [17]. We observed a slightly higher maternal 25(OH)D increment during vitamin D supplementation (5.5 ng/ml in the 400 IU/d group and 11 ng/ml in the 1200 IU/d) due to additional input from diet and endogenous skin synthesis [37,43]. McDonnell's et al. revealed that every intake of 1 serving per day increases serum 25(OH)D by about 2 ng/ml for eggs and 1 ng/ml for meat and total protein [43]. Interestingly, the fish intake was not associated with serum 25(OH)d level in that study, despite fish being considered a rich source of vitamin D. On the other hand, a mean skin synthesis of vitamin D was 200–650 IU/d at the summer peak, but it accounted for only 10–25% of total basal vitamin D input [37]. In the light of the aforementioned studies, vitamin D supplements seems to be more effective as a source of vitamin D in many contemporary industrialized populations suffering from

Table 4. Serum iPTH and calcium concentrations, and urinary Ca/Cr ratio during 6 months of vitamin D supplementation.

Parameter	Time	400 IU/d group	1200 IU/d group	*P*-value between groups
Mothers		n = 67	n = 70	
iPTH, pg/ml	Baseline	30.4 (20.2–43.5)	28.6 (20–42)	0.54
ΔiPTH, pg/ml	Baseline to 3 months	−8.7±18.2	−9.0±15.9	0.70
	3 to 6 months	4.1±10.4	3.5±10.3	0.75
Serum Ca, mmol/l	3 months	2.43 (2.36–2.49)	2.44 (2.38–2.52)	0.54
	6 months	2.37 (2.33–2.43)	2.40 (2.36–2.47)	0.13
UCa/Cr ratio, mmol/mmol	3 months	0.22 (0.12–0.38)	0.3 (0.16–0.43)	0.17
	6 months	0.19 (0.08–0.34)	0.23 (0.11–0.41)	0.27
Infants		n = 67	n = 70	
iPTH, pg/ml	Baseline	4.8 (3.7–7.1) (n = 61)	4.5 (3.8–5.8) (n = 60)	0.69
ΔiPTH, pg/ml	Baseline to 3 months	10.7±10.0	11.5±6.3	0.80
	3 to 6 months	5.1±8.4	3.0±6.4	0.08
Serum Ca, mmol/l	3 months	2.66 (2.61–2.73)	2.67 (2.62–2.74)	0.76
	6 months	2.62 (2.57–2.68)	2.65 (2.62–2.7)	0.009
UCa/Cr ratio, mmol/mmol	3 month	1.58 (1.02–2.40)	1.51 (0.89–2.47)	0.55
	6 months	1.26 (0.87–1.81)	1.47 (0.86–2.27)	0.17

Data presented as median (interquartile range: Q1–Q3) or mean ± SD. *P-value*<0.05 are highlighted.
Ca- calcium, UCa/Cr ratio- urinary calcium creatinine ratio in spot urine, ΔiPTH- increment of iPTH concentration between the study visits.

Table 5. Maternal anthropometry and body composition throughout the study.

Parameter	Time	400 IU/d group	1200 IU/d group	*P*-value between groups
Mothers		(n = 67)	(n = 70)	
Weight (kg)	Baseline	66.3 (59.1–77)	65.3 (58–73)	0.35
	3 months	64.5 (58–74)	62.8 (57–70)	0.25
	6 months	63 (55–71)	61.5 (55–68)	0.33
BMI (kg/m^2)	Baseline	24.4 (22.2–27.3)	23.8 (22.1–26.8)	0.49
	3 months	23.5 (21.4–25.6)	22.8 (21.1–25.7)	0.26
	6 months	23.3 (20.8–25.5)	22.6 (20.1–24.7)	0.59
Total body BMC (g)	Baseline	2545 (2227–2800)	2490 (2201–2741)	0.31
	3 months	2517 (2212–2724) (n = 66)	2456 (2164–2596)	0.29
	6 months	2569 (2161–2764) (n = 59)	2410 (2141–2595) (n = 62)	0.19
Lumbar BMC (g)	Baseline	48.3 (44.1–57.2)	47.5 (43.9–53.8)	0.34
	3 months	47.2 (42.0–55.6) (n = 66)	47.0 (41.6–52.2)	0.46
	6 months	48.8 (42.1–56.3) (n = 59)	47.0 (42.8–53.3) (n = 62)	0.21
Total body BMD (g/cm^2)	Baseline	1.14 (1.09–1.18)	1.12 (1.07–1.17)	0.23
	3 months	1.13 (1.07–1.18) (n = 66)	1.12 (1.06–1.17)	0.41
	6 months	1.13 (1.08–1.19) (n = 59)	1.11 (1.06–1.16) (n = 62)	0.16
FM (kg)	Baseline	24.25 (19.84–32.57)	23 10 (18.89–29.17)	0.39
	3 months	23.03 (17.39–29.29) (n = 66)	21.47 (17.27–26.29)	0.44
	6 months	21.54 (16.07–27.60) (n = 59)	20.12 (15.11–25.90) (n = 62)	0.46
LBM (kg)	Baseline	39.21 (36.50–42.93)	38.69 (36.64–41.30)	0.43
	3 months	38.81 (35.76–41.84) (n = 66)	37.57 (35.84–40.91)	0.20
	6 months	39.01 (36.79–41.63) (n = 59)	38.39 (35.92–40.49) (n = 62)	0.16

Data presented as median (interquartile range: Q1–Q3). No significant differences between groups, all *P-value*>0.05. (*BMD* - bone mineral density, less head BMD - total body less head mineral density, BMC -bone mineral content, less head BMC - total body less head mineral content, LBM - total lean body mass, BMI - body mass index, FM- total fat, android FM – android fat mass, gynoid FM – gynoid fat mass).

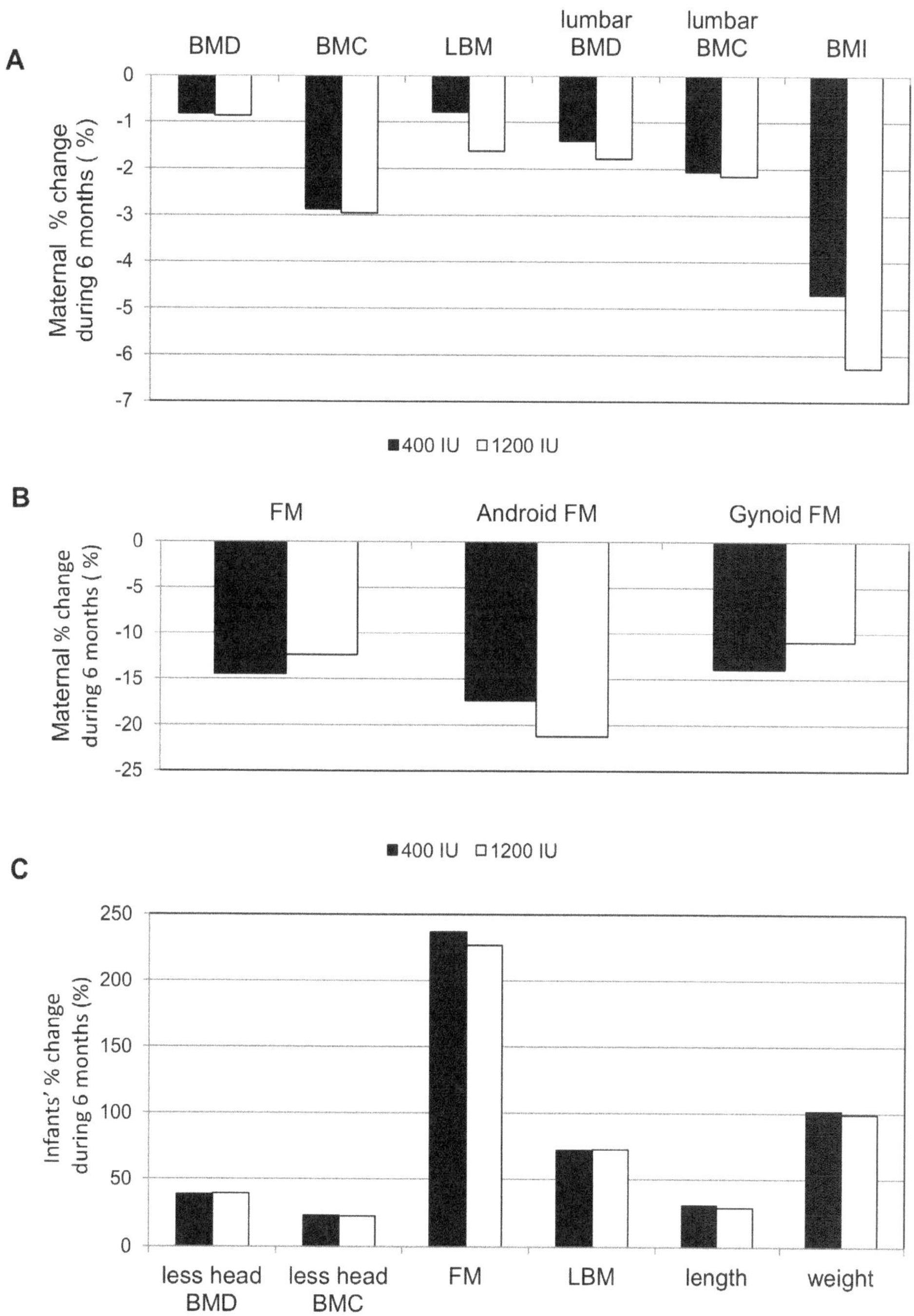

Figure 4. Maternal (A, B) and infants' (C) % change (between baseline and 6 months visit) in body composition and anthropometric parameters in the study groups during vitamin D3 supplementation. No significant difference between the study groups for all variables (*P*-values>*0.05)*. BMD - bone mineral density, less head BMD - total body less head mineral density, BMC -bone mineral content, less head BMC - total body less head mineral content, LBM - total lean body mass, BMI - body mass index, FM - total fat, android FM – android fat mass, gynoid FM – gynoid fat mass.

changing lifestyles (restricted sun exposure, obesity, unhealthy diet).

Another interesting observation relates to PTH as a functional marker of vitamin D status in adults, children and infants but not necessarily in neonates [44–47]. We found no correlation between 25(OH)D and iPTH in cord blood, which is in agreement with previous reports [44,48,49]. However, a weak correlation between cord blood 25(OH)D level and PTH was also reported [50]. During vitamin D supplementation in our infants, an increasing infants' 25(OH)D level coincided with an increase in iPTH. However, the inverse association between serum 25(OH)D levels and PTH was noted, as also reported by others [46]. On the other hand, stable and comparable PTH concentrations were reported by Greer in infants supplemented with vitamin D or receiving a placebo, despite significantly lower 25(OH)D levels in the placebo group [45]. Our results indicate that the PTH concentration

Table 6. Infants' anthropometry and body composition throughout the study.

Parameter	Time	400 IU/d group	1200 IU/d group	*P*-value between groups
		n = 67	n = 70	
Weight (g)	Baseline	3880 (3555–4198)	3715 (3415–4045)	0.12
Δ Weight (g)	Baseline- 3 months	2205 (1870–2650)	2200 (1770–2625)	0.68
	Baseline- 6 months	3940 (3364–4408	3650 (3275–4185)	0.17
Length (cm)	Baseline	52.5 (49.6–54.0)	52.0 (48.5–54.0)	0.36
Δ Length (cm)	Baseline- 3 months	8.6 (6.5–11)	8.5 (6–11.5)	0.81
	Baseline- 6 months	15.5 (13.0–18.7)	15 (12.7–19.0)	0.77
Ponderal Index (kg/m^3)	Baseline	26.2 (23.8–31.9)	26.4 (24.1–33.0)	0.60
	3 months	26.8 (24.5–30.4)	27.0 (24.8–30.2)	0.67
	6 months	24.5 (23.0–27.1)	24.2 (22.6–26.6)	0.61
Head circumference (cm)	Baseline	36.0 (35.5–37.0)	36.0 (35–36.5)	0.18
Δ Head circumference (cm)	Baseline- 3 months	4 (3.5–5)	4.2 (3.5–4.6)	0.94
	Baseline- 6 months	7.1 (6–8)	7 (6.5–7)	0.64
Less head BMC (g)	Baseline	48 (44–53)	47 (41–51)	0.15
Δ Less head BMC (g)	Baseline- 3 months	−1 ((5)–4)	1.5 ((−5)–5)	0.48
	Baseline- 6 months	10 (4–15)	9 (1–19)	0.62
Less head BMD (g/cm^2)	Baseline	0.33 (0.30–0.35)	0.31 (0.29–0.35)	0.19
Δ Less head BMD (g/cm^2)	Baseline- 3 months	0.10 (0.07–0.13)	0.11 (0.08–0.12)	0.36
	Baseline- 6 months	0.12 (0.09–0.15)	0.13 (0.09–0.14)	0.50
FM (g)	Baseline	662 (557–780)	640 (581–737)	0.37
Δ FM (g)	Baseline- 3 months	934 (723–1171)	919 (730–1128	0.65
	Baseline- 6 months	1606 (1264–2002)	1514 (1234–1837)	0.32
LBM (g)	Baseline	3444 (3162–3672)	3277 (3017–3523)	0.10
Δ LBM (g)	Baseline- 3 months	1337 (1101–1727)	1335 (1080–1669)	0.66
	Baseline- 6 months	2469 (2129–2947)	2340 (2094–2748)	0.41

Data presented as median (interquartile range: Q1–Q3). No significant differences between groups, all *P-value*>0.05. (Δ - increment (change) of the study variable between baseline and next visit, *BMD* - bone mineral density, less head BMD - total body less head mineral density, BMC - bone mineral content, less head BMC - total body less head mineral content, LBM - total lean body mass, BMI - body mass index, FM - total fat, android FM – android fat mass, gynoid FM – gynoid fat mass).

should not be considered a reliable functional marker of vitamin D status in newborn infants. In contrast, fluctuations in iPTH in breastfeeding mothers during supplementation were in agreement with changes in 25(OH)D. Although a statistically significant negative correlation between maternal 25(OH)D level and iPTH was found, the clinical relevance of such an association is questionable due to its weakness.

We did not find significant differences in any of the body composition variables between intervention groups during supplementation. Keeping in mind the diminutive differences in 25(OH)D levels among the study groups, we assumed that the vitamin D status in nursing women had no impact on bone mass and body composition. On the other hand, a weak negative correlation between maternal 25(OH)D and maternal BMC at the end of the study was noted, but maternal 25(OH)D levels were not associated with maternal total body BMD, lumbar spine BMD, or lumbar spine BMC. The influence of vitamin D status and bone mass in nursing women might be evaluated further but higher vitamin D doses are necessary. The negative impact of maternal fat mass on 25(OH)D level was distinct. The role of android mass should be underlined [51], as the observed increment in maternal 25(OH)D inversely correlated with android fat mass, only. Furthermore, postpartum changes in maternal body composition observed in both intervention groups are in agreement with most previous findings in nursing women [18,19,52]. Interestingly, some changes in bone structure geometry also occur, but with minimal impact on bending or compressive strength [52]. The adaptation mechanism during human lactation is still under study. Animal data demonstrate that, instead of vitamin D, calcitriol, or the vitamin D receptor, the increase in intestinal calcium absorption is likely due to the pregnancy-related increase in duodenal expression of the calcium transporter gene *Trpv6* [53]. If the same mechanism exists in humans, increasing the vitamin D intake of lactating women can be presumed to have no beneficial effect on bone mineral content and density. The afore-mentioned speculation is another possible explanation for the lack of intergroup differences in maternal DXA results in our study. Additionally, the dose of maternal vitamin D supplementation had no impact on their infants' measured DXA variables despite the fact that infants received vitamin D at a dose of 400 IU/d. Gallo et al, also found no differences in BMC between infants supplemented with diverse doses of vitamin D (400–1600 IU/d) [26].

This study has some limitations. First, a small difference was achieved in the 25(OH)D level during supplementation, making it difficult to prove/exclude a positive effect of vitamin D supplementation on bone mass in nursing women. In addition, differences in compliance, maternal education level and final rate of exclusive breastfeeding were observed between study groups, which may have influenced the primary outcome. Finally, dietary vitamin D intake was based solely on fish consumption, not overall food frequency. However, diet is not an important source of vitamin D in Poland [5].

Conclusions

In summary, our study showed a very high prevalence (~65%) of postpartum vitamin D deficiency among Caucasian mothers and their newborn offspring living at latitude 52°N. We have demonstrated that vitamin D3 supplementation at a dose of 400 IU/d is not sufficient for nursing women to maintain 25(OH)D > 20 ng/ml. Vitamin D3 supplementation at a dose of 1200 IU/d is more effective at improving vitamin D status of nursing women, but still seems too low to fully replenish vitamin D deficiency/ insufficiency. Furthermore, maternal vitamin D3 supplementation during lactation at a dose up to 1200 IU/d had no influence on maternal and infant body composition or infant vitamin D status. Further studies of vitamin D supplementation during lactation are necessary to determine the optimal dosing for nursing women when taking into account maternal needs.

Supporting Information

Checklist S1 The CONSORT 2010 checklist of information to include when reporting a randomized trial.

Protocol S1 The study protocol.

Protocol S2 The study protocol in the original language (Polish).

Acknowledgments

We would like to thank the nurses who were responsible for blood and urine sample collection and Agata Pleskaczynska, Justyna Lygas, Dorota Maksym-Gasiorek, and Monika Nowakowska – Rysz for participants assessment.

Author Contributions

Conceived and designed the experiments: JCK AD EK. Performed the experiments: JCK JLG DB. Analyzed the data: JCK MJ PP EK. Contributed reagents/materials/analysis tools: JCK DB JLG MJ EC EK BC BP GW AZ MKB. Wrote the paper: JCK PP.

References

1. Pludowski P, Holick MF, Pilz S, Wagner CL, Hollis BW, et al. (2013) Vitamin D effects on musculoskeletal health, immunity, autoimmunity, cardiovascular disease, cancer, fertility, pregnancy, dementia and mortality-a review of recent evidence. Autoimmun Rev 12: 976–989.
2. Specker BL, Tsang RC, Ho ML (1991) Changes in calcium homeostasis over the first year postpartum: effect of lactation and weaning. Obstet Gynecol 78: 56–62.
3. Milman N, Hvas AM, Bergholt T (2011) Vitamin D status during normal pregnancy and postpartum. A longitudinal study in 141 Danish women. J Perinat Med 40: 57–61.
4. Narchi H, Kochiyil J, Zayed R, Abdulrazzak W, Agarwal M (2010) Maternal vitamin D status throughout and after pregnancy. J Obstet Gynaecol 30: 137–142.
5. Wawrzyniak A, Hamulka J, Gorzel K (2009) [Assessment of vitamins and minerals intake with supplements during breast-feeding]. Rocz Panstw Zakl Hig 60: 353–356.
6. Czech-Kowalska J, Dobrzanska A, Gruszfeld D, Zochowska A, Malinowska E, et al. (2008) High prevalence of neonatal vitamin D deficiency - rationale for reevaluation of vitamin D supplementation during pregnancy. Arch Perinatal Med 14: 18–22.
7. Holick MF, Binkley NC, Bischoff-Ferrari HA, Gordon CM, Hanley DA, et al. (2011) Evaluation, treatment, and prevention of vitamin D deficiency: an Endocrine Society clinical practice guideline. J Clin Endocrinol Metab 96: 1911–1930.
8. Basile LA, Taylor SN, Wagner CL, Horst RL, Hollis BW (2006) The effect of high-dose vitamin D supplementation on serum vitamin D levels and milk calcium concentration in lactating women and their infants. Breastfeed Med 1: 27–35.
9. Wagner CL, Hulsey TC, Fanning D, Ebeling M, Hollis BW (2006) High-dose vitamin D3 supplementation in a cohort of breastfeeding mothers and their infants: a 6-month follow-up pilot study. Breastfeed Med 1: 59–70.
10. Saadi HF, Dawodu A, Afandi B, Zayed R, Benedict S, et al. (2009) Effect of combined maternal and infant vitamin D supplementation on vitamin D status of exclusively breastfed infants. Matern Child Nutr 5: 25–32.
11. Oberhelman SS, Meekins ME, Fischer PR, Lee BR, Singh RJ, et al. (2013) Maternal Vitamin D Supplementation to Improve the Vitamin D Status of Breast-fed Infants: A Randomized Controlled Trial. Mayo Clin Proc 88: 1378–1387. doi:1310.1016/j.mayocp.2013.1309.1012.
12. IOM (2011) *Dietary Reference Intakes for Calcium and Vitamin D.* Washington, DC: The National Academies Press.
13. Paxton GA, Teale GR, Nowson CA, Mason RS, McGrath JJ, et al. (2013) Vitamin D and health in pregnancy, infants, children and adolescents in Australia and New Zealand: a position statement. Med J Aust 198: 142–143.
14. Godel J, Irvine J, Onyett H, Saylor K, Schroter H, et al. (2007) Vitamin D supplementation: Recommendations for Canadian mothers and infants. Paediatrics & Child Health: 583–589.
15. Department of Health (2012) Vitamin D - advice on supplements for at risk groups - letter from UK Chief Medical Officers. Available: www.gov.uk/government/publications/vitamin-d-advice-on-supplements-for-at-risk-groups/.
16. Płudowski P, Karczmarewicz E, Bayer M, Carter G, Chlebna-Sokół D, et al. (2013) Practical guidelines for the supplementation of vitamin D and the treatment of deficits in Central Europe - recommended vitamin D intakes in the general population and groups at risk of vitamin D deficiency. Endokrynol Pol 64: 319–327.
17. Heaney RP, Davies KM, Chen TC, Holick MF, Barger-Lux MJ (2003) Human serum 25-hydroxycholecalciferol response to extended oral dosing with cholecalciferol. Am J Clin Nutr 77: 204–210.
18. Costa ML, Krupa FG, Rehder PM, Sousa MH, Costa-Paiva L, et al. (2012) Forearm bone mineral density changes during postpartum and the effects of breastfeeding, amenorrhea, body mass index and contraceptive use. Osteoporos Int 23: 1691–1698.
19. Moller UK, Vieth Streym S, Mosekilde L, Rejnmark L (2012) Changes in bone mineral density and body composition during pregnancy and postpartum. A controlled cohort study. Osteoporos Int 23: 1213–1223.
20. Kalkwarf HJ (1999) Hormonal and dietary regulation of changes in bone density during lactation and after weaning in women. J Mammary Gland Biol Neoplasia 4: 319–329.
21. Kalkwarf HJ, Specker BL, Bianchi DC, Ranz J, Ho M (1997) The effect of calcium supplementation on bone density during lactation and after weaning. N Engl J Med 337: 523–528.
22. Kovacs CS (2012) The role of vitamin D in pregnancy and lactation: insights from animal models and clinical studies. Annu Rev Nutr 32: 97–123.
23. Møller UK, Streym S, Mosekilde L, Heickendorff L, Flyvbjerg A, et al. (2013) Changes in calcitropic hormones, bone markers and insulin-like growth factor I (IGF-I) during pregnancy and postpartum: a controlled cohort study. Osteoporos Int 24: 1307–1320.
24. Kull M, Kallikorm R, Lember M (2012) Vitamin D as a possible independent predictor of bone mineral density in Estonian adults: a cross-sectional population-based study. Intern Med J 42: e89–94.
25. Al-Shaar L, Nabulsi M, Maalouf J, El-Rassi R, Vieth R, et al. (2013) Effect of vitamin D replacement on hip structural geometry in adolescents: a randomized controlled trial. Bone 56: 296–303.
26. Gallo S, Comeau K, Vanstone C, Agellon S, Sharma A, et al. (2013) Effect of different dosages of oral vitamin D supplementation on vitamin D status in healthy, breastfed infants: a randomized trial. JAMA 309: 1785–1792.
27. Specker BL, Tsang RC, Hollis BW (1985) Effect of race and diet on human-milk vitamin D and 25-hydroxyvitamin D. Am J Dis Child 139: 1134–1137.
28. Czech-Kowalska J, Dobrzanska A, Janowska J, Pleskaczynska A, Niezgoda A, et al. (2004) [Neonatal vitamin D status and calcium-phosphorus homeostasis in the third week of life]. Med Wieku Rozwoj 8: 115–124.
29. Dawson-Hughes B, Heaney RP, Holick MF, Lips P, Meunier PJ, et al. (2005) Estimates of optimal vitamin D status. Osteoporos Int 16: 713–716.
30. Gillings D, Koch G (1991) The Application of the Principle of Intention-to-Treat to the Analysis of Clinical Trials. Drug Inf J 25: 411–424.
31. Hollis BW, Wagner CL (2004) Vitamin D requirements during lactation: high-dose maternal supplementation as therapy to prevent hypovitaminosis D for both the mother and the nursing infant. Am J Clin Nutr 80: 1752S–1758S.
32. Rosen CJ, Abrams SA, Aloia JF, Brannon PM, Clinton SK, et al. (2012) IOM committee members respond to Endocrine Society vitamin D guideline. J Clin Endocrinol Metab 97: 1146–1152. doi:1110.1210/jc.2011-2218. Epub 2012 Mar 1122.

33. Holick MF, Binkley NC, Bischoff-Ferrari HA, Gordon CM, Hanley DA, et al. (2012) Guidelines for preventing and treating vitamin D deficiency and insufficiency revisited. J Clin Endocrinol Metab 97: 1153–1158.
34. Hollis BW, Wagner CL (2013) Vitamin D and pregnancy: skeletal effects, nonskeletal effects, and birth outcomes. Calcif Tissue Int 92: 128–139. doi:110.1007/s00223-00012-09607-00224. Epub 02012 May 00224.
35. Hollis BW, Johnson D, Hulsey TC, Ebeling M, Wagner CL (2011) Vitamin D supplementation during pregnancy: double-blind, randomized clinical trial of safety and effectiveness. J Bone Miner Res 26: 2341–2357.
36. Garland CF, French CB, Baggerly LL, Heaney RP (2011) Vitamin D supplement doses and serum 25-hydroxyvitamin D in the range associated with cancer prevention. Anticancer Res 31: 607–611.
37. Heaney RP, Armas LA, French C (2013) All-source basal vitamin D inputs are greater than previously thought and cutaneous inputs are smaller. J Nutr 143: 571–575.
38. Ala-Houhala M, Koskinen T, Terho A, Koivula T, Visakorpi J (1986) Maternal compared with infant vitamin D supplementation. Arch Dis Child 61: 1159–1163.
39. Hollis BW, Wagner CL (2004) Assessment of dietary vitamin D requirements during pregnancy and lactation. Am J Clin Nutr 79: 717–726.
40. Saadi HF, Dawodu A, Afandi BO, Zayed R, Benedict S, et al. (2007) Efficacy of daily and monthly high-dose calciferol in vitamin D-deficient nulliparous and lactating women. Am J Clin Nutr 85: 1565–1571.
41. Anderson DM, Hollis BW, LeVine BR, Pittard WB (1988) Dietary assessment of maternal vitamin D intake and correlation with maternal and neonatal serum vitamin D concentrations at delivery. J Perinatol 8: 46–48.
42. Wagner CL, Taylor SN, Johnson DD, Hollis BW (2012) The role of vitamin D in pregnancy and lactation: emerging concepts. Womens Health (Lond Engl) 8: 323–340. doi:310.2217/whe.2212.2217.
43. McDonnell SL, French CB, Heaney RP (2013) Quantifying the food sources of basal vitamin d input. J Steroid Biochem Mol Biol.
44. Czech-Kowalska J, Pludowski P, Dobrzanska A, Kryskiewicz E, Karczmarewicz E, et al. (2012) Impact of vitamin D supplementation on markers of bone mineral metabolism in term infants. Bone 51: 781–786.
45. Greer FR (2008) 25-Hydroxyvitamin D: functional outcomes in infants and young children. Am J Clin Nutr 88: 529S–533S.
46. Cranney A, Horsley T, O'Donnell S, Weiler H, Puil L, et al. (2007) Effectiveness and safety of vitamin D in relation to bone health. Evid Rep Technol Assess (Full Rep): 1–235.
47. Sai AJ, Walters RW, Fang X, Gallagher JC (2011) Relationship between vitamin D, parathyroid hormone, and bone health. J Clin Endocrinol Metab 96: E436–446.
48. Bowyer L, Catling-Paull C, Diamond T, Homer C, Davis G, et al. (2009) Vitamin D, PTH and calcium levels in pregnant women and their neonates. Clin Endocrinol (Oxf) 70: 372–377.
49. Young BE, McNanley TJ, Cooper EM, McIntyre AW, Witter F, et al. (2012) Maternal vitamin D status and calcium intake interact to affect fetal skeletal growth in utero in pregnant adolescents. Am J Clin Nutr 95: 1103–1112. doi:1110.3945/ajcn.1111.023861. Epub 022012 Apr 023864.
50. Dror DK, King JC, Fung EB, Van Loan MD, Gertz ER, et al. (2012) Evidence of associations between feto-maternal vitamin D status, cord parathyroid hormone and bone-specific alkaline phosphatase, and newborn whole body bone mineral content. Nutrients 4: 68–77. doi:10.3390/nu4020068. Epub 4022012 Feb 4020066.
51. Greco EA, Francomano D, Fornari R, Marocco C, Lubrano C, et al. (2013) Negative association between trunk fat, insulin resistance and skeleton in obese women. World J Diabetes 4: 31–39.
52. Laskey M, Price R, Khoo B, Prentice A (2011) Proximal femur structural geometry changes during and following lactation. Bone 48: 755–759.
53. Fudge NJ, Kovacs CS (2010) Pregnancy up-regulates intestinal calcium absorption and skeletal mineralization independently of the vitamin D receptor. Endocrinology 151: 886–895.

4

Maternal Vitamin D Status in Preeclampsia: Seasonal Changes Are Not Influenced by Placental Gene Expression of Vitamin D Metabolizing Enzymes

Carolin Lechtermann[1], Berthold P. Hauffa[1], Ralf Herrmann[1,2], Michael M. Schündeln[3], Alexandra Gellhaus[4], Markus Schmidt[5], Corinna Grasemann[1]*

1 Department of Pediatric Endocrinology and Diabetology, Kinderklinik II, Universitätsklinikum-Essen and the University of Duisburg-Essen, Essen, Germany, **2** Department of Neonatology, Kinderklinik I, Universitätsklinikum -Essen and the University of Duisburg-Essen, Essen, Germany, **3** Department of Pediatric Oncology and Hematology, Kinderklinik III, Universitätsklinikum -Essen and the University of Duisburg-Essen, Essen, Germany, **4** Institute of Molecular Biology, Universitätsklinikum -Essen and the University of Duisburg-Essen, Essen, Germany, **5** Department of Gynecology and Obstetrics, Klinikum Duisburg and the University of Duisburg-Essen, Duisburg, Germany

Abstract

Preeclampsia, a hypertensive disorder in pregnancy develops in 2–8% of pregnancies worldwide. Winter season and vitamin D deficiency have been associated with its onset.

Objective: To investigate the influence of season on maternal vitamin D status and placental vitamin D metabolism.

Methods: 25-OH vitamin D and 1,25-$(OH)_2$ vitamin D were measured in maternal serum obtained during the winter or summer months from 63 pregnant women at delivery (43 healthy, 20 preeclampsia). In a subgroup, mRNA expression of CYP24A1 (24-hydroxylase), CYP27B1 (1α-hydroxylase) and VDR (vitamin D receptor) were quantified by real time PCR in placental samples of 14 women with normal pregnancies and 13 with preeclampsia.

Results: In patients with preeclampsia,25-OH vitamin D levels were lower, but differed significantly from controls only in summer (18.21 ± 17.1 vs 49.2 ± 29.2 ng/mL, $P<0.001$), whereas 1,25-$(OH)_2$ vitamin D levels were significantly lower only in winter (291 ± 217 vs 612.3 ± 455 pmol/mL, $P<0.05$). A two-factorial analysis of variance produced a statistically significant model ($P<0.0001$) with an effect of season ($P<0.01$) and preeclampsia ($P=0.01$) on maternal 25-OH vitamin D levels, as well as a significant interaction between the two variables ($P=0.02$). Placental gene expression of CYP24A1, CYP27B1, and VDR did not differ between groups or seasons. A negative correlation between placental gene expression of CYP24A1 and CYP27B1 was observed only in healthy controls ($r=-0.81$, $P<0.0001$).

Summary: Patients with preeclampsia displayed lower vitamin D serum levels in response to seasonal changes.The regulation of placental CYP24A1, but not of the VDR or CYP27B1 might be altered in preeclampsia.

Editor: Ana Claudia Zenclussen, Medical Faculty, Otto-von-Guericke University Magdeburg, Medical Faculty, Germany

Funding: CG and MS were supported by an IFORES stipend of the 'Faculty of Medicine, University of Duisburg-Essen'. The funders had no role in study design, data collection and analysis, decision to publish, or preparation of the manuscript.

Competing Interests: The authors have declared that no competing interests exist.

* Email: corinna.grasemann@uk-essen.de

Introduction

Preeclampsia, a hypertensive disorder of pregnancy, affects about 2–8% of pregnancies worldwide [1]. It poses a threat to maternal and fetal health and often results in premature delivery of the child. The development of preeclampsia is linked to altered vitamin D metabolism [2], and might be a result from placental dysfunction [24]. However, the underlying cause of the development of preeclampsia remains elusive.

Worldwide, the onset of preeclampsia is more frequent during winter months, which in tropical countries corresponds to the rain season, than during any other season [3]. Since vitamin D deficiency is also more frequent during winter months, these findings point towards a potential role of vitamin D in the development of preeclampsia. Indeed, studies found lower 25-OH vitamin D serum levels as well as lower 1,25-$(OH)_2$ vitamin D levels in patients with preeclampsia compared to healthy pregnant women of the same gestational age [2].

Vitamin D deficiency itself is common during pregnancy in the European and North American populations [4–6] and is associated with complications during the perinatal period [2] [7].

In the non-pregnant state, vitamin D status is regulated mainly by the enzymatic activity of the '1α-hydroxylase' (CYP27B1), which converts 25-OH vitamin D to its active form 1,25-$(OH)_2$ vitamin D (also called calcitriol), mostly at the renal site, and the '1,25-$(OH)_2$ vitamin D 24-hydroxylase' (24-hydroxylase, CYP24A1), which converts 1,25-$(OH)_2$ vitamin D to the inactive 24,25-vitamin D.

During pregnancy, maternal 1,25-$(OH)_2$ vitamin D levels are elevated [8]. It has been suggested that the physiological feedback regulation is uncoupled during pregnancy due to placenta-specific methylation of the promoter region of the 24-hydroxylase (CYP24A1), to allow for an increase in 1,25-$(OH)_2$ vitamin D levels during the period of fetal development [9].

The placenta is thought to be the major site of vitamin D metabolism in pregnancy. The 1α-hydroxylase, the 24-hydroxylase, the 25-hydroxylase (CYP2R1), the vitamin D binding protein (VDB), and the vitamin D receptor (VDR) have all been detected either in trophoblast cultures or in freshly obtained, placental tissue [10–13]. Undoubtedly, the placenta is able to metabolize vitamin D, providing active 1,25-$(OH)_2$ vitamin D *in vitro*. However, it is unclear to what extent placental vitamin D metabolism contributes to maternal vitamin D status in pregnancy.

Since placental dysfunction in preeclampsia might affect placental vitamin D metabolism, we aimed to investigate maternal and placental vitamin D metabolism in vitamin D deficient (winter) and sufficient (summer) season in women with and without preeclampsia.

Results

Maternal vitamin D and calcium status

Both delivery season and preeclampsia had a significant effect on maternal 25-OH vitamin D serum concentration ($P<0.0001$).

In patients with preeclampsia maternal 25-OH vitamin D serum levels were significantly lower compared to healthy controls during summer (18.21±17.1 vs 49.2±29.2 ng/mL, $P<0.001$).

In healthy controls, serum 25-OH vitamin D levels were higher in the summer than in the winter (49.2±29.2 vs 19.5±16 ng/mL). Surprisingly, these seasonal changes in 25-OH vitamin D levels were not present in patients with preeclampsia (18.21±17.1 vs 17.6±23.5 ng/mL), indicating a significant interaction between seasonality and pregnancy outcome on 25-OH vitamin D ($P=0.02$, Regression Model). (Figure 1)

Maternal 1,25 -$(OH)_2$ vitamin D levels were differently affected by season than 25-OH vitamin D levels: While no seasonal changes were detected in healthy controls (612.3±455.7 in winter vs.748.5±462 pmol/L in summer), patients with preeclampsia had significantly lower 1,25-$(OH)_2$ vitamin D levels in the winter compared to the summer months (291±217 vs 815±478 pmol/L, $P<0.01$), and also compared to the levels of healthy controls ($P<0.01$) (Figure 1).

Maternal serum calcium levels did not differ between healthy controls (2.23±0.18 mmol/L) and patients with preeclampsia (2.13±0.17 mmol/L, Table 1). In both groups individual cases displayed serum calcium levels below the lower norm. Maternal serum calcium correlated positively with 25-OH vitamin D levels in healthy controls ($r=0.42$, $P=0.015$), but not in patients with preeclampsia. In the group of preeclampsia, maternal calcium levels correlated positively with the child-BMI at birth ($r=0.59$, $P=0.023$).

Placental gene expression of CYP24A1, CYP27B1, and VDR

The lowest mRNA levels between the three genes were found for CYP27B1. In few samples, CYP27B1 expression was below the detection limit. This affected 3of the 14 non-PE samples (21%), and 2 of the 13 PE samples (18%). Placental gene expression of neither CYP24A1 nor CYP27B1 nor VDR differed between seasons or between patients with preeclampsia and healthy controls (as determined by the Mann-Whitney test). Results are displayed in table 2.

However, in healthy controls, placental gene expression of CYP24A1 negatively correlated with CYP27B1 expression ($r=-0.81$, $P<0.0001$) (Figure 2) and with maternal serum calcium levels ($r=-0.8$, $P<0.01$). This finding was not detectable in patients with preeclampsia (Figure 2).

Instead, in patients with preeclampsia, a negative correlation between placental gene expression of CYP24A1 with maternal 25-OH vitamin D levels ($r=-0.76$, $P=0.01$) was observed (Figure 2).

In a stepwise regression analysis, adding placental CYP24A1, CYP27B1, and VDR gene expression to a model already containing season and pregnancy status, an additional effect of placental gene expression of CYP24A1 on maternal 25-OH vitamin D serum levels (partial $r^2=0{,}12$) was detected. No such effects were seen on serum 1,25-$(OH)_2$ vitamin D levels. Delivery-season and preeclampsia combined had no significant effect on maternal 1,25-$(OH)_2$ vitamin D serum concentration.

Discussion

Alterations in vitamin D metabolism in preeclampsia have been documented by many studies.

In this study, we report evidence supporting a role for vitamin D deficiency in the development of preeclampsia.

Maternal vitamin D-status

Consistent with previous studies, we found significantly lower maternal 25-OH vitamin D serum levels in patients with preeclampsia than in healthy pregnant controls. Surprisingly, this was most apparent during the summer months, when 25-OH vitamin D levels increased in women with healthy pregnancies, but remained at deficient levels in patients with preeclampsia. It is feasible that low 25-OH vitamin D levels are a contributing factor to the development of preeclampsia. Conversely, it is also feasible that vitamin D deficiency is a result of preeclampsia.

Serum 1,25-$(OH)_2$ vitamin D levels were higher (643.5±452.4 pmol/L) in this cohort of pregnant women compared to levels in non-pregnant females [8]. Other studies have demonstrated both lowered maternal 1,25-$(OH)_2$ vitamin D and 25-OH vitamin D levels in preeclampsia compared to healthy controls [16] [17] [18]. In our study, maternal 1,25-$(OH)_2$ vitamin D levels were significantly lower only during winter months in patients with preeclampsia. There was an impressive difference between summer and winter 1,25-$(OH)_2$ vitamin D levels in this group. This finding may indicate that during winter months vitamin D deficiency becomes more severe in patients with preeclampsia resulting in the inability of the vitamin D metabolizing sites to provide sufficient levels of 1,25-$(OH)_2$ vitamin D.

In the non-pregnant state, the kidney is the major site of calcitriol synthesis. During pregnancy, 1,25-$(OH)_2$ vitamin D synthesis is uncoupled, resulting in increased amounts of the active hormone in maternal serum in healthy pregnancies [19]. Whether the high 1,25-$(OH)_2$ vitamin D output is achieved entirely by the kidney or whether placental sites contribute to the production is not clear.

However, since both placenta and kidney are affected by preeclampsia, the pathophysiological changes in both these organs might result in an impairment of 1,25-$(OH)_2$ vitamin D synthesis. This would be consistent with higher PTH levels in women affected by preeclampsia, indicating a chronic impairment of renal function [20]. It is a shortcoming of this study that no PTH levels of the participants were available. However, an impairment of kidney function resulting in elevated creatinine levels was not observed in this cohort.

Maternal 25-OH vitamin D levels did not correlate to any of the clinical data we assessed. However, maternal serum calcium levels

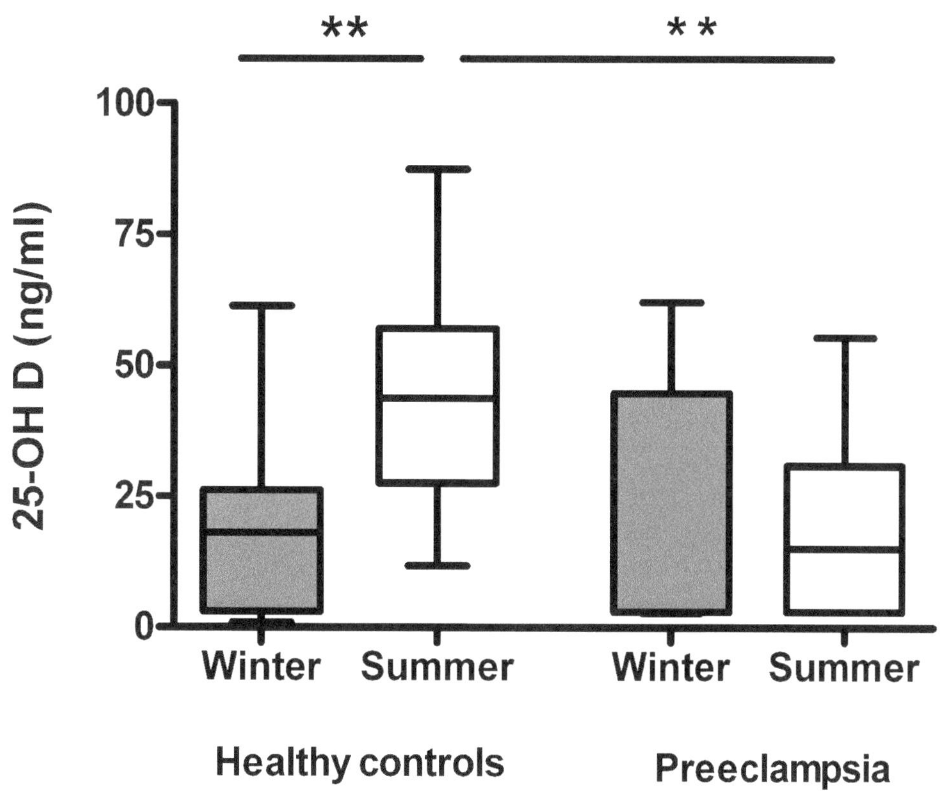
**
**
100
75
50
25
0
25-OH D (ng/ml)
Winter
Summer
Winter
Summer
Healthy controls
Preeclampsia

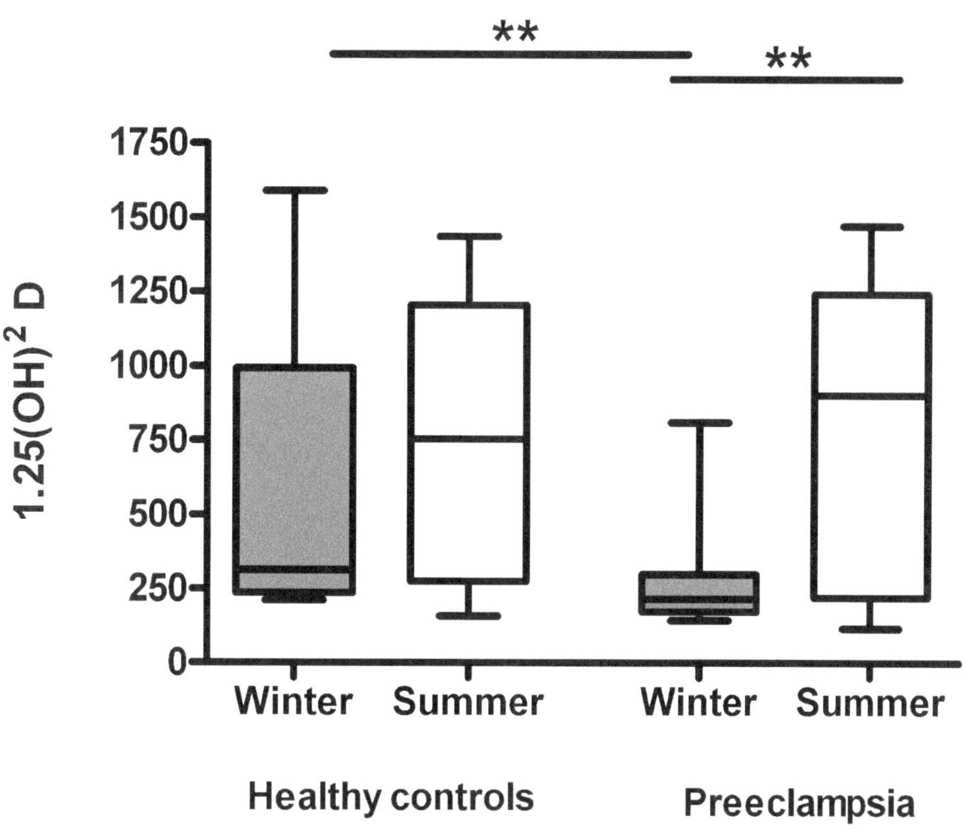
**
**
1750
1500
1250
1000
750
500
250
0
1.25(OH)2 D
Winter
Summer
Winter
Summer
Healthy controls
Preeclampsia

Figure 1. Boxplots showing the smallest observation (lower bar), lower and upper quartile (box), median (line in the box) and largest observation (upper bar) of a) maternal 25-OH vitamin D serum levels (ng/mL) in winter (grey box) and summer (open box). Maternal 25-OH vitamin D levels differ between patients with preeclampsia and healthy controls in the summer (** $p<0.01$). b) Maternal $1,25\text{-}(OH)_2$ vitamin D (pmol/mL) serum levels are similar in both groups, but significantly lower during winter months in patients with preeclampsia (** $p<0.01$).

positively correlated with child BMI at birth in pregnancies complicated by preeclampsia, indicating that calcium may have a beneficial role for fetal outcome in this condition.

Placental gene expression of CYP24A1, CYP27B1, and VDR

There was no difference in placental gene expression of vitamin D metabolizing enzymes between patients with preeclampsia and healthy controls. Neither were differences detectable between samples that were taken during summer or winter respectively.

Particularly, no differences in CYP27B1 placental gene expression were found between healthy controls and patients with preeclampsia. It has previously been suggested that placental activity of the 1-αlpha hydroxylase, the product of CYP27B1, is responsible for the synthesis of $1,25(OH)_2$-vitamin D by the placenta. [9]. However, in about 20% of our samples, CYP27B1 mRNA expression was below the detections limits by real time PCR. In the remaining samples CYP27B1 mRNA was detectable, but at much lower levels than in e.g. in lymphocytes. This is a surprising finding and might point towards additional enzymatic pathways in the placenta, allowing for $1,25(OH)_2$-vitamin D synthesis.

Quantification of vitamin D metabolizing enzyme mRNA in freshly obtained placental tissue is rarely reported in published studies. Few studies show decreased CYP27B1 expression in cultured syncytiothrophoblasts of preeclampsia placentas compared to controls [11], and increased CYP27B1 protein levels in freshly obtained placentas from preeclamptic pregnancies compared to healthy pregnancies [10]. Increased mRNA expression of CYP27B1 was detected in placentas of preeclamptic women

Table 1. Patient characteristics (mean + SD and (range)) for age, pre-pregnancy BMI, maternal calcium, 25- OH vitamin D, 1,25-$(OH)_2$ vitamin D levels in serum, systolic (SBP) and diastolic (DBP) blood pressure on admission to the hospital, as well as child length, weight, and BMI standard deviation scores (SDS) at birth.

	All	Healthy controls	Preeclampsia
Maternal AGE (y)	31.9±5.6	32.2±5.4	31.3±6.1
	(20–43, 63)	(20–43, 43)	(21–41, 20)
BMI	28.5±6.6	28.5±7.1	28.5±5.3
	(18.5–44.1, 34)	(18.5–44.1, 24)	(22–36.8, 10)
Calcium (mmol/L)	2.19±0.18	2.23±0.18	2.13±0.17
	(1.7–2.9, 49)	(1.7–2.9, 32)	(1.9–2.4, 17)
25-OHD (ng/mL)	28.5±26.0	**33.3±27.3**	**18.2±20.0***
	(0.98–132.8, 63)	**(0.1–132.8, 43)**	**(2.9–62.1, 20)**
1,25-(OH)^2 D (pmol/mL)	643.5±456.4	671.7±457.5	582.6±461.2
	(118–1590, 57)	(158–1590, 39)	(118–1473, 18)
SBP mmHG	NA	**119.2 ± 6.**	**172.3 ± 22.6****
		0 (105–131, 21)	**(135#–220, 16)**
DBP mmHG	NA	**74.0 ± 8.4**	**99.1 ± 10.1****
		(60–88, 21)	**(82#–118, 16)**
Gestational week (weeks)	37.6±2.7	**38.8±1.5**	**35.0±2.9****
	(29–42, 63)	**(35.3–42, 43)**	**(29–40.3, 20)**
Child Birth-Weight (g)	2965±695	**3271±418**	**2269±782****
	(4270–740, 63)	**(2050–4270, 43)**	**(740–3780, 20)**
Child Birth-Weight SDS	-0.50±1.	**−0.13±0.87**	**−0.15±1.15****
	13 (−3.6–1.8, 60)	**(−2.5–1.8, 43)**	**(−3.6–0.8, 20)**
Child Birth-Length (cm)	49.7±3.6	**51±2**	**46±5****
	(35–55, 60)	**(47–54, 43)**	**(35–55, 17)**
Child Birth-Length SDS	−0.51±1.13	**−0.16±0.73**	**−0.15±1.5****
	(−4.7–1.43, 60)	**(−2.5–1.0, 43)**	**(−4.6–1.4, 17)**
Child Birth-BMI SDS	−0.30±1.12	**0.0±1**	**−1.16±1 ****
	(−3.0–2.25, 60)	**(−2.5–2.5, 43)**	**(−3–0.1, 17)**

In patients with preeclampsia, maternal 25-OH vitamin D levels are significantly lower than in healthy controls. * differs from healthy controls (*$P<0.05$, ** $P<0.01$)
#blood pressure obtained on admission to hospital was below the criterion for preeclampsia in one patient, despite preeclampsia with proteinuria and elevated blood pressure readings before and after admission.

Table 2. mRNA expression of placental CYP24A1, CYP27B1 and VDR (mean ± SD and (range) do not differ between patients with preeclampsia and healthy controls.

	All	Healthy controls	Preeclampsia
Placental:			
CYP 24A1 (fold change)	1.2±0.7	1.2±0.7	1.1±0.7
	(0.1–2.8, 27)	(0.1–2.2, 14)	(0.3–2.8, 13)
CYP 27B1 (fold change)	1.09±0.7	1.14±0.6	1.03±0.8
	(0.3–3.4, 22)	(0.4–2.1, 11)	(0.3–3.4, 11)
VDR (fold change)	1.2±0.6	1.1±0.4	1.3±0.8
	(0.5–2.7, 27)	(0.5–1.8, 14)	(0.5–2.7, 13)

compared to at-term placentas of women with normal pregnancies. However, when compared to placentas of the appropriate gestational age, CYP27B1 expression was unaltered [21]. It is possible that CYP27B1 gene expression is differentially regulated across gestational age and that the time point chosen in our sampling protocol was not one during which aberrant expression levels between patients with preeclampsia and controls were present.

In healthy pregnancies, placental gene expression of CYP27B1 negatively correlates with CYP24A1 expression, indicating a functional regulation of the two opposing enzymes. In preeclampsia, this correlation is not detectable. Instead, there is a strong negative correlation between placental CYP24A1 gene expression and maternal 25-OH vitamin D serum levels in this condition. If the lowered maternal vitamin D status in preeclampsia is not solely attributable to reduced vitamin D intake and reduced renal activation of vitamin D, these findings may indicate that activation of the 25-hydroxylase, the product of CYP24A1, could play a role in the reduced serum levels of 25-OH vitamin D and 1,25-$(OH)_2$ vitamin D in patients with preeclampsia. Halhali et al. (2014) showed a decrease in the production of 1,25-$(OH)_2$ vitamin D in homogenates of preeclamptic placentas. As the authors discuss, this might be due to the fact that CYP24A1 is active and shifts vitamin D metabolism towards inactive forms (24,25 VDH) in preeclampsia [22].

Since placenta specific methylation of the promoter of CYP24A1 has been reported [9], alterations in methylation could be responsible for these changes. Further work investigating methylation status in placentas from pregnancies complicated by preeclampsia is needed.

Alternatively, inconsistencies in findings regarding the expression levels of vitamin D regulating enzymes in the placenta might be explained by their involvement in local immunological functions. Instead of contributing to maternal vitamin D levels, synthesis and metabolism of vitamin D in the placenta may serve placental requirements only. In the future, it would be valuable to assess 24,25-OH vitamin D levels in healthy versus preeclamptic pregnancies to investigate whether activation of CYP24A1 is related to the diminished 1,25-$(OH)_2$ vitamin D levels observed in winter in patients with preeclampsia.

Limitations of the study. Preeclampsia poses a threat to maternal and fetal health. Delivery of the child is the only curative measure, and thus pregnancies affected by preeclampsia frequently result in premature delivery of the child. In our study, the mean gestational age at birth was 35.0 (29–40.3) gestational weeks in the group with preeclampsia, compared to 38.8 (35.3–42.4) gestational weeks in the group of healthy controls. It was not possible for us to investigate gestational-age matched placental samples from healthy pregnancies. Therefore – some of the differences reported in this study might be founded in the different gestational ages of the investigated groups.

Summary

In summary, our study confirms that women with preeclampsia exhibit vitamin D deficiency compared to healthy controls. Interestingly, changes in maternal vitamin status are mediated by season, and seasonal changes differ in preeclampsia and healthy controls. Whether that is due to aberrant placental vitamin D metabolism is unknown. It is likely that the placental mRNA expression of CYP24A1 is dysregulated in preeclampsia and responsible for the observed seasonal differences in maternal vitamin D status.

Our study also indicates that higher levels of maternal serum calcium may have a beneficial effect on child BMI in preeclampsia. Since vitamin D deficiency during pregnancy is detrimental to maternal and fetal health, [6] [23] a sufficient vitamin D supplementation should be recommended for pregnant women.

Patients and Methods

Samples and clinical data were obtained from a study cohort of 600 patients living in the Northern hemisphere. These patients were enrolled to identify prognostic markers for the development of preeclampsia at the Department of Gynecology and Obstetrics, UK-Essen, University of Duisburg-Essen, Germany during *January 2005 – December 2008*. The clinical data of the patients can be found in Gellhaus et al. [14]. Preeclampsia (PE) was diagnosed according to international criteria [15] [1]. Generally, PE was defined as a blood pressure of at least 140/90 mmHg on two occasions at least 6 h apart occurring after 20 weeks of gestation in women known to be normotensive beforehand and detectable urinary protein (proteinuria: ≥30 mg/dl or >1 by dipstick).

All included patients carried an intact singleton pregnancy. Patients were included after written informed consent was obtained. The study was approved by the local ethics committee [Ehik-Kommission der Medizinischen Fakultät Essen, votum No. 03-2157 (April 2003) and 08-3684 (July 2008)].

From this cohort, serum samples of all women who delivered during the summer months (June, July, and August) or during the winter months (December, January, and February) were included into the analyses (N = 63). Of the 63 women, 20 had developed

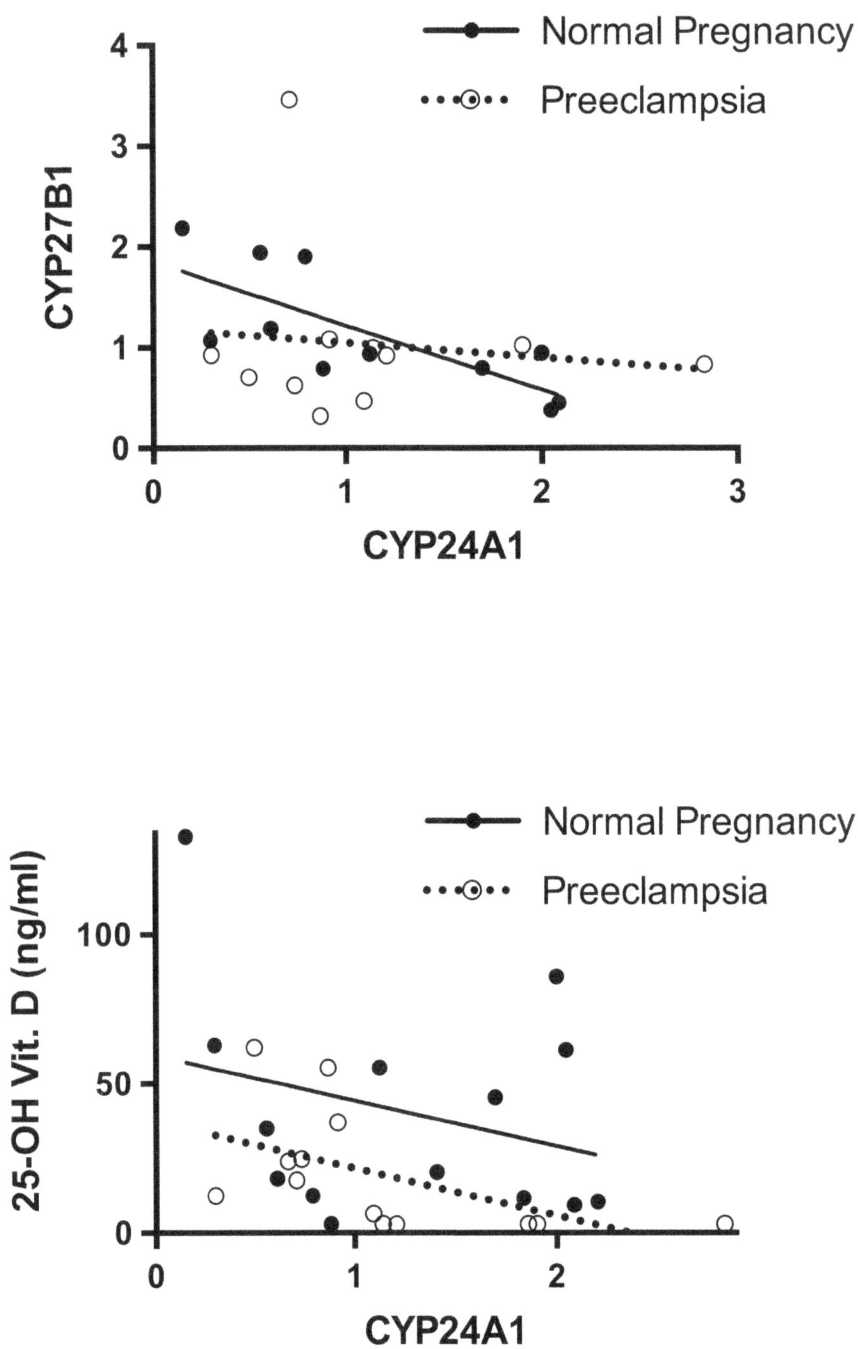

Figure 2. Correlation of placental mRNA expression of CYP24A1 (x-axis) and a) CYP27B1 or b) maternal 25-OH vitamin D (ng/ml) in healthy controls (black circles) and patients with preeclampsia (transparent circles). a) Placental gene expression of CYP24A1 correlates negatively with CYP27B1 expression in healthy controls (r = −0.81, $P<0.0001$, solid line) but not in the patients with preeclampsia (dotted line). b) CYP24A1 correlates negatively with maternal 25-OH vitamin D levels (r = −0.76, $P = 0.01$) in patients with preeclampsia (dotted line).

preeclampsia during pregnancy (PE) and 43 had normal pregnancies (non-PE).

Clinical data, including: biochemical data (maternal serum calcium, phosphate, alkaline phosphatase, creatinine), parity, ethnicity, maternal pre-pregnancy weight, maternal height, maternal blood pressure, presence of proteinuria, birth modus, child birth weight, child birth height, and Apgar scores, were retrieved from patient charts.

Patient characteristics

Patients with preeclampsia did not differ from healthy controls with respect to age, pre-pregnancy BMI, parity, or serum levels of calcium, alkaline phosphatase, or creatinine.

As expected, birth occurred at an earlier gestational age in patients with preeclampsia and, accordingly, child birth weight, child birth length, and child birth BMI were significantly lower in offspring of these mothers ($P<0.001$, Table 1).

33% of the infants born to mothers with PE were small for gestational age (SGA) as defined by a birth weight below the 3rd percentile for the appropriate gestational age (vs 4% in the non-PE group) and 60% displayed a birth weight below the 10th percentile for the appropriate gestational week, versus 9% in the non-PE group. Apgar scores at 5 minutes were lower in infants of PE mothers (8.6±1.5) vs non-PE mothers (9.6±0.7, $P<0.001$)

Blood pressure was significantly higher in women with preeclampsia compared to healthy controls ($P<0.001$, Table 1). All patients with preeclampsia displayed proteinuria (99±68.6, range 35–255 mg/dl). Of the 43 healthy controls, 39 were Caucasian and 4 of African descent. Of the 20 women with preeclampsia, 18 were Caucasian and 2 of African descent. See Table 1 for patient characteristics.

Immunoassays

Maternal 25 OH-vitamin D serum levels were assessed using a commercial enzyme-linked immunosorbent assay (25-OH-vitamin D ELISA, Immundiagnostik, Bensheim, Germany). Intra-assay variation was 9.6% at 20.1 nmol/l, inter-assay variation was below 13% for samples measuring 33–110 nmol/l.

Maternal 1,25-$(OH)_2$ vitamin D serum levels were assessed using a commercial enzyme immunoassay [1,25-$(OH)_2$ vitamin D EIA, Immunodiagnostic Systems Limited (IDS Ltd.), Boldon, UK]. Intra-assay variation was below 11% and inter-assay variation was below 17% for samples measuring 19–152 pmol/l.

Real time PCR

Total placental RNA was isolated from the placental tissues of 14 normal pregnancies and 13 pregnancies complicated by preeclampsia. Only chorionic tissue from the central part of the placenta, close to the center of the insertion of the umbilical cord, was collected and contamination with maternal decidua and amniotic membranes was excluded by morphological observation. Tissues were frozen in liquid nitrogen and stored at −80°C until extraction of total RNA was performed using the E.Z.N.A.Total RNA kit (Omega Bio-Tek, Norcross, USA). For the removal of DNA contaminants, 2 µg RNA was incubated with 1 U/µl DNase I (Invitrogen, Karlsruhe, Germany) and 2 µg RNA was used as a template for cDNA synthesis using the SuperScript II pre-amplification system, according to manufacturer instructions (Invitrogen, Life Technologies, CA, USA).

Placental expression of CYP24A, CYP27B, and VDR was assessed using real time PCR and quantified against the β-actin signal. The following primer sequences (sense-antisense) were used for Cyp27B1: ggaaggcgaagaatggcaaagg – tcgcagactacgttgttcagggttc; CYP24A1: tctggaaagggggtctcaagaaaca – accgactcaaaggaacccaacttca; VDR: ggacctgtggcaaccaagactacaa – ttcagtcccacctggaacttgatga; and Actin: catcctcaccctgaagtaccccatc – agccacacgcagctcattgtagaag. Fold change was calculated by normalizing to the mean gene expression of healthy controls.

Statistical analysis

The effect of season and preeclampsia on serum vitamin D metabolite concentrations was tested by a two-factorial ANOVA. The influence of placental expression of CYP24A1, CYP27B1, and VDR was assessed by a multiple stepwise regression analysis, adding these variables to a model containing season and pregnancy outcome. The Shapiro Wilk test was used to test for normal distribution of the data. The hypothesis for normal distribution was rejected at $\alpha<0.1$ (Proc univariate, SAS 9.4 SAS Institute Inc., Carey, NC, USA, 2008). Associations between single variables were described by the Spearman correlation. Differences between group means and reference cohorts were assessed by the Mann-Whitney test. Statistical significance was assumed at $P<0.05$. Data are given as mean ±1 SD. Data analysis was performed using SAS statistical software (SAS System, release 9.2, SAS Institute Inc., Carey, NC, USA, 2008).

Acknowledgments

The authors thank Wiebke Diesner, Kinderklinik II, University of Essen-Duisburg, for exceptional technical support.

Author Contributions

Conceived and designed the experiments: CG RH. Performed the experiments: CL. Analyzed the data: BPH CG M. Schuendeln RH CL. Contributed reagents/materials/analysis tools: AG M. Schmidt BPH. Wrote the paper: CL CG BPH AG M. Schmidt.

References

1. Sibai B, Dekker G, Kupferminc M (2005) Pre-eclampsia. Lancet 365: 785–799.
2. Tabesh M, Salehi-Abargouei A, Tabesh M, Esmaillzadeh A (2013) Maternal vitamin D status and risk of pre-eclampsia: a systematic review and meta-analysis. J Clin Endocrinol Metab 98: 3165–3173.
3. TePoel MR, Saftlas AF, Wallis AB (2011) Association of seasonality with hypertension in pregnancy: a systematic review. J Reprod Immunol 89: 140–152.
4. Sharma S, Khan N, Khadri A, Julies P, Gnanasambandam S, et al. (2009) Vitamin D in pregnancy-time for action: a paediatric audit. BJOG 116: 1678–1682.
5. Bodnar LM, Simhan HN, Powers RW, Frank MP, Cooperstein E, et al. (2007) High prevalence of vitamin D insufficiency in black and white pregnant women residing in the northern United States and their neonates. J Nutr 137: 447–452.
6. Weisse K, Winkler S, Hirche F, Herberth G, Hinz D, et al. (2013) Maternal and newborn vitamin D status and its impact on food allergy development in the German LINA cohort study. Allergy 68: 220–228.
7. Aghajafari F, Nagulesapillai T, Ronksley PE, Tough SC, O'Beirne M, et al. (2013) Association between maternal serum 25-hydroxyvitamin D level and pregnancy and neonatal outcomes: systematic review and meta-analysis of observational studies. BMJ 346: f1169.
8. Seki K, Makimura N, Mitsui C, Hirata J, Nagata I (1991) Calcium-regulating hormones and osteocalcin levels during pregnancy: a longitudinal study. Am J Obstet Gynecol 164: 1248–1252.
9. Novakovic B, Sibson M, Ng HK, Manuelpillai U, Rakyan V, et al. (2009) Placenta-specific methylation of the vitamin D 24-hydroxylase gene: implications for feedback autoregulation of active vitamin D levels at the fetomaternal interface. J Biol Chem 284: 14838–14848.
10. Ma R, Gu Y, Zhao S, Sun J, Groome LJ, et al. (2012) Expressions of vitamin D metabolic components VDBP, CYP2R1, CYP27B1, CYP24A1, and VDR in placentas from normal and preeclamptic pregnancies. Am J Physiol Endocrinol Metab 303: E928–E935.
11. Díaz L, Arranz C, Avila E, Halhali A, Vilchis F, et al. (2002) Expression and activity of 25-hydroxyvitamin D-1 alpha-hydroxylase are restricted in cultures of human syncytiotrophoblast cells from preeclamptic pregnancies. J Clin Endocrinol Metab 87: 3876–3882.
12. Pospechova K, Rozehnal V, Stejskalova L, Vrzal R, Pospisilova N, et al. (2009) Expression and activity of vitamin D receptor in the human placenta and in choriocarcinoma BeWo and JEG-3 cell lines. Mol Cell Endocrinol 299: 178–187.
13. Slominski AT, Kim TK, Shehabi HZ, Semak I, Tang EK, et al. (2012) In vivo evidence for a novel pathway of vitamin D_3 metabolism initiated by P450scc and modified by CYP27B1. FASEB J 26: 3901–3915.
14. Gellhaus A, Schmidt M, Dunk C, Lye SJ, Kimmig R, et al. (2006) Decreased expression of the angiogenic regulators CYR61 (CCN1) and NOV (CCN3) in human placenta is associated with pre-eclampsia. Mol Hum Reprod 12: 389–399.
15. Roberts JM, Redman CW (1993) Pre-eclampsia: more than pregnancy-induced hypertension. Lancet 341: 1447–1451.
16. August P, Marcaccio B, Gertner JM, Druzin ML, Resnick LM, et al. (1992) Abnormal 1,25-dihydroxyvitamin D metabolism in preeclampsia. Am J Obstet Gynecol 166: 1295–1299.
17. Halhali A, Tovar AR, Torres N, Bourges H, Garabedian M, et al. (2000) Preeclampsia is associated with low circulating levels of insulin-like growth factor I and 1,25-dihydroxyvitamin D in maternal and umbilical cord compartments. J Clin Endocrinol Metab 85: 1828–1833.

18. Frølich A, Rudnicki M, Storm T, Rasmussen N, Hegedüs L (1992) Impaired 1,25-dihydroxyvitamin D production in pregnancy-induced hypertension. Eur J Obstet Gynecol Reprod Biol 47: 25–29.
19. Kovacs CS, Kronenberg HM (1997) Maternal-fetal calcium and bone metabolism during pregnancy, puerperium, and lactation. Endocr Rev 18: 832–872.
20. Lalau JD, Jans I, el Esper N, Bouillon R, Fournier A (1993) Calcium metabolism, plasma parathyroid hormone, and calcitriol in transient hypertension of pregnancy. Am J Hypertens 6: 522–527.
21. Fischer D, Schroer A, Lüdders D, Cordes T, Bücker B, et al. (2007) Metabolism of vitamin D3 in the placental tissue of normal and preeclampsia complicated pregnancies and premature births. Clin Exp Obstet Gynecol 34: 80–84.
22. Halhali A, Díaz L, Barrera D, Avila E, Larrea F (2013) Placental calcitriol synthesis and IGF-I levels in normal and preeclamptic pregnancies. J Steroid Biochem Mol Biol.
23. Liu NQ, Ouyang Y, Bulut Y, Lagishetty V, Chan SY, et al. (2013) Dietary vitamin D restriction in pregnant female mice is associated with maternal hypertension and altered placental and fetal development. Endocrinology 154: 2270–2280.
24. Burton GJ, Yung HW, Cindrova-Davies T, Charnock-Jones DS (2009) Placental endoplasmic reticulum stress and oxidative stress in the pathophysiology of unexplained intrauterine growth restriction and early onset preeclampsia. Placenta. 2009 Suppl A:S43–8.

5

RNA-Seq Analysis of the Effect of Kanamycin and the ABC Transporter AtWBC19 on *Arabidopsis thaliana* Seedlings Reveals Changes in Metal Content

Ayalew Mentewab[1]*, Kinnari Matheson[1,2], Morayo Adebiyi[1,3], Shanice Robinson[1], Brianna Elston[1,4]

1 Biology Department, Spelman College, Atlanta, Georgia, United States of America, **2** Molecular Biology Department, Princeton University, Princeton, New Jersey, United States of America, **3** The Graduate School of Biomedical Sciences, University of Texas Health Science Center at Houston, Houston, Texas, United States of America, **4** College of Health Care Sciences, Nova Southeastern University, Davie, Florida, United States of America

Abstract

Plants are exposed to antibiotics produced by soil microorganisms, but little is known about their responses at the transcriptional level. Likewise, few endogenous mechanisms of antibiotic resistance have been reported. The *Arabidopsis thaliana* ATP Binding Cassette (ABC) transporter AtWBC19 (ABCG19) is known to confer kanamycin resistance, but the exact mechanism of resistance is not well understood. Here we examined the transcriptomes of control seedlings and *wbc19* mutant seedlings using RNA-seq analysis. Exposure to kanamycin indicated changes in the organization of the photosynthetic apparatus, metabolic fluxes and metal uptake. Elemental analysis showed a 60% and 80% reduction of iron uptake in control and *wbc19* mutant seedlings respectively, upon exposure to kanamycin. The drop in iron content was accompanied by the upregulation of the gene encoding for FERRIC REDUCTION OXIDASE 6 (FRO6) in mutant seedlings but not by the differential expression of other transport genes known to be induced by iron deficiency. In addition, *wbc19* mutants displayed a distinct expression profile in the absence of kanamycin. Most notably the expression of several zinc ion binding proteins, including ZINC TRANSPORTER 1 PRECURSOR (ZIP1) was increased, suggesting abnormal zinc uptake. Elemental analysis confirmed a 50% decrease of zinc content in *wbc19* mutants. Thus, the antibiotic resistance gene WBC19 appears to also have a role in zinc uptake.

Editor: John R. Battista, Louisiana State University and A & M College, United States of America

Funding: This study was supported by grants from the National Science Foundation (www.nsf.gov; Molecular and Cellular Biology grant #1052172) and Quality Education for Minorities Network (qemnetwork.qem.org; Professional Development and Mentoring program) to AM and the Howard Hughes Medical Institute (www.hhmi.org; Educational grant #52006930) to the Biology Department at the Massachusetts Institute of Technology. The funders had no role in study design, data collection and analysis, decision to publish, or preparation of the manuscript.

Competing Interests: The authors have declared that no competing interests exist.

* Email: mayalew@spelman.edu

Introduction

Plants are exposed to a variety of antibiotics produced by soil microorganisms. One such antibiotic is kanamycin, originally isolated from the soil bacterium *Streptomyces kanamyceticus*. Many plant species display exquisite sensitivity to a number of antibiotics, hence their usefulness as selection agents in plant genetic engineering. Kanamycin belongs to the aminoglycoside class of antibiotics. Aminoglycosides are multifunctional hydrophilic sugars that possess several amino and hydroxy groups. Aminoglycosides directly bind to the A site of the 16S rRNA of prokaryotic ribosomes causing codon misreading and inhibiting translocation [1,2,3]. The presence of an adenosine at position 1408 of the 16S rRNA is a key feature of prokaryotic ribosomes that allows binding of aminoglycosides. In the eukaryotic rRNA, the corresponding position is occupied by a guanine resulting in a lowered affinity for aminoglycosides [4]. Based on the similarity of their ribosomes to those of prokaryotes, plastids and mitochondria may represent the primary targets of aminoglycoside antibiotics in plants.

Plant responses to antibiotics have been poorly characterized. Nonetheless, several observations support the notion that chloroplasts are a major target of aminoglycosides. When plants are exposed to kanamycin, a characteristic symptom is the bleaching of the leaves indicating the breakdown of cholorophyll in choloroplasts [5]. When the chloroplast transporter MAR1 is mutated [6] or silenced [7], plants become resistant to kanamycin and several other aminoglycosides. MAR1 has a role in iron homeostasis and is thought to allow the passage of aminoglycosides into the chloroplast given their structural resemblance with chelated iron molecules [8].

Despite their sensitivity, *Arabidopsis* plants harbor at least one gene that confers antibiotic resistance – that encoding for the ABC transporter WBC19 (ABCG19). ABC transporters are defined by the presence of the highly conserved ATP Binding Cassette (ABC) domain responsible for the hydrolysis of ATP and a transmembrane domain (TMD) responsible for solute movement across the phospholipid bilayer. With a single ABC domain and a single TMD domain encompassing six predicted alpha helices, WBC19 is categorized as a half ABC molecule. Such half ABC molecules are thought to dimerize to form functional transporters. When WBC19 is mutated, kanamycin sensitivity of seedlings is exacerbated while expression of WBC19 in tobacco resulted in increased levels of antibiotic resistance [9]. In tobacco (*Nicotiana tabacum*), WBC19 was found to be specific to kanamycin, but in hybrid aspen (*Populus canescens x P. grandidentata*) it also showed resistance to three other aminoglycoside antibiotics - neomycin, geneticin, and paromomycin [10]. Further investigation in bacteria showed WBC19 did not confer resistance to kanamycin in *E. coli* [11]. A direct role of WBC19 in transport was not investigated as it was not localized in a membrane compartment. Thus the mechanism of antibiotic resistance associated with WBC19 has not been fully characterized.

The presence of several hydroxyl and amine groups makes kanamycin a polar compound. As a result, it poorly diffuses through membranes. Before reaching chloroplasts it has to first enter root cells, get mobilized through the vascular system and unloaded - most likely by co-opting other transporters. Given the previously reported association between antibiotic resistance and metal transport [6,8], we postulate that endogenous mechanisms of antibiotic resistance, specifically the one associated with WBC19 is also linked to the transport of metals. Here we examined the transcriptomes and analyzed the metal content of control and *wbc19* mutant seedlings. We report that kanamycin induces transcriptional changes revealing an adaptation of the photosynthetic apparatus, metabolic fluxes and metal uptake. Most significantly, the iron content of seedling exposed to kanamycin is drastically reduced and the zinc content of *wbc19* mutants is lower even under normal conditions. Overall, our findings suggest that the antibiotic resistance gene WBC19 has a role in zinc homeostasis and to a lesser extent that of the other metals examined, copper and manganese.

Materials and Methods

RNA-seq transcriptome analysis

Plant Material. Control (SALK_064816C) and *wbc19* mutant (SALK_107731) lines generated by Alonso et al. [12] were previously obtained from the Arabidopsis Biological Resource Center (Columbus, OH). Homozygous seeds were plated under sterile conditions on MS media with or without kanamycin 50 mg/l. SALK_064816C mutants served as controls as they carry a T-DNA insertion that does not disrupt a gene. The T-DNA insertion is located in the vicinity of the TRANSPARENT TESTA 4 gene, 260 bp upstream of the start codon and the mutants have no visible phenotype. After stratification (3 days at 4°C), plates were transferred to a controlled-environment cabinet (23°C, 16 h light; 18°C, 8 h dark) and plant material was harvested and flash frozen 5 days later.

Library Preparation. Total RNA was extracted using a Plant RNeasy Mini Kit (Qiagen) and poly(A) mRNA isolated using oligo(dT) DynaBeads (Life Technologies). Messenger RNA fragmentation and RNA-seq library generation was according to [13]. Briefly, after alkaline fragmentation of mRNA, ~25–45 mer fragments were gel purified on a 10% denaturing polyacrylamide-urea gel. After 3′-dephosphorylation with polynucleotide kinase (PNK, New England Biolabs) a 3′ adaptor was ligated to the fragments. Following a second gel purification step, the fragments were 5′phosphorylated with PNK and the 5′ adapter ligated. Each library was then amplified for 21 cycles and gel purified on a 90% formamide, 8% acrylamide denaturing gel. Four libraries, one per treatment condition were submitted for single-end sequencing on the Illumina GAII high throughput sequencing platform.

Analysis pipeline. Sequence analysis was carried out in the iPlant Collaborative Discovery Environment (www.iplantcollaborative.org). Reads were processed with FASTX clipper (version 0.0.6) to remove adapter sequences and keep sequences of 36 mer. Processed reads were aligned to the *Arabidopsis* thaliana reference genome (TAIR10) using TopHat2 (version 2.0.5) [14,15]. The minimum read length was set to 18 and up to 2 mismatches were tolerated. Mapped reads were assembled and merged using Cufflinks (version 2.0.2) and Cuffmerge (version 2.0.2) respectively [16]. Transcript abundance and differential expression was analyzed using Cuffdiff (version 1.3.0) [16] whenever a minimum of 10 reads were available. Differential gene expression across samples was deemed significant when expression differences reached 2 fold and $p<0.001$. Gene descriptions and GO classifications were obtained from The Arabidopsis Information Resource (TAIR). The Functional Classification SuperViewer tool (http://bar.utoronto.ca/ntools/cgi-bin/ntools_classification_superviewer.cgi) was used to identify gene groups that were significantly over-represented under each treatment condition compared with their relative amount in the whole genome. GO Classifications were further mined for the words photosynthesis, oxidoreduction, electron carrier and various metals to identify specific transcripts among those that were differentially expressed.

Real-Time PCR

Two sets of Real-Time PCR assays were performed. To validate the RNA-seq results, a set of 11 genes were randomly selected among those with the GO classifications of interest as listed in **Tables 1–6**. The second set of genes consisted of a panel of 5 iron homeostasis genes. Both sets of genes are listed in **Table S1**. To perform Real-Time PCRs, homozygous *wbc19* mutants (SALK_107731) and controls (SALK_064816C) seedlings were grown with or without kanamycin as above, RNA was extracted using the Plant RNeasy Mini Kit (Qiagen) and treated with DNAseI (Life Technologies). The cDNA was then synthesized using the SuperScript VILO cDNA synthesis kit (Life Technologies). Samples were diluted 200 fold before use for real-time assays. The TaqMan Universal Master Mix II with Uracil-N-Glycosylase (Life Technologies) was used along with predesigned TaqMan Assays (Life Technologies) as listed in **Table S1**. All selected assays featured probes that span exons. Target genes were FAM labeled whereas the control RAD23C was labeled with VIC for use in multiplex reactions. For each gene, Real-Time PCR assays were performed with samples representing all 4 experimental conditions and included 4 biological replicates and 3 technical replicates. Data was analyzed using the Pfaffl method [18]; comparisons between experimental conditions were carried out using a Student T-test and deemed significant when $P<0.05$.

Metal Analysis

To evaluate the effect of kanamycin, 5 day old seedlings from homozygous *wbc19* mutants (SALK_107731) and controls (SALK_064816C) were grown on media with or without kanamycin 50 mg/l as above. Seedlings were collected from plates and rinsed 3 times with 18 mΩ distilled water and dried for 2 d at 70°C. The plant material was weighed before shipping to the Lab for Environmental Analysis at the University of Georgia, Athens (UGA) where samples were digested with nitric acid before metal analysis by Inductively Coupled Plasma- Mass Spectrometry (ICP-MS) for Fe, Zn, Mn and Cu. For each treatment condition, metal content was analyzed using 3 biological replicates.

Expression pattern of WBC19

The promoter region of WBC19 (2130 bp upstream of the start codon) was amplified from genomic DNA extracts of WT Arabidopsis plants using the forward 5′ CACCTTTGGGACCCC-CAAAATCTC 3′ and reverse 5′ TCCCGGACGGCGTCGTT-TAGA 3′ primers. The resulting fragment was cloned in the pENTR-D-TOPO vector (LifeTechnologies) and checked by restriction digestion. It was subsequently recombined with the pMDC162 vector designed for the expression of promoter-β-glucuronidase (GUS) fusions [19] and again checked by restriction digestion.

WT Arabidopsis plants were transformed with *Agrobacterium tumefaciens* strain GV3850 containing the construct using the floral dip method [20]. Seven transgenic plants were recovered and grown to maturity. Seeds were collected, sterilized and germinated on MS media and plants were transferred to soil after 2 weeks. Plant material was collected throughout development, fixed in 90% cold acetone for 20 minutes on ice and stained for histochemical localization of GUS activity [21].

Accession number

The RNA-seq data used in this study is available in the Gene Expression Omnibus(GEO) database under accession number GSE58662.

Results

RNA-seq analysis was conducted to capture the effect of kanamycin on *Arabidopsis* seedlings and examine how the response was modulated by WBC19. Control and *wbc19* mutant seedlings were grown with or without 50 mg/l kanamycin. The *wbc19* mutants used were T-DNA insertional knockouts in which the bacterial kanamycin resistance gene, neomycin phosphotransferase type II (NPTII) is expressed at a relatively high level [9]. Yet, because of the disruption of *wbc19* they are sensitive to kanamycin at 50 mg/l. To compensate for the confounding effect that might be added by the NPTII gene, a line with an insertion of the same T-DNA, but where no gene is disrupted was used as control. This line and all other T-DNA insertional mutants from the same collection we have tested are resistant to kanamycin 50 mg/l. In this experiment, all seedlings developed long roots in the absence of kanamycin, but in the presence of kanamycin, *wbc19* mutants exhibited their characteristic stunted root growth, although their leaves remained green.

Sequencing libraries were prepared from the seedlings and resulted in an average of 2.3 million reads per library uniquely mapping to the *Arabidopsis* genome (**Table S2**). The differential expression of genes was analyzed using Cuffdiff and deemed significant when $p<0.001$ and two fold differences were observed. To validate the RNA-seq results, 11 genes were randomly selected among those with a GO classification of interest as listed in Tables 1–6. Their transcript levels were examined by Real-Time PCR under all 4 experimental conditions and 3 sets of comparisons were made (control vs. control + kanamycin; control vs. mutant; control + kanamycin vs. mutant + kanamycin). The overlap between the 3 sets of comparisons from Real-Time data and RNA-seq data was examined. For the total of 30 comparisons where statistical significance could be assessed, a good overlap between Real-Time results and RNA-seq results was observed. For the 13 instances where significant differences were found in the RNA-seq experiment, 11 (84.6%) were also found to be differentially expressed in the Real-Time PCR assays (**File S1**). Thus the false positive discovery rate was at 15.4%. Among the 17 comparisons that were found non-significant in the RNA-seq experiment, 14 (82.3%) remained non-significant when Real-Time PCR assays were done. Thus the false negative rate is estimated at 17.6%. Overall the Real-Time PCR results validate the RNA-seq data although the amplitude of the observed differences were more modest. For Real-Time PCR assays, the highest fold difference was observed for FERRIC REDUCTION OXIDASE 6 (FRO6) where five times more transcripts are expressed in the mutant seedlings exposed to kanamycin compared to the control.

Transcriptional response of control Arabidopsis seedlings to kanamycin

Although control plants exposed to kanamycin were visually asymptomatic, a total of 116 genes were differentially regulated, of which 88 were upregulated and 28 were downregulated (**File S2**). Examination of over-represented categories (**Figure S1**) indicated that photosynthesis light reaction components were more frequent among the differentially regulated transcripts than might be expected by chance. Further detailed analysis of the GO classification of differentially expressed genes allowed us to identify three overlapping sets of transcripts, given our interest in metal homeostasis. The first set is represented by genes with a direct or indirect role in photosynthesis. For example, increased transcripts of the P subunit of photosystem I (PSI-P) and that of the chlorophyll a/b-binding protein 2 (CAB2), a component of the light harvesting complex associated with photosystem II (PSII) denote changes taking place in both photosystems (**Table 1**). The upregulation of both transcripts was confirmed in Real-Time PCR assays. These changes are accompanied by the upregulation of ALBINO3 which is essential for the efficient assembly of photosystem II [22] as well as DEGP PROTEASE 7 (DegP7) which is involved in the repair of photodamaged PSII via cleavage of its D1 protein [23]. In addition the differential regulation of a number of plastid genes involved in transcription and translation (plastid transcriptionally active 6, Ts translation elongation factor, chloroplastic ribosomal protein L9) further highlight changes taking place in plastids.

A second set of transcripts is represented by redox enzymes. Two enzymes enabling the exchange of electrons with ferredoxins were differentially regulated. The mitochondrial ferredoxin reductase (AtMFDR) was found to be upregulated which was confirmed in Real-Time PCR assays. AtMFDR enables the transfer of electron from NADP(H) to ferredoxin most likely for Fe-S cluster assembly and biotin synthesis in the mitochondria [24,25]. On the other hand, NAD(P)H dehydrogenase C1(NDC1) was downregulated. NDC1 can localize to both mitochondria and chloroplasts [26,27,28] and was shown to reduce the pool of plastoquinone (PQ) in plastoglobules, thereby playing a role in the synthesis of prenylquinones such as vitamin K1 [29]. These changes suggest the presence of alternative pathways of electron flow as these enzymes were shown to have variable metabolic roles. More specifically, biosynthetic pathways in the chloroplast appear to be reduced while biosynthetic pathways in the mitochondria especially Fe-S cluster containing proteins are promoted. Taken together these changes likely reflect an adaptation of the photosynthetic apparatus and metabolic fluxes upon plant exposure to kanamycin.

A third set of differentially expressed genes encode for metal binding proteins (**Table 2**). Among these, the best characterized gene is the Magnesium transporter MGT4 (MRS2-3). Our Real-Time PCR assays also confirmed the upregulation of MGT4 transcripts. MGT4 was initially identified as a candidate locus in a search for quantitative trait loci affecting seed concentrations of Mg^{2+} [30] and later confirmed to transport Mg^{2+} [31]. MRS2-3 could complement yeast deficient in Mg^{2+} transport but direct

Table 1. Differentially expressed transcripts encoding for proteins involved in photosynthesis and oxidoreduction upon seedling germination on kanamycin containing media.

GO ID	Description	Gene ID	Description	control rpkm	Control + kan rpkm	log2 (fold change)
GO:0015979	photosynthesis	AT2G46820	PHOTOSYSTEM I P SUBUNIT (PSI-P)	339.20	732.37	1.11
GO:0015979	photosynthesis	AT1G29920	CHLOROPHYLL A/B-BINDING PROTEIN 2 (CAB2) (LHCB1.1)	122.61	979.94	2.99
GO:0016491	oxidoreductase activity	AT5G08740	NAD(P)H dehydrogenase C1 (NDC1)	22.47	0.34	−6.01
GO:0016491	oxidoreductase activity	AT4G32360	Mitochondrial Ferredoxin reductase (AtMFDR)	0.63	24.83	5.29
GO:0016491	oxidoreductase activity	AT2G40370	LACCASE 5 (LAC5) *	0.81	28.42	5.12
GO:0016491	oxidoreductase activity	AT5G66920	SKU5 similar 17 (sks17) *	4.21	75.98	4.17
GO:0016491	oxidoreductase activity	AT2G37240	Thioredoxin superfamily protein	25.53	0.57	−5.48
GO:0015035	protein disulfide oxidoreductase activity	AT5G18600	Thioredoxin superfamily protein	18.50	207.63	3.48

The terms photosynthesis and oxidoreduction were searched in the GO IDs associated with genes differentially expressed when comparing transcripts from control seedlings germinating on MS media to transcripts from control seedlings germinating on MS media with 50 mg/l kanamycin (minimum 2 fold difference in expression, $P<0.001$). * denotes genes also identified as encoding for metal binding proteins in **Table 2**.

uptake was not found to be considerably higher than the background level in the mutant. It was therefore suggested that MRS2-3 may act as a slow transporter for Mg^{2+} requiring long time intervals for achieving homeostasis and thus represent a high affinity Mg^{2+} transporter. Further, a number of genes encoding for copper binding proteins were found to be differentially regulated, including the gene encoding for LACCASE 5 (LAC5). Real-Time PCR assays confirmed significantly higher levels of LAC5 transcripts in control plants exposed to kanamycin and generally lower levels in mutants. LAC5 is a member of the laccase-like multicopper oxidases generally viewed as phenoloxidases enabling the polymerization of lignin. However, members of the family were shown to have a ferroxidase activity and thus LAC5 might play a role in iron metabolism [32,33]. More specifically, they are thought to function in iron-uptake systems similar to FET3 in *Saccharomyces cerevisiae*. In the FET3 system, the strict coupling of Fe^{2+} oxidation by Fet3p with transport of Fe^{3+} by Ftr1p allows for a high affinity transport of iron [34,35,36]. Thus, the upregulation of LAC5 may signify that plants exposed to kanamycin switch to a higher affinity iron transport system. These changes along with the decrease in the expression of heavy metal transport/detoxification superfamily protein and increased transcripts from the molybdenum cofactor sulfurase family suggest that plants exposed to kanamycin alter their uptake of metals.

Differences between control plants and wbc19 knockout mutants

In the absence of kanamycin exposure, no visual differences were observed between control and *wbc19* mutant plants, however the RNA-seq analysis revealed significant differences, with 26 genes being downregulated and 69 genes upregulated in the mutant. These changes were subtle as minor effects on the over-representation of the various functional categories were observed (**Figure S2**). The detailed analysis of GO classifications, however, indicated that a number of transcripts are again found to encode for photosynthesis and oxidoreduction related proteins (**Table 3**). In mutant plants, transcripts of one isoform of the PsbP protein (At1g76450) are downregulated while those of its most similar isoform (At3g05410) are upregulated. PsbP is one of extrinsic proteins on the luminal side of PSII involved in the oxidation of water to molecular oxygen by using light energy. The reaction is catalized by a cluster of three inorganic ions, manganese (Mn), calcium (Ca), and chloride (Cl) and PsbP participates in the regulation of the unique redox environment of this inorganic catalytic center (Debus, 2000). Specifically, PsbP is involved in Ca^{2+} and Cl^{-} retention in PSII as well as the protection of the Mn cluster from a wide range of small (H_2O_2, NH_2NH_2, NH_2OH, Fe^{2+}) and bulky (benzidine, hydroquinone) reductants [37,38]; and is essential for normal PSII function [39,40]. The observed shift from one isoform of PsbP to another in *wbc19* mutants suggests an adaptation of PSII to a new ionic or redox environment.

Ferredoxin 3 (Fd3) is expressed at a much lower level in *wbc19* mutants compared to control plants, a finding that was confirmed in Real-Time PCR assays. While ferredoxins primarily contribute to photosynthesis by shuttling electrons from photosystem I (PSI) to the enzyme ferredoxin:$NADP^+$ oxidoreductase (FNR) for reduction of $NADP^+$ and eventually provide reducing power for CO_2 assimilation, they can also contribute to a wide range of metabolic reactions such as nitrogen assimilation [41]. Fd3 is a root type or heterotrophic isoform of ferredoxin [42]. Its redox potential favors electron transfer from NADPH to ferredoxin in a predominantly heterotrophic pathway. A decreased expression of Fd3 in mutants once again suggests changes in metabolic fluxes.

When examining transcripts of metal binding proteins differentially expressed in the mutant, six out of eight encode for zinc binding proteins (**Table 4**). All six transcripts are upregulated in *wbc19* mutant seedlings compared to control seedlings. Most notably, the expression of ZINC TRANSPORTER 1 PRECURSOR (ZIP1) was increased. ZIP1 is a highly specific zinc transporter. It can functionally complement the zrt1/zrt2 yeast double mutant deficient in zinc transport but not the fet3/fet4 mutant indicating that it does not transport iron [43]. Although it

Table 2. Transcripts encoding for metal binding proteins differentially expressed upon seedling germination on kanamycin containing media.

GO ID	Description	Gene ID	Description	control rpkm	control + kan rpkm	log2 (fold change)
GO:0008270	zinc ion binding	AT2G29580	MOS4-ASSOCIATED COMPLEX SUBUNIT 5B (MAC5B)	31.66	0.35	−6.49
GO:0008270	zinc ion binding	AT1G09920	TRAF-type zinc finger protein	2.57	100.45	5.28
GO:0004222	Metalloendo peptidase	AT5G65620	Zincin-like metalloprotease	20.76	0.25	−6.32
GO:0005507	copper ion binding	AT2G36950	Heavy metal transport/ detoxification superfamily protein	24.80	0.37	−6.05
GO:0005507	copper ion binding	AT4G33680	L,L-diaminopimelate aminotransferase	54.00	1.29	−5.37
GO:0005507	copper ion binding	AT5G66920	SKU5 SIMILAR 17 (sks17) *	4.21	75.98	4.17
GO:0005507	copper ion binding	AT2G40370	LACCASE 5 (LAC5) *	0.81	28.42	5.12
GO:0005507	copper ion binding	AT5G55200	MITOCHONDRIAL GRPE 1 (MGE1)	1.03	71.28	6.10
GO:0015095	magnesium ion transmembrane transporter activity	AT3G19640	MAGNESIUM TRANSPORTER 4 (MGT4)	0.70	28.06	5.32
GO:0030151	molybdenum ion binding	AT1G30910	Molybdenum cofactor sulfurase family protein	1.17	53.01	5.49

The terms metal, iron, zinc, copper, manganese, magnesium, cobalt, molybdenum etc were searched in the GO terms associated with genes differentially expressed when comparing transcripts from control seedlings germinating on MS media to transcripts from control seedlings germinating on MS media with 50 mg/l kanamycin (minimum 2 fold difference in expression, $P<0.001$). * denotes genes also identified as encoding for oxidoreductases in **Table 1.**

is normally expressed in roots and induced upon zinc deficiency [43], it can be activated in shoots in IRT1 mutants which are severely iron and zinc deprived [44]. This upregulation of ZIP1 in mutants suggested an altered Zn homeostasis, similar to Zn deficiency responses.

Additionally, transcripts of a cytochrome B561 are also increased in mutants compared to control seedlings. Cytochrome B561s are typically membrane proteins that catalize a transmembrane electron transport from ascorbate to an extracellular substrate. Although the first well-charaterized cytochrome B561 from chromaffin granules of neuroendocrine tissues reduced intravesicular ascorbic acid [45] many cytochrome B561 proteins were later found to have a ferric and cupric reductase activity [46,47,48,49]. The upregulation of cytochrome B561 transcripts in mutants suggested an altered iron and or copper homeostasis.

Overall the comparison of transcripts from *wbc19* mutants and control seedling suggest differences in the architecture of their photosynthetic apparatus, their metabolic fluxes and their metal uptake. These differences are observed while seedlings were grown in the absence of kanamycin, indicating that WBC19 has a physiological role under normal conditions and therefore one that is not strictly adaptive upon exposure to kanamycin.

Effect of WBC19 on the response to kanamycin

To examine how the lack of WBC19 affects responses to kanamycin, we compared transcript abundance between control plants exposed to kanamycin and mutant plants exposed to kanamycin. We found that 38 genes were upregulated and 98 genes were downregulated in the mutant. The functional categories 'photosystem', 'metal handling' and 'transport' were found to be over-represented (**Figure S3**). Twenty-two of the differentially expressed genes were found to be significantly upregulated in the controls upon exposure to kanamycin but failed to be upregulated in the mutants exposed to kanamycin (**Figure S4**). Most notably, LHCb1.1 and the Magnesium transporter MGT4 failed to be upregulated (**Table 5**). Conversely, transcripts of genes such as the Heavy Metal Transporter and NAD(P)H dehydrogenase C1 (NDC1) that were significantly downregulated in the control upon kanamycin exposure, failed to be downregulated in the mutant. Thus mutant plants did not exhibit the signature responses of the control plants. Instead, among genes encoding for photosynthesis related proteins, we observe a reduced amount of transcripts of PHOTOSYSTEM II REACTION CENTER PROTEIN D2 (PSBD). PSII reaction center proteins D1 and D2 are two chlorophyll binding proteins at the core of the site for oxygen evolution. Under conditions of high light and abiotic stress D1 and D2 are photodamaged and repair consists of disassembly of PSII, synthesis of the proteins and reassembly [50]. The low levels of PSII reaction center protein D2 transcripts detected in mutants exposed to kanamycin suggests a lower rate of PSII repair. In addition, the upregulation of the O subunit of PLASTOQUINONE DEHYDROGENASE COMPLEX (NDH-O) suggests increased cyclic electron flow around PSI. The NDH complex catalyzes the transfer of electrons from

Table 3. Transcripts encoding for proteins involved in photosynthesis and oxidoreduction differentially expressed in *wbc19* mutant seedlings.

GO ID	Description	Gene ID	Description	control rpkm	mutant rpkm	log2 (fold change)
GO:0015979	photosynthesis	AT1G76450	Photosystem II reaction center PsbP family protein	50.43	0.83	−5.92
GO:0015979	photosynthesis	AT3G05410	Photosystem II reaction center PsbP family protein	1.29	128.25	6.63
GO:0015979	photosynthesis	AT3G53920	RNAPOLYMERASE SIGMA-SUBUNIT C (SIGC)	3.54	82.28	4.54
GO:0015979	photosynthesis	AT2G18790	PHYTOCHROME B (PHYB)	14.70	0.19	−6.27
GO:0009055	electron carrier activity	AT2G27510	FERREDOXIN 3 (FD3) *	75.02	1.11	−6.08
GO:0016491	oxidoreductase activity	AT1G34200	Glyceraldehyde-3-phosphate dehydrogenase-like family protein	0.83	85.45	6.68
GO:0015035	protein disulfide oxidoreductase activity	AT2G32920	ARABIDOPSIS THALIANA PROTEIN DISULFIDE ISOMERASE 9 (ATPDI9)	30.76	0.48	−6.02
GO:0016705	oxidoreductase activity, acting on paired donors, with incorporation or reduction of molecular oxygen	AT3G14650	CYTOCHROME P450, FAMILY 72, SUBFAMILY A, POLYPEPTIDE 11" (CYP72A11) *	19.93	0.36	−5.77

The terms photosynthesis, oxidoreduction and electron carrier were searched in the GO associated with genes differentially expressed when comparing transcripts from control seedlings to transcripts from *wbc19* mutant seedlings germinating on MS media (minimum 2 fold difference in expression; $P<0.001$). * denotes genes also identified as encoding for metal binding proteins in **Table 4.**

Table 4. Transcripts encoding for metal binding proteins differentially expressed in *wbc19* mutant seedlings.

GO ID	Description	Gene ID	Description	control rpkm	mutant rpkm	log2 (fold change)
GO:0008270	zinc ion binding	AT5G59820	RESPONSIVE TO HIGH LIGHT 41 (RHL41)	6.28	197.89	4.98
GO:0008270	zinc ion binding	AT4G21350	PLANT U-BOX 8 (PUB8)	2.23	110.71	5.63
GO:0008270	zinc ion binding	AT5G01450	RING/U-box superfamily protein	0.71	45.47	6.00
GO:0008270	zinc ion binding	AT1G68190	B-box zinc finger family protein	1.00	107.51	6.74
GO:0008270	zinc ion binding	AT3G46090	C2H2-type zinc finger protein ZAT7	1.88	211.01	6.81
GO:0006829	zinc ion transport	AT3G12750	ZINC TRANSPORTER 1 PRECURSOR (ZIP1)	0.91	100.73	6.79
GO:0005506	iron ion binding	AT3G14650	CYTOCHROME P450, FAMILY 72, SUBFAMILY A, POLYPEPTIDE 11 (CYP72A11) *	19.93	0.36	−5.77
GO:0051536	iron-sulfur cluster binding	AT2G27510	FERREDOXIN 3 (FD3) *	75.02	1.10	−6.08

The terms metal, iron, zinc, copper, manganese, magnesium, cobalt, molybdenum etc were searched in the GO terms associated with genes differentially expressed when comparing transcripts from control seedlings to transcripts from *wbc19* mutant seedlings germinating on MS media (minimum 2 fold difference in expression; $P< 0.001$). * denotes genes also identified as encoding for oxidoreductases in **Table 3.**

ferredoxin and NADH back to plastoquinone [51,52]. This role of the NDH complex is not crucial under normal conditions as mutants do not exhibit a phenotype, but appears important under conditions of stress [53,54,55,56,57,58,59]. Thus, the response of mutant seedlings to kanamycin suggests an adaptation of photosynthetic apparatus to stress, with a disassembly of PSII and cyclic electron flow around PSI.

When transcripts for metal binding proteins were examined, a total of 20 genes were found to be differentially expressed between control and mutant seedlings exposed to kanamycin (**Table 6**). The majority are downregulated, however the expression of FRO6 is increased by about 5 fold in the mutant exposed to kanamycin. FRO6 is a ferric reductase found in the plasma membrane of mesophyll cells in the shoots [60,61]. Its expression is light inducible and is thought to coordinate iron uptake with photosynthetic activity. The increase of FRO6 transcripts in mutant seedlings exposed to kanamycin is accompanied by significantly lower levels of NICOTIANAMINE SYNTHASE 1 (NAS1) transcripts and for both genes, Real-Time PCR results confirmed RNA-seq findings. NAS1 enables the synthesis of nicotianamine (NA), a low molecular weight chelator of transition metal cations, including Fe^{2+}, Fe^{3+}, Cu and Zn [62,63,64]. NA facilitates the transport of Fe from the phloem to sink organs via YELLOW-STRIPE1-LIKE (YSL) transporters [65,66]. These findings suggest iron deficiency in leaves and decreased mobilization of metals via the phloem.

Plant Metal Content

The RNA-seq results supported our hypothesis that plants' responses to the antibiotic kanamycin would affect metal homeostasis. Mutation of the kanamycin resistance gene WBC19 further indicated metal uptake deficiencies. We therefore quantified the Fe, Zn, Mn and Cu content of control and mutant plants grown in the presence or absence of kanamycin. Exposure to kanamycin resulted in the reduction of iron content in control seedlings by approximately 60% (**Figure 1**). The reduction in iron content was accompanied by a significant increase in the Cu content by about 50%. As predicted, these results indicate that a major response of plants exposed to kanamycin is to limit their Fe

Table 5. Transcripts encoding for proteins involved in photosynthesis and oxidoreduction differentially expressed when comparing control and *wbc19* mutant seedlings geminating on MS media with 50 mg/l kanamycin.

GO ID	Description	Gene ID	Description	Control + kan rpkm	Mutant + kan rpkm	log2 (fold change)
GO:0015979	photosynthesis	AT1G29920	CHLOROPHYLL A/B-BINDING PROTEIN 2 (CAB2) (LHCB1.1)	979.95	0.01	−16.58
GO:0015979	photosynthesis	ATCG00270	PHOTOSYSTEM II REACTION CENTER PROTEIN D (PSBD)	1000.97	334.95	−1.58
GO:0015979	photosynthesis	AT1G74880	NADH DEHYDROGENASE-LIKE COMPLEX) (NdhO)	5.85	113.43	4.28
GO:0009055	electron carrier activity	AT5G49730	FERRIC REDUCTION OXIDASE 6 (FRO6)	7.18	75.65	3.40
GO:0009055	electron carrier activity	AT5G08740	NAD(P)H DEHYDROGENASE C1 (NDC1)	0.35	16.69	5.58
GO:0009055	electron carrier activity	AT1G06820	CAROTENOID ISOMERASE (CRTISO)	1.34	36.41	4.76
GO:0009055	electron carrier activity	AT1G64640	EARLY NODULIN-LIKE PROTEIN 8 (ENODL8)	97.44	2.04	−5.58
GO:0009055	electron carrier activity	AT2G47470	UNFERTILIZED EMBRYO SAC 5 (UNE5)	6.31	85.77	3.77
GO:0016491	oxidoreductase activity	AT2G37240	Thioredoxin superfamily protein	0.57	28.75	5.65
GO:0016616	oxidoreductase activity, acting on the CH-OH group of donors, NAD or NADP as acceptor	AT4G29010	ABNORMAL INFLORESCENCE MERISTEM (AIM1)	7.05	61.77	3.13
GO:0016627	oxidoreductase activity, acting on the CH-CH group of donors	AT5G65110	ACYL-COA OXIDASE 2 (ACX2)	1.49	36.79	4.62
GO:0016639	oxidoreductase activity, acting on the CH-NH2 group of donors, NAD or NADP as acceptor	AT5G07440	GLUTAMATE DEHYDROGENASE 2 (GDH2)	147.51	39.11	−1.92

The terms photosynthesis, oxidoreduction and electron carrier were searched in the GO IDs associated with genes differentially expressed when comparing transcripts from control and *wbc19* mutant seedlings germinating on MS media with 50 mg/l of kanamycin (minimum 2 fold difference in expression; $P<0.001$).

Table 6. Transcripts encoding for metal binding proteins differentially expressed when comparing control and *wbc19* mutant seedlings geminating on MS media with 50 m/l kanamycin.

GO ID	Description	Gene ID	Description	control + kan rpkm	Mutant + kan rpkm	log2 (fold change)
GO:0000041	transition metal ion transport	AT2G36290	alpha/beta-Hydrolases superfamily protein	49.93	0.94	−5.73
GO:0005506	iron ion binding	AT5G49730	FERRIC REDUCTION OXIDASE 6 (FRO6)	7.18	75.65	3.4
GO:0071281	cellular response to iron ion	AT5G04950	NICOTIANAMINE SYNTHASE 1 (NAS1)	46.06	1.24	−5.22
GO:0005507	copper ion binding	AT2G36950	Heavy metal transport/ detoxification superfamily	0.37	17.67	5.56
GO:0005507	copper ion binding	AT5G07440	GLUTAMATE DEHYDROGENASE 2 (GDH2)	147.51	39.11	−1.92
GO:0005507	copper ion binding	AT5G55200	MITOCHONDRIAL GRPE 1 (MGE1)	71.29	2.15	−5.05
GO:0008270	zinc ion binding	AT1G76950	(PRAF1)	31.11	2.03	−3.94
GO:0008270	zinc ion binding	AT3G42790	ALFIN-LIKE 3 (AL3)	45.02	1.18	−5.26
GO:0008270	zinc ion binding	AT3G43240	ARID/BRIGHT DNA-binding domain-containing protein	0.25	13.69	5.78
GO:0008270	zinc ion binding	AT5G48250	B-box type zinc finger protein with CCT domain	33.25	0.77	−5.44
GO:0004222	metalloendopeptidase activity	AT5G65620	Zincin-like metalloproteases family protein	0.26	35.28	7.09
GO:0008237	metallopeptidase activity	AT4G20070	ALLANTOATE AMIDOHYDROLASE (AAH)	0.35	19.08	5.77
GO:0015095	magnesium ion transmembrane transporter activity	AT3G19640	MAGNESIUM TRANSPORTER 4 (MGT4)	28.06	0.72	−5.29
GO:0070838	divalent metal ion transport	AT4G23890	NADH DEHYDROGENASE-LIKE COMPLEX S (NdhS)	45.4	1.21	−5.23
GO:0051539	4 iron, 4 sulfur cluster binding	AT5G04560	DEMETER (DME)	22.58	1.34	−4.08
GO:0016226	iron-sulfur cluster assembly	AT1G14030	LYSINE METHYLTRANSFERASE (LSMT)-LIKE (LSMT-L)	51.02	1.57	−5.03
GO:0030145	manganese ion binding	AT4G29490	Metallopeptidase M24 family protein	54.69	1.56	−5.13
GO:0046872	metal ion binding	AT1G65290	MITOCHONDRIAL ACYL CARRIER PROTEIN 2 (mtACP2)	2.01	90.61	5.49
GO:0046872	metal ion binding	AT4G00900	ER-TYPE CA2+-ATPASE 2 (ECA2)	21.46	0.4	−5.75
GO:0010038	response to metal ion	AT5G26240	CHLORIDE CHANNEL D (CLC-D)	0.25	19.85	6.34

uptake. This in turn may result in secondary effects on the uptake of other metals.

When metal levels of control and *wbc19* mutant plants grown in the absence of kanamycin are compared, significant differences were observed for Zn and Cu. Mutant plants had about 50% less Zn and Cu than control plants while Fe and Mn levels remained unaffected. These results suggested that, WBC19 plays a role in metal uptake even in the absence of kanamycin. Surprisingly, it was not the Fe content that was altered, but that of Zn and Cu.

In mutant plants exposed to kanamycin, Fe levels were even lower than in control seedlings; Cu and Zn levels reach their lowest points and Mn levels reach significantly lower concentrations. Thus mutants exhibit the same response as control plants in reducing their Fe uptake and their overall lower metal content is exacerbated by the exposure to kanamycin. This may be in part due to the stunted roots which further compromised the uptake of nutrients from the media.

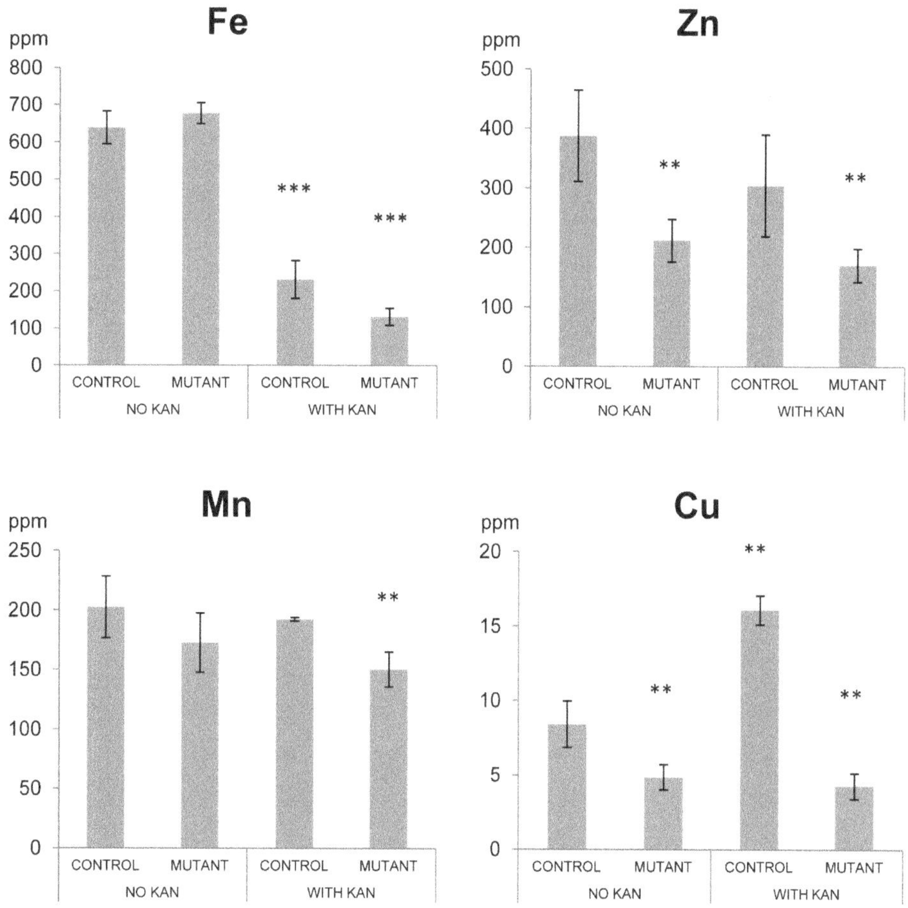

Figure 1. Metal content of seedlings grown in the presence or absence of kanamycin (50mg/l). Iron, zinc, manganese and copper contents from control and *wbc19* mutant seedlings were measured by ICP-MS five days after germination and shown in parts per million (ppm). Error bars represent ± standard deviation from 3 biological replicates. **, *** indicate significant difference with the control on media with no kanamycin at $P<0.01$ and 0.001 respectively (*t*- test).

Transcript abundance of iron homeostasis genes

To further analyze the effect of kanamycin on iron homeostasis, a panel of six well characterized genes was selected for real-time PCR analysis (**Figure 2**). These include genes known to be involved in iron uptake in roots (IRON REGULATED TRANSPOTER 1 (IRT1), FERRIC REDUCTION OXIDASE 2, (FRO2)), iron loading and transport in xylem (IRON REGULATED PROTEIN 1 (IREG1/FPN1), FERRIC REDUCTASE DEFECTIVE 3 (FRD3)), iron unloading and remobilization (YELLOW STRIPE LIKE 1 and 3(YSL1, YSL3)), iron uptake in mesophyll cells (FRO6). The latter was already found to be upregulated in mutant plants exposed to kanamycin and inclusion of this gene would further serve to confirm results from the transcriptome profiling. When control seedlings were exposed to kanamycin, no significant changes in transcript levels were observed for all genes studied except for a small decrease in transcript levels of YSL3. This finding indicates that despite their low levels iron, seedlings exposed to kanamycin do not induce genes known to be upregulated during iron deficiency. On the other hand, there were no differences in iron content between control and mutant seedlings grown in the absence of kanamycin, but transcript levels of IREG1/FPN1 were found to be significantly different. IREG1/FPN1 transcripts were about 30% higher in mutants and increased further upon kanamycin exposure. IREG1/FPN1 is not responsive to iron but is thought to be involved in iron loading in the xylem [67].

In mutant plants exposed to kanamycin several iron homeostasis genes were found to be differentially regulated. Transcripts of IRT1, FRD3 and YSL1 were significantly less abundant. This likely reflected the fact that mutant seedlings had stunted roots as all three transcripts are mainly expressed in roots of seedlings [68,69,70]. Transcripts of IREG1 and FRO6 were significantly more abundant when mutant plants were exposed to kanamycin. The results obtained for FRO6 in Real-Time assays corroborated findings from RNA-seq experiments. Mutants exhibited a five-fold increase of FRO6 transcripts, but not controls despite low levels of iron in both lines after germination in the presence of kanamycin. FRO6 encodes for an iron chelate reductase expressed in green tissues [60,61]. It is was found to be mainly regulated by light rather than iron and thought to coordinate iron needs with photosynthesis. In light of this expression pattern, it is difficult to attribute difference in FRO6 induction between mutant and control plants to the differences in iron content after exposure to kanamycin. Nonetheless, our results show that kanamycin is a potent inducer of FRO6 in *wbc19* mutants. Likewise, a more modest increase in the transcript levels of IREG1 (FPN1) was detected. Previous experiments have shown that IREG1 is mainly expressed in the vasculature of the root and shoot [67] and not

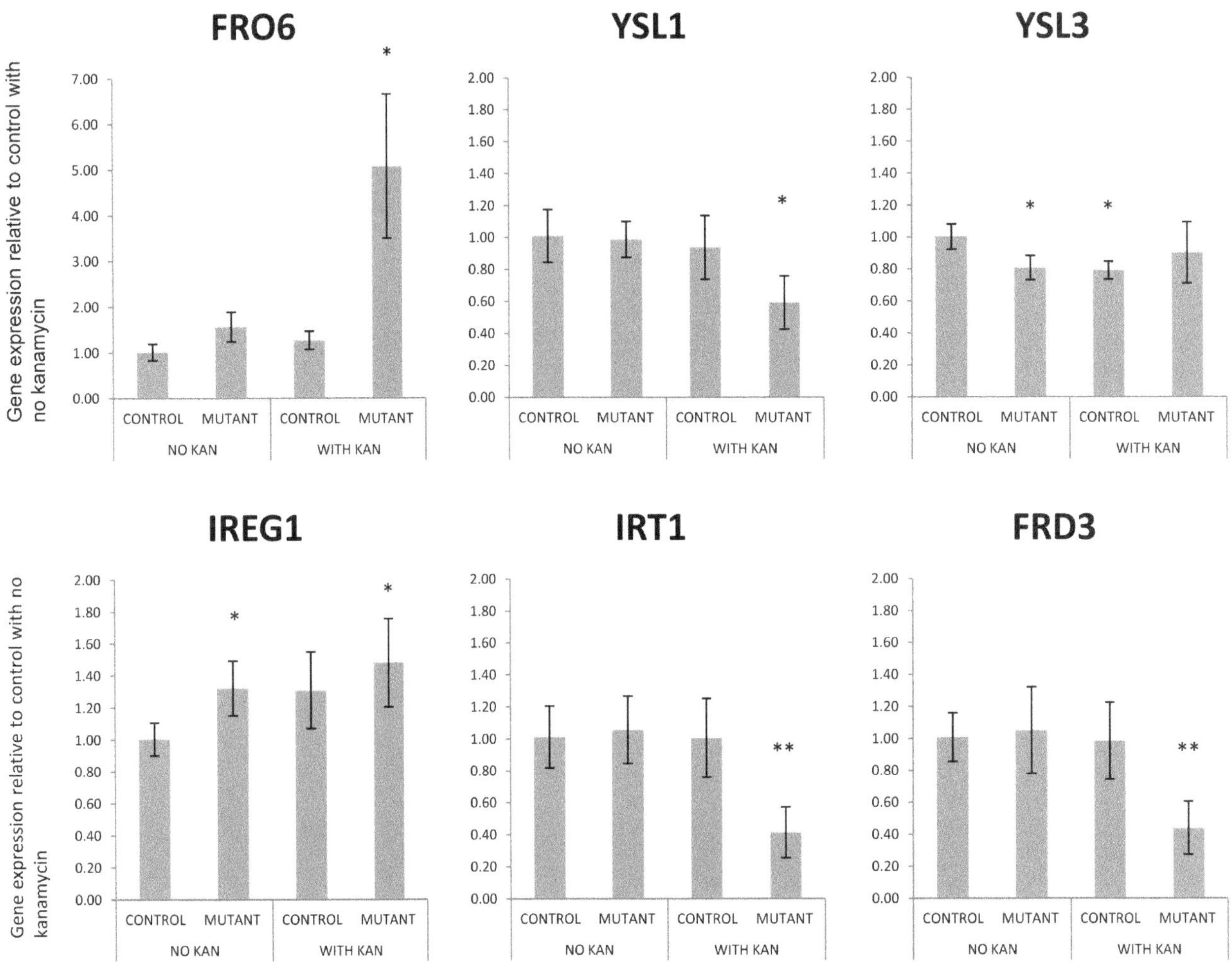

Figure 2. Real-Time RT-PCR analysis of transcript levels of iron homeostasis genes. Multiplexed TaqMan assays were performed for the quantification of iron homeostasis genes as indicated (FAM labeled) and the control, RAD23-3 (VIC labeled) after reverse-transcription of mRNA extracts from control and *wbc19* mutant plants germinated on MS media with or without 50 mg/l kanamycin. Data shown are from 4 biological replicates and 3 technical replicates. Error bars indicate standard deviation.

iron regulated [71,72]. It likely effluxes metals from the cytoplasm into the vasculature, allowing movement of metals from root to shoot [67].

WBC19 is predominantly expressed in vascular tissues

To gain further insight on the role of WBC19 in antibiotic resistance, we analyzed the expression pattern of its native promoter. A 2.1 kb DNA fragment upstream of the start codon was cloned in front of a GUS gene and *Arabidopsis* plants containing the constructs assayed for histochemical GUS activity. Strong GUS expression was observed in leaves and stele of 10 day old seedlings (**Figure 3**. A, B, C). Actively dividing cells of the pericycle also showed GUS expression. Once the secondary root emerges, the new meristematic region no longer showed GUS expression. In contrast to what is seen in young leaves, GUS expression in older leaves is restricted to the veins. Similarly in flowers, GUS staining is prominent in the vascular tissue of the sepals, petals and anther filaments (**Figure 3** D, E). Overall, GUS expression was predominantly vascular, a pattern characteristic of genes with a role in the long distance transport of nutrients.

Discussion

Plants are exposed to a variety of antibiotics produced by soil microorganisms. Therefore understanding how plants have adapted to this prevalent, yet less recognized form of stress is important not only at the fundamental level but also for its implications in plant nutrition, productivity and in genetic engineering. In this study we undertook a large-scale analysis of the effect of kanamycin and examined the role of WBC19 in resistance using the RNA-seq technique. In conjunction with metal analysis and expression profiling with a promoter-GUS fusion, important insights were gained on the physiology of plants exposed to kanamycin and the role of WBC19.

Plant exposure to kanamycin leads to reduced iron uptake

The elemental analysis showed that *Arabidopsis* seedlings exposed to kanamycin reduced their iron uptake by 60%. Chloroplasts represent the major reservoir of iron in plants where it is needed as a component of PSI and PSII and serves as a co-factor in the electron transport chain during the light reactions of

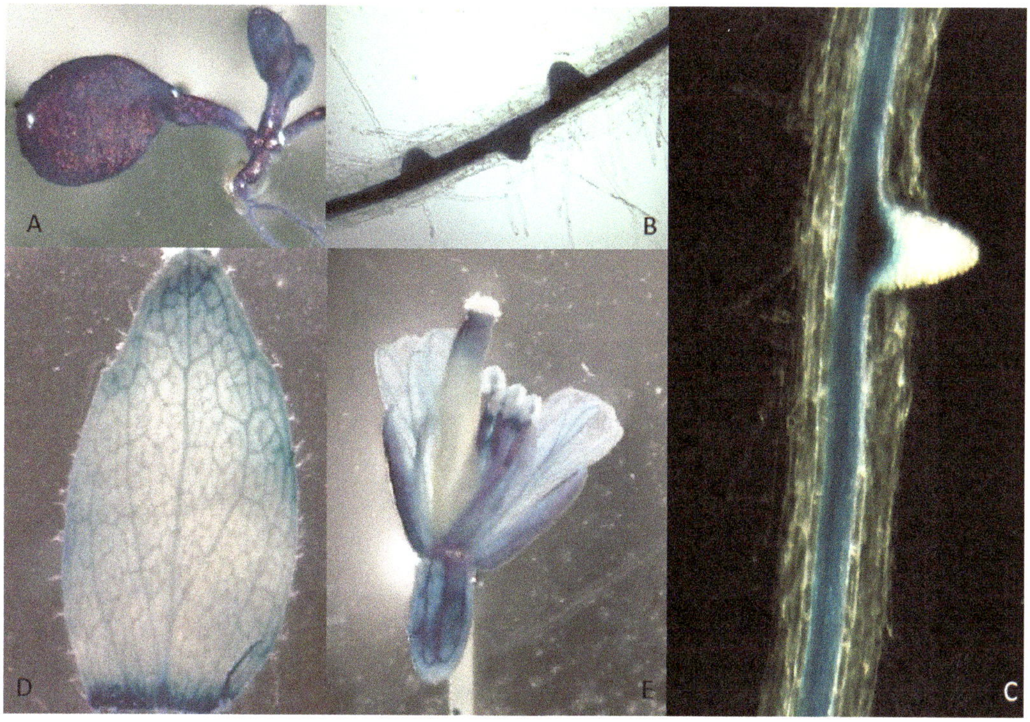

Figure 3. Expression pattern of WBC19. A wbc19 promoter-GUS fusion construct was generated to examine the endogenous expression pattern of wbc19. GUS stained 10 days old seedling showing leaf (A) and roots (B,C); older leaf (D) and flower (E).

photosynthesis. It is also used for the assembly of Fe-S clusters and the synthesis of chlorophyll [73,74]. Iron deficiency primarily affects PSI function, probably because of its high requirement for iron (12 Fe atoms per PSI unit) [75]. In turn, the decline in PSI function affects electron transport from PSII to PSI, leading to the generation of reactive oxygen species and photo-oxidative damage. Adaptive responses vary in different organisms but generally involve the dissipation of light energy and optimization of photosynthetic function [75,76,77,78]. In plants, the LHCII plays a critical role in the dissipation of light energy [79] and specific isoforms of LHCII subunits were shown to be induced by iron deficiency [78].

In our experiments, the increase of transcripts encoding for components of PSI and PSII (PSI-P and CAB2/LHCB1.1) and the repair of photodamaged PSII (ALBINO3 and DegP7) captured the adaptation of the photosynthetic apparatus to kanamycin and emulated a response to reduced iron. Overall, the observed changes were limited considering the large reduction in iron content. It is possible that a limited response is observed at the transcript level but more significant changes might take place at the protein level. Previous studies in *Chlamydomonas reinhardtii* have revealed that protein levels of many PS I components decrease under iron limitation [77], but changes in the transcript levels of these proteins were not detected [75]. Thus transcript profiling might only provide a partial portrayal of all the changes that are taking place upon plant exposure to kanamycin.

Prior to its arrival in chloroplasts, iron is acquired from the soil and mobilized to the leaves. Iron acquisition in roots, especially in response to iron deficiency has been well characterized. In *Arabidopsis*, Fe^{3+} in the soil is typically reduced to Fe^{2+} by a ferric oxidase reductase (FRO2) found in root epidermal cells. It is then taken-up by the iron regulated transporter IRT1 that belongs to the ZIP family of metal transporters [70,71,80,81]. Iron moves symplastically in root cells and is loaded into the xylem by IRON REGULATED1 (IREG1/FPN1) [67]. Concomitant loading of citrate by FERRIC REDUCTASE DEFECTIVE3 (FRD3) allows the long-distance transport of iron as an Fe^{3+}-citrate chelate [68,82,83]. Iron is also mobilized in the phloem as an Fe^{2+}-nicotinamine chelate where it can be transported by members of the YSL family of transporters [65,66,69,84]. We examined transcript levels of these genes involved in iron acquisition and mobilization using TaqMan real-time PCR assays. Our results indicated that transcript levels of most genes were not affected by exposure to kanamycin in control plants. This observation indicated that the reduction in iron content was not accompanied by changes resembling iron deficiency responses. Thus, the physiological state induced by kanamycin is distinct from that caused by iron deficiency alone.

Nonetheless, control plants exposed to kanamycin appear to be upregulating a high-affinity iron transport system represented by LAC5. In *Chlamydomonas reinhardtii* a similar multicopper oxidase, FOX1, involved in high-affinity iron uptake is dramatically upregulated under iron limited conditions. FOX1 is upregulated before growth of cells is inhibited such that it used as a sentinel marker in iron deficiency studies [85,86]. Similarly LAC5 could represents a high-affinity transporter upregulated in response to reduced levels of iron in control plants exposed to kanamycin. The upregulation of LAC5 and transcripts of two other copper binding proteins (SKS17, MGE1) in control plants exposed to kanamycin was concomitant with an increase of the copper content of seedlings. Copper is known to play a role in iron homeostasis as a cofactor in multicopper oxidases such as FOX1, FET3 and caeruploplasmin responsible for high-affinity iron transport in green algae, yeast and humans [34,35,36,85,86,87]. More recently copper was also shown to play a role in iron homeostasis in *Arabidopsis*, but specific copper dependent oxidases have not identified [88,89]. Under our experimental conditions control plants exposed to kanamycin significantly increased their copper uptake. Aside from possibly participating in a high-affinity iron uptake system, increased copper levels may help mitigate oxidative stress under low iron. An increase in copper uptake is generally observed in plants grown under iron limiting conditions and is thought to represent an adaptive response to minimize oxidative stress damage by supplying Cu to Cu Superoxide Dismutases (CuSODs) and compensate for the lack of functional FeSODs [89]. Overall, based on the observed transcriptional changes in control plants exposed to kanamycin, the reduction in iron content could either be a direct consequence of the stress caused by kanamycin on choloroplasts, but could also represent, at least partially, an adaptive response to limit iron uptake.

WBC19 and zinc homeostasis

Important insights on the role of WBC19 were gained from the comparison of control and mutant plants in the absence of kanamycin. *wbc19* mutants contain about half the amount of zinc and copper compared to control plants suggesting that WBC19 plays an important role in zinc and copper uptake under normal conditions. The low levels of zinc in mutants were accompanied by increased expression of the zinc transporter ZIP1 as well as a number of zinc binding proteins. We sought to confirm increased expression of ZIP1 by real-time RT-PCR, however adequate custom or predesigned primer and probe sets could not be generated for our Taq-Man assays. This was in part due to the fact that ZIP1 transcripts overlapped with ALIS1 transcripts. Zinc is the second most abundant microelement found in plants. In *Arabidopdsis*, zinc is initially taken-up by IRT1 in root epidermal cells along with iron and other metals. Once in the root symplast, it can either be loaded into the xylem mainly by two P-type ATPases, HEAVY METAL ATPASE 2 and 4 (HMA2 and HMA4) [90,91,92] sequestered in root vacuoles via two transporters of the cation diffusion facilitator family, the METAL TOLERANCE PROTEIN 1 and 3 (MTP1 and MTP3) [93,94,95] or extruded by PLANT CADMIUM RESISTANCE 2 (PCR2) from root epidermal cells under conditions of excess zinc [96]. The presence, transport and compartmentalization of zinc chelators especially nicotianamine (NA) also play an important role in the uptake and distribution of zinc [64,97,98,99].

It is not clear how WBC19 contributes to zinc homeostasis. The phenotype observed for *wbc19* mutants bares similarities with the phenotypes of the *hma2 hma4* double mutants and *hma4* single mutants [90] but also the ZINC-INDUCED FACILITATOR1 (ZIF1) overexpressing lines [64] and the NICOTIANAMINE SYNTHASE (NAS) mutants [99]. ZIF1 is an NA transporter that localizes to the vacuolar membranes. Its overexpression leads to the enhanced sequestration of zinc in root cell vacuoles and therefore a decrease in the mobilization of zinc from roots to shoots. The dramatic effect of ZIF1 on zinc mobilization, but limited effect on iron mobilization is explained by the differences in the stability of Fe-NA and Zn-NA complexes in the vacuole [64,97,100]. Fe-NA complexes are not stable at vacuolar pH, whereas Zn-NA complexes are. Similarly, *nas* mutants are deficient in their ability to mobilize zinc from root to shoot but not iron [99]. Although NA has a high affinity for copper, differences in the mobilization of Cu were not observed with ZIF1 overexpressing lines [64] nor *nas* mutants [99]. Our study however also points to a decrease in the uptake of copper by *wbc19* mutants. Given the phenotypic similarities between *wbc19* mutants with *hma2 hma4* double mutants and *hma4* single on one hand and ZIF1 overexpressors and *nas* mutants on the other, WBC19 could have a function in zinc or NA movement. Since WBC19 has a role in antibiotic resistance, a function linked to NA movement is more likely.

NA allows the long-distance transport of iron in the phloem and probably that of zinc and copper in both the xylem and phloem [66,100,101]. NA is a non proteinogenic amino acid synthesized by a condensation reaction of three molecules of *S*-adenosyl-Met by nicotianamine synthase (NAS) [102]. Four NAS genes are encoded in the *Arabidopsis* genome and their transcript levels are upregulated in response to iron, zinc and copper deficiency [103,104]. With the optimal spacing of its six functional groups, the structure of NA allows octahedral coordination and formation of chelate rings, making it a high affinity chelator of several metals [101]. It is also thought that the structure of NA or metal-NA complexes bears similarities with that of aminoglycoside antibiotics such that they can move through the same transporters [6,8]. In *wbc19* mutants, defects in zinc deficiency are coupled to kanamycin sensitivity. One possible explanation is that mutants have increased expression of NA transporters for xylem loading. In turn this leads to increased transport of kanamycin. Conversely, when WBC19 is functional, lower levels of NA transporters are present and thus result in decreased kanamycin movement. Our analysis of the expression pattern of WBC19 further support the notion that it might have a role in long-distance transport as expression was predominantly vascular. Future studies will examine the relationship between NA, zinc and WBC19.

Conclusion

Plants mine the soil to obtain essential nutrients and in so doing can take-up antibiotics produced by soil microorganisms. Our study supports the view that chloroplasts are an important target of aminoglycosides as several transcripts of the photosynthetic apparatus were differentially expressed upon seedling exposure to kanamycin. Another consequence of the exposure to kanamycin is a significant decrease in iron content. It is unknown whether this is due to a decreased requirement for iron or an adaptive response to limit iron uptake and possibly restrict kanamycin movement. We also observed notable differences between control and *wbc19* mutants. The fact that mutant seedlings upregulate FRO6 while control seedlings do not highlights a major difference in the way kanamycin affects iron homeostasis in the two lines. Hence, aside from lower levels of zinc observed in mutant, more subtle differences with regard to iron homeostasis are affected by WBC19.

Supporting Information

Figure S1 Over-represented functional categories for transcripts differentially expressed upon germination of control seedlings on media with kanamycin. The normalized representation relative to the frequency of group members in the *Arabidopsis* genome (± bootstrap StdDev) is shown. Significantly overrepresented groups ($P<0.05$) are in bold.

Figure S2 Over-represented functional categories for transcripts differentially expressed in *wbc19* mutant seedlings. The normalized representation relative to the frequency of group members in the *Arabidopsis* genome (±bootstrap StdDev) is shown. Significantly overrepresented groups ($P<0.05$) are in bold.

Figure S3 Over-represented functional categories for transcripts differentially expressed when comparing control and *wbc19* mutant seedlings germinating on

media with kanamycin. The normalized representation relative to the frequency of group members in the *Arabidopsis* genome (±bootstrap StdDev) is shown. Significantly overrepresented groups ($P<0.05$) are in bold.

Figure S4 Venn Diagram showing the overlap between genes found to be significantly up or downregulated in the control exposed to kanamycin compared to the control, and genes differentially expressed between control and mutant plants exposed to kanamycin (fold change>2; $P<0.001$).

Table S1 Pre-Designed TaqMan Assays from Life Technologies used in multiplex Real-Time PCRs for the quantification of various iron homeostasis genes (FAM labeled) and the control, RAD23-3 (VIC labeled).

Table S2 Mapping efficiency of reads obtained for each RNA-seq library. An average of 2.3 million reads per library uniquely mapped to the Arabidopsis genome.

File S1 Real-Time PCR validation of RNA-seq data on a random selection of eleven genes across the four treatment conditions.

File S2 RNA-seq analysis and differentially expressed genes. The columns were color coded as follows: yellow: gene descriptions retrieved from TAIR, blue: CuffDiff output when comparing control no kan and mutant no kan samples, pink: CuffDiff output when comparing control + kan and mutant + kan samples, green: CuffDiff output when comparing control no kan and control + kan samples, orange: CuffDiff output when comparing mutant no kan and mutant + kan samples.

Acknowledgments

We thank David Bartel for hosting MA as a visiting assistant professor at the Whitehead Institute, Massachusetts Institute of Technology as well as lab members Huili Guo, Michael Nodine for their help and discussions. Finally, we are grateful to Casonya Johnson for her comments on the manuscript.

Author Contributions

Conceived and designed the experiments: AM. Performed the experiments: AM MA SR BE. Analyzed the data: AM KM. Contributed to the writing of the manuscript: AM.

References

1. Fourmy D, Recht MI, Blanchard SC, Puglisi JD (1996) Structure of the A site of Escherichia coli 16S ribosomal RNA complexed with an aminoglycoside antibiotic. Science 274: 1367–1371.
2. Mingeot-Leclercq MP, Glupczynski Y, Tulkens PM (1999) Aminoglycosides: activity and resistance. Antimicrob Agents Chemother 43: 727–737.
3. Recht MI, Fourmy D, Blanchard SC, Dahlquist KD, Puglisi JD (1996) RNA sequence determinants for aminoglycoside binding to an A-site rRNA model oligonucleotide. J Mol Biol 262: 421–436.
4. Recht MI, Douthwaite S, Puglisi JD (1999) Basis for prokaryotic specificity of action of aminoglycoside antibiotics. EMBO J 18: 3133–3138.
5. Machold O (1971) Lamellar proteins of green and chlorotic chloroplasts as affected by iron deficiency and antibiotics. Biochim Biophys Acta 238: 324–331.
6. Conte S, Stevenson D, Furner I, Lloyd A (2009) Multiple antibiotic resistance in Arabidopsis is conferred by mutations in a chloroplast-localized transport protein. Plant Physiol 151: 559–573.
7. Aufsatz W, Nehlin L, Voronin V, Schmidt A, Matzke AJ, et al. (2009) A novel strategy for obtaining kanamycin resistance in Arabidopsis thaliana by silencing an endogenous gene encoding a putative chloroplast transporter. Biotechnol J 4: 224–229.
8. Conte SS, Lloyd AM (2010) The MAR1 transporter is an opportunistic entry point for antibiotics. Plant Signal Behav 5: 49–52.
9. Mentewab A, Stewart CN Jr (2005) Overexpression of an Arabidopsis thaliana ABC transporter confers kanamycin resistance to transgenic plants. Nat Biotechnol 23: 1177–1180.
10. Kang BG, Ye X, Osburn LD, Stewart CN Jr, Cheng ZM (2010) Transgenic hybrid aspen overexpressing the Atwbc19 gene encoding an ATP-binding cassette transporter confers resistance to four aminoglycoside antibiotics. Plant Cell Rep 29: 643–650.
11. Burris K, Mentewab A, Ripp S, Stewart CN Jr (2008) An Arabidopsis thaliana ABC transporter that confers kanamycin resistance in transgenic plants does not endow resistance to Escherichia coli. Microb Biotechnol 1: 191–195.
12. Alonso JM, Stepanova AN, Leisse TJ, Kim CJ, Chen H, et al. (2003) Genome-wide insertional mutagenesis of Arabidopsis thaliana. Science 301: 653–657.
13. Guo H, Ingolia NT, Weissman JS, Bartel DP (2010) Mammalian microRNAs predominantly act to decrease target mRNA levels. Nature 466: 835–840.
14. Trapnell C, Pachter L, Salzberg SL (2009) TopHat: discovering splice junctions with RNA-Seq. Bioinformatics 25: 1105–1111.
15. Kim D, Pertea G, Trapnell C, Pimentel H, Kelley R, et al. (2013) TopHat2: accurate alignment of transcriptomes in the presence of insertions, deletions and gene fusions. Genome Biol 14: R36.
16. Trapnell C, Williams BA, Pertea G, Mortazavi A, Kwan G, et al. (2010) Transcript assembly and quantification by RNA-Seq reveals unannotated transcripts and isoform switching during cell differentiation. Nat Biotechnol 28: 511–515.
17. Provart N, Zhu T (2003) A Browser-based Functional Classification Super-Viewer for Arabidopsis Genomics. Currents in Computational Molecular Biology 271–272.
18. Pfaffl MW (2001) A new mathematical model for relative quantification in real-time RT-PCR. Nucleic Acids Res 29: e45.
19. Curtis MD, Grossniklaus U (2003) A gateway cloning vector set for high-throughput functional analysis of genes in planta. Plant Physiol 133: 462–469.
20. Clough SJ, Bent AF (1998) Floral dip: a simplified method for Agrobacterium-mediated transformation of Arabidopsis thaliana. Plant J 16: 735–743.
21. Jefferson RA, Kavanagh TA, Bevan MW (1987) GUS fusions: beta-glucuronidase as a sensitive and versatile gene fusion marker in higher plants. EMBO J 6: 3901–3907.
22. Ossenbuhl F, Gohre V, Meurer J, Krieger-Liszkay A, Rochaix JD, et al. (2004) Efficient assembly of photosystem II in Chlamydomonas reinhardtii requires Alb3.1p, a homolog of Arabidopsis ALBINO3. Plant Cell 16: 1790–1800.
23. Sun X, Fu T, Chen N, Guo J, Ma J, et al. (2010) The stromal chloroplast Deg7 protease participates in the repair of photosystem II after photoinhibition in Arabidopsis. Plant Physiol 152: 1263–1273.
24. Takubo K, Morikawa T, Nonaka Y, Mizutani M, Takenaka S, et al. (2003) Identification and molecular characterization of mitochondrial ferredoxins and ferredoxin reductase from Arabidopsis. Plant Mol Biol 52: 817–830.
25. Picciocchi A, Douce R, Alban C (2003) The plant biotin synthase reaction. Identification and characterization of essential mitochondrial accessory protein components. J Biol Chem 278: 24966–24975.
26. Michalecka AM, Svensson AS, Johansson FI, Agius SC, Johanson U, et al. (2003) Arabidopsis genes encoding mitochondrial type II NAD(P)H dehydrogenases have different evolutionary origin and show distinct responses to light. Plant Physiol 133: 642–652.
27. Elhafez D, Murcha MW, Clifton R, Soole KL, Day DA, et al. (2006) Characterization of mitochondrial alternative NAD(P)H dehydrogenases in Arabidopsis: intraorganelle location and expression. Plant Cell Physiol 47: 43–54.
28. Carrie C, Murcha MW, Kuehn K, Duncan O, Barthet M, et al. (2008) Type II NAD(P)H dehydrogenases are targeted to mitochondria and chloroplasts or peroxisomes in Arabidopsis thaliana. FEBS Lett 582: 3073–3079.
29. Eugeni Piller L, Besagni C, Ksas B, Rumeau D, Brehelin C, et al. (2011) Chloroplast lipid droplet type II NAD(P)H quinone oxidoreductase is essential for prenylquinone metabolism and vitamin K1 accumulation. Proc Natl Acad Sci U S A 108: 14354–14359.
30. Waters BM, Grusak MA (2008) Quantitative trait locus mapping for seed mineral concentrations in two Arabidopsis thaliana recombinant inbred populations. New Phytol 179: 1033–1047.
31. Gebert M, Meschenmoser K, Svidova S, Weghuber J, Schweyen R, et al. (2009) A root-expressed magnesium transporter of the MRS2/MGT gene

family in Arabidopsis thaliana allows for growth in low-Mg^{2+} environments. Plant Cell 21: 4018–4030.

32. Hoopes JT, Dean JF (2004) Ferroxidase activity in a laccase-like multicopper oxidase from Liriodendron tulipifera. Plant Physiol Biochem 42: 27–33.
33. McCaig BC, Meagher RB, Dean JF (2005) Gene structure and molecular analysis of the laccase-like multicopper oxidase (LMCO) gene family in Arabidopsis thaliana. Planta 221: 619–636.
34. Taylor AB, Stoj CS, Ziegler L, Kosman DJ, Hart PJ (2005) The copper-iron connection in biology: structure of the metallo-oxidase Fet3p. Proc Natl Acad Sci U S A 102: 15459–15464.
35. Kwok EY, Severance S, Kosman DJ (2006) Evidence for iron channeling in the Fet3p-Ftr1p high-affinity iron uptake complex in the yeast plasma membrane. Biochemistry 45: 6317–6327.
36. Askwith C, Eide D, Van Ho A, Bernard PS, Li L, et al. (1994) The FET3 gene of S. cerevisiae encodes a multicopper oxidase required for ferrous iron uptake. Cell 76: 403–410.
37. Ghanotakis DF, Topper JN, Babcock GT, Yocum CF (1984) Water-soluble 17 and 23 kDa polypeptides restore oxygen evolution activity by creating a high-affinity binding site for Ca^{2+} on the oxidizing side of Photosystem II. FEBS Letters 170: 169–173.
38. Ghanotakis DF, Topper JN, Youcum CF (1984) Structural organization of the oxidizing side of photosystem II. Exogenous reductants reduce and destroy the Mn-complex in photosystems II membranes depleted of the 17 and 23 kDa polypeptides. Biochimica et Biophysica Acta (BBA) - Bioenergetics 767: 524–531.
39. Ifuku K, Yamamoto Y, Ono TA, Ishihara S, Sato F (2005) PsbP protein, but not PsbQ protein, is essential for the regulation and stabilization of photosystem II in higher plants. Plant Physiol 139: 1175–1184.
40. Yi X, Hargett SR, Liu H, Frankel LK, Bricker TM (2007) The PsbP protein is required for photosystem II complex assembly/stability and photoautotrophy in Arabidopsis thaliana. J Biol Chem 282: 24833–24841.
41. Hanke G, Mulo P (2013) Plant type ferredoxins and ferredoxin-dependent metabolism. Plant Cell Environ 36: 1071–1084.
42. Hanke GT, Kimata-Ariga Y, Taniguchi I, Hase T (2004) A post genomic characterization of Arabidopsis ferredoxins. Plant Physiol 134: 255–264.
43. Grotz N, Fox T, Connolly E, Park W, Guerinot ML, et al. (1998) Identification of a family of zinc transporter genes from Arabidopsis that respond to zinc deficiency. Proc Natl Acad Sci U S A 95: 7220–7224.
44. Henriques R, Jasik J, Klein M, Martinoia E, Feller U, et al. (2002) Knock-out of Arabidopsis metal transporter gene IRT1 results in iron deficiency accompanied by cell differentiation defects. Plant Mol Biol 50: 587–597.
45. Dhariwal KR, Shirvan M, Levine M (1991) Ascorbic acid regeneration in chromaffin granules. In situ kinetics. J Biol Chem 266: 5384–5387.
46. Berczi A, Su D, Asard H (2007) An Arabidopsis cytochrome b561 with trans-membrane ferrireductase capability. FEBS Lett 581: 1505–1508.
47. Wyman S, Simpson RJ, McKie AT, Sharp PA (2008) Dcytb (Cybrd1) functions as both a ferric and a cupric reductase in vitro. FEBS Lett 582: 1901–1906.
48. Tsubaki M, Takeuchi F, Nakanishi N (2005) Cytochrome b561 protein family: expanding roles and versatile transmembrane electron transfer abilities as predicted by a new classification system and protein sequence motif analyses. Biochim Biophys Acta 1753: 174–190.
49. Cenacchi L, Busch M, Schleidt PG, Muller FG, Stumpp TV, et al. (2012) Heterologous production and characterisation of two distinct dihaem-containing membrane integral cytochrome b(561) enzymes from Arabidopsis thaliana in Pichia pastoris and Escherichia coli cells. Biochim Biophys Acta 1818: 679–688.
50. Melis A (1999) Photosystem-II damage and repair cycle in chloroplasts: what modulates the rate of photodamage ? Trends Plant Sci 4: 130–135.
51. Munekage Y, Shikanai T (2005) Cyclic electron transport through photosystem I. Plant Biotech 22: 361–369.
52. Ifuku K, Endo T, Shikanai T, Aro EM (2011) Structure of the chloroplast NADH dehydrogenase-like complex: nomenclature for nuclear-encoded subunits. Plant Cell Physiol 52: 1560–1568.
53. Horvath EM, Peter SO, Joet T, Rumeau D, Cournac L, et al. (2000) Targeted inactivation of the plastid ndhB gene in tobacco results in an enhanced sensitivity of photosynthesis to moderate stomatal closure. Plant Physiol 123: 1337–1350.
54. Endo T, Shikanai T, Takabayashi A, Asada K, Sato F (1999) The role of chloroplastic NAD(P)H dehydrogenase in photoprotection. FEBS Lett 457: 5–8.
55. Hashimoto M, Endo T, Peltier G, Tasaka M, Shikanai T (2003) A nucleus-encoded factor, CRR2, is essential for the expression of chloroplast ndhB in Arabidopsis. Plant J 36: 541–549.
56. Munekage Y, Hashimoto M, Miyake C, Tomizawa K, Endo T, et al. (2004) Cyclic electron flow around photosystem I is essential for photosynthesis. Nature 429: 579–582.
57. Li XG, Duan W, Meng QW, Zou Q, Zhao SJ (2004) The function of chloroplastic NAD(P)H dehydrogenase in tobacco during chilling stress under low irradiance. Plant Cell Physiol 45: 103–108.
58. Wang P, Duan W, Takabayashi A, Endo T, Shikanai T, et al. (2006) Chloroplastic NAD(P)H dehydrogenase in tobacco leaves functions in alleviation of oxidative damage caused by temperature stress. Plant Physiol 141: 465–474.
59. Rumeau D, Becuwe-Linka N, Beyly A, Louwagie M, Garin J, et al. (2005) New subunits NDH-M, -N, and -O, encoded by nuclear genes, are essential for plastid Ndh complex functioning in higher plants. Plant Cell 17: 219–232.
60. Li LY, Cai QY, Yu DS, Guo CH (2011) Overexpression of AtFRO6 in transgenic tobacco enhances ferric chelate reductase activity in leaves and increases tolerance to iron-deficiency chlorosis. Mol Biol Rep 38: 3605–3613.
61. Feng H, An F, Zhang S, Ji Z, Ling HQ, et al. (2006) Light-regulated, tissue-specific, and cell differentiation-specific expression of the Arabidopsis Fe(III)-chelate reductase gene AtFRO6. Plant Physiol 140: 1345–1354.
62. Haydon MJ, Cobbett CS (2007) Transporters of ligands for essential metal ions in plants. New Phytol 174: 499–506.
63. Palmer CM, Guerinot ML (2009) Facing the challenges of Cu, Fe and Zn homeostasis in plants. Nat Chem Biol 5: 333–340.
64. Haydon MJ, Kawachi M, Wirtz M, Hillmer S, Hell R, et al. (2012) Vacuolar nicotianamine has critical and distinct roles under iron deficiency and for zinc sequestration in Arabidopsis. Plant Cell 24: 724–737.
65. DiDonato RJ Jr, Roberts LA, Sanderson T, Eisley RB, Walker EL (2004) Arabidopsis Yellow Stripe-Like2 (YSL2): a metal-regulated gene encoding a plasma membrane transporter of nicotianamine-metal complexes. Plant J 39: 403–414.
66. Schuler M, Rellan-Alvarez R, Fink-Straube C, Abadia J, Bauer P (2012) Nicotianamine functions in the Phloem-based transport of iron to sink organs, in pollen development and pollen tube growth in Arabidopsis. Plant Cell 24: 2380–2400.
67. Morrissey J, Baxter IR, Lee J, Li L, Lahner B, et al. (2009) The ferroportin metal efflux proteins function in iron and cobalt homeostasis in Arabidopsis. Plant Cell 21: 3326–3338.
68. Rogers EE, Guerinot ML (2002) FRD3, a member of the multidrug and toxin efflux family, controls iron deficiency responses in Arabidopsis. Plant Cell 14: 1787–1799.
69. Waters BM, Chu HH, Didonato RJ, Roberts LA, Eisley RB, et al. (2006) Mutations in Arabidopsis yellow stripe-like1 and yellow stripe-like3 reveal their roles in metal ion homeostasis and loading of metal ions in seeds. Plant Physiol 141: 1446–1458.
70. Eide D, Broderius M, Fett J, Guerinot ML (1996) A novel iron-regulated metal transporter from plants identified by functional expression in yeast. Proc Natl Acad Sci U S A 93: 5624–5628.
71. Colangelo EP, Guerinot ML (2004) The essential basic helix-loop-helix protein FIT1 is required for the iron deficiency response. Plant Cell 16: 3400–3412.
72. Dinneny JR, Long TA, Wang JY, Jung JW, Mace D, et al. (2008) Cell identity mediates the response of Arabidopsis roots to abiotic stress. Science 320: 942–945.
73. Ravet K, Pilon M (2013) Copper and iron homeostasis in plants: the challenges of oxidative stress. Antioxid Redox Signal 19: 919–932.
74. Yruela I (2013) Transition metals in plant photosynthesis. Metallomics 5: 1090–1109.
75. Moseley JL, Allinger T, Herzog S, Hoerth P, Wehinger E, et al. (2002) Adaptation to Fe-deficiency requires remodeling of the photosynthetic apparatus. EMBO J 21: 6709–6720.
76. Naumann B, Stauber EJ, Busch A, Sommer F, Hippler M (2005) N-terminal processing of Lhca3 Is a key step in remodeling of the photosystem I-light-harvesting complex under iron deficiency in Chlamydomonas reinhardtii. J Biol Chem 280: 20431–20441.
77. Naumann B, Busch A, Allmer J, Ostendorf E, Zeller M, et al. (2007) Comparative quantitative proteomics to investigate the remodeling of bioenergetic pathways under iron deficiency in Chlamydomonas reinhardtii. Proteomics 7: 3964–3979.
78. Saito A, Iino T, Sonoike K, Miwa E, Higuchi K (2010) Remodeling of the major light-harvesting antenna protein of PSII protects the young leaves of barley (Hordeum vulgare L.) from photoinhibition under prolonged iron deficiency. Plant Cell Physiol 51: 2013–2030.
79. Ruban AV, Berera R, Ilioaia C, van Stokkum IH, Kennis JT, et al. (2007) Identification of a mechanism of photoprotective energy dissipation in higher plants. Nature 450: 575–578.
80. Vert G, Grotz N, Dedaldechamp F, Gaymard F, Guerinot ML, et al. (2002) IRT1, an Arabidopsis transporter essential for iron uptake from the soil and for plant growth. Plant Cell 14: 1223–1233.
81. Robinson NJ, Procter CM, Connolly EL, Guerinot ML (1999) A ferric-chelate reductase for iron uptake from soils. Nature 397: 694–697.
82. Durrett TP, Gassmann W, Rogers EE (2007) The FRD3-mediated efflux of citrate into the root vasculature is necessary for efficient iron translocation. Plant Physiol 144: 197–205.
83. Green LS, Rogers EE (2004) FRD3 controls iron localization in Arabidopsis. Plant Physiol 136: 2523–2531.
84. Chu HH, Chiecko J, Punshon T, Lanzirotti A, Lahner B, et al. (2010) Successful reproduction requires the function of Arabidopsis Yellow Stripe-Like1 and Yellow Stripe-Like3 metal-nicotianamine transporters in both vegetative and reproductive structures. Plant Physiol 154: 197–210.
85. La Fontaine S, Quinn JM, Nakamoto SS, Page MD, Gohre V, et al. (2002) Copper-dependent iron assimilation pathway in the model photosynthetic eukaryote Chlamydomonas reinhardtii. Eukaryot Cell 1: 736–757.
86. Glaesener AG, Merchant SS, Blaby-Haas CE (2013) Iron economy in Chlamydomonas reinhardtii. Front Plant Sci 4: 337.

87. Vashchenko G, MacGillivray RT (2013) Multi-copper oxidases and human iron metabolism. Nutrients 5: 2289–2313.
88. Bernal M, Casero D, Singh V, Wilson GT, Grande A, et al. (2012) Transcriptome sequencing identifies SPL7-regulated copper acquisition genes FRO4/FRO5 and the copper dependence of iron homeostasis in Arabidopsis. Plant Cell 24: 738–761.
89. Waters BM, McInturf SA, Stein RJ (2012) Rosette iron deficiency transcript and microRNA profiling reveals links between copper and iron homeostasis in Arabidopsis thaliana. J Exp Bot 63: 5903–5918.
90. Hussain D, Haydon MJ, Wang Y, Wong E, Sherson SM, et al. (2004) P-type ATPase heavy metal transporters with roles in essential zinc homeostasis in Arabidopsis. Plant Cell 16: 1327–1339.
91. Verret F, Gravot A, Auroy P, Leonhardt N, David P, et al. (2004) Overexpression of AtHMA4 enhances root-to-shoot translocation of zinc and cadmium and plant metal tolerance. FEBS Lett 576: 306–312.
92. Eren E, Arguello JM (2004) Arabidopsis HMA2, a divalent heavy metal-transporting P(IB)-type ATPase, is involved in cytoplasmic Zn^{2+} homeostasis. Plant Physiol 136: 3712–3723.
93. Arrivault S, Senger T, Kramer U (2006) The Arabidopsis metal tolerance protein AtMTP3 maintains metal homeostasis by mediating Zn exclusion from the shoot under Fe deficiency and Zn oversupply. Plant J 46: 861–879.
94. Desbrosses-Fonrouge AG, Voigt K, Schroder A, Arrivault S, Thomine S, et al. (2005) Arabidopsis thaliana MTP1 is a Zn transporter in the vacuolar membrane which mediates Zn detoxification and drives leaf Zn accumulation. FEBS Lett 579: 4165–4174.
95. Kobae Y, Uemura T, Sato MH, Ohnishi M, Mimura T, et al. (2004) Zinc transporter of Arabidopsis thaliana AtMTP1 is localized to vacuolar membranes and implicated in zinc homeostasis. Plant Cell Physiol 45: 1749–1758.
96. Song WY, Choi KS, Kim DY, Geisler M, Park J, et al. (2010) Arabidopsis PCR2 is a zinc exporter involved in both zinc extrusion and long-distance zinc transport. Plant Cell 22: 2237–2252.
97. Sinclair SA, Kramer U (2012) The zinc homeostasis network of land plants. Biochim Biophys Acta 1823: 1553–1567.
98. Clemens S, Deinlein U, Ahmadi H, Horeth S, Uraguchi S (2013) Nicotianamine is a major player in plant Zn homeostasis. Biometals 26: 623–632.
99. Klatte M, Schuler M, Wirtz M, Fink-Straube C, Hell R, et al. (2009) The analysis of Arabidopsis nicotianamine synthase mutants reveals functions for nicotianamine in seed iron loading and iron deficiency responses. Plant Physiol 150: 257–271.
100. von Wiren N, Klair S, Bansal S, Briat JF, Khodr H, et al. (1999) Nicotianamine chelates both FeIII and FeII. Implications for metal transport in plants. Plant Physiol 119: 1107–1114.
101. Rellan-Alvarez R, Abadia J, Alvarez-Fernandez A (2008) Formation of metal-nicotianamine complexes as affected by pH, ligand exchange with citrate and metal exchange. A study by electrospray ionization time-of-flight mass spectrometry. Rapid Commun Mass Spectrom 22: 1553–1562.
102. Shojima S, Nishizawa NK, Mori S (1989) Establishment of a Cell-Free System for the Biosynthesis of Nicotianamine. Plant Cell Physiol 30: 673–677.
103. Wintz H, Fox T, Wu YY, Feng V, Chen W, et al. (2003) Expression profiles of Arabidopsis thaliana in mineral deficiencies reveal novel transporters involved in metal homeostasis. J Biol Chem 278: 47644–47653.
104. Bauer P, Thiel T, Klatte M, Bereczky Z, Brumbarova T, et al. (2004) Analysis of sequence, map position, and gene expression reveals conserved essential genes for iron uptake in Arabidopsis and tomato. Plant Physiol 136: 4169–4183.

6

Abnormal Calcium Handling and Exaggerated Cardiac Dysfunction in Mice with Defective Vitamin D Signaling

Sangita Choudhury[1], Soochan Bae[1], Qingen Ke[1], Ji Yoo Lee[1], Sylvia S. Singh[1], René St-Arnaud[2], Federica del Monte[1], Peter M. Kang[1]*

1 Cardiovascular Institute, Beth Israel Deaconess Medical Center and Harvard Medical School, Boston, Massachusetts, United States of America, **2** Shriners Hospital and Departments of Surgery and Human Genetics, McGill University, Montreal, Canada

Abstract

Aim: Altered vitamin D signaling is associated with cardiac dysfunction, but the pathogenic mechanism is not clearly understood. We examine the mechanism and the role of vitamin D signaling in the development of cardiac dysfunction.

Methods and Results: We analyzed 1α-hydroxylase (1α-OHase) knockout (1α-OHase$^{-/-}$) mice, which lack 1α-OH enzymes that convert the inactive form to hormonally active form of vitamin D. 1α-OHase$^{-/-}$ mice showed modest cardiac hypertrophy at baseline. Induction of pressure overload by transverse aortic constriction (TAC) demonstrated exaggerated cardiac dysfunction in 1α-OHase$^{-/-}$ mice compared to their WT littermates with a significant increase in fibrosis and expression of inflammatory cytokines. Analysis of calcium (Ca^{2+}) transient demonstrated profound Ca^{2+} handling abnormalities in 1α-OHase$^{-/-}$ mouse cardiomyocytes (CMs), and treatment with paricalcitol (PC), an activated vitamin D_3 analog, significantly attenuated defective Ca^{2+} handling in 1α-OHase$^{-/-}$ CMs. We further delineated the effect of vitamin D deficiency condition to TAC by first correcting the vitamin D deficiency in 1α-OHase$^{-/-}$ mice, followed then by either a daily maintenance dose of vitamin D or vehicle (to achieve vitamin D deficiency) at the time of sham or TAC. In mice treated with vitamin D, there was a significant attenuation of TAC-induced cardiac hypertrophy, interstitial fibrosis, inflammatory markers, Ca^{2+} handling abnormalities and cardiac function compared to the vehicle treated animals.

Conclusions: Our results provide insight into the mechanism of cardiac dysfunction, which is associated with severely defective Ca^{2+} handling and defective vitamin D signaling in 1α-OHase$^{-/-}$ mice.

Editor: Sudhiranjan Gupta, Texas A & M University Health Science Center, United States of America

Funding: This work was supported in part by NIH Grants R01 HL65742 (P.M.K.) and the World Class University program (R31-20029) from the Ministry of Education, Science and Technology, South Korea (P.M.K.). Support for generating the 1α-OHase -/- mice was provided by a grant from Shriners Hospitals for Children, Canada (R.St-A.). The funders had no role in study design, data collection and analysis, decision to publish, or preparation of the manuscript.

Competing Interests: The authors have declared that no competing interests exist.

* Email: pkang@bidmc.harvard.edu

Introduction

Cardiovascular disease (CVD) is the most common cause of mortality and morbidity in the United States and other developed nations. Clinical and epidemiological studies suggest an association between vitamin D deficiency and various cardiovascular disorders [1,2], and vitamin D therapy has been shown to improve cardiovascular function [3]. Particularly, in patients with chronic renal failure (CRF), vitamin D deficiency is uniformly present because the critical conversion of nutritional vitamin D_3 ($25(OH)D_3$) to the hormonally active form of vitamin D_3 ($1,25(OH)_2D_3$) occurs primarily in the kidney by 1α-hydroxylase (1α-OHase)[4]. CRF has been shown to be an independent risk factor for CVD, with 10–20 times greater incidence of cardiovascular disease in CRF patients [5]. Clinical studies have also demonstrated that there is an association between improved survival and decreased cardiovascular mortality in hemodialysis patients treated with an activated vitamin D analog, paricalcitol (PC) [6,7]. In fact, similar to CRF patients, 1α-OHase knockout (1α-OHase$^{-/-}$) mice show baseline hypertension, cardiac hypertrophy, and impaired cardiac function [8]. Despite these associations between vitamin D deficiency and cardiac dysfunction, the pathogenic mechanism of cardiac dysfunction associated with vitamin D deficiency is not fully elucidated.

Cardiomyocyte (CM) contractility is regulated by Ca^{2+} handling contractile proteins via regulation of intracellular levels of Ca^{2+} [9]. Thus, abnormalities in Ca^{2+} homeostasis, as seen in vitamin D deficiency, may lead to a chronic defect in E–C coupling, which may in turn lead to cardiac dysfunction. Delays in Ca^{2+} transients, for example, have been observed in myocardial tissue obtained from failing hearts [10]. Although it might not be surprising to find abnormal Ca^{2+} handling in a vitamin D deficiency state, the exact mechanism of vitamin D deficiency affecting the Ca^{2+} handling in CMs, however, is poorly understood. In this study, we examined whether abnormal Ca^{2+} homeostasis and Ca^{2+} handling may mediate structural and functional cardiac abnormalities and examined the relationship between vitamin D deficiency and the development of cardiac hypertrophy in 1α-OHase$^{-/-}$ mice. We hypothesize that restoration of vitamin D signaling improves cardiac functions by restoring Ca^{2+} homeostasis.

Methods

Animal care

Experiments were conducted using 8–10-week old male 1α-OH$^{-/-}$ mice and their littermates in a C57BL/6 background. 1α-OHase$^{+/-}$ and 1α-OHase$^{-/-}$ mice were produced from 1α-OHase$^{+/-}$ [11]. All mice, breeders and offspring were housed at the Animal Research Facility at Beth Israel Deaconess Medical Center (BIDMC) under pathogen-free conditions with a reverse daily 12:12 h light: dark cycle. Euthanasia was performed by CO_2 via a gas cylinder. All experimental procedures were approved by the Institutional Animal Care and Use Committee of BIDMC.

Animal surgery and hemodynamic measurement

TAC was performed in 8–10 week old male C57BL/6 mice and in 1α-OHase$^{-/-}$ [12,13] mice. Cardiac function was analyzed using echocardiography (for baseline cardiac function) and left ventricular (LV) pressure-volume loop measurement (after TAC) as described previously [14,15]. Detailed method is provided in Text S1.

Morphometric analysis of isolated CMs

CMs were enzymatically dissociated from 12 weeks old male mouse hearts according to previously described protocol [16,17]. Detailed method is provided in Text S1.

Serum Ca^{2+} and vitamin D metabolite analysis

Serum 1, $25(OH)_2$ D_3 (n = 8–10 replicates per group) was analyzed via enzyme immunoassays using commercial kits (Immunodiagnostic Systems). Serum Ca^{2+} (n = 8–10) was analyzed via a quantitative Calcium Colorimetric Detection Kit (Bio Vision).

Serum PTH analysis

Serum PTH (n = 8–10 replicates per group) was analyzed via enzyme immunoassays using commercial kits (Immunooptics Inc.)

Ca^{2+} transients and cell shortening measurements of isolated CMs

Measurement of Ca^{2+} transient and cell shortening in isolated CMs [18]. Briefly, CMs were isolated and contraction parameters and Ca^{2+} transient $[Ca^{2+}]$ i were measured in response to electrical stimulation. Caffeine induced $[Ca^{2+}]$ i release was measured after a 10-second pause following steady-state stimulation at increasing rates. Detailed methods are described in Text S1.

Histology and Western Blots

Hearts were fixed in 10% formalin and paraffin-embedded. Sections were stained with hematoxylin and eosin and Masson Trichrome (MT) at the Histology Core facility at BIDMC [14,15]. Quantification of fibrosis was performed as described previously [16]. To compare the levels of the major proteins involved in Ca^{2+} handling, Western blot analysis was performed on total protein from WT and 1α-OHase$^{-/-}$ mice as described previously [14,15].

Statistical Analysis

Data are reported as mean SEM. Statistical significance was determined by one-way or two-way ANOVA and Student-Newman-Keuls post hoc test. Values of $p<0.05$ were considered significant.

Results

Exaggerated hypertrophic responses after transverse aortic constriction (TAC) in 1α-OHase$^{-/-}$ mice

At baseline, 1α-OHase$^{-/-}$ mice demonstrated a modest 5% increase in heart weight compared to their WT littermates at 12 weeks of age (**Fig. 1A**). Corresponding isolated adult CMs also demonstrated modest increase in surface areas of 1α-OHase$^{-/-}$ mice compared to the age and gender matched WT mice (**Fig. 1B and 1C**). Cross sectional area of the CMs further confirmed these findings (**Fig. 1D and 1E**). We also observed that baseline systolic cardiac function was modestly reduced in 1α-OHase$^{-/-}$ mice compared with the WT mice (**Fig. 1F**). In addition, the mean arterial pressure (MAP) of 1α-OHase$^{-/-}$ was significantly higher than that of WT littermate mice (**Fig. 1G**). These findings suggested that there is baseline mild cardiac hypertrophy and cardiac dysfunction in 1α-OHase$^{-/-}$ mice compared to the WT mice.

To elucidate the effect of defective vitamin D signaling under pathological conditions, we imposed pressure overload on the heart using TAC. Morphometric analysis demonstrated significant increases in heart weight/body weight (HW/BW) ratio in both 1α-OHase$^{-/-}$ and WT mice compared with the corresponding sham-operated groups after 4 weeks of TAC (**Fig. 2A and 2B**). However, there were exaggerated hypertrophic responses to TAC in 1α-OHase$^{-/-}$ mice heart compared to the WT mice. Cardiac functional analysis using pressure-volume (PV) loop measurement revealed that 1α-OHase$^{-/-}$ mice demonstrated significantly greater cardiac dysfunction after TAC, as observed by reduction in stroke volume and cardiac output, compared to their WT littermates (**Fig. 2C and 2D**).

We further analyzed these hearts for the presence of interstitial fibrosis using Masson-Trichrome staining We found that both WT and 1α-OHase$^{-/-}$ mice showed presence of fibrosis after TAC, (**Fig. 2E**) which was significantly increased in 1α-OHase$^{-/-}$ mice compared with those in WT mice (WT = 11.9±1.5% vs. 1α-OHase$^{-/-}$ = 21.5±1.2%; $p<0.05$). These findings demonstrated that there were exaggerated pathological responses to TAC in 1α-OHase$^{-/-}$ mice that are associated with greater decreased cardiac function and more aggressive development of cardiac fibrosis.

Increased fetal gene activation and inflammatory responses after TAC in 1α-OHase$^{-/-}$ mice

We determined the biochemical markers for cardiac hypertrophy and heart failure by measuring the level of "fetal" genes, such as atrial natriuretic factor (ANF) and brain natriuretic peptide (BNP). Ventricular ANF was significantly expressed in all TAC groups. However, there was a 8-fold greater increase in ANF mRNA levels after TAC in 1α-OHase$^{-/-}$ mice compared to the WT littermates (**Fig. 3A**). Similarly, there was also a greater increase in BNP expression in 1α-OHase$^{-/-}$ mice compared to the WT mice hearts after TAC (**Fig. 3B**). Another marker for cardiac hypertrophy, the ratio of ß-MHC to total MHC mRNA expression, was also increased after TAC in both groups. Yet, there were again dramatic and exaggerated increases observed in 1α-OHase$^{-/-}$ mice compared to the WT mice after TAC (**Fig. 3C**).

It's known that vitamin D, a steroid hormone, affects immune regulation by preventing excessive expression of inflammatory cytokines and increasing the 'oxidative burst' potential of macrophages [19]. Interestingly, we observed a reduction in

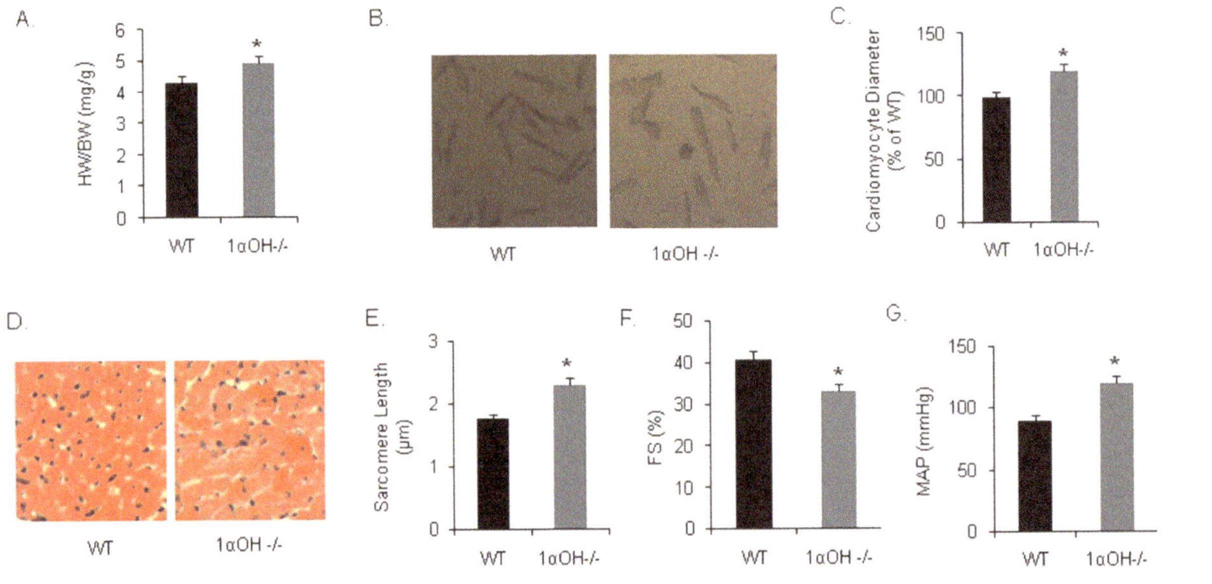

Figure 1. Physiological, echocardiographic, and hemodynamic parameters in 1αOHase−/− mice at baseline: (A) Baseline HW/BW of 1α-OHase −/− mice. *, $p<0.05$ compared to WT. N = 8–10. (B and C) Isolated adult CMs from 1α-OHase$^{-/-}$ mice showing increased surface area compared to WT CMs. *, $p<0.05$ compared to WT. N = 8–10. (D) Cross sectional area of mice heart showing CM surface area. (E) Resting sarcomere length of 1α-OHase$^{-/-}$ and WT CMs. *, $p<0.05$ compared to WT. N = 8–10. (F) Baseline fractional shortening (FS) of WT and KO mice. *, $p<0.05$ compared to WT. N = 8–10. (G) MAP of WT and 1α-OHase−/− mice at baseline. *, $p<0.05$ compared to WT. N = 8–10.

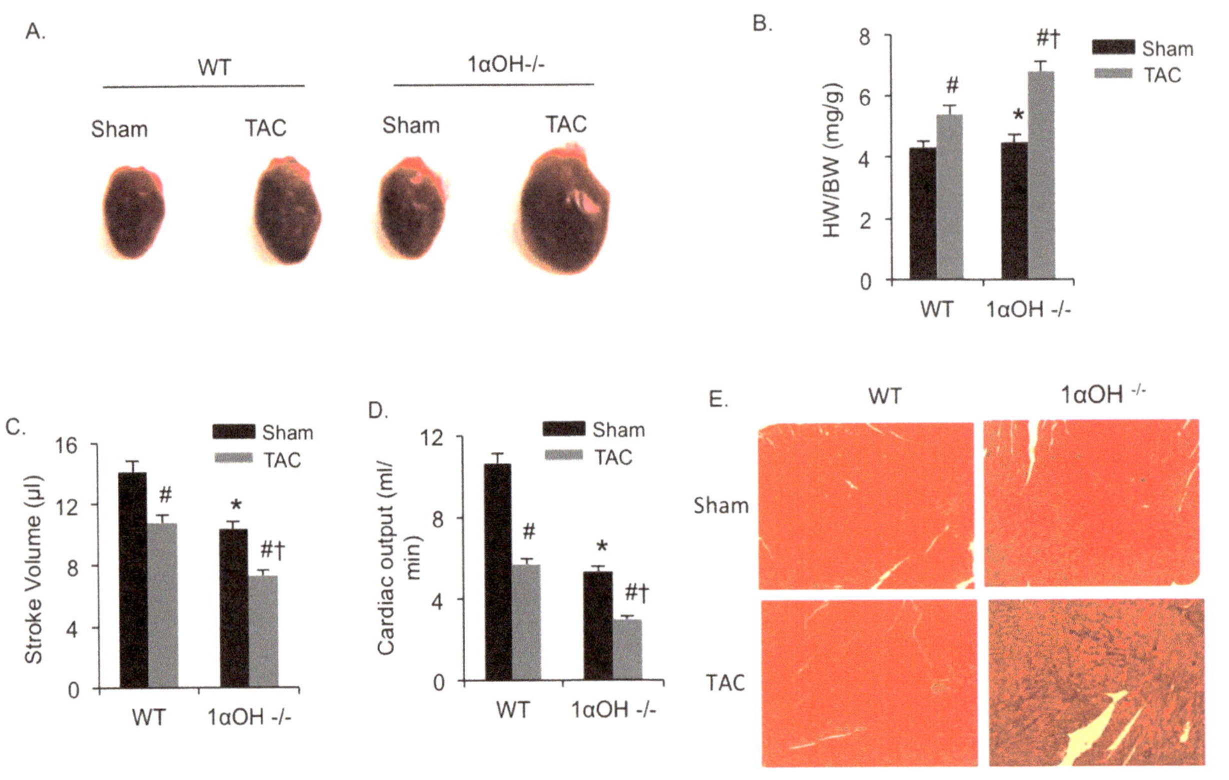

Figure 2. In response to pressure overload mutant mice showing exaggerated hypertrophy. (A) Representative hearts after 4 weeks of sham or TAC in WT and 1α-OHase$^{-/-}$ mice. (B) HW/BW after 4 weeks of sham or TAC in WT and 1α-OHase$^{-/-}$ mice. *, $p<0.05$ compared to WT. #, $p<0.05$ compared to sham. †, $p<0.05$ compared to WT TAC. N = 8–10. (C and D) Stroke volume (C) and cardiac output (D) in WT and 1α-OHase$^{-/-}$ mice after 4 weeks of sham or TAC. *, $p<0.05$ compared to WT. #, $p<0.05$ compared to sham. †, $p<0.05$ compared to WT TAC. N = 8–10. (E) Representative Masson-Trichrome heart staining in 1α-OHase$^{-/-}$ mice after 4 weeks of sham or TAC.

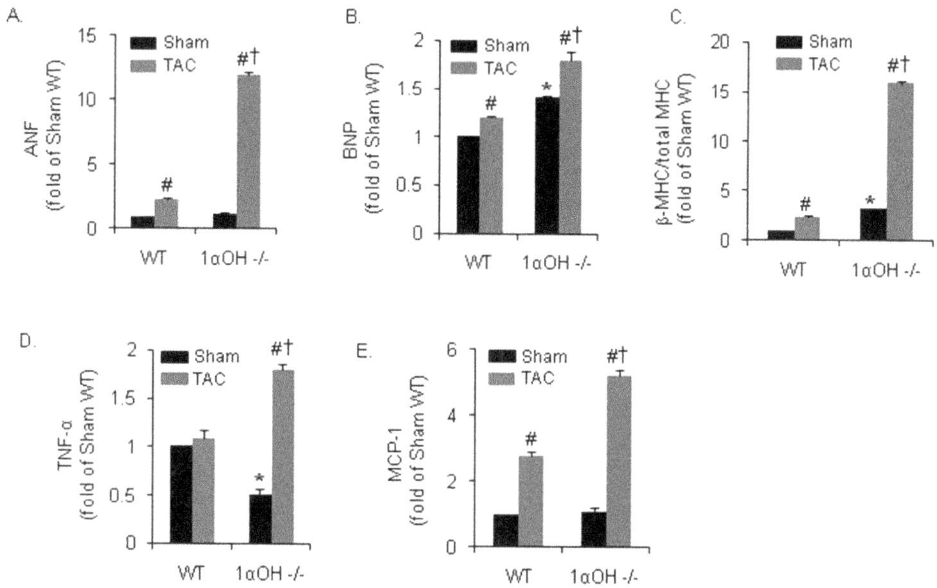

Figure 3. Biochemical findings after 4 weeks of Pressure overload in 1αOHase$^{-/-}$ mice. (A–C) Real-time PCR mRNA expression of ANF (A), BNP (B) and of ß-MHC to total MHC ratio (C) in WT and 1α-OHase$^{-/-}$ mice after 4 weeks of sham or TAC. *, $p<0.05$ compared to WT. #, $p<0.05$ compared to sham. †, $p<0.05$ compared to WT TAC. N = 8–10. (D and E) Real-time PCR mRNA expression of inflammatory cytokines TNF-α (D) and MCP-1 (E) in WT and 1α-OHase -/- mice after 4 weeks of sham or TAC. *, $p<0.05$ compared to WT. #, $p<0.05$ compared to sham. †, $p<0.05$ compared to WT TAC. N = 8–10.

tumor necrosis factor-α (TNF-α) expression at baseline in 1α-OHase$^{-/-}$ mice compared to WT mice. Although no significant differences were observed in TNF-α expression after TAC in WT mice, 1α-OHase$^{-/-}$ mice hearts showed enhanced activation of TNF-α after TAC (**Fig. 3D**). Another inflammatory marker, monocyte chemotactic protein-1 (MCP-1), was activated by TAC in both mice, but with significantly greater activation was observed in 1α-OHase$^{-/-}$ mice after TAC (**Fig. 3E**). These findings demonstrated that there is an exaggerated biochemical evidence of cardiac dysfunction and uncontrolled immune response associated with TAC in 1α-OHase$^{-/-}$ mice.

Defective Ca^{2+} handling and modulation of Ca^{2+} regulatory protein expressions in 1α-OHase$^{-/-}$ mice CMs

We found that the circulating 1, 25(OH) vitamin D_3 level was undetectable in 1α-OHase$^{-/-}$ mice and significantly reduced in heterozygous 1α-OHase$^{+/-}$ littermates (**Fig. 4A**), which coincide with previous findings [20,21]. Without vitamin D supplementation, 1α-OHase$^{-/-}$ mice at 12 weeks showed severe hypocalcemia with plasma Ca^{2+} concentrations as low as 1.2 mmol/L in contrast to the WT littermates, which exhibited normal plasma Ca^{2+} concentrations (WT = 2.5 mmol/L vs. 1α-OHase$^{-/-}$ = 1.2 mmol/L; $P<0.05$). Supplementation of vitamin D using injection of PC (200 ng/kg), an activated vitamin D_3 analog, starting at 4 weeks after birth normalized the plasma Ca^{2+} concentration in 1α-OHase mice by 12 weeks (**Fig. 4B**).

To examine the effect of the vitamin D deficiency in CMs, contraction parameters of individual isolated CM from 1α-OHase$^{-/-}$ mice and their WT littermates were studied by measuring sarcomere shortening (contraction) and relengthening (relaxation) in response to electrical stimulation (**see Text S1 for detail**). Baseline 1α-OHase$^{-/-}$ CM sarcomeres were significantly larger compared to WT (**Fig. 4C, Table S1**). Additionally, 1α-OHase$^{-/-}$ CMs showed a significant decrease in peak shortening, as well as the rate of cell shortening and rate of cell relengthening compared to WT CMs (**Fig. 4D and 4E**). Peak shortening is calculated from the percent shortening of length data (**Fig. 4D**). The highest and lowest value reached by the transient.

We then investigated Ca^{2+} handling properties of individual CM from 1α-OHase$^{-/-}$ mice (**see Text S1 for detail**). Analysis of Ca^{2+} transients indicated decreased peak systolic Ca^{2+}, measured as Fura-2 ratios in CM from 1α-OHase$^{-/-}$ compared to WT group CM (**Fig. 4F**). The rate of Ca^{2+} transient decay (*tau*, exponential decay of time constant, the speed of relaxation/calcium uptake) was also significantly reduced in 1α-OHase$^{-/-}$ CMs (**Fig. 4G**) which was calculated by the ionoptix program from the transient, with a reduced time to peak (TTP) and a decrease in relaxation rate (Ca^{2+} efflux) (**Fig. 4H and 4I**). Caffeine causes Ca^{2+} release from the sarcoplasmic reticulum (SR) of mammalian muscle. Thus, to evaluate the SR Ca^{2+} load, we tested caffeine-induced Ca^{2+} release amount from SR in WT and 1α-OHase$^{-/-}$ CMs. We found that CMs from 1α-OHase$^{-/-}$ mice presented a decreased caffeine-induced Ca^{2+} transient compared to WT CMs (**Fig. 4J**). These findings demonstrated profound Ca^{2+} handling abnormalities in 1α-OHase$^{-/-}$ mice CMs, which may contribute to the development of fulminant heart failure after TAC.

The expression level and the activity of sarcoplasmic reticulum Ca^{2+} ATPase (SERCA) is significantly decreased in pressure overload-induced hypertrophy and during heart failure in animals and human, which correlate with decreased myocardial dysfunction [22,23]. To further elucidate the mechanism underlying the defective Ca^{2+} handling, we examined the SERCA2a protein expression level in these mice. We found that 1α-OHase$^{-/-}$ mice showed significant decreased SERCA2a expression after TAC compared to WT mice (**Fig. 5A and 5B**). Phospholamban (PLB) interacts with SERCA and inhibits its Ca^{2+} transport rate, and the relative abundance of SERCA and PLB maintains Ca^{2+} homeostasis and CM contractility. Therefore, SERCA/PLB ratio reflects Ca^{2+} transport capacity of the SR [24]. At baseline, 1α-OHase$^{-/-}$

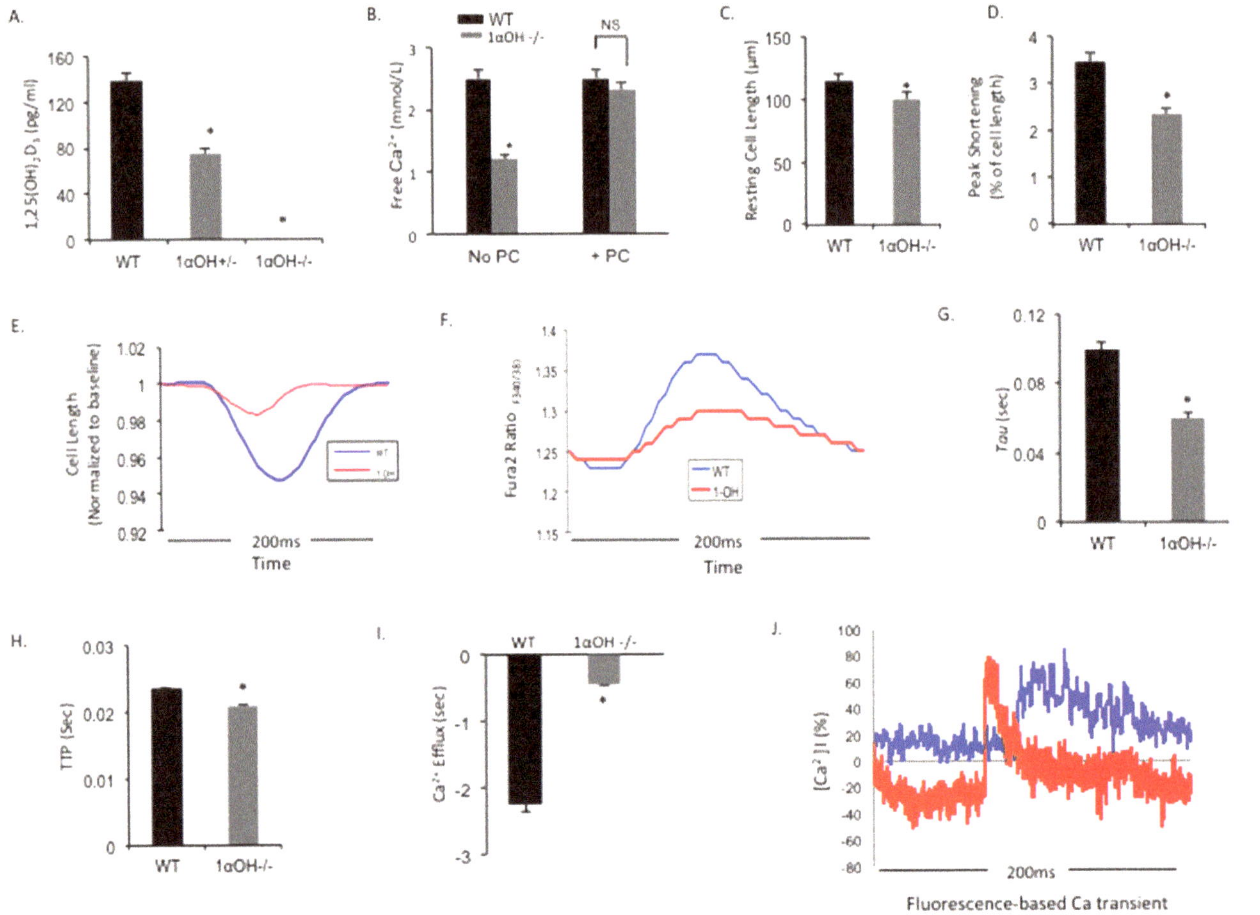

Figure 4. Contractile function and Ca^{2+} transient parameters in isolated CMs from 1αOHase −/− mice. (A and B) Baseline 1, 25(OH)$_2$D$_3$ (A) and free Ca^{2+} (B) level in WT and 1αOHase −/− mice serums. *, $p<0.05$ compared to WT, N = 6–8 mice. (C) Resting cell length (D) and peak shortening (% of cell length) from isolated CMs obtained from WT and 1αOHase −/− mice. *, $p<0.05$ compared to WT. Ten twitches per CMs were collected for each mouse heart. N = 6–8 mice/group. (E) Continuous measurement of cell contractility from isolated CMs obtained from WT (blue line) and 1αOHase$^{-/-}$ (red line) mice. *, $p<0.05$ compared to WT. Ten twitches per CMs were collected for each mouse heart. N = 6–8 mice/group. (F) Representative Fura 2 ratio (F340/380) from isolated CMs obtained from WT (blue line) and 1αOHase -/- (red line) mice. Data shows that the twitch peak amplitudes are significantly different between WT and 1αOHase -/- CMs, which indicate severely defective Ca^{2+} handling in 1αOHase$^{-/-}$ CMs. (G–I) The rate of Ca^{2+} transient decay (*Tau*) (G), time to peak contraction (TTP) (H), and return velocity to baseline or Ca^{2+} efflux in WT and 1αOHase$^{-/-}$ CMs. *, $p<0.05$ compared to WT. N = 10 CMs/mouse heart. N = 6–8 mice/group. (J) Representative traces of Ca^{2+} transients evoked by 10 mM caffeine recorded in WT (blue line) and 1αOHase$^{-/-}$ (red line) mice CMs.

mouse hearts showed significant increase in PLB, which decreased after TAC (**Fig. 5A and 5B**). SERCA/PLB ratio was also significantly decreased in 1α-OHase$^{-/-}$ mice compared to WT mice (**Fig. 5C**). This may explain the difference in SR Ca^{2+} load and contractile function between WT and 1α-OHase$^{-/-}$ mice CMs, and the depressed levels of SERCA2a may contribute to the severity of heart failure after TAC in 1α-OHase$^{-/-}$ mice.

The Na^{+}- Ca^{2+}-exchanger (NCX) is the dominant myocardial Ca^{2+} efflux mechanism. Ca^{2+} removal from the cytosol occurs by activity of the SR Ca^{2+} pump and by exchange of Ca^{2+} for sodium by the sarcolemmal NCX [25]. The decrease in PLB might lead to a higher activation of the remaining SERCA pumps and increase the activity of NCX [26]. At baseline, there were no significant difference in expression of NCX between the WT and 1α-OHase$^{-/-}$ mice (**Fig. 5A and 5B**). However, we found significant up-regulation of NCX expression in banded WT and 1α-OHase$^{-/-}$ mice with significant 4-folds increase seen in 1α-OHase$^{-/-}$ mice. A relative increase in NCX is expected when SR function is impaired [27]. The function of ryanodine receptor 2 (RyR2) (the cardiac isoform) is to allow Ca^{2+}-induced Ca^{2+} release that brings about contraction, while myocyte relaxation results in RyR2 closure accompanied by the Ca^{2+} re-uptake into SR through the SERCA [28]. After TAC, there was a moderate decrease in RyR2 expression in both WT and 1α-OHase$^{-/-}$ mice (**Fig. 5A and 5B**).

Treatment with PC attenuates cardiac dysfunction after TAC in 1α-OHase -/- mice

The responses of 1α-OHase$^{-/-}$ mice to TAC in our previous experiments may be compounded by their baseline cardiac hypertrophy. Thus, we further determined the specific role of defective vitamin D to pathological conditions by first using "rescue" vitamin D protocol as described previously in 1α-OHase$^{-/-}$ mice, where vitamin D deficiency and its non-cardiac phenotype were both corrected [29]. From 28–30 days of life, 1-α-OHase$^{-/-}$ mice were treated with an initial "rescue" dose of 500 ng/kg of PC, followed by a daily "maintenance" dose of 200 ng/kg from 5 to 8 weeks of age. At 8 weeks, the animals were

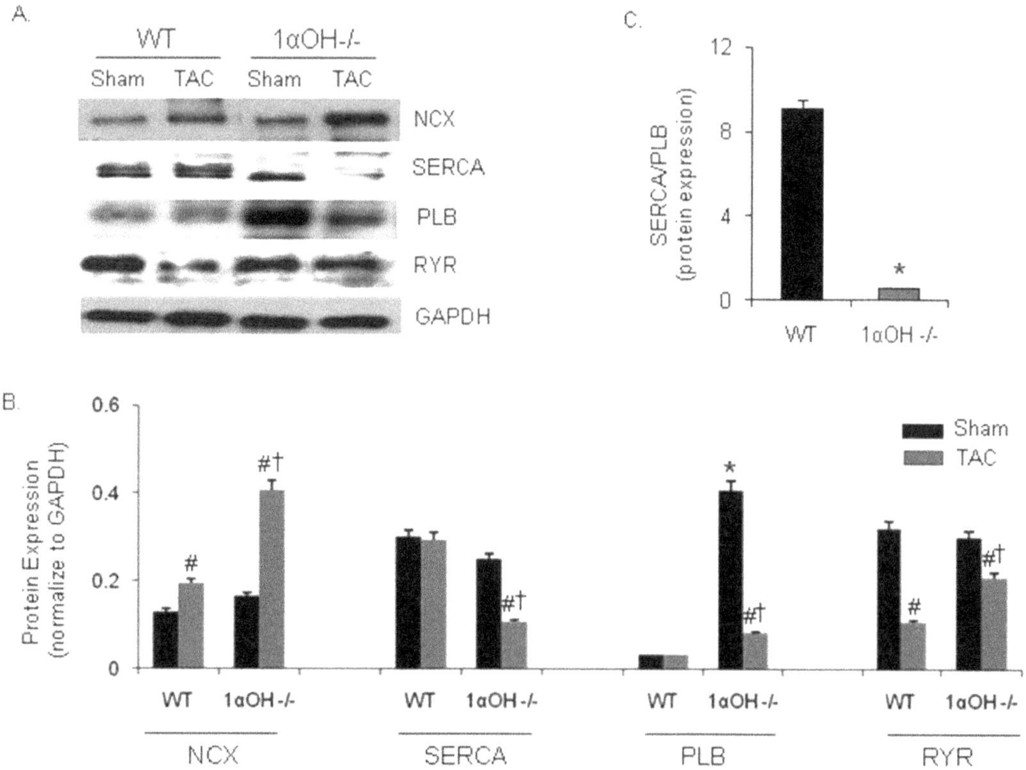

Figure 5. Expressions of Ca^{2+} regulatory protein in mice with altered metabolism of Vitamin D. (A) Representative western blots of various Ca^{2+} handling proteins. (B) Quantitative analysis of various Ca^{2+} handling proteins. NCX = Na^+/Ca^{2+} exchanger, SERCA2a = sarcoplasmic reticulum Ca^{2+} ATPase, PLB = phospholamban, and RYR = ryanodine receptor. GAPDH = glyceraldehyde 3-phosphate dehydrogenase. GAPDH was used as internal loading control. *, $p<0.05$ compared to WT. #, $p<0.05$ compared to sham. †, $p<0.05$ compared to WT TAC. N = 8–10. (C) Quantitative analysis of SERCA/PLB protein expression ratio. *, $p<0.05$ compared to WT. #, $p<0.05$ compared to sham, N = 8–10.

divided into the following groups: 1) Vehicle + Sham, 2) Vehicle + TAC, 3) PC + Sham, and 4) PC+TAC. For the vehicle conditions, maintenance doses of PC were changed to vehicle injections, while the PC dose was maintained for PC groups. TAC resulted in a significant increase in HW/BW and LW/BW ratios in mice receiving vehicle for 4 weeks compared to the sham operated mice (**Fig. 6A and 6B**). In mice treated with PC, there was a significant 18% attenuation of TAC-induced HW/BW ratio increase compared to the vehicle treated animals. Histological examination demonstrated that interstitial fibrosis induced by TAC in vehicle-administered 1α-OHase$^{-/-}$ mice were significantly inhibited in PC treated group after TAC (**Fig. 6C**). TAC-induced increases in ANF and β-MHC gene expression, which were both attenuated by PC treatment (**Fig. 6D and 6E**).

We found that decreased fractional shortening after TAC in vehicle treated mice was significantly improved with vitamin D replacement in 1α-OHase$^{-/-}$ mice (**Fig. 6G**). In addition, we observed reduced stroke volume and cardiac output in vehicle treated group after TAC. These parameters also improved after vitamin D replacement (**Fig. 6G and 6H**). Thus, vitamin D replacement resulted in significant attenuation of cardiac dysfunction after TAC in 1α-OHase$^{-/-}$ mice.

Treatment with PC attenuates defective Ca^{2+} handling associated with defective vitamin D signaling

To further assess the effect of vitamin D replacement on CMs contractility in 1α-OHase$^{-/-}$ mice contraction parameters, we performed Ca^{2+} handling analysis of isolated CMs in1α-OHase$^{-/-}$ mice with or without PC treatment. We found that vitamin D replacement attenuated hypocontractility and increased peak shortening in PC treated 1α-OHase$^{-/-}$ mice (**Fig. 6I and 6J**). Rate of relaxation was significantly increased with PC treatment and the rate of Ca^{2+} transient decay (*tau*) was significantly improved (**Fig. 6K and 6L**). Treatment with PC also normalized the PTH level in 1α-OHase$^{-/-}$ mice (**Fig. 7**). These findings suggest that the pathological response in 1α-OHase$^{-/-}$ mice is mainly due to defective vitamin D signaling and associated Ca^{2+} handling, and correcting these abnormalities could rescue these pathological responses.

Discussion

In this study, we demonstrated that vitamin D deficiency is associated with cardiac hypertrophy at baseline results in an exaggerated progression to heart failure after pressure overload in 1α-OHase$^{-/-}$ mice. We also found that there is defective Ca^{2+} handling in 1α-OHase$^{-/-}$ mice, with structural and functional cardiac abnormalities in these mice. These cardiac Ca^{2+} handling abnormalities were completely corrected with vitamin D replacement in 1α-OHase$^{-/-}$ mice. Thus, our studies strongly support the notion that vitamin D deficiency is an under-recognized, non-classic risk factor for developing heart failure that is readily correctable.

Vitamin D is known for its primary role in Ca^{2+} and bone homeostasis [30]. Biological activities of vitamin D are mediated by a hormonally active 1, 25-dihydroxyvitamin D_3 that is converted from 25-hydroxyvitamin D_3 by 1α-OHase. It binds to

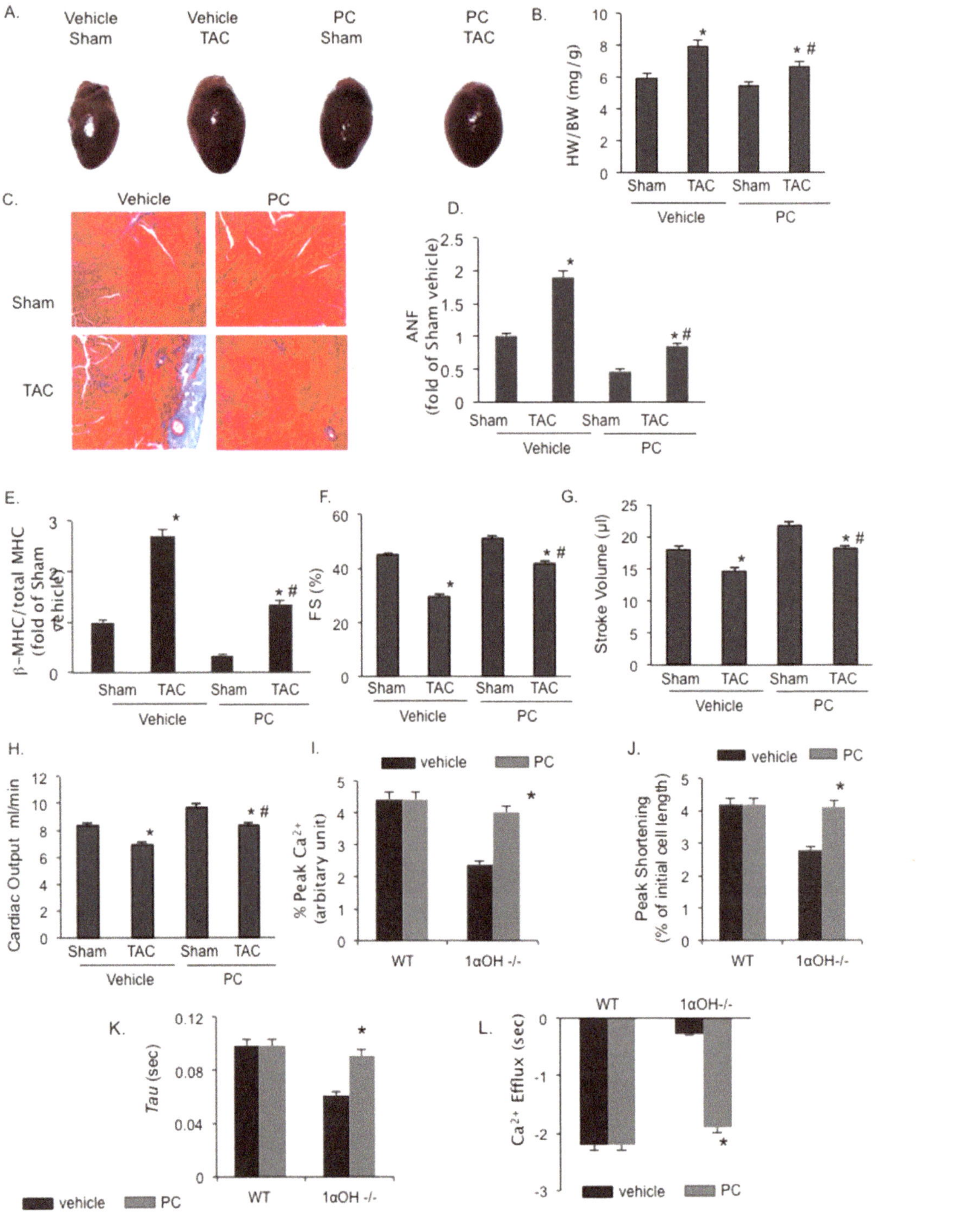

Figure 6. Effect of paricalcitol on cardiac dysfunction parameters. (A) Representative hearts in 1α-OHase$^{-/-}$ mice with or without PC treatment after 4 weeks of sham or TAC. (B) HW/BW ratio in 1α-OHase$^{-/-}$ mice with or without PC treatment after 4 weeks of sham or TAC. *, $p<0.05$ compared to Sham. #, $p<0.05$ compared to vehicle TAC. N = 8–10. (C) Representative Masson-Trichrome heart staining in 1α-OHase$^{-/-}$ mice with or without PC treatment after 4 weeks of sham or TAC. (D and E) Real-time PCR mRNA expression of ANF (D) and of ß-MHC to total MHC ratio (E) after 4 weeks of sham or TAC in 1α-OHase$^{-/-}$ mice with or without PC treatment. *, $p<0.05$ compared to Sham. #, $p<0.05$ compared to vehicle TAC. N = 8–10. (F–H) Fractional shortening (F), stroke volume (G) and cardiac output (H) in 1α-OHase -/- mice with or without PC treatment after 4 weeks of sham or TAC. *, $p<0.05$ compared to Sham. #, $p<0.05$ compared to vehicle TAC. N = 8–10. Effect of paricalcitol on defective calcium handling in 1αOHase −/− mice. (I–L). The % peak Ca^{2+} (I), % peak shortening (J), the rate of Ca^{2+} transient decay (*Tau*) (K), and the return velocity to baseline or Ca^{2+} efflux (L) in 1α-OHase$^{-/-}$ mice with or without PC treatment. *, $p<0.05$ compared to vehicle treated mice group, N = 20 CMs/mouse from 6–8 mice/group.

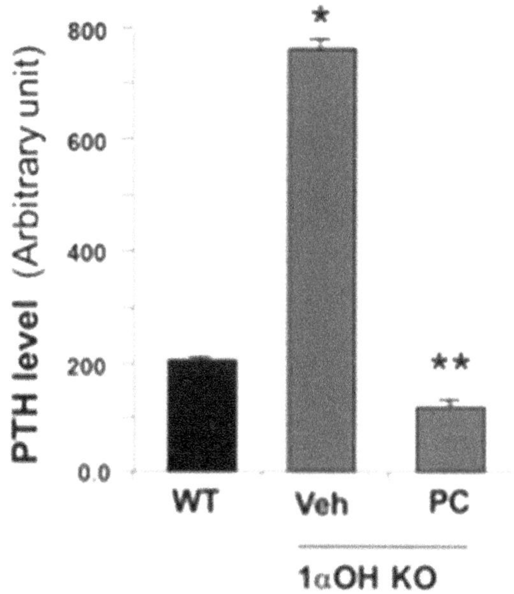

Figure 7. Paricalcitol restore the parathyroid hormone in 1α-OHase$^{-/-}$ mice this model. PTH level in 1α-OHase$^{-/-}$ mice with or without PC treatment. *, $p<0.05$ compared to WT. **, $p<0.05$ compared to vehicle. N = 8–10.

a specific high-affinity vitamin D receptor (VDR), a member of the superfamily of nuclear receptors for steroid hormones [4]. Vitamin D plays an important physiological role in controlling cardiac functions and vitamin D-dependent signaling systems are present in cardiac myocytes and fibroblasts [31]. Vitamin D deficiency has been associated with abnormal cardiac relaxation, proliferation, and increased cardiac renin gene expression [32,33]. Previously, we showed that vitamin D therapy prevents the progression to cardiac hypertrophy [34], and attenuates the development of heart failure in salt sensitive rat model [35]. In addition, 1α-OHase -/- mice developed hypertension, cardiac hypertrophy, and impaired cardiac systolic function, possibly due to the activation of the RAS [8]. Clinically, vitamin D deficiency has been associated with the increased prevalence of myocardial dysfunctions and heart failure [36,37]. Since the critical conversion of the storage form to the active form of vitamin D by 1α-OHase occurs in the kidney, patients with CKD are typically vitamin D deficient. In fact, the prevalence of cardiac hypertrophy and cardiac dysfunction is over 80% in these patients [38,39], and vitamin D therapy has been shown to improve survival and decrease cardiovascular mortality [6,7]. These findings suggest that the role of vitamin D signaling may be significant in the heart, and vitamin D deficiency may offer novel therapeutic target in the treatment of heart failure.

CM contraction is regulated by the interplay between Ca^{2+}, contractile proteins, and the intracellular handling of Ca^{2+}, whereas abnormal Ca^{2+} homeostasis is primarily responsible for depression of CM contractility [22,23]. In several animal and human models of cardiac hypertrophy and heart failure, the whole-cell $[Ca^{2+}]_i$ transient is altered [40,41]. Decreases in SERCA pump expression and activity have been observed in a variety of animal and human models of heart failure and a degree of decrease in SERCA level and its activity, closely correlate with a decreased myocardial function [27]. Thus, these data suggest that alterations in Ca^{2+} handling proteins are important contributors to cardiac dysfunction and heart failure. We found profound Ca^{2+} transient abnormalities, contractile abnormalities and altered expression of various Ca^{2+} handling regulatory proteins in vitamin D deficient CMs, which became exaggerated after TAC. Abnormalities in Ca^{2+} homeostasis, as seen in vitamin D deficiency, may lead to a chronic defect in E–C coupling, which may in turn lead to cardiac dysfunction. Particularly, decreased SERCA and SERCA/PLB expression in 1α-OHase$^{-/-}$ mice supports the hypothesis that alterations in abundance or activity of molecules that regulate systolic and diastolic Ca^{2+} are centrally involved in depressed contractility in hypertrophied and failing hearts.

The key role of cardiac hypertrophy in the pathogenesis of heart disease underscores the need to identify the cellular and molecular mechanisms responsible for both cardiac hypertrophy and its progression to heart failure. A better understanding of disease progression may facilitate the development of novel therapeutic modalities, as well as the development of better guidelines for the prevention of cardiac hypertrophy. Our findings contribute to a better understanding of disease progression that are involved in vitamin D signaling and the development of heart failure. Our finding provides evidences that Ca^{2+} homeostasis and Ca^{2+} handling mediate structural and functional cardiac abnormalities in vitamin D deficient 1α-OHase$^{-/-}$ mice and development of cardiac hypertrophy.

Supporting Information

Table S1 Comparison of cardiomyocytes resting sarcomere length in 0.5 Hz paced cells in WT and 1αOH$^{-/-}$. Sarcomere length of 1α-OHase$^{-/-}$ and WT CMs, raw value in 0.5 Hz paced.

Author Contributions

Conceived and designed the experiments: SC RSA PMK. Performed the experiments: SC SB QK JYL SSS. Analyzed the data: SC FdM. Contributed reagents/materials/analysis tools: SC SB QK JYL SSS. Wrote the paper: SC PMK.

References

1. Wang TJ, Pencina MJ, Booth SL, Jacques PF, Ingelsson E, et al. (2008) Vitamin D deficiency and risk of cardiovascular disease. Circulation 117: 503–511.
2. Zittermann A (2006) Vitamin D and disease prevention with special reference to cardiovascular disease. Prog Biophys Mol Biol 92: 39–48.
3. Park CW, Oh YS, Shin YS, Kim CM, Kim YS, et al. (1999) Intravenous calcitriol regresses myocardial hypertrophy in hemodialysis patients with secondary hyperparathyroidism. Am J Kidney Dis 33: 73–81.
4. Demay MB (2006) Mechanism of vitamin D receptor action. Ann N Y Acad Sci 1068: 204–213.
5. McCullough PA, Jurkovitz CT, Pergola PE, McGill JB, Brown WW, et al. (2007) Independent components of chronic kidney disease as a cardiovascular risk state: results from the Kidney Early Evaluation Program (KEEP). Arch Intern Med 167: 1122–1129.
6. Teng M, Wolf M, Lowrie E, Ofsthun N, Lazarus JM, et al. (2003) Survival of patients undergoing hemodialysis with paricalcitol or calcitriol therapy. N Engl J Med 349: 446–456.
7. Teng M, Wolf M, Ofsthun MN, Lazarus JM, Hernan MA, et al. (2005) Activated injectable vitamin D and hemodialysis survival: a historical cohort study. J Am Soc Nephrol 16: 1115–1125.
8. Zhou C, Lu F, Cao K, Xu D, Goltzman D, et al. (2008) Calcium-independent and 1,25(OH)2D3-dependent regulation of the renin-angiotensin system in 1alpha-hydroxylase knockout mice. Kidney Int 74: 170–179.

9. Wehrens XH, Lehnart SE, Reiken SR, Marks AR (2004) Ca2+/calmodulin-dependent protein kinase II phosphorylation regulates the cardiac ryanodine receptor. Circ Res 94: e61–70.
10. Chien KR, Ross J, Jr., Hoshijima M (2003) Calcium and heart failure: the cycle game. Nat Med 9: 508–509.
11. Dardenne O, Prud'homme J, Arabian A, Glorieux FH, St-Arnaud R (2001) Targeted inactivation of the 25-hydroxyvitamin D(3)-1(alpha)-hydroxylase gene (CYP27B1) creates an animal model of pseudovitamin D-deficiency rickets. Endocrinology 142: 3135–3141.
12. McMullen JR, Sherwood MC, Tarnavski O, Zhang L, Dorfman AL, et al. (2004) Inhibition of mTOR signaling with rapamycin regresses established cardiac hypertrophy induced by pressure overload. Circulation 109: 3050–3055.
13. McMullen JR, Shioi T, Zhang L, Tarnavski O, Sherwood MC, et al. (2003) Phosphoinositide 3-kinase(p110alpha) plays a critical role for the induction of physiological, but not pathological, cardiac hypertrophy. Proc Natl Acad Sci U S A 100: 12355–12360.
14. Bae S, Siu PM, Choudhury S, Ke Q, Choi JH, et al. (2010) Delayed activation of caspase-independent apoptosis during heart failure in transgenic mice overexpressing caspase inhibitor CrmA. Am J Physiol Heart Circ Physiol 299: H1374–1381.
15. Choudhury S, Bae S, Ke Q, Lee JY, Kim J, et al. (2011) Mitochondria to nucleus translocation of AIF in mice lacking Hsp70 during ischemia/reperfusion. Basic Res Cardiol 106: 397–407.
16. Rigor DL, Bodyak N, Bae S, Choi JH, Zhang L, et al. (2009) Phosphoinositide 3-kinase Akt signaling pathway interacts with protein kinase Cbeta2 in the regulation of physiologic developmental hypertrophy and heart function. Am J Physiol Heart Circ Physiol 296: H566–572.
17. Shioi T, Kang PM, Douglas PS, Hampe J, Yballe CM, et al. (2000) The conserved phosphoinositide 3-kinase pathway determines heart size in mice. EMBO J 19: 2537–2548.
18. Bassani JW, Bassani RA, Bers DM (1995) Calibration of indo-1 and resting intracellular [Ca]i in intact rabbit cardiac myocytes. Biophys J 68: 1453–1460.
19. Di Rosa M, Malaguarnera M, Nicoletti F, Malaguarnera L (2011) Vitamin D3: a helpful immuno-modulator. Immunology 134: 123–139.
20. Hoenderop JG, Dardenne O, Van Abel M, Van Der Kemp AW, Van Os CH, et al. (2002) Modulation of renal Ca2+ transport protein genes by dietary Ca2+ and 1,25-dihydroxyvitamin D3 in 25-hydroxyvitamin D3-1alpha-hydroxylase knockout mice. FASEB J 16: 1398–1406.
21. Xue Y, Karaplis AC, Hendy GN, Goltzman D, Miao D (2005) Genetic models show that parathyroid hormone and 1,25-dihydroxyvitamin D3 play distinct and synergistic roles in postnatal mineral ion homeostasis and skeletal development. Hum Mol Genet 14: 1515–1528.
22. Del Monte F, Hajjar RJ (2008) Intracellular devastation in heart failure. Heart Fail Rev 13: 151–162.
23. Morgan JP (1991) Abnormal intracellular modulation of calcium as a major cause of cardiac contractile dysfunction. N Engl J Med 325: 625–632.
24. Pieske B, Kretschmann B, Meyer M, Holubarsch C, Weirich J, et al. (1995) Alterations in intracellular calcium handling associated with the inverse force-frequency relation in human dilated cardiomyopathy. Circulation 92: 1169–1178.
25. Bers DM (2000) Calcium fluxes involved in control of cardiac myocyte contraction. Circ Res 87: 275–281.
26. Kubo H, Margulies KB, Piacentino V, 3rd, Gaughan JP, Houser SR (2001) Patients with end-stage congestive heart failure treated with beta-adrenergic receptor antagonists have improved ventricular myocyte calcium regulatory protein abundance. Circulation 104: 1012–1018.
27. Hasenfuss G (1998) Alterations of calcium-regulatory proteins in heart failure. Cardiovasc Res 37: 279–289.
28. Asahi M, Sugita Y, Kurzydlowski K, De Leon S, Tada M, et al. (2003) Sarcolipin regulates sarco(endo)plasmic reticulum Ca2+-ATPase (SERCA) by binding to transmembrane helices alone or in association with phospholamban. Proc Natl Acad Sci U S A 100: 5040–5045.
29. Dardenne O, Prudhomme J, Hacking SA, Glorieux FH, St-Arnaud R (2003) Rescue of the pseudo-vitamin D deficiency rickets phenotype of CYP27B1-deficient mice by treatment with 1,25-dihydroxyvitamin D3: biochemical, histomorphometric, and biomechanical analyses. J Bone Miner Res 18: 637–643.
30. Dusso AS, Brown AJ, Slatopolsky E (2005) Vitamin D. Am J Physiol Renal Physiol 289: F8–28.
31. Chen S, Glenn DJ, Ni W, Grigsby CL, Olsen K, et al. (2008) Expression of the vitamin d receptor is increased in the hypertrophic heart. Hypertension 52: 1106–1112.
32. Lee W, Kang PM (2010) Vitamin D deficiency and cardiovascular disease: Is there a role for vitamin D therapy in heart failure? Curr Opin Investig Drugs 11: 309–314.
33. Xiang W, Kong J, Chen S, Cao L-P, Qiao G, et al. (2005) Cardiac hypertrophy in vitamin D receptor knockout mice: role of the systemic and cardiac renin-angiotensin systems. American Journal of Physiology - Endocrinology And Metabolism 288: E125–E132.
34. Bodyak N, Ayus JC, Achinger S, Shivalingappa V, Ke Q, et al. (2007) Activated vitamin D attenuates left ventricular abnormalities induced by dietary sodium in Dahl salt-sensitive animals. Proc Natl Acad Sci U S A 104: 16810–16815.
35. Bae S, Yalamarti B, Ke Q, Choudhury S, Yu H, et al. (2011) Preventing progression of cardiac hypertrophy and development of heart failure by paricalcitol therapy in rats. Cardiovasc Res 91: 632–639.
36. Gotsman I, Shauer A, Zwas DR, Hellman Y, Keren A, et al. (2012) Vitamin D deficiency is a predictor of reduced survival in patients with heart failure; vitamin D supplementation improves outcome. Eur J Heart Fail 14: 357–366.
37. Holick MF (2007) Vitamin D deficiency. N Engl J Med 357: 266–281.
38. Pilz S, Tomaschitz A, Marz W, Drechsler C, Ritz E, et al. (2011) Vitamin D, cardiovascular disease and mortality. Clin Endocrinol (Oxf) 75: 575–584.
39. Vacek JL, Vanga SR, Good M, Lai SM, Lakkireddy D, et al. (2012) Vitamin D Deficiency and Supplementation and Relation to Cardiovascular Health. Am J Cardiol 109: 359–363.
40. Beuckelmann DJ, Nabauer M, Erdmann E (1992) Intracellular calcium handling in isolated ventricular myocytes from patients with terminal heart failure. Circulation 85: 1046–1055.
41. Perreault CL, Shannon RP, Komamura K, Vatner SF, Morgan JP (1992) Abnormalities in intracellular calcium regulation and contractile function in myocardium from dogs with pacing-induced heart failure. J Clin Invest 89: 932–938.

7

Four Weeks of IV Iron Supplementation Reduces Perceived Fatigue and Mood Disturbance in Distance Runners

Amy Woods[1], Laura A. Garvican-Lewis[1,2]*, Philo U. Saunders[2], Greg Lovell[2], David Hughes[2], Ruth Fazakerley[2], Bev Anderson[2], Christopher J. Gore[2], Kevin G. Thompson[1]

1 University of Canberra, Research Institute for Sport and Exercise, Canberra, Australia, **2** Australian Institute of Sport, Canberra, Australia

Abstract

Purpose: To determine the effect of intravenous iron supplementation on performance, fatigue and overall mood in runners without clinical iron deficiency.

Methods: Fourteen distance runners with serum ferritin 30–100 $\mu g \cdot L^{-1}$ were randomly assigned to receive three blinded injections of intravenous ferric-carboxymaltose (2 ml, 100 mg, IRON) or normal saline (PLACEBO) over four weeks (weeks 0, 2, 4). Athletes performed a 3,000 m time trial and 10×400 m monitored training session on consecutive days at week 0 and again following each injection. Hemoglobin mass (Hbmass) was assessed via carbon monoxide rebreathing at weeks 0 and 6. Fatigue and mood were determined bi-weekly until week 6 via Total Fatigue Score (TFS) and Total Mood Disturbance (TMD) using the Brief Fatigue Inventory and Brunel Mood Scale. Data were analyzed using magnitude-based inferences, based on the unequal variances t-statistic and Cohen's Effect sizes (ES).

Results: Serum ferritin increased in IRON only (Week 0: 62.8±21.9, Week 4: 128.1±46.6 $\mu g \cdot L^{-1}$; $p = 0.002$) and remained elevated two weeks after the final injection (127.0±66.3 $\mu g \cdot L^{-1}$, $p = 0.01$), without significant changes in Hbmass. Supplementation had a moderate effect on TMD of IRON (ES -0.77) with scores at week 6 lower than PLACEBO (ES -1.58, $p = 0.02$). Similarly, at week 6, TFS was significantly improved in IRON vs. PLACEBO (ES −1.54, $p = 0.05$). There were no significant improvements in 3,000 m time in either group (Week 0 vs. Week 4; Iron: 625.6±55.5 s vs. 625.4±52.7 s; PLACEBO: 624.8±47.2 s vs. 639.1±59.7 s); but IRON reduced their average time for the 10×400 m training session at week 2 (Week 0: 78.0±6.6 s, Week 2: 77.2±6.3; ES–0.20, $p = 0.004$).

Conclusion: During 6 weeks of training, intravenous iron supplementation improved perceived fatigue and mood of trained athletes with no clinical iron deficiency, without concurrent improvements in oxygen transport capacity or performance.

Editor: Stephen E Alway, West Virginia University School of Medicine, United States of America

Funding: Funding for the study was received from a University of Canberra grant for Post-doctoral Fellowship Research. The funder had no role in study design, data collection and analysis, decision to publish, or preparation of the manuscript.

Competing Interests: The authors have declared that no competing interests exist.

* Email: laura.garvican@ausport.gov.au

Introduction

Iron is an essential nutrient for the optimal functioning of the human body [1]. Integral for hemoglobin synthesis, iron also plays an important role in many cellular processes; particularly, oxygen transport and storage, generation of energy through oxidative phosphorylation [1] and enzyme function affecting intracellular metabolism [2]. In addition, iron assists immune function, DNA synthesis, the functioning of neurotransmitters and the formation of myelin, and is therefore critical for normal brain function and cognitive development [3].

Iron status is influenced by both intake from dietary sources and iron loss through sweat and urine [4], gastrointestinal bleeding, menstruation and trauma. In athletes, exercise stress may exacerbate iron loss due to foot-strike hemolysis associated with running [5]. Iron deficiencies are common in athletic populations, and frequently manifest through feelings of lethargy, a lack of energy and lowered perceived ability to train and perform [4]. In clinical terms, iron deficiency is often classified as serum ferritin values below $<22\ \mu g \cdot L^{-1}$, with iron deficiency anemia diagnosed when iron stores are exhausted (serum ferritin $<15\ \mu g \cdot L^{-1}$), and consequently hemoglobin (Hb) levels fall below $12\ g \cdot L^{-1}$ [6]. However, even amongst the medical literature there remains wide debate as to the most appropriate thresholds for diagnosis and when to begin supplementation, particularly in athletes [7].

Iron supplementation, typically via the oral route, is commonly used for the treatment of iron deficiency. Recently, carbohydrate-encased intravenous (IV) compounds such as ferric carboxymaltose have proven successful in treating iron-deficiency anemia [8] and improving fatigue [9] in an outpatient setting. Krayenbuehl et al. [10] examined the effect of IV iron (III)-hydroxide sucrose on fatigue in non-anemic, premenopausal women with serum ferritin $<50\ \mu g \cdot L^{-1}$ using a placebo-controlled blinded design. Reduced feelings of perceived fatigue were observed following treatment but without concomitant changes in hemoglobin concentration ([Hb]), leading the authors to speculate that the non-hematological functions of iron, namely its involvement in the formation of key enzymes involved in oxidative metabolism [11–13], were responsible for the observed benefits of the iron treatment.

Indeed, the chosen delivery route (intravenous as opposed to oral), and subsequent bioavailability of the supplemented iron may also be a contributing factor to relatively novel findings of the Krayenbuehl study [14]. Recently, Garvican et al. [15] compared the efficacy of 6 weeks of oral versus IV iron supplementation in distance runners with "low" (initial serum ferritin $<35\ \mu g.L^{-1}$ and transferrin saturation $<20\%$, or serum ferritin $<15\ \mu g.L^{-1}$) or "suboptimal" (serum ferritin $<65\ \mu g.L^{-1}$) iron status. Whilst both forms of supplementation improved iron status, the increase in serum ferritin was greater in the IV treated group and improvements in hemoglobin mass (Hbmass), maximal aerobic power (VO_2max) and run time to exhaustion were evident only in the IV treated athletes with initial "low" iron status. Increases in Hbmass were not observed in the "suboptimal" group suggesting that their iron stores did not limit erythropoiesis or aerobic capacity. Unfortunately, neither subjective measures nor performance *per se* were formally assessed by Garvican et al. [15], so conclusions about any other potential benefits (non-hematological or otherwise) of IV iron therapy for an athletic population could not be drawn.

At present, the optimal iron status for overall wellbeing and training ability (that is, over and above that which is required for erythropoiesis) in athletic populations is unclear. Previous investigations of the benefit of oral supplementation for endurance performance in athletes without a clinical iron deficiency, i.e. "normal" iron status, have been equivocal [4] and as a result, routine supplementation for iron-replete individuals is not encouraged. However the recent findings of Krayenbuehl et al. (2011) suggest that IV iron supplementation may afford some potential benefits unrelated to erythropoiesis or oxygen transport, due to its high bioavailability [16] compared with oral supplements [15], which may have consequences for athletic performance and thus permit the topic to be revisited. Nonetheless, the ethical and potential health implications (both long and short term) of IV iron supplementation for athletes considered "clinically normal" in terms of iron status should also be considered, particularly in regard to risk of toxicity and iron overload, and notwithstanding the difficulty in determining the appropriate IV iron dose for such individuals.

Given the efficacy of the newer formulations of iron (as opposed to oral supplementation) at improving fatigue in clinical settings [14,17], the aim of the present study was to assess the impact of intravenous iron supplementation on perceived fatigue, mood disturbance, training ability and running performance in non-anemic athletes with clinically normal serum ferritin levels.

Methods

Ethics Statement

The study was approved by both the Australian Institute of Sport Human Ethics Committee and the University of Canberra Human Research Ethics Committee. All athletes provided written informed consent prior to participation.

Study design

Highly trained distance runners with clinically normal iron status (serum ferritin 30–100 $\mu g.L^{-1}$) were randomly assigned to receive either 2 ml (100 mg) of ferric carboxymaltose (IRON) or normal saline (PLACEBO) intravenously every fortnight for four weeks. Each IV injection was closely followed by a 3000 m time trial run and a monitored training session consisting of an all-out 400 m time trial and 10×400 m training session, performed on consecutive evenings during the months of June and July in Canberra, Australia, with mean environmental temperature of 10.4°C. Iron status, mood and fatigue were examined throughout, with Hbmass assessed pre and post the intervention period (Figure 1).

Inclusion/Exclusion criteria

Non-anemic athletes ([Hb]$>$ 12 $g.d{\cdot}L^{-1}$) with serum ferritin between 30–100 $\mu g{\cdot}L^{-1}$ (determined in duplicate prior to inclusion in the study) were screened by a medical doctor to determine their suitability for participation. Athletes excluded from participation were those currently taking oral supplementation or presenting with iron deficiency anemia, anemia not related to simple iron deficiency, serum ferritin $<30\ \mu g.L^{-1}$ or$>$ 100 $\mu g.L^{-1}$, previously documented hypersensitivity to iron, iron overload, acute illness, renal and endocrine disorders, pregnancy, or those having completed altitude training within one month prior.

Participants

Fourteen trained distance runners (six males, eight females) were recruited from local distance running groups (Table 1). All athletes had a minimum three-year consistent training history, and were competitive at State level or above. All athletes were familiar with the running tests employed, since similar training sessions were performed regularly within their training groups.

Hemoglobin Mass

Hemoglobin mass was measured prior to the study, and two weeks following the final injection (week 6) using the optimized carbon monoxide (CO) rebreathing method of Schmidt and Prommer [18], whereby a 1.2 $ml{\cdot}kg^{-1}$ bolus of CO was rebreathed through a closed-system spirometer for two minutes. A CO-oximeter (OSM3, Radiometer, Copenhagen, Denmark) measured the percent carboxyhemoglobin of capillary blood at 0 and 7 minutes post-rebreathing, with five replicates of each sample performed where possible. Typical error, calculated previously from duplicate measures on a separate group of distance runners was 1.6 % (90% CL 1.3 to 2.2%) [15].

Familiarization

One to two weeks before the study commenced, two 3000 m time trials and one 400 m time trial were performed within one week on a synthetic 400 m running track for familiarization.

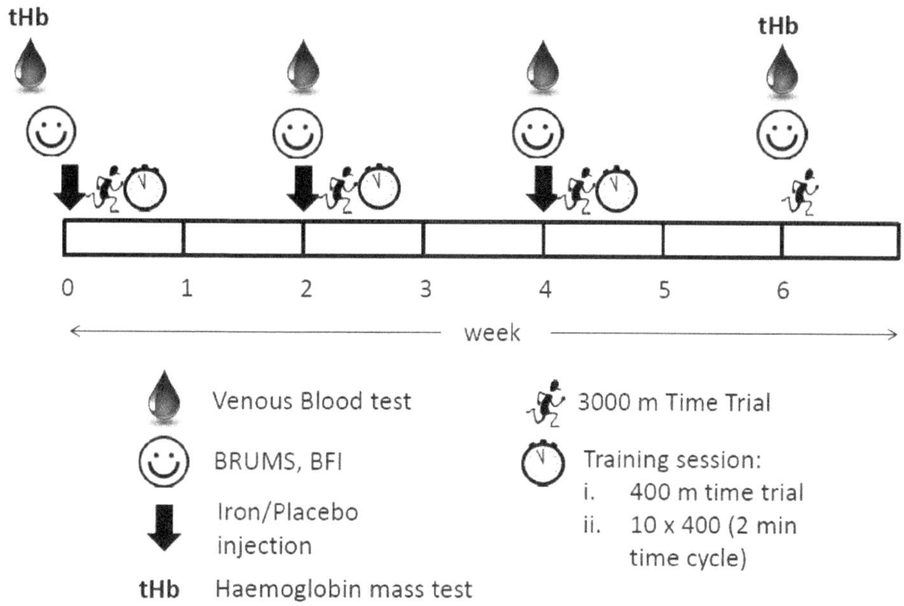

Figure 1. Schematic outline of the study design and testing sessions. BRUMS: Brunel mood Scale; BFI: Brief fatigue Inventory. Weekly injections performed on day 1, followed by 3000 m time trial on day 2 and monitored training session (400 m time trial/10 min recovery/10×400 m) on day 3.

Intervention

Participants were pair-matched by an independent researcher based on their initial serum ferritin level, Hbmass, personal best time for 3000 m and aerobic fitness (VO_2max, assessed at the start of the study as described previously [15]). Individuals were then randomly assigned to either the IRON (n = 7) or PLACEBO (n = 7) group to receive three fortnightly injections over four weeks (weeks 0, 2, 4). The IRON group received 2 ml (100 mg) of ferric carboxymaltose solution (Ferinject©, Vifor Pharma Ltd, Switzerland), whilst the corresponding PLACEBO group received 2 ml of 0.9% saline solution (Sodium chloride 0.9%).

Prior to each injection, and at least 12 h since the last training session, a venous blood sample (5 ml) was obtained via venepuncture by a trained phlebotomist to assess [Hb], hematocrit (Hct), and iron status (serum ferritin, soluble iron, transferrin and percent transferrin saturation (TSAT). Whole blood was analyzed within four hours of collection (XT-2000i, Sysmex Corporation, Japan), whilst iron status was assessed from serum (Integra 400 biochemistry analyzer, Roche Diagnostics, Switzerland). If Hct values exceeded 50%, or serum ferritin values exceeded 200 $\mu g \cdot L^{-1}$ for females, or 300 $\mu g \cdot L^{-1}$ for males, then iron supplementation would not be performed and instead replaced by saline. Each injection was performed by a medical practitioner via an indwelling venous cannula in the forearm after first flushing with 2 ml of 0.9% saline. All participants were monitored for heart rate, blood pressure, oxygen saturation and temperature by medical staff prior to administration, and every five minutes for 15 minutes afterwards in case of any adverse reactions. Throughout each injection, the participant's arm was shielded using a screen with the injection solution prepared out of sight. In addition to all athletes, all research staff associated with the testing and training sessions were blinded to the treatment groups and were unable to access blood results, nor preside over the injections. Thus, only the medical staff administering the injections had access to grouping allocation information.

Fatigue and Mood Questionnaires

Participants were assessed fortnightly for six weeks for their perceptions of fatigue and mood disturbance using the Brief Fatigue Inventory (BFI) [19] and Brunel Mood Scale (BRUMS) [20,21] (Figure 1). The BFI consists of nine standardized questions that participants answered on a scale of 1 "No fatigue" to 10 "As bad as you can imagine", as previously detailed [10]. The resulting scores from each question were averaged to produce a Total Fatigue Score.

Mood was assessed using the Brunel Mood Scale (BRUMS) [20,21], a 24-item questionnaire for assessment of mood descriptors including Tension, Depression, Anger, Fatigue, Vigor and Confusion. Each item was anchored by a 5-point Likert scale from 0 "Not at all" to 4 "Extremely" according to how participants feel "right now". Raw scores for each question and the related mood descriptor were converted to standard T-scores using normative data [22] to produce a final score, with Total Mood Disturbance then calculated by adding each of the scores for the mood descriptors and subtracting the score for Vigor [23].

Performance Testing Set: 3000 m Time Trial

The day following each injection (week 0, 2, and 4), and approximately two weeks after the completion of the supplementation period (week 6 follow-up), participants completed a maximal effort 3000 m time trial individually on a synthetic outdoor 400 m (7.5 laps) running track (Figure 1) to assess their maximal running performance capability. The 3000 m distance was chosen since it is run at speeds associated with VO_2max, and has been shown previously to be a reliable indicator of running performance in trained runners [24]. Athletes were familiar with the protocol and were blinded to pace and time during the effort. Total time was recorded via a manual stopwatch (S056-4000, Seiko, Japan). BLa was measured one minute post-trial, as well as RPE using the 6-20 Borg Scale [25].

Table 1. Participant characteristics used to pair match groups at the start of the study (means ± standard deviations).

Group	Male/Female (M/F)	Age (y)	Height (cm)	Mass (kg)	Training ($km \cdot wk^{-1}$)	3000 m PB (s)	VO_2max ($ml \cdot kg \cdot min^{-1}$)	Hbmass (g)	Relative Hbmass ($g \cdot kg^{-1}$)	Serum ferritin ($\mu g \cdot L^{-1}$)
IRON	3M/4F	29±10	170±7	59.0±6.3	86±22	606±49	60.9±6.9	703±154	11.7±1.9	62.8±21.9
PLACEBO	3M/4F	28±10	172±7	62.6±8.7	70±25	606±76	59.4±6.2	760±157	12.0±1.6	62.8±26.4

IRON = iron supplemented group; PLACEBO = saline supplemented group; PB = personal best running time.

Monitored Training Set: 10×400 m

In order to assess the athletes' ability to recover from the time trial, and their subsequent readiness to train, a monitored training session was completed 22–24 hours after the 3000 m time trial at week 0, 2 and 4. The timeframe between the time trial and monitored training session was "24 h shorter than typically experienced by the athletes, but is reflective of competition schedules at major championship meets where athletes may be required to complete heats and finals on consecutive days. After a standardized self-selected warm-up, participants completed an all-out 400 m time trial individually. BLa and RPE were recorded three minutes post-trial. After 10 minutes of active recovery, athletes undertook as a group a training session consisting of 10×400 m, on a two minute time cycle (Figure 1), with individual lap times recorded via manual stopwatch. Mean lap time was calculated as the average of the 10 lap times. BLa was measured one minute after completion of the final 400 m lap. After 10 min, session RPE was obtained using the 1–10 Borg Scale for Session RPE (sRPE) [26].

Training and Lifestyle

Participants were asked to record their training daily using an electronic training diary for the duration of the study period. In addition to recording total distance and training time, they were asked to rate their feelings related to "*How ready do you feel to train today? How easy was it to get out of bed this morning? How energized do you feel today? How much did you give in your training today? How sore are you feeling?*" on a scale of 1–5. Athletes were also instructed not to change their normal dietary practices, and to refrain from taking any oral iron supplements.

Statistics

Potential differences between groups at baseline were assessed using a Student's t-test, with significance set to $p \leq 0.05$. Otherwise, magnitude-based inferences were used in order to define the practical significance of the results using the unequal variances t-statistic and Cohen's Effect Sizes (ES) [27,28]. The differences and associated 90% confidence limits (CL) for changes in hematological, physiological and performance characteristics were examined *within* each group over the duration of the study, as well as *between* the groups for the differences in their respective changes from baseline measures. Prior to analysis, raw data were log transformed to reduce non-uniformity of errors. The magnitude of an effect and the associated P-value was presented as percent change and standardized mean differences (ES); calculated as the difference in mean divided by the between-subject standard deviation (SD); where a small effect is> 0.2, moderate> 0.6 and large> 1.2 [27]. The reference threshold for the smallest worthwhile change was set to 0.2, which is Cohen's smallest standardized effect calculated from the between-subject SD at baseline. Effects were deemed *unclear* if the confidence interval overlapped the thresholds for the smallest positive and negative effects. Data are reported as mean ± SD unless otherwise stated.

The overall change in the subjective parameters of the training diaries was assessed with within-individual linear regressions (change/day, with 90% CL) as described by others [29]. Trends were deemed substantial if the 90% CL did not overlap zero. Differences of the slopes between the IRON and PLACEBO groups were also assessed using magnitude based inferences as described above [27].

Table 2. Iron parameters, Hbmass,[Hb] and fatigue scores of IRON and PLACEBO groups pre-supplementation and at 2, 4 and 6 weeks post-supplementation.

	IRON				PLACEBO			
	Week 0	**Week 2**	**Week 4**	**Week 6**	**Week 0**	**Week 2**	**Week 4**	**Week 6**
Serum ferritin ($\mu g \cdot L^{-1}$)	62.8±21.9	104.1±31.7 *†	128.1±46.6 *†	127.0±66.3 *†	62.8±26.4	65.7±30.1	65.8±26.4	57.3±17.7
Hbmass (g)	703±154	-	-	709±148	759±157	-	-	758±170
Relative Hbmass ($g \cdot kg^{-1}$)	11.7±1.9	-	-	11.8±1.6	12.0±1.6	-	-	12.1±1.6
[Hb] ($g \cdot dL^{-1}$)	14.6±1.6	14.2±1.3	14.3±1.5	14.4±1.1	14.6±1.0	14.3±1.2	14.4±1.0	14.3±1.0
Hct	42.8±3.8	41.7±2.9	41.9±3.8	42.0±2.4	42.5±2.8	42.5±2.7	42.2±1.8	41.6±2.2
Iron ($\mu mol \cdot L^{-1}$)	19.8±4.3	18.2±7.0	16.1±3.8	17.2±6.6	17.5±3.5	15.1±4.2	18.5±4.6	16.6±7.5
Transferrin ($g \cdot L^{-1}$)	3.3±0.4	2.8±0.4 *	2.8±0.6 *	2.7±0.4 *	3.1±0.3	2.8±0.2	2.9±0.2	2.8±0.3
TSAT (%)	23.0±4.6	25.0±9.1	23.1±7.0	23.6±8.3	21.7±5.7	20.6±6.1	24.3±6.7	22.0±9.3

Mean ± SD; * denotes significant difference ($p \leq 0.05$) from week 0 values within a group.
†significant difference ($p \leq 0.05$) between groups at matched time point.
Hbmass: haemoglobin mass, [Hb]: haemoglobin concentration, Hct: Haematocrit, TSAT: percent transferrin saturation.

Results

Study Population

There were no significant differences between the IRON and PLACEBO groups at the start of the study in terms of baseline characteristics (Table 1), hematological parameters (Table 2), or mood scores associated with the BRUMS (Figure 2A). However at baseline, IRON had a significantly higher Total Fatigue Score than PLACEBO on the BFI (Figure 2B, $p = 0.04$).

Supplementation, Hematology and Iron profile

Each scheduled injection was administered without incident. Serum ferritin values did not change significantly in PLACEBO but increased two-fold from baseline in the IRON group at week 4 (Week 0: 62.8±21.9, Week 4: 128.1±46.6 $\mu g \cdot L^{-1}$; $p = 0.002$) and remained elevated two weeks after the final injection (127.0± 66.3 $\mu g \cdot L^{-1}$; $p = 0.01$; Table 2). There were no statistically

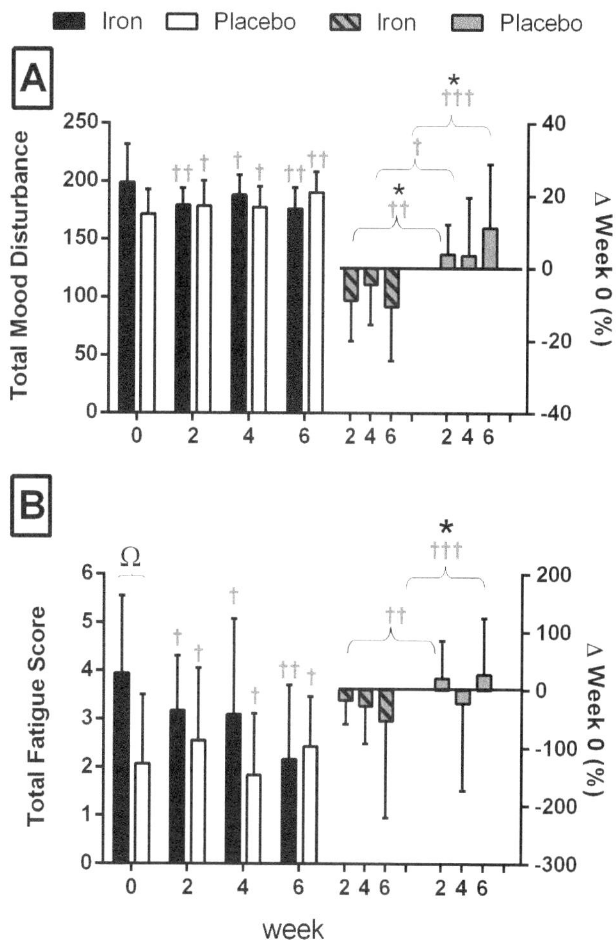

Figure 2. Changes in mood and fatigue scores during the study. A) Total Mood Disturbance from the Brunel Mood Scale and **B)** Total Fatigue Score from the Brief Fatigue Inventory. Data are presented in raw form on the Left Y-axis and as percent change from week 0 on the Right Y-axis (mean ± SD). Within a group change from Week 0: † small effect (Effect size> 0.2), †† moderate effect (Effect size>0.6); between group percent change from week 0 at matched time; * p≤ 0.05; † small effect (Effect size> 0.2), †† moderate effect (Effect size> 0.6), ††† Large effect (Effect size> 1.2); Ω denotes difference between groups at week 0.

significant changes in Hbmass, [Hb] or Hct in either group over the course of the investigation (Table 2).

Fatigue Scores

Brunel Mood Scale. Iron supplementation had a moderate (but not significant) effect on Total Mood Disturbance (Figure 2A), with values within the IRON group tending to be lower than baseline at week 2 (ES -0.64, $p = 0.06$) and 6 (ES -0.77, $p = 0.08$). Between the groups, Total Mood Disturbance significantly improved in IRON compared with PLACEBO (Figure 2A), at both week 2 (% change compared with PLACEBO; 90% CL, ES, p value: −12.3%; −19.8 to −4.1%, −0.95, $p = 0.02$) and week 6 (−19.6%; −30.4 to −7.1%, −1.58, $p = 0.02$).

Brief Fatigue Inventory. Within the IRON group, supplementation resulted in a trend to decrease the Total Fatigue Score at week 6 (ES -1.35, $p = 0.09$), but the latter large effect size failed to attain statistical significance (Figure 2B). Between the groups, Total Fatigue Score in the IRON group significantly improved at week 6 compared to PLACEBO (−63.0%; −83.7 to −16.1%, −1.54, $p = 0.05$).

Running performance

3000 m Time Trial. Mean 3000 m run time did not change significantly within IRON during the study but PLACEBO were slower than week 0 at week 4 ($p = 0.04$). Therefore, at week 4 there was a small effect on 3000 m time between the groups, with IRON faster than PLACEBO (−2.1 %; −3.8 to 0.3 %, 0.22; $p = 0.05$); Table 3). Compared with PLACEBO, the BLa of IRON was reduced at week 2 (−29.5%; −43.7 to −11.7%, −1.00, $p = 0.02$), week 4 (−30.8%; −44.0 to −14.5%, −1.06, $p = 0.01$) and week 6 (−35.8%; −48.4 to −20.1%, −1.27, $p = 0.003$; Figure 3A). Between the groups, iron supplementation had no significant effect on RPE.

All-out 400 m Time Trial. All-out 400 m time did not change significantly within or between either group over the course of the study (Table 3). Differences between the groups for changes in BLa and RPE were not significant (Figure 3B).

10×400 m Training Session. The average time for the 10×400 m session of the IRON group was faster at week 2 (−0.8%; −1.2 to −0.5%, −0.09, $p = 0.004$) compared with week 0. There were no significant differences within PLACEBO over time (Table 3), nor were there any significant differences between groups. Between the groups, iron supplementation had no significant effect on RPE or BLa (Figure 3C).

Training Diaries

Day-to-day mean training diary scores improved in the following areas within the IRON group only: "How easy was it to get out of bed this morning?", "How ready do you feel to train today?", and "How energized do you feel today?" (Figure 4). The observed positive effects for these questions were greater in IRON compared with PLACEBO (Effect size; 90CL: "How easy was it to get out of bed this morning?"0.88; 0.04 to 1.71; "How ready do you feel to train today?"1.12; 0.38 to 1.86, and "How energized do you feel today?" 1.04; 0.11 to 1.97).

Discussion

The main finding of the present study was that, compared with PLACEBO, three fortnightly IV injections of ferric carboxymaltose over 4 weeks improved self-reported perceptions of fatigue and reduced mood disturbance in trained distance runners with "clinically normal"serum ferritin levels between 30 and 100 $\mu g \cdot L^{-1}$, without concomitant changes in Hbmass or [Hb]. Supplementation had no acute effects on 3000 m running performance; however iron supplemented athletes decreased their 10×400 m training set time at week 2, and recorded improvements in their perceptions about their preparedness to train, which collectively may indicate a potential training benefit of IV iron for the treatment group.

The most widely accepted clinical threshold for iron deficiency is 22 $\mu g \cdot L^{-1}$ [30], where storage iron is exhausted but transport and functional compounds are maintained. When ferritin stores fall below 22 $\mu g \cdot L^{-1}$, functional compounds become compromised, including but not limited to hemoglobin, myoglobin and cytochromes [30]. However, the "optimal" level for serum ferritin is still unknown in terms of athletic performance and an athlete's ability to train and recover between sessions over weeks or months. Uncertainty is due largely to discrepancies in the literature regarding the effect of iron supplementation, particularly in athletes with 'normal' iron status [2], and hampered by a wide variety of supplementation methods and protocols [7]. In the present study, we specifically recruited subjects with clinically normal ferritin levels (30–100 $\mu g \cdot L^{-1}$), whose Hbmass was therefore unlikely to be compromised [15], in order to investigate possible non-hematological effects of IV iron supplementation; that is, those unrelated to erythropoiesis or oxygen transport, such as subjective wellbeing and training ability.

Intravenous ferric carboxymaltose supplementation increased serum ferritin throughout the supplementation period. Further, serum ferritin remained elevated by approximately double the pre-treatment levels two weeks following the final injection. However, Hbmass and [Hb] did not change, confirming previous research [15] but also indicating that the observed reductions in fatigue and mood disturbance in the iron treatment group, compared to placebo, were unlikely to be related to oxygen-carrying capacity.

When storage iron is> 35 $\mu g \cdot L^{-1}$, erythropoiesis and thereby oxygen transport, are unlikely to be affected [15]. However, it is possible that if the amount of iron available for the formation of enzymes and compounds associated with muscle metabolism is insufficient, then endurance performance may also become impaired [31]. Since it would appear that the supplemental iron provided in the present study was not required for the formation of Hb, it is possible that the available iron may have been shuttled towards oxidative enzymes for intracellular metabolism and electron transport [1]. However, in the present study, 3000 m running time was not acutely improved following each injection; indicating neither a direct performance advantage following IV iron administration nor a placebo effect of an injection. Further, although subtle improvements in the 10×400 m training set were observed in the IRON group at week 2, overall our results do not provide compelling evidence for any performance advantage arising from increasing ferritin stores. Of note, however, is the observation that 3000 m performance was worse in the PLACEBO group at week 4, and as a result the IRON group performed significantly better. These findings provide tentative evidence that the IRON group performed more consistently throughout the study, and may be related to improved perceptions of fatigue and well-being as opposed to effects at a metabolic level.

The presence of blood lactate, a gross indirect measure of anaerobic metabolism, reflects the contribution of each of the body's energy systems with which an exercise effort is undertaken. A decrease in BLa within the IRON group was observed following the week 2 and week 6, 3000 m time trials, which is similar to previous findings [32–34], whilst PLACEBO recorded higher BLa for comparable run times. Hinton et al. [35] report that as a result of iron deficits, the oxidative capacity of the muscle is reduced and therefore the workload at which the ventilatory threshold and

Table 3. Performance test times (mean ± SD) and mean difference (with 90% CL) between groups (IRON vs. PLACEBO) for the respective percent change from week 0.

Performance test	Group	Week 0	Week 2	Week 4	Week 6 (Follow-up)	Week 2 Difference in change between groups (%)	Week 4 Difference in change between groups (%)	Week 6 Difference in change between groups (%)
3000 m time trial (s)	Iron	625.6±55.5	627.1±55.3	625.4±52.7	631.3±49.7	−1.2 (−2.8 to 0.3)	−2.1 (−3.8 to −0.3) †	−0.9 (−3.7 to 1.9)
	Placebo	624.8±47.2	634.9±55.2	639.1±59.7 * Ω	638.0±63.2 †			
All-out 400 m time trial (s)	Iron	67.5±6.2	68.0±6.6	68.8±6.1	-	0.6 (−2.9 to 4.2)	−0.1 (−2.7 to 2.6)	-
	Placebo	66.9±9.8	66.7±7.5	68.2±9.4	-			
10×400 m Average time (s)	Iron	78.0±6.6	77.2±6.3 *	77.1±5.7	-	−0.7 (−4.3 to 2.0)	−1.8 (−5.5 to 2.1) †	-
	Placebo	78.4±7.3	78.2±6.2	78.9±7.6	-			

Within group change from Week 0: * $p \leq 0.05$, Ω small effect (Effect size > 0.2).
Between groups change from Week 0: † small effect (Effect size > 0.2).

blood lactate accumulation occurs is lower [35]. Some studies have reported no change in BLa following supplementation [36,37], but discrepancies in time course of treatment and the chosen modality (most have involved oral supplementation), dosage and study design may have influenced these results. The iron recipients in the present study may thus have improved aspects of their lactate metabolism [1,34] as a result of treatment effects at a metabolic level, although further investigation is required to confirm this notion.

Iron deficiency without anemia can result in a greater energy expenditure during a simulated time trial [38] as well as lower exercise tolerance and a more prolonged recovery from exercise [39]. The IRON group decreased their average 10×400 m time shortly after the second injection, even though their 3000 m and all-out 400 m times did not improve. These results partially support the notion of resilience to an exercise bout and weakly suggest the iron supplemented group may have displayed a greater ability to complete consecutive training sessions whilst carrying potential fatigue from a prior effort. It is possible that improved iron stores may result in greater coping ability and enhanced recovery before the next session, which may in turn facilitate augmented wellbeing and ability to train more effectively, although further research is required.

There is evidence that iron insufficiencies impact mental function and emotional health as a result of reduced neurotransmitter activity in the brain and central nervous system [1]. Iron therapy can result in improved cognitive function [40] and has been associated with improvements in memory, energy and mood [41], as well as improvement in subjective feelings of physical fitness and performance [42,43]. This is supported by data in the present study where the recipients of IV iron reported improvement in total fatigue and total mood disturbance, in addition to an improvement in their training diary scores relating to readiness to train, energy levels and ease of getting out of bed. By contrast, some studies have reported that iron supplementation has no significant effect on deficiency symptoms, mood state [44] or quality of life [45]. The discrepancy may be due to the oral treatment modality examined by earlier researchers, which may not deliver enough bioavailable iron for substantial cognitive improvements.

Limitations

Despite careful pair matching of subjects based on initial ferritin, Hbmass and performance characteristics, the PLACEBO group reported lower fatigue scores on the one of the two questionnaire scales (BFI) at the start of the study. The BFI is a tool typically used to assess cancer-related fatigue but has been used previously in a non-athletic population to assess iron related fatigue [14]; whereas the BRUMS was developed for assessment of mood (including fatigue) in performance environments. The difference in baseline scores using the BFI highlights that the presence of fatigue symptoms is not solely related to initial ferritin level. Nonetheless, when the difference in change scores of both scales (BRUMS and BFI) was analyzed, a superiority of the IRON group over the PLACEBO group was observed, indicating a possible role of supplemental iron in the reduction of perceived fatigue and an improvement in overall mood. It should also be noted that whilst improvements were observed in the self-reported training diary scores of the IRON group, this method of reporting is only typically used in an applied sport model as opposed to a clinical setting.

No clear acute or chronic benefits of iron supplementation on 3000 m running performance were observed although consistently similar performances were evident throughout which was not the

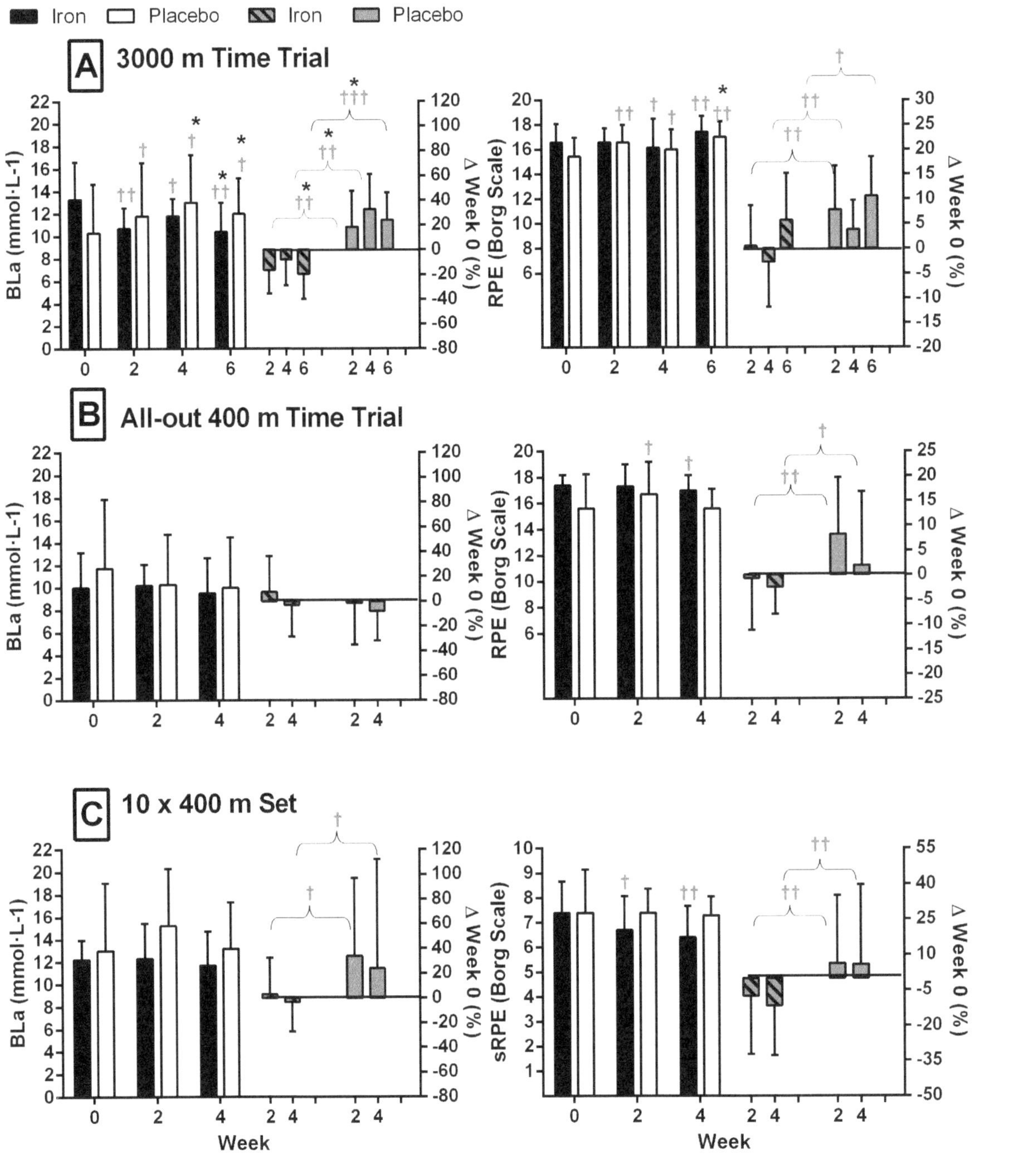

Figure 3. Blood lactate concentration (Bla) and Rating of Perceived Exertion (RPE) from the run trials over the course of the study. **A)** 3000 m time trial; **B)** All-out 400 m time trial; **C)** 10×400 m session. Data are presented in raw form on the Left Y-axis and as % change from week 0 on the Right Y-axis (mean ± SD). Within a group change from Week 0: * $p \le 0.05$; † small effect (Effect size> 0.2), †† moderate effect (Effect size> 0.6); between group percent change from PRE at matched time; † small effect (Effect size> 0.2), †† moderate effect (Effect size> 0.6).

case in the PLACEBO group. Measuring a true maximal effort of an individual as well as obtaining optimal performance on a particular day, remain inherently difficult [46]. The very nature of simulated performance testing means that is nearly impossible to mimic real-life competition through a time trial or simulated laboratory test, which may explain some early research reporting no improvement in performance post-supplementation even in iron-deficient participants [36,37,47]. A further limitation to consider is that our total monitoring period was possibly too short, particularly since we did not follow the 10×400 m training set at two weeks post injection.

Implications

This study demonstrated improvements in fatigue and mood disturbance in the IRON group during a 6 week training period. Whether or not such improvements in fatigue and mood (potentially arising from elevated ferritin levels) may lead to better training quality and subsequently improved performance over a

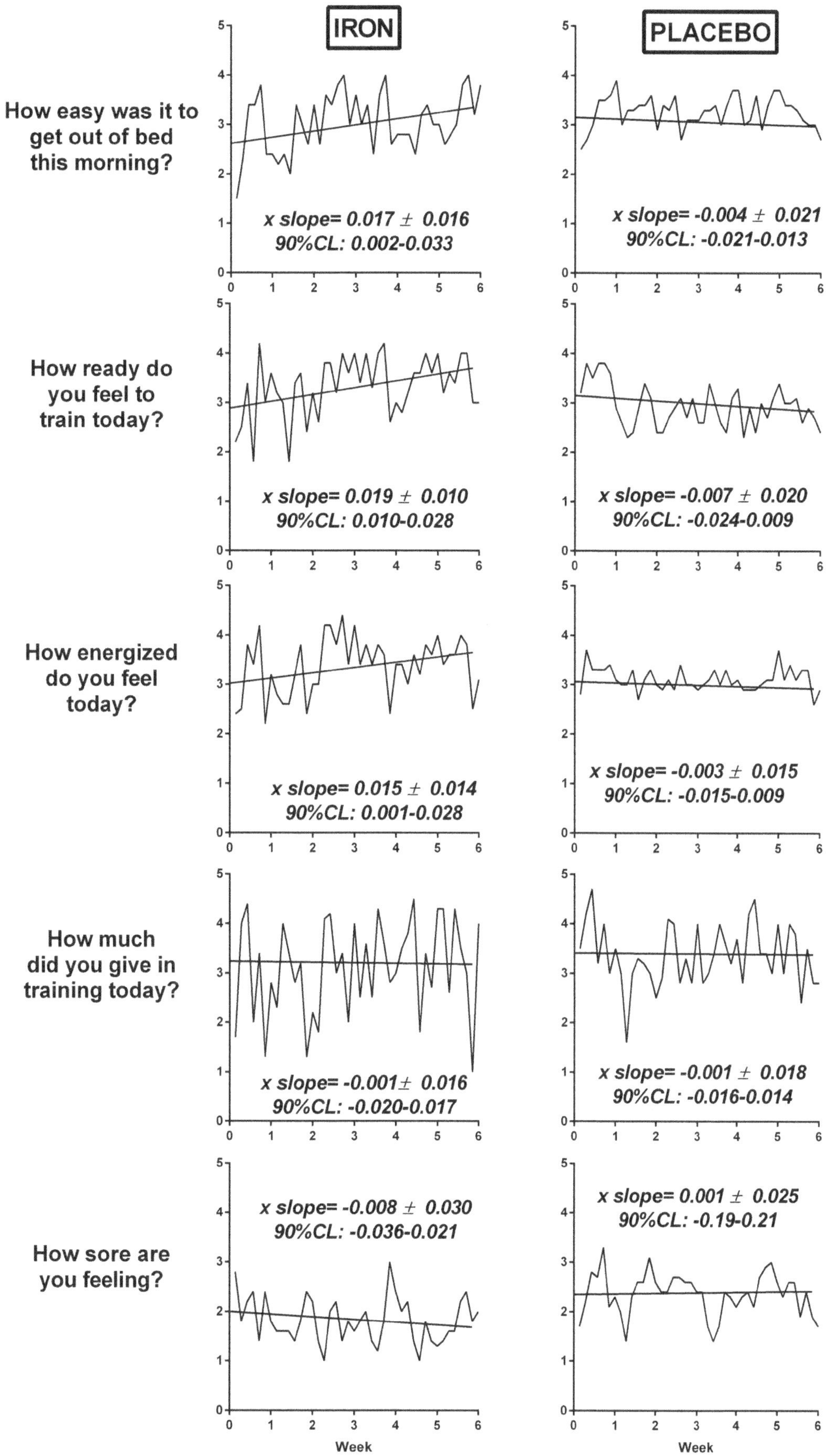
IRON
PLACEBO
How easy was it to get out of bed this morning?
x slope= 0.017 ± 0.016
90%CL: 0.002-0.033
x slope= -0.004 ± 0.021
90%CL: -0.021-0.013
How ready do you feel to train today?
x slope= 0.019 ± 0.010
90%CL: 0.010-0.028
x slope= -0.007 ± 0.020
90%CL: -0.024-0.009
How energized do you feel today?
x slope= 0.015 ± 0.014
90%CL: 0.001-0.028
x slope= -0.003 ± 0.015
90%CL: -0.015-0.009
How much did you give in training today?
x slope= -0.001± 0.016
90%CL: -0.020-0.017
x slope= -0.001 ± 0.018
90%CL: -0.016-0.014
How sore are you feeling?
x slope= -0.008 ± 0.030
90%CL: -0.036-0.021
x slope= 0.001 ± 0.025
90%CL: -0.19-0.21
Week
Week

Figure 4. Mean perceptual daily training diary ratings for IRON and PLACEBO during the study (rated 1 to 5). X slope (90%CL): derived as the mean of individual regression analysis for each subject.

longer period of time cannot be determined from this study. However, the long term or repeated use of iron supplementation in athletes who are not iron deficient should not be advocated. In the short-term, the efficacy of IV Iron supplementation for athletes with moderate ferritin levels also requires careful consideration, because a performance improvement remains unclear. For this reason the data in this study do not provide strong evidence for IV iron supplementation in athletes with clinically normal ferritin levels, especially when taking into account the ethical and potential health implications of sustained iron supplementation for iron replete individuals. Specifically, the potential risk of toxicity and iron overload following IV administration must be acknowledged, particularly since the primary route for regulating whole body iron stores is bypassed using this method, allowing ferritin levels to be elevated rapidly. Therefore, IV injections should not be administered without first assessing existing iron stores, and careful consideration of the total dose to be given, and its likely impact on whole body iron stores, is required. IV iron should only be administered under medical supervision, with patients closely monitored for adverse reactions. Follow-up tests should also be conducted to ensure ferritin levels do not exceed healthy limits. Lastly, researchers need to be acutely up to date with any changes to the World Anti-Doping Agency code when planning future research with elite athletes [48].

Conclusion

Four weeks of IV ferric carboxymaltose supplementation doubled serum ferritin, and decreased feelings of fatigue and mood disturbance in non-anemic athletes with initial ferritin levels in the clinically normal range of 30–100 $\mu g \cdot L^{-1}$ without associated changes in Hbmass. Running performance was not acutely affected by iron supplementation, but there was some evidence from self-reported training diaries that participants felt more able to train. Together, these results indicate a potential psychobiological influence of iron supplementation on feelings of mood and fatigue in athletic populations with clinically normal serum ferritin.

Acknowledgments

We would sincerely like to thank the staff from AIS Physiology, AIS Medicine, and AIS Biochemistry for their assistance during data collection, as well as the athletes for their participation in the study.

Author Contributions

Conceived and designed the experiments: LGL AW PS GL DH RF BA CG KT. Performed the experiments: LGL AW PS GL DH RF BA. Analyzed the data: LGL AW PS CG KT. Wrote the paper: LGL AW PS GL DH CG KT.

References

1. Beard JL (2001) Iron biology in immune function, muscle metabolism and neuronal functioning. J Nutr 131: 568–580.
2. Deli CK, Fatouros IG, Koutedakis Y, Jamurtas AZ (2013) Iron supplementation and physical performance In: A. P. M. . Hamlin, editor editors. Current Issues in Sports and Exercise Medicine.
3. Rattehalli D, Pickard L, Tselepis C, Sharma N, Iqbal TH (2013) Iron deficiency without anaemia: Do not wait for the haemoglobin to drop? Health Policy Technol 2: 45–58.
4. Nielsen P, Nachtigall D (1998) Iron supplementation in athletes: current recommendations. Sports Med 26: 207–216.
5. Telford RD, Sly GJ, Hahn AG, Cunningham RB, Bryant C, et al. (2003) Footstrike is the major cause of hemolysis during running J Appl Physiol 94: 38–42.
6. Suominen P, Punnonen K, Rajamaki A, Irjala K (1998) Serum transferrin receptor and transferrin receptor-ferritin index identify healthy subjects with subclinical iron deficits. Blood 92: 2934–2939.
7. Nielsen P, Nachtigall D (1998) Iron supplementation in athletes. Current recommendations. Sports Med 26: 207–216.
8. Lyseng-Williamson K, Keating G (2009) Ferric Carboxymaltose. Drugs 69: 739–756.
9. Favrat B, Balck K, Gasche C, Hedenus M, Mezzacasa A, et al. (2012) W472 A single 1000 mg iron dose of Ferric Carboxymaltose improves fatigue in iron deficient, non-anaemic premenopausal women - Results of the randomised, placebo-controlled PREFER study. Int J Gynecol Obstet 119: S858–S859.
10. Krayenbuehl PA, Battegay E, Breymann C, Furrer J, Schulthess G (2011) Intravenous iron for the treatment of fatigue in nonanemic, premenopausal women with low serum ferritin concentration. Blood 118: 3222–3227.
11. Ackrell BA, Kearney EB, Mims WB, Peisach J, Beinert H (1984) Iron-sulfur cluster 3 of beef heart succinate-ubiquinone oxidoreductase is a 3-iron cluster. The Journal of biological chemistry 259: 4015–4018.
12. Finch CA, Miller LR, Inamdar AR, Person R, Seiler K, et al. (1976) Iron deficiency in the rat. Physiological and biochemical studies of muscle dysfunction. The Journal of clinical investigation 58: 447–453.
13. McLane JA, Fell RD, McKay RH, Winder WW, Brown EB, et al. (1981) Physiological and biochemical effects of iron deficiency on rat skeletal muscle. The American journal of physiology 241: C47–54.
14. Krayenbuehl PA, Battegay E, Breymann C, Furrer J, Schulthess G (2011) Intravenous iron for the treatment of fatigue in nonanemic, premenopausal women with low serum ferritin concentration. Blood 118: 3222–3227.
15. Garvican LA, Saunders PU, Cardoso T, Macdougall IC, Lobigs LM, et al. (2014) Intravenous iron supplementation in distance runners with low or suboptimal ferritin. Medicine and science in sports and exercise 46: 376–385.
16. Macdougall IC (1999) Strategies for iron supplementation: oral versus intravenous. Kidney Int 55: 61–66.
17. Favrat B, Balck K, Gasche C, Hedenus M, Mezzacasa A, et al. (2012) A single 1,000 mg iron dose of ferric carboxymaltose improves fatigue in iron deficient, non-anaemic premenopausal women – Results of the randomised, placebo-controlled PREFER study. XX FIGO World Congress of Gynecology and Obstetrics. Rome, Italy.
18. Schmidt W, Prommer N (2005) The optimised CO-rebreathing method: a new tool to determine total haemoglobin mass routinely. Eur J Appl Physiol 95: 486–495.
19. Mendoza TR, Wang XS, Cleeland CS, Morrissey M, Johnson BA, et al. (1999) The rapid assessment of fatigue severity in cancer patients: use of the Brief Fatigue Inventory. Cancer 85: 1186–1196.
20. Terry PC, Lane AM, Lane HJ, Keohane L (1999) Development and validation of a mood measure for adolescents. J Sport Sci 17: 861–872.
21. Terry PC, Lane AM, Fogarty GJ (2003) Construct validity of the Profile of Mood States - Adolescents for use with adults. Psych Sport Exerc 4: 125–139.
22. Terry PC, Lane AM (2010) User Guide for the Brunel Mood Scale (BRUMS). [Obtained from Author].
23. Lane AM, Jackson A, Terry PC (2005) Preferred modality influences on exercise-induced mood changes. J Sports Sci Med 4: 195–200.
24. Robertson EY, Saunders PU, Pyne DB, Gore CJ, Anson JM (2010) Effectiveness of intermittent training in hypoxia combined with live high/train low. European journal of applied physiology 110: 379–387.
25. Borg G (1990) Psychophysical scaling with applications in physical work and the perception of exertion. Scand J Work Environ Health 16: 55–58.
26. Foster C, Florhaug JA, Franklin J, Gottschall L, Hrovatin LA, et al. (2001) A new approach to monitoring exercise training. Journal of strength and conditioning research/National Strength & Conditioning Association 15: 109–115.
27. Hopkins WG, Marshall SW, Batterham AM, Hanin J (2009) Progressive statistics for studies in sports medicine and exercise science. Medicine and science in sports and exercise 41: 3–13.
28. Ploutz-Snyder RJ, Fiedler J, Feiveson AH (2014) Justifying small-n research in scientifically amazing settings: Challenging the notion that only "big-n" studies are worthwhile. J Appl Physiol (1985).
29. Buchheit M, Racinais S, Bilsborough JC, Bourdon PC, Voss SC, et al. (2013) Monitoring fitness, fatigue and running performance during a pre-season training camp in elite football players. Journal of science and medicine in sport/Sports Medicine Australia 16: 550–555.
30. Suominen P, Punnonen K, Rajamaki A, Irjala K (1998) Serum transferrin receptor and transferrin receptor-ferritin index identifies healthy subjects with subclinical iron deficits Blood 92: 2934–2939.
31. DellaValle DM (2013) Iron supplementation for female athletes: Effects on iron status and performance outcomes. Curr Sports Med Rep 12: 234–239.
32. LaManca JJ, Haymes EM (1993) Effects of iron repletion on VO2max, endurance, and blood lactate in women. Med Sci Sports Exerc 25: 1386–1392.

33. Schoene RB, Escourrou P, Robertson HT, Nilson KL, Parsons JR, et al. (1983) Iron repletion decreases maximal exercise lactate concentrations in female athletes with minimal iron-deficiency anemia. J Lab Clin Med 102: 306–312.
34. Pedlar CR, Whyte GP, Burden R, Moore B, Horgan G, et al. (2013) A case study of an iron deficient female Olympic 1500 m runner. Int J Sports Physiol Perf [Ahead of Print].
35. Hinton PS, Sinclair L (2007) Iron supplementation maintains ventilatory threshold and improves energetic efficiency in iron-deficient nonanemic athletes. Eur J Clin Nutr 61: 30–39.
36. Klingshirn LA, Pate RR, Bourque SP, Davis JM, Sargent RG (1992) Effect of iron supplementation on endurance capacity in iron-depleted female runners. Med Sci Sports Exerc 24: 819–824.
37. Fogelholm M, Jaakkola L, Lampisjärvi T (1992) Effects of iron supplementation in female athletes with low serum ferritin concentration. Int J Sports Med 13: 158–162.
38. Zhu YI, Haas JD (1998) Altered metabolic response of iron-depleted nonanemic women during a 15-km time trial. J Appl Physiol 84: 1768–1775.
39. Newhouse I, Clement D (1988) Iron status in athletes. Sports Med 5: 337–352.
40. Murray-Kolb LE, Beard JL (2007) Iron treatment normalizes cognitive functioning in young women. Am J Clin Nutr 85: 778–787.
41. Yehuda S, Youdim MB (1989) Brain iron: a lesson from animal models. Am J Clin Nutr 50: 618–629.
42. Nachtigall D, Nielsen P, Fischer R, Engelhardt R, Gabbe E (1996) Iron deficiency in distance runners: a reinvestigation using 59Fe-Labelling and non-invasive liver iron quantification. J Sports Med 17: 473–479.
43. Martin DE, et al. (1986) Physiological changes in elite male distance runners training for Olympic competition. Phys Sportsmed 14: 152–161, 154–167,171.
44. Risser WL, Lee EJ, Poindexter HB, West MS, Pivarnik JM, et al. (1988) Iron deficiency in female athletes: its prevalence and impact on performance. Med Sci Sports Exerc 20: 116–121.
45. Vaucher P, Druais P-L, Waldvogel S, Favrat B (2012) Effect of iron supplementation on fatigue in nonanemic menstruating women with low ferritin: a randomized controlled trial. Can Med Assoc J 184: 1247–1254.
46. Gore CJ (2014) The challenge of assessing athlete performance after altitude training. J Appl Physiol (1985).
47. Peeling P, Blee T, Goodman C, Dawson B, Claydon G, et al. (2007) Effect of iron injections on aerobic-exercise performance of iron-depleted female athletes. Int J Sports Nutr Exerc Metabol 17: 221–231.
48. Howman D (2013) Scientific research using elite athletes: WADA point of view. J Appl Physiol (1985) 114: 1365.

The Effect of S-Adenosylmethionine on Cognitive Performance in Mice

Sarah E. Montgomery[1]*, Amir A. Sepehry[2,3], John D. Wangsgaard[1], Jeremy E. Koenig[4¶]

[1] Department of Applied Human Nutrition, Mount Saint Vincent University, Halifax, Nova Scotia, Canada, [2] College for Interdisciplinary Studies, Graduate program in Neuroscience, University of British Columbia (UBC), Vancouver, BC, Canada, [3] UBC Division of Neurology, Department of Medicine, University of British Columbia (UBC), Vancouver, BC, Canada, [4] Faculty of Computer Science, Dalhousie University, Halifax, NS, Canada

Abstract

Background: Alzheimer's disease (AD) is the most frequently diagnosed form of dementia resulting in cognitive impairment. Many AD mouse studies, using the methyl donor S-adenosylmethionine (SAM), report improved cognitive ability, but conflicting results between and within studies currently exist. To address this, we conducted a meta-analysis to evaluate the effect of SAM on cognitive ability as measured by Y maze performance. As supporting evidence, we include further discussion of improvements in cognitive ability, by SAM, as measured by the Morris water maze (MWM).

Methods: We conducted a comprehensive literature review up to April 2014 based on searches querying MEDLINE, EMBASE, Web of Science, the Cochrane Library and Proquest Theses and Dissertation databases. We identified three studies containing a total of 12 experiments that met our inclusion criteria and one study for qualitative review. The data from these studies were used to evaluate the effect of SAM on cognitive performance according to two scenarios: 1. SAM supplemented folate deficient (SFD) diet compared to a folate deficient (FD) diet and 2. SFD diet compared to a nutrient complete (NC) diet. Hedge's g was used to calculate effect sizes and mixed effects model meta-regression was used to evaluate moderating factors.

Results: Our findings showed that the SFD diet was associated with improvements in cognitive performance. SFD diet mice also had superior cognitive performance compared to mice on an NC diet. Further to this, meta-regression analyses indicated a significant positive effect of study quality score and treatment duration on the effect size estimate for both the FD vs SFD analysis and the SFD vs NC analysis.

Conclusion: The findings of this meta-analysis demonstrate efficacy of SAM in acting as a cognitive performance-enhancing agent. As a corollary, SAM may be useful in improving spatial memory in patients suffering from many dementia forms including AD.

Editor: Bart O. Williams, Van Andel Institute, United States of America

Funding: Funding was provided by Mount Saint Vincent University (JK). The funders had no role in study design, data collection and analysis, decision to publish, or preparation of the manuscript.

Competing Interests: The authors have declared that no competing interests exist.

* Email: sarah.montgomery@msvu.ca

¶ JEK is the supervising author on this work.

Introduction

As of 2013, approximately 44.4 million people suffer from dementia [1]. Alzheimer's disease is the most widely recognized and diagnosed form of dementia [2]. It is a neurodegenerative disease characterized by severe cognitive impairment, with learning, memory, and visuospatial abilities being three of the most prominent behavioral processes to deteriorate [3].

S-adenosylmethionine (SAM), has gained considerable attention for its enhancing effect on cognitive performance in both human and animal model research [4–9]. SAM is a naturally occurring compound in the human body that carries out numerous metabolic reactions. SAM plays an integral role as methyl donor in the metabolism of Methionine (Met) to homocysteine (Hcy). In this conversion, SAM regulates epigenetic processes via DNA methylation [10] that have been implicated in its efficacy for the treatment of depression, osteoarthritis and liver support in humans [7,11,12].

There have been a few promising human studies evaluating the effects of SAM on improving cognitive performance in patients with AD [7,8,12]. However, there has been more extensive research on SAM using AD mouse models [5,13–15]. To date, many of the animal studies exhibit differences in methodology protocols between studies as well as conflicting results. These differences have presented challenges in drawing definitive conclusions on the efficacy of SAM in improving cognitive performance.

Animal models commonly used in AD research, as it relates to metabolism, are used to evaluate the relationship between nutrient status and gene expression. Two mouse models used in the studies included in this meta-analysis are the apolipoprotein E4 (APOE4) model and the methylenetetrahydrofolate reductase deficiency (MTHFR −/−) model [13]. These two models have been associated with a greater risk for AD development, particularly in combination with a folate deficient diet [16]. It has previously been established that SAM confers a positive effect on cognitive performance in these two genotypes under folate deficient conditions [11]. Alternatively, Apolipoprotein E2 and E3 genotypes present protective and neutral effects on risk of developing AD, respectively [9]. All of these models, combined, provide a comprehensive illustration of SAM's effect on cognitive performance across varying genotypic backgrounds.

The outcome of this research is particularly important in the consideration of treatments for other conditions such as cardiovascular diseases and low bone mineral density since these diseases have frequently been associated with high levels of plasma Hcy and corresponding hypomethylation [17–19]. The widespread theory that elevated Hcy and corresponding hypomethylation are risk factors for multiple diseases and disorders suggests that many populations may benefit from these findings.

The purpose of this research is to evaluate the effect of SAM as a novel nutraceutical treatment for halting the progression of cognitive decline in both healthy and AD mouse models through a meta-analysis research design. We hope to further substantiate the evidence that SAM can exhibit a restorative effect on cognitive performance by evaluating the performance of various mouse strains in the Y maze and Morris Water Maze (MWM). Both mazes are well-established tools for measuring spatial learning and memory in mice and widely recognized and used in AD research [20]. Specifically, the studies in this meta-analysis evaluated the effect of a folate deficient (FD) diet and a SAM supplemented folate deficient (SFD) diet on percent spontaneous alternations in the Y maze and latency to swim, swimming speed and number of annulus crossings in the MWM using healthy and transgenic mice. Firstly, we tested the hypothesis that SAM supplementation improves cognitive performance in mice fed a folate deficient diet. Secondly, we tested the hypothesis that S-adenosylmethionine can raise cognitive performance to the level of mice fed a nutrient complete (NC) diet.

Methods

Search criteria

The Preferred Reporting Items for Systematic Reviews and Meta-Analyses (PRISMA, 2009) search strategy flow chart and checklist were used as guides in identifying and selecting relevant studies [21]. MEDLINE, EMBASE, Web of Science, the Cochrane Library and Proquest Theses and Dissertations database were used to search for articles containing a combination of the following words: s-adenosylmethionine, adomet, cognitive, cognition, dementia and Alzheimer's. Following these searches, MeSH terms were used to further extend the search. Study selection was restricted to the English language and all relevant papers published up until April 2014 were included in the analysis. Refer to Table S2 for an example of a more detailed search summary.

Reference lists of the selected articles from the original search were reviewed for additional relevant papers. The journals, of the articles that were selected from the primary search, were manually searched as well. A search of Proquest Dissertations and Theses was included to ensure that any unpublished theses were identified for relevant use. Correspondence authors were contacted for unpublished studies when possible; however, no unpublished works were available to us for two reasons: 1. There were no unpublished results that met the inclusion criteria or 2. The authors preferred not to disclose their work until it was submitted for publication.

Inclusion and Exclusion Criteria

The following criteria were used in the selection of studies for our meta-analysis: 1. All data must be of mouse model origin, 2. Studies must have a cognitive performance outcome as measured by the Y maze or MWM, which are commonly used tools in evaluating spatial learning/memory test in both mice and rats [20], 3. Studies were required to have both a SFD diet group and one or two of the following additional groups: a FD diet and/or a NC diet. Both healthy strains and transgenic mouse models of AD were used in the analysis (Table 1). The measure of interest was cognitive performance in the Y maze as measured by % of spontaneous alternations and latency, swim speed and number of annulus crossing as measured by the MWM.

Data extraction and management

Two researchers independently reviewed and selected studies based on the inclusion criteria. Mouse strains, ages, diets/interventions, duration of intervention and cognitive outcomes were identified and extracted from the methods sections of each study (Table 1). Authors were contacted for original data when possible. Means and standard errors of Y maze percent alternation scores were extracted from bar graphs using GraphClick 3.0.2 if authors preferred not to share data. Standard errors were converted to standard deviations for calculation of effect sizes. MWM data was not subject to quantitative data extraction as this data was used as a qualitative contribution in comparing meta-analyses results.

Study Quality Assessment

A modified version of the gold standard publication checklist (GSPC) developed by Hooijmans et al (2010) was used to assess the quality of the studies included in this analysis [22]. It should be noted that all studies, with the exception of Fuso et al 2012, were published prior to the publication of the GSPC; the GSPC was developed in response to insufficient detail provided in publications. The GSPC is a comprehensive and high quality tool for assessing quality of studies; however, its use in evaluating the quality of papers written prior to its publication may not be appropriate. Scores were re-scaled such that each study was ranked in comparison with the Fuso et al 2012 paper (the highest ranked paper in the overall analysis); Fuso et al 2012 was scaled to 100%.

Statistical Analysis

Comprehensive Meta Analysis (Version 2.0) was used to analyze the data and generate forest plots and funnel plots [23]. Means and standard deviations were used to generate the effect size estimates (i.e., Hedge's g). The Hedges's g effect-size estimate was generated given that it adjusts for the variation in sample sizes [24]. A random effects model was used to summarize the data; random effects models account for methodological and in part statistical variability. Tests of heterogeneity including the Q-statistic and I^2 statistic were calculated; I^2 scores of 25%, 50%, and 75% were considered low, moderate, and high heterogeneity, respectively [25]. Heterogeneity was further investigated using categorical data variables including type of mouse model (healthy vs. transgenic) and specific genotypes (ApoE4). Mixed-effect model

Table 1. Characteristics of mouse studies used in meta-analysis and qualitative analysis.

Study	Intervention	Sample size	Mouse model	Duration of treatment (months)	Age (months)	Favored Group: 1. FD vs SFD 2. NC vs SFD	Quality assessment score (%)[F]
1. Chan et al 2008A[A]	1. NC diet	1. n = 7[C]	Normal (C57B/6)	1	9–12	1. SFD	62
	2. FD diet	2. n = 7[C]				2. SFD	
	3. SFD diet (100 mg/kg)	3. n = 7[C]					
2. Chan et al 2008B[A]	1. NC diet	1. n = 7[C]	ApoE −/−	1	9–12	1. SFD	62
	2. FD diet	2. n = 7[C]				2. SFD	
	3. SFD diet (100 mg/kg)	3. n = 7[C]					
3. Chan et al 2008C[A]	1. NC diet	1. n = 7[C]	ApoE2	1	9–12	1. SFD	62
	2. FD diet	2. n = 7[C]				2. SFD	
	3. SFD diet (100 mg/kg)	3. n = 7[C]					
4. Chan et al 2008D[A]	1. NC diet	1. n = 7[C]	ApoE3	1	9–12	1. FD	62
	2. FD diet	2. n = 7[C]				2. NC	
	3. SFD diet (100 mg/kg)	3. n = 7[C]					
5. Chan et al 2008E[A]	1. NC diet	1. n = 7[C]	ApoE4	1	9–12	1. SFD	62
	2. FD diet	2. n = 7[C]				2. SFD	
	3. SFD diet (100 mg/kg)	3. n = 7[C]					
6. Chan et al 2008F[A]	1. NC diet	1. n = 7[C]	Healthy, Aged (C57B/6)	1	2–2.5 (years)	1. SFD	62
	2. FD diet	2. n = 7[C]				2. SFD	
	3. SFD diet (100 mg/kg)	3. n = 7[C]					
7. Chan et al 2008G[A]	1. NC diet	1. n = 7[C]	MTHFR +/+	1	9–12	1. SFD	62
	2. FD diet	2. n = 7[C]				2. NC	
	3. SFD diet (100 mg/kg)	3. n = 7[C]					
8. Chan et al 2008H[A]	1. NC diet	1. n = 7[C]	MTHFR +/−	1	9–12	1. SFD	62
	2. FD diet	2. n = 7[C]				2. SFD	
	3. SFD diet (100 mg/kg)	3. n = 7[C]					
9. Shea et al 2007A[A]	1. NC diet	1. n = 12	ApoE4	1 month SAM fortification for group 3 started 2 weeks after experiment started	9–12	1. SFD	66
	2. FD diet	2. n = 6				2. SFD	
	3. SFD diet (100 mg/kg)	3. n = 6					
10. Shea et al 2007B[A]	1. NC diet	1. n = 16	Normal (C57B/6)	1 month SAM fortification for group 3 started 2 weeks after experiment started	9–12	1. No comparison	66
	2. No group	2. N/A				2. SFD	
	3. SFD diet (100 mg/kg)	3. n = 8					

Table 1. Cont.

Study	Intervention	Sample size	Mouse model	Duration of treatment (months)	Age (months)	Favored Group: 1. FD vs SFD 2. NC vs SFD	Quality assessment score (%)^{F}
11. Tchantchou et al 2004A^{A}	1. NC diet	1. n = 11^{D}	ApoE−/−	1	9–12	1. FD	58
	2. FD diet	2. n = 11^{D}				2. NC	
	3. SFD diet (80 mg/kg)	3. n = 11^{D}					
12. Fuso et al 2012A^{B}	1. NC diet	1. n = 10	TgCRND8	3	3+3 weeks	Not included for quantitative analysis^{E}	100
	2. FD diet	2. n = 10					
	3. SFD diet (400 μg/mouse)	3. n = 9					
13. Fuso et al 2012B^{B}	1. NC diet	1. n = 8	129SV	3	3+3 weeks	Not included for quantitative analysis^{E}	100
	2. FD diet	2. n = 15					
	3. SFD diet (400 μg/mouse)	3. n = 12					

[A] Y maze used to measure spatial memory outcome.
[B] Morris Water Maze (MWM) used to measure spatial memory outcome.
[C] Sample size reported in original article as 3–4 mice in 2 independent experiments.
[D] Sample size reported as 3–4 mice/diet/experiment × 2–4 experiments for a total of 6–16 mice per treatment group.
[E] Data not included in quantitative analysis due to differences in measures, included in qualitative analysis for discussion.
[F] Quality assessment conducted using the Gold Standard Publication Checklist by Hooijmans (2010); quality assessment scores re-scaled such that the study with the highest quality score was set at 100 (% scale).

Study	Hedge's g	Standard Error	Variance	Lower Limit	Upper Limit	Z Value	P Value
Chan 2008A	1.8951	0.6154	0.3787	0.6890	3.1011	3.0796	0.0021
Chan 2008B	1.4648	0.5719	0.3270	0.3440	2.5857	2.5614	0.0104
Chan 2008C	0.7724	0.5213	0.2717	-0.2493	1.7940	1.4817	0.1384
Chan 2008D	-0.2005	0.5018	0.2518	-1.1841	0.7831	-0.3995	0.6895
Chan 2008E	4.6089	1.0045	1.0090	2.6401	6.5777	4.5882	0.0000
Chan 2008F	0.6084	0.5134	0.2636	-0.3979	1.6148	1.1850	0.2360
Chan 2008G	0.8205	0.5239	0.2744	-0.2063	1.8472	1.5661	0.1173
Chan 2008H	0.4845	0.5087	0.2588	-0.5125	1.4816	0.9524	0.3409
Tchantchou 2004A	-0.0497	0.4103	0.1683	-0.8538	0.7545	-0.1210	0.9037
Shea 2007A	4.2065	1.0106	1.0213	2.2257	6.1872	4.1624	0.0000
Random Effects	1.2104	0.3768	0.1420	0.4719	1.9489	3.2122	0.0013

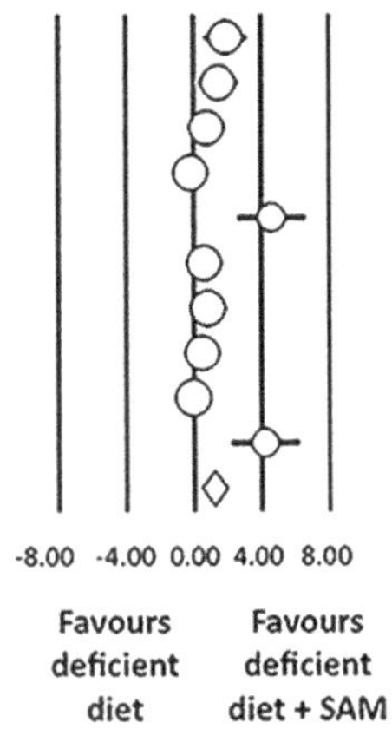

1A

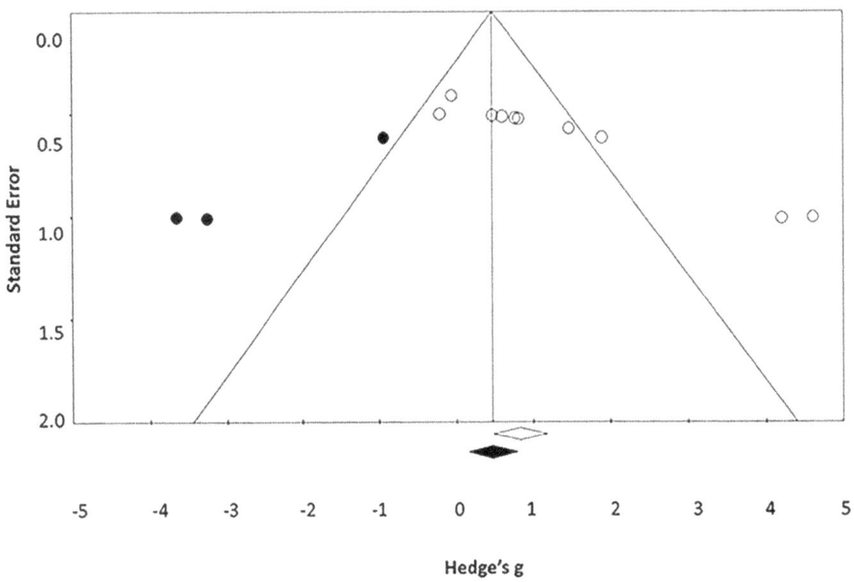

1B

Figure 1. A) Effect size estimate: Comparison of a folate deficient diet and a folate deficient diet supplemented with S-adenosylmethionine (SAM) using Hedge's g as the effect size estimate statistic. B) Funnel Plot representation of potential publication bias in the comparison of a folate deficient diet supplemented with S-adenosylmethionine (SAM).

meta-regression was utilized to examine the effect of potential *a priori* selected moderating factors including age, duration of treatment, and study quality assessment, on the overall effect-size estimate [26]. Funnel plots were used to examine the overall heterogeneity via visual presentation.

Results and Discussion

Search Results

A total of 2563 articles were found across all searches combined (Figure S1). A total of 1037 unique titles remained, after duplicates were removed. After reviewing article titles and/or abstracts, 19 articles were selected for further review. After full text review, 14 articles were eliminated because there was no cognitive performance outcome included in the study design or because the study did not incorporate a SAM intervention. Five articles remained, three were used in the meta-analysis, one was included as a qualitative accompaniment in the discussion of the results (Fuso et al 2012) and one was eliminated on the basis of previously published results (Tchantchou et al 2006). The Fuso et al 2012 paper was excluded from the quantitative analysis because the learning/memory tests were different and had different scoring outcomes; these discrepancies would have led to increase methodological heterogeneity. The cognitive performance tasks in the Fuso study measured latency, swim speed and annulus crossings on the Morris water maze; neither of these three measures could be combined with the other studies in a quantitative analysis without disrupting the integrity of the results. Data from the Tchantchou et al 2006 study came from the same sample as data in the Tchantchou et al 2004 study. The Tchantchou et al 2006 publication was excluded because it did not contain Y maze data; therefore, the Tchantchou et al 2004 paper was used for its Y maze data.

A total of 3 studies including 12 experiments comprised of 12 complete diet groups, 11 deficient diet groups and 11 deficient+ SAM groups were included in the meta-analysis (Table 1). The following sample sizes represent the summative sample size for each group: control (n = 100), FD (n = 84) and SFD (n = 81). Despite a low, but sufficient number of studies included in this meta-analysis, the number of mouse experiments contributed by

Study	Hedge's g	Standard Error	Variance	Lower Limit	Upper Limit	Z Value	P Value
Chan 2008A	0.0971	0.5007	0.2507	-0.8844	1.0785	0.1939	0.8463
Chan 2008B	0.5934	0.5128	0.2630	-0.4117	1.5985	1.1571	0.2472
Chan 2008C	0.6100	0.5135	0.2637	-0.3965	1.6164	1.1878	0.2349
Chan 2008D	-0.2603	0.5028	0.2528	-1.2458	0.7252	-0.5178	0.6046
Chan 2008E	1.8020	0.6053	0.3664	0.6156	2.9883	2.9770	0.0029
Chan 2008F	-0.3479	0.5047	0.2547	-1.3371	0.6413	-0.6893	0.4906
Chan 2008G	0.5206	0.5100	0.2601	-0.4789	1.5202	1.0209	0.3073
Chan 2008H	0.0531	0.5005	0.2505	-0.9279	1.0341	0.1061	0.9155
Tchantchou 2004A	-0.2710	0.4122	0.1699	-1.0790	0.5369	-0.6575	0.5109
Shea 2007A	2.0624	0.5873	0.3449	0.9113	3.2135	3.5117	0.0004
Shea 2007B	3.5209	0.6581	0.4331	2.2311	4.8107	5.3503	0.0000
Random Effects	0.7016	0.3251	0.1057	0.0645	1.3388	2.1584	0.0309

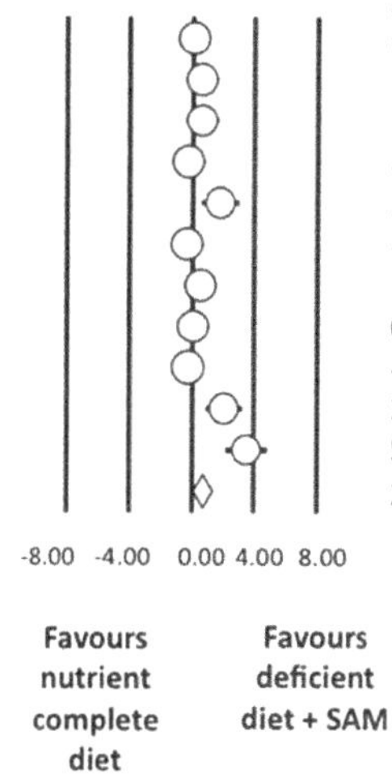

2A

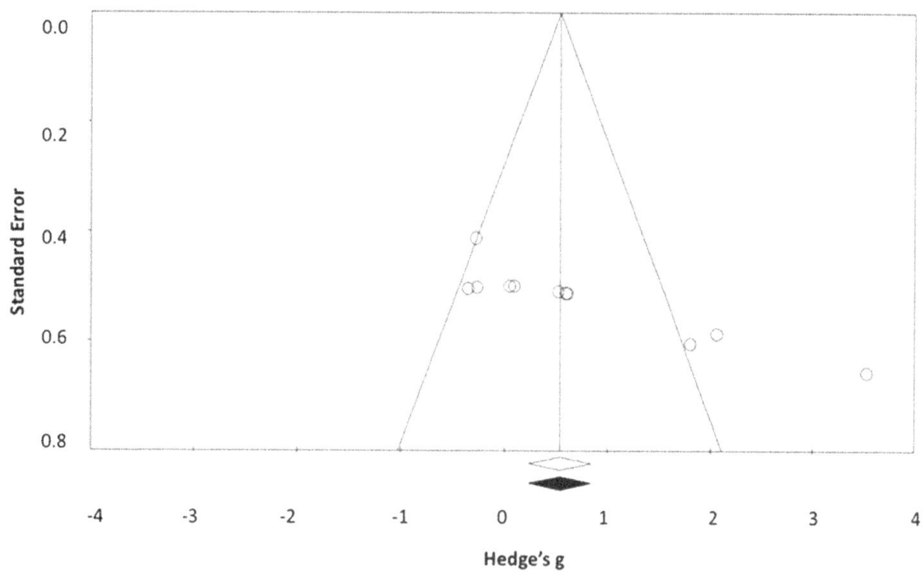

2B

Figure 2. A) Effect size estimate: Comparison of a nutrient complete diet and folate deficient diet supplemented with S-adenosylmethionine (SAM) using Hedge's g as the effect size estimate statistic. B) Funnel Plot representation of potential publication bias in the comparison of a nutrient complete diet with a folate deficient diet supplemented with S-adenosylmethionine (SAM).

these three studies made for sufficient power to conduct this meta-analysis. Finally, two studies including 4 subgroups comprised of 4 complete diet groups, 4 deficient diet groups and 2 deficient+SAM groups were included for qualitative review.

Study Characteristics

The mice receiving a SAM supplemented diet were treated with 80–100 g/kg of SAM or a nutraceutical formula containing 80–100 g/kg of SAM (Table 1). Duration of treatment ranged from 2 weeks to 1 month and mice were between 9 and 12 months of age except for one group, which were 2–2.5 years of age [13]. All studies utilized a folate deficient framework to assess the effects of SAM on cognitive performance. The deficient diet in two studies also included a vitamin E deficiency and addition of iron as a pro-oxidant [13,27]. Further to this, two of the studies used a nutraceutical formula comprised of a blend of several compounds including SAM, all of which have demonstrated to have neuroprotective properties [14,15]. Table 1 summarizes the genotypes of the transgenic animals.

Chan et al (2008) and Tchantchou et al (2004) reported sample sizes as a range for each experiment (ie. 3–4 mice were used for each group in a single study). It was not possible to obtain individual sample sizes for each group from the authors and therefore, an average of the range was calculated for the sample size in order to obtain effect sizes. Publication bias was minimized by contacting authors for unpublished data; however, no further relevant data was identified following communication with authors.

Effect of a SFD diet versus FD diet on cognitive performance

Three studies, including 10 subgroups, studied the effect of SAM supplementation on cognitive performance, within the context of a folate deficient diet. There was a significant effect of SAM supplementation on cognitive performance (Figure 1A, Table S3). Mice fed a SFD diet performed better than mice consuming a FD diet only ($g = 1.2104$[95%CI: 0.4719–1.9489], $p = 0.0013$). Heterogeneity was significant in the evaluation of the effects of a FD diet versus a SFD diet on cognitive performance ($I^2 = 76.9\%$, $p<0.001$). Healthy mice were analyzed separately from transgenic mice to further assess heterogeneity. In healthy mice, there was no difference between the groups ($g = 0.9399$[95%CI: −0.0184–1.8981], $p = 0.0546$). However, there was a significant effect of the SFD diet on cognitive performance in transgenic mice ($g = 1.3272$[95%CI: 0.3967–2.2577], $p = 0.0052$).

Heterogeneity was significant for the transgenic mouse analysis ($I^2 = 81.2\%$, $p<0.001$), but not for the healthy mouse analysis ($I^2 = 39.0\%$, $p = 0.2003$). The heterogeneity in the transgenic subgroup may be attributed to variations in performance response to FD diets across genotypes. There were three healthy mouse subgroups and seven transgenic mouse subgroups; therefore, the difference in sample size would no doubt contribute to differences in heterogeneity in the two analyses. There were not enough subgroups to apply genotype as a moderating variable to further evaluate heterogeneity; however, this would be a worthwhile analysis to consider in future meta-analyses when more data is available. Treatment effect size was associated with quality assessment ($p<0.05$) and treatment duration ($p<0.05$). Finally, a funnel plot of the 11 studies is presented in Figure 1B. The asymmetrical appearance of this plot suggests the potential presence of publication bias; however, it is difficult to assess this condition as none of these data come from unpublished work. With all studies coming from the same lab, there may or may not be an element of publication bias.

In comparison with results from the Fuso lab, there was a significant difference between the FD mice and the SFD mice in number of annulus crossings with the SFD group having a higher number of annulus crossings than the FD group. This result is in agreement with the Shea lab, in which, SAM supplementation improves cognitive performance in the Y maze in mice fed folate deficient diets. The increase in number of annulus crossings made by the TgCRND8 mice was not observed in wild type mice and, in fact, the opposite was observed, in which, mice consuming a SFD diet made fewer crossings than mice consuming a FD diet. The large differences between strains, across both labs, suggest substantial genotypic responses to folate deficiencies.

Quality assessment and diet duration both interacted with diet type ($p<0.001$ and $p<0.001$ respectively), accounting for a proportion of the variance in cognitive performance (Table S4). There was only one group of mice that differed in age from the other groups [13]; no association of age with diet type on cognitive performance was observed ($p = 0.7533$).

SFD diet versus a NC diet and cognitive performance

There was a significant difference between mice fed a SFD diet and mice consuming a NC diet (Figure 2A, Table S3). Mice fed a SFD diet performed better on the Y maze than mice fed a NC diet ($g = 0.7016$[95%CI: 0.0645–1.3388], $p = 0.0309$). Heterogeneity was significant ($I^2 = 76.7\%$, $p<0.001$) and an asymmetrical funnel plot suggested the possibility of publication bias (Figure 2B). None of the studies included in this analysis were unpublished; however, all efforts to contact authors were made. Therefore, we believe that publication bias is minimal.

Healthy animals and transgenic animals were analyzed separately to further investigate heterogeneity; despite separation of the groups, heterogeneity was still significant (Healthy: $I^2 = 89.4\%$, $p< 0.001$; Transgenic: $I^2 = 65.9\%$, $p = 0.0046$). Healthy mice and transgenic mice, consuming the SFD diet, did not perform any better than mice consuming the NC diet for either group (Healthy: $g = 1.3461$[95%CI: −0.5743–3.2665], $p = 0.1695$; Transgenic: $g = 0.4716$[95%CI: −0.1357–1.0788], $p = 0.1280$). The heterogeneity in the healthy animal analysis may be explained, in part, by the substantial variability found among a small number of studies.

There was an association between diet type and quality assessment ($p = 0.0116$) and diet type and diet duration ($p = 0.0164$); however, there was no association between mouse age and diet type ($p = 0.7533$) on cognitive performance (Table S5). The impact of quality assessment and diet duration would inevitably contribute to the heterogeneity in this analysis. All of the mice from each subgroup were placed on their diets for 1 month except for the mice in the Shea (2007) study who were on diets for 2 weeks. Interestingly, the effect size for the Shea (2007) study was much greater than effect sizes for the other studies despite the 2-week diet duration; however, the sample size for the Shea 2007 study was much greater than the other studies and may partially explain this result (refer to table 1 for sample sizes).

In considering these findings, it is important to recognize that while all of the mice in the treatment group received SAM, one of the mouse groups received a nutraceutical formula containing SAM combined with other compounds; Shea (2007) included N-acetyl cysteine and acetyl-L-carnitine in their SAM-containing nutraceutical preparations. While SAM was the intervention of interest in this analysis, it is possible that other compounds in the formulation may have contributed to the positive result found in this analysis via an addition or synergistic mechanism. In addition, although all diets studied SAM supplementation within the context of a folate deficient diet, the Fuso lab deficient diet was also deficient in vitamins B6 and B12. The differences in study design of these experiments may contribute to variability between study results and this should be taken into consideration in the interpretation of these results. The small number of studies, containing other ingredients besides SAM, did not allow for further analysis of nutraceutical compounds as a moderating variable. However, evaluating clinical significance and efficacy of these neuroprotective compounds would be a worthwhile investigation in future reviews.

Additionally, it is important to note that while every effort was taken to increase accuracy of reported sample sizes, this error cannot be overlooked in the interpretation of these results. Underreporting methodological details in animal model studies is prevalent and more recently, publication reporting guidelines and checklists have been developed in response to these issues [22,28]. It is imperative that future studies include these details in published work, either in the body of the paper or as supplementary material. In addition, publication bias has been demonstrated to be substantial in animal model literature. Registering animal model studies has been suggested as a means of reducing publication bias in meta-analyses; however, at this time there is no policy concerning this matter [29].

Although the literature search was extensive, all of the studies that were selected for this analysis and review came from only two labs; therefore, the diversity of this research, at this time, is limited. However, this meta-analysis allows for comparison of results within the Shea lab and between the Shea and Fuso labs and demonstrates that although there are some differences among findings within and between the labs, there appears to be evidence to support the use of SAM as a nutraceutical treatment for cognitive decline. Given the findings of this analysis, further research is warranted, particularly at the randomized controlled trial stage. Although it was not possible to include the Fuso et al (2012) study in the quantitative analysis, the trend of improved cognitive performance associated with SAM supplementation continues throughout the Fuso lab. The results of this meta-analysis substantiate the claim that SAM can improve cognitive performance in mice with compromise cognitive abilities. However, the number of studies, sample size accuracy and heterogeneity are substantial limitations and should be addressed in future studies.

The findings of this analysis suggest that there is evidence that SAM can improve spatial memory and learning in both healthy and transgenic mice fed a nutrient deficient diet. In combination, with human data from the Shea lab [12,13,30] and others [7,8,31], it is reasonable to expect that SAM could benefit those with reduced folate status or genotypes at higher risk for AD development.

Implications for clinical practice and research

Further research concerning the roles of SAM and folate in human cognition should consider the relationship between folate fortification and SAM. Folate fortification, in North America, has resulted in a substantial improvement in folate status in North Americans; however, it appears that the effect of folate fortification on homocysteine concentrations is still unclear [32]. There is some evidence that an increase in folate status is not associated with a reduction in homocysteine; however, it is difficult to make this conclusion since B12 and B6 also play key roles in clearing plasma homocysteine [32]. This evidence, in conjunction with the theory that homocysteine may have no direct role in cognitive performance, suggests that the relationship between folate and SAM are still unclear. If dysfunction of the homocysteine-methionine cycle is not the direct cause of cognitive decline, then it is plausible that SAM exhibits an effect on cognitive performance separate from this cycle, which likely involves more complex epigenetic mechanisms.

Despite folic acid fortification, many people struggle to maintain sufficient folate status due to nutrient-drug/nutrient-gene interactions or poor intake of folate fortified foods [33]. Individuals taking "anti-folate drugs" such as oral contraceptives, anti-convulsants and anti-cancer drugs may be at an increased risk for poor folate status and subsequent risk for cognitive decline later in life [34,35]. If there is a substantial impact of folate on SAM and vice versa, in relation to cognitive performance, then these populations stand to benefit from this supplement. SAM may also be an appropriate alternative for people who are unable to absorb and/or metabolize B vitamins from food or supplements. Of particular importance is decreased absorption of vitamin B12 in the elderly [36].

In addition to the effects of nutrient-drug interactions on folate metabolism, the differences in the ApoE4 mice, between the treatment and control groups, is noteworthy. It would be interesting to evaluate the effects of SAM supplementation on CpG methylation in these mice compared to ApoE2, ApoE3 and MTHFR −/− mice. If it is true that Apoe4 mice respond more strongly to SAM supplementation than other genotypes, then SAM may be more appropriate in the prevention of cognitive decline in the ApoE4 genotype than other genotypes. Further research using mouse and human models are needed to capture a more comprehensive analysis of the effects of this gene variant on SAM and cognitive performance.

Future research should consider the effect of SAM supplementation on healthy individuals consuming a healthy diet and individuals with gene variants who also consume a healthy diet. Investigation into the effects of SAM on disease risk in individuals taking anti-folate medications is also warranted. Finally, evaluation of the clinical significance and effectiveness of SAM as a supplement for cognitive performance is also important.

Authors' conclusions

Supplementing a folate deficient diet with SAM appears to improve performance in spatial memory tasks on the Y maze. These results can be observed in transgenic mice, but not in healthy mice, when analyzed separately. More data with clear and consistent methodologies are required to substantiate these claims. Finally, genotypes with a higher risk for AD, such as the ApoE4 mouse, demonstrated greater responses to SAM supplementation than other genotypes, suggesting an epigenetic affinity by SAM for this animal model.

Supporting Information

Figure S1 PRISMA search strategy flow diagram.

Table S1 PRISMA checklist.

Table S2 Effect size estimates: 1. FD diet versus SFD diet, 2. NC diet versus SFD diet (n = 3).

Table S3 Meta-regression analysis: FD diet versus SFD diet (N represents number of mouse studies).

Table S4 Meta-regression analysis: NC diet versus SFD diet (N represents number of mouse studies).

Table S5 Full search strategy for Cochrane Review search.

Table S6 Raw data file.

Acknowledgments

We wish to thank Mount Saint Vincent University and the Tula Foundation for funding this research.

Author Contributions

Conceived and designed the experiments: SEM JEK. Performed the experiments: SEM JDW. Analyzed the data: AAS. Wrote the paper: SEM AAS JDW JEK.

References

1. Batsch NL, Mittelman MS, Blankman K, Ellenbogen M, Graham N, et al. (2012) World alzheimer report 2012: Overcoming the stigma of dementia.
2. Anonymous (2012) A new way of looking at the impact of dementia in canada.
3. Graham N, Emery T, Hodges J. (2004) Distinctive cognitive profiles in alzheimer's disease and subcortical vascular dementia. Journal of Neurology, Neurosurgery & Psychiatry 75: 61–71.
4. Cavallaro RA, Fuso A, Nicolia V, Scarpa S. (2010) S-adenosylmethionine prevents oxidative stress and modulates glutathione metabolism in TgCRND8 mice fed a B-vitamin deficient diet. J Alzheimer's Dis 20: 997–1002.
5. Fuso A, Nicolia V, Ricceri L, Cavallaro RA, Isopi E, et al. (2012) S-adenosylmethionine reduces the progress of the alzheimer-like features induced by B-vitamin deficiency in mice. Neurobiol Aging 33: 1482. e1–1482. e16.
6. Hooijmans CR, Blom HJ, Oppenraaij-Emmerzaal D, Ritskes-Hoitinga M, Kiliaan AJ. (2009) S-adenosylmethionine and S-adenosylhomocysteine levels in the aging brain of APP/PS1 alzheimer mice. Neurol Sci 30: 439–445.
7. Rudolph ML, Rabinoff M, Kagan BL. (2011) A prospective, open-label, 12 week trial of S-adenosylmethionine in the symptomatic treatment of alzheimer's disease. Neuroscience & Medicine 2: 222–225.
8. Thompson MA, Bauer BA, Loehrer LL, Cha SS, Mandrekar JN, et al. (2009) Dietary supplement S-adenosyl-L-methionine (AdoMet) effects on plasma

homocysteine levels in healthy human subjects: A double-blind, placebo-controlled, randomized clinical trial. Journal of Alternative and Complementary Medicine 15: 523–529.
9. Chan A, Rogers E, Shea TB. (2009) Dietary deficiency in folate and vitamin E under conditions of oxidative stress increases phospho-tau levels: Potentiation by ApoE4 and alleviation by S-adenosylmethionine. J Alzheimer's Dis 17: 483–487.
10. Coppedè F. (2010) One-carbon metabolism and alzheimer's disease: Focus on epigenetics. Curr Genomics 11: 246.
11. Chan A, Tchantchou F, Rogers EJ, Shea TB. (2009) Dietary deficiency increases presenilin expression, gamma-secretase activity, and abeta levels: Potentiation by ApoE genotype and alleviation by s-adenosyl methionine. J Neurochem 110: 831–836.
12. Remington R, Chan A, Paskavitz J, Shea TB. (2009) Efficacy of a vitamin/nutriceutical formulation for moderate-stage to later-stage alzheimer's disease: A placebo-controlled pilot study. Am J Alzheimers Dis Other Demen 24: 27–33.
13. Chan A, Tchantchou F, Graves V, Rozen R, Shea T. (2008) Dietary and genetic compromise in folate availability reduces acetylcholine, cognitive performance and increases aggression: Critical role of S-adenosyl methionine. The Journal of Nutrition, Health and Aging 12: 252–261.
14. Shea TB. (2007) Effects of dietary supplementation with N-acetyl cysteine, acetyl-L-carnitine and S-adenosyl methionine on cognitive performance and aggression in normal mice and mice expressing human ApoE4. Neuromolecular medicine 9: 264–269.
15. Tchantchou F, Graves M, Ortiz D, Rogers E, Shea TB. (2004) Dietary supplementation with 3-deaza adenosine, N-acetyl cysteine, and S-adenosyl methionine provide neuroprotection against multiple consequences of vitamin deficiency and oxidative challenge. Neuromol Med 6: 93–103.
16. Huang Y. (2011) Roles of apolipoprotein E4 (ApoE4) in the pathogenesis of alzheimer's disease: Lessons from ApoE mouse models. *
*. Biochem Soc Trans 39: 924.
17. Herrmann M, Tami A, Wildemann B, Wolny M, Wagner A, et al. (2009) Hyperhomocysteinemia induces a tissue specific accumulation of homocysteine in bone by collagen binding and adversely affects bone. Bone 44: 467–475.
18. Veeranna V, Zalawadiya SK, Niraj A, Pradhan J, Ference B, et al. (2011) Homocysteine and reclassification of cardiovascular disease risk. J Am Coll Cardiol 58: 1025–1033.
19. Ordovás JM, Smith CE. (2010) Epigenetics and cardiovascular disease. Nature Reviews Cardiology 7: 510–519.
20. Stewart S, Cacucci F, Lever C. (2011) Which memory task for my mouse? A systematic review of spatial memory performance in the tg2576 alzheimer's mouse model. J Alzheimer's Dis 26: 105–126.
21. Moher D, Liberati A, Tetzlaff J, Altman DG. (2009) Preferred reporting items for systematic reviews and meta-analyses: The PRISMA statement. Ann Intern Med 151: 264–269.
22. Hooijmans C, de Vries R, Leenaars M, Ritskes-Hoitinga M. (2011) The gold standard publication checklist (GSPC) for improved design, reporting and scientific quality of animal studies GSPC versus ARRIVE guidelines. Lab Anim 45: 61–61.
23. Borenstein M, Hedges LV, Higgins JP, Rothstein HR. (2011) Comprehensive meta analysis. 2.0.
24. Hedges LV, Olkin I, Statistiker M, Olkin I, Olkin I. (1985) Statistical methods for meta-analysis.: Academic Press New York.
25. Higgins JP, Thompson SG, Deeks JJ, Altman DG. (2003) Measuring inconsistency in meta-analyses. BMJ: British Medical Journal 327: 557.
26. DerSimonian R, Laird N. (1986) Meta-analysis in clinical trials. Control Clin Trials 7: 177–188.
27. Tchantchou F, Graves M, Ortiz D, Rogers E, Shea TB. (2004) Dietary supplementation with 3-deaza adenosine, N-acetyl cysteine, and S-adenosyl methionine provide neuroprotection against multiple consequences of vitamin deficiency and oxidative challenge. Neuromolecular medicine 6: 93–103.
28. Kilkenny C, Browne W, Cuthill IC, Emerson M, Altman DG. (2010) Animal research: Reporting in vivo experiments: The ARRIVE guidelines. Br J Pharmacol 160: 1577–1579.
29. Perel P, Roberts I, Sena E, Wheble P, Briscoe C, et al. (2007) Comparison of treatment effects between animal experiments and clinical trials: Systematic review. BMJ 334: 197.
30. Chan A, Remington R, Kotyla E, Lepore A, Zemianek J, et al. (2010) A vitamin/nutriceutical formulation improves memory and cognitive performance in community-dwelling adults without dementia. The Journal of Nutrition Health and Aging 14: 224–230.
31. Bottiglieri T, Godfrey P, Flynn T, Carney M, Toone B, et al. (1990) Cerebrospinal fluid S-adenosylmethionine in depression and dementia: Effects of treatment with parenteral and oral S-adenosylmethionine. Journal of Neurology, Neurosurgery & Psychiatry 53: 1096–1098.
32. Enquobahrie DA, Feldman HA, Hoelscher DH, Steffen LM, Webber LS, et al. (2012) Serum homocysteine and folate concentrations among a US cohort of adolescents before and after folic acid fortification. Public Health Nutrition 15: 1818.
33. Shuaibi AM, House JD, Sevenhuysen GP. (2008) Folate status of young canadian women after folic acid fortification of grain products. J Am Diet Assoc 108: 2090–2094.
34. Sener U, Zorlu Y, Karaguzel O, Ozdamar O, Coker I, et al. (2006) Effects of common anti-epileptic drug monotherapy on serum levels of homocysteine, vitamin B12, folic acid and vitamin B6. Seizure 15: 79–85.
35. Wani NA, Hamid A, Kaur J. (2008) Folate status in various pathophysiological conditions. IUBMB Life 60: 834–842.
36. Andrès E, Loukili NH, Noel E, Kaltenbach G, Abdelgheni MB, et al. (2004) Vitamin B12 (cobalamin) deficiency in elderly patients. Can Med Assoc J 171: 251–259.

Prevalence of Goiter and Thyroid Nodules before and after Implementation of the Universal Salt Iodization Program in Mainland China from 1985 to 2014

Wei Zhao[9], Cheng Han[9], Xiaoguang Shi[9], Chuhui Xiong, Jie Sun, Zhongyan Shan, Weiping Teng*

Department of Endocrinology and Metabolism, Institute of Endocrinology, Liaoning Provincial Key Laboratory of Endocrine Diseases, the First Affiliated Hospital of China Medical University, Shenyang, Liaoning Province, People's Republic of China

Abstract

Objectives: We comprehensively estimated the prevalence of goiter and thyroid nodules (TNs) before and after the implementation of the Universal Salt Iodization (USI) program in mainland China and provided information for creating effective health policies.

Methods: PubMed, Google Scholar, CNKI, Chinese Wanfang and Chongqing VIP databases were searched for relevant studies from Jan 1985 to Feb 2014. Data from eligible citations were extracted by two independent reviewers. All analyses were performed with Stata 11.0 and SPSS 17.0.

Results: Eligible articles (N = 31; 4 in English and 27 in Chinese) included 52 studies (15 about goiter rates made before 1996 and 14 afterwards, and 23 about TNs). Our meta-analysis suggests a pooled prevalence for goiter before and after 1996 and for TNs of 22.8% (95% CI: 15.3%, 30.3%), 12.6% (95% CI: 9.4%, 15.8%) and 22.7% (95% CI: 18.3%, 27.0%), respectively. Egger's test of three independent categories revealed no evidence of publication bias ($p = 0.101$, 0.148 and 0.113, respectively).

Conclusions: The prevalence of goiter was reduced by almost half after 1996 in mainland China, so the USI program was considered beneficial. However, subgroup analysis suggests that both insufficient and excess iodine may be associated with goiter. The prevalence of goiter and TNs increased significantly after 2002, suggesting a risk of excessive iodine intake. Thus, salt iodization standardizations should be set according to local conditions.

Editor: Yue Wang, National Institute for Viral Disease Control and Prevention, CDC, China, China

Funding: This work was supported by the National Natural Science Foundation (81370893, URL: http://npd.nsfc.gov.cn/fundingProjectSearchAction.action). The funders had no role in study design, data collection and analysis, decision to publish, or preparation of the manuscript.

Competing Interests: The authors have declared that no competing interests exist.

* Email: twp@vip.163.com

[9] These authors contributed equally to this work.

Introduction

Iodine is an essential trace element required for the normal thyroid hormone activity, specifically that of thyroxine and triiodothyronine. Both insufficient and excessive iodine intake can cause thyroid-hormone disorders [1–4] and the presence of goiter and thyroid nodules (TNs) represents thyroid diseases. The term *goiter* describes the enlargement of the thyroid gland and the goiter prevalence of this condition is considered an important and sensitive long-term indicator of iodine intake [1,5]. The prevalence of goiter in school-age children is related to the severity of iodine deficiency. For example, a prevalence of 0.0–4.9% suggests no iodine deficiency; 5.0–19.9% indicates mild deficiency; 20.0–29.9% reveals moderate deficiency; and severe deficiency is observed at ≥30% [1]. Excessive iodine, however, can also lead to goiter [1].

TNs are discrete structurally distinct lesions within the thyroid gland, separate from the surrounding parenchyma [6]. Previous work indicates that the frequency of TNs vary considerably among the general population—4–7% are detected by palpation [7], 20–76% are found with ultrasound [8,9], and 19–67% are documented from autopsy data [10–12]. Although most TNs are benign, cancer should be suspected with the presence of TNs [6,13], because 5–15% may be malignant (carcinomas) [14]. Thus, goiter and TNs are

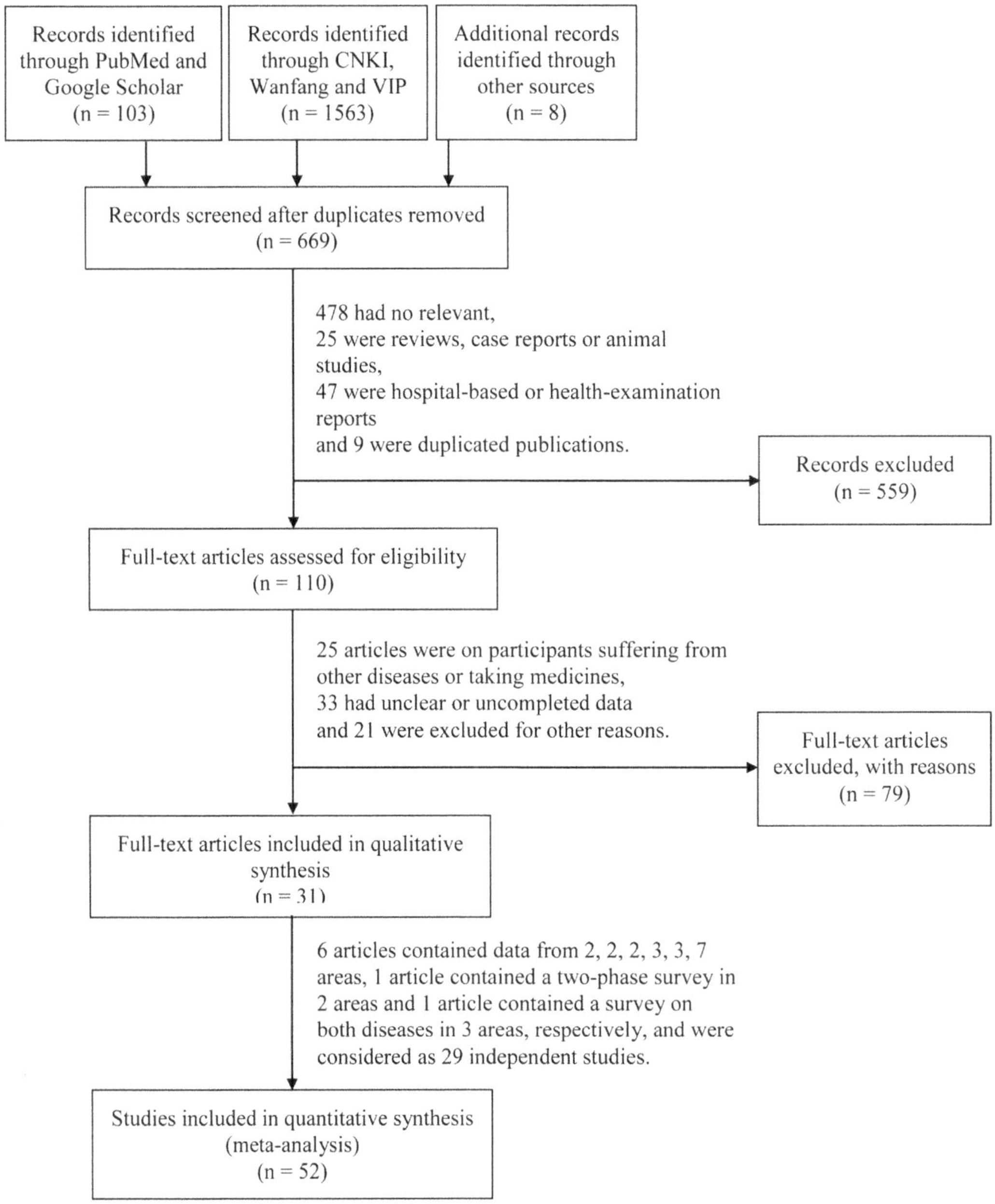

Figure 1. Flow diagram of the literature-search process.

common thyroid disorders with an intimate association with iodine intake.

China was once an iodine-deficient country; prior to the 1970s, 370 million people lived in iodine-deficient areas [15]. Iodine deficiencies manifested various ways, including goiter, cretinism, endemic mental retardation, and decreased fertility rates [1], all of which are generally classified as iodine deficiency disorders (IDDs) [1,16]. To reduce IDDs, in 1979, a program of local iodine fortification was introduced into these iodine-deficient areas; and in 1996, China launched the Universal Salt Iodization (USI) program [17]. Although the USI program reduced the prevalence of goiter, the median urinary iodine concentration (UIC) in school-age children simultaneously rose sharply—reaching 330 µg/L in 1997 and 306 µg/L in 1999. For this reason, in 2002, national standards for iodized salt were revised to reduce the iodine concentration at the production level [5]. In 2012, global data identified China as a region with more than adequate iodine intake [18]. Meanwhile, since the implementation of the USI program, a growing number of Chinese clinical endocrinologists have reported an increasing incidence of thyroid diseases, especially in recent years [19–25].

China has diverse environments with varied populations and socio-economic conditions, complicating unified epidemiological investigations for prevalence of goiter and TNs, most of which were limited to specific geographic areas or populations. Thus, data may not accurately represent these two diseases especially in light of the implementation of the USI program which may skew data for the epidemiology of goiter and TNs. Thus, to formulate appropriate local public health policies and

Table 1. Characteristics of studies on the prevalence of goiter and TNs.

First author	Publication year	Area	Rural/Urban	Inland/Coastal	Study year	Sample size	Case	Prevalence (%)
Prevalence of goiter before 1996								
Wang LF [29]	1992	Kunlun Plain, Xinjiang	Rural	Inland	1987	1236	629	50.89
Wang LF [29]	1992	Kunlun Plain, Xinjiang	Rural	Inland	1987	3686	1223	33.18
Wang LF [29]	1992	Kunlun Plain, Xinjiang	Rural	Inland	1987	2351	415	17.65
Dou DX [30]	1992	Zhaoguan, Anhui	Rural	Inland	1986	398	71	17.84
Chen HM [31]	2000	Puyang, Henan	Rural	Inland	1990	1589	336	21.15
Zhang JL [32]	1992	Linyi, Shandong	Mixed	Inland	1985	48083	2324	4.83
Zhang JL [32]	1992	Linyi, Shandong	Mixed	Inland	1989	110609	3445	3.11
Wu WY [33]	2002	Qingyuan, Zhejiang	Rural	Inland	1985	154451	60434	39.13
Zhang Z [34]	2002	Fuzhou, Fujian	Urban	Coastal	1989	10454	584	5.59
Zhang Z [34]	2002	Wuyishan, Fujian	Urban	Inland	1989	1032	253	24.52
Bao Y [35]	1994	Xuzhou, Jiangsu	Rural	Inland	1990	81548	16720	20.50
Bao Y [35]	1994	Xuzhou, Jiangsu	Urban	Inland	1990	3999	732	18.30
Su MY [36]	1989	Tekesi, Xinjiang	Rural	Inland	1987	202	92	45.54
Su MY [36]	1989	Tekesi, Xinjiang	Rural	Inland	1987	220	54	24.55
Zheng HB [37]	1988	Cangzhou, Hebei	Rural	Inland	1985	16324	2631	16.12
Prevalence of goiter after 1996								
Yu J [38]	2004	Huachuan, Heilongjiang	Rural	Inland	2002	112	21	18.75
Yu XH [39]	2008	Panshan, Liaoning	Rural	Inland	1999	815	189	23.19
Yu XH [39]	2008	Zhangwu, Liaoning	Rural	Inland	1999	1514	256	16.91
Yu XH [39]	2008	Huanghua, Hebei	Rural	Inland	1999	1056	80	7.58
Zhao SH [40]	2004	Yantai, Shandong	Rural	Coastal	2000	554	60	10.83
Zhao SH [40]	2004	Weihai, Shandong	Rural	Coastal	2000	543	54	9.94
Zhao SH [40]	2004	Weihai, Shandong	Rural	Coastal	2000	437	32	7.32
Zhao SH [40]	2004	Rizhao, Shandong	Rural	Coastal	2000	610	51	8.36
Zhao SH [40]	2004	Rizhao, Shandong	Rural	Coastal	2000	330	43	13.03
Zhao SH [40]	2004	Qingdao, Shandong	Rural	Coastal	2000	570	49	8.60
Zhao SH [40]	2004	Wulian, Shandong	Rural	Inland	2000	562	24	4.27
Zhang Z [34]	2002	Fuzhou, Fujian	Urban	Coastal	1999	3473	272	7. 83
Zhang Z [34]	2002	Wuyishan, Fujian	Urban	Inland	1999	2394	277	11.57
Zhu WY [41]	2009	Zhoushan, Zhejiang	Mixed	Coastal	2007	1389	421	30.31
Prevalence of TNs								
Yu XH [39]	2008	Panshan, Liaoning	Rural	Inland	1999	815	103	12.64
Yu XH [39]	2008	Zhangwu, Liaoning	Rural	Inland	1999	1514	154	10.17
Yu XH [39]	2008	Huanghua, Hebei	Rural	Inland	1999	1056	114	10.80
Chen ZX [42]	2013	Hangzhou, Zhejiang	Mixed	Inland	2010	9412	2822	29.98
Lou XM [43]	2011	Daishan, etc, Zhejiang	Mixed	Coastal	2009	456	66	14.47
Lou XM [43]	2011	Haining, etc, Zhejiang	Mixed	Coastal	2009	321	48	14.95
Lou XM [43]	2011	Xiangshan, etc, Zhejiang	Mixed	Coastal	2009	280	59	21.07
Feng SY [44]	2006	Gaochun and Chuzhou, Jiangsu	Rural	Inland	2005	2280	407	17.85
Li SJ [45]	2012	Fenghua, Zhejiang	Rural	Coastal	2010	781	160	20.49
Chi HY [46]	2013	Weihai, Shandong	Urban	Coastal	2008	4405	1390	31.56
Chen LD [47]	2011	Lishui, Zhejiang	Rural	Inland	2006	638	245	38.40
Wang XD [48]	2008	Wuxi, Jiangsu	Urban	Inland	2005	750	169	22.53
Liu F [49]	2012	Ruian, Zhejiang	Urban	Inland	2010	5060	1166	23.04
Yang NZ [50]	2012	Taizhou, Zhejiang	Mixed	Inland	2010	793	182	22.95
Liu ZY [51]	2012	Zhoushan, Zhejiang	Mixed	Coastal	2010	3206	926	28.88
Zhu WY [52]	2010	Zhoushan, Zhejiang	Mixed	Coastal	2006	3284	831	25.30

Table 1. Cont.

First author	Publication year	Area	Rural/Urban	Inland/Coastal	Study year	Sample size	Case	Prevalence (%)
Zou SR [27]	2012	Shanghai	Mixed	Coastal	2009	7369	2011	27.29
Guo HW [53]	2014	Nanjing, Jiangsu	Urban	Inland	2011	9533	4439	46.56
Zhang JL [54]	2013	Yan'an, Shanxi	Mixed	Inland	2012	2970	822	27.68
Liu Y [55]	2012	Chengdu, Sichuan	Urban	Inland	2009	1500	255	17.00
Yang YX [56]	2011	Guiyang, Guizhou	Urban	Inland	2009	1512	153	10.12
Shen Y [57]	2013	Shanghai	Mixed	Coastal	2010	695	159	22.88
Zhang SG [58]	2010	Xuzhou, Jiangsu	Rural	Inland	2008	468	117	25.00

criteria, we must document the epidemiology and distribution of both diseases and use the few previous studies to provide comprehensive analyses of detailed explorations and secular trends, geographic properties, and iodine status.

Here, we describe a systematic review and meta-analysis of the prevalence of goiter and TNs before and after implementation of the USI program in mainland China from 1985 to 2014.

Materials and Methods

Search Strategy

Goiter and TNs are independent diseases and iodine intake in China changed markedly after 1996 after the implementation of USI. Therefore, we conducted three meta-analyses—one on the prevalence of goiter before 1996 and one after 1996 and one analysis of the prevalence of TNs. We searched all English-

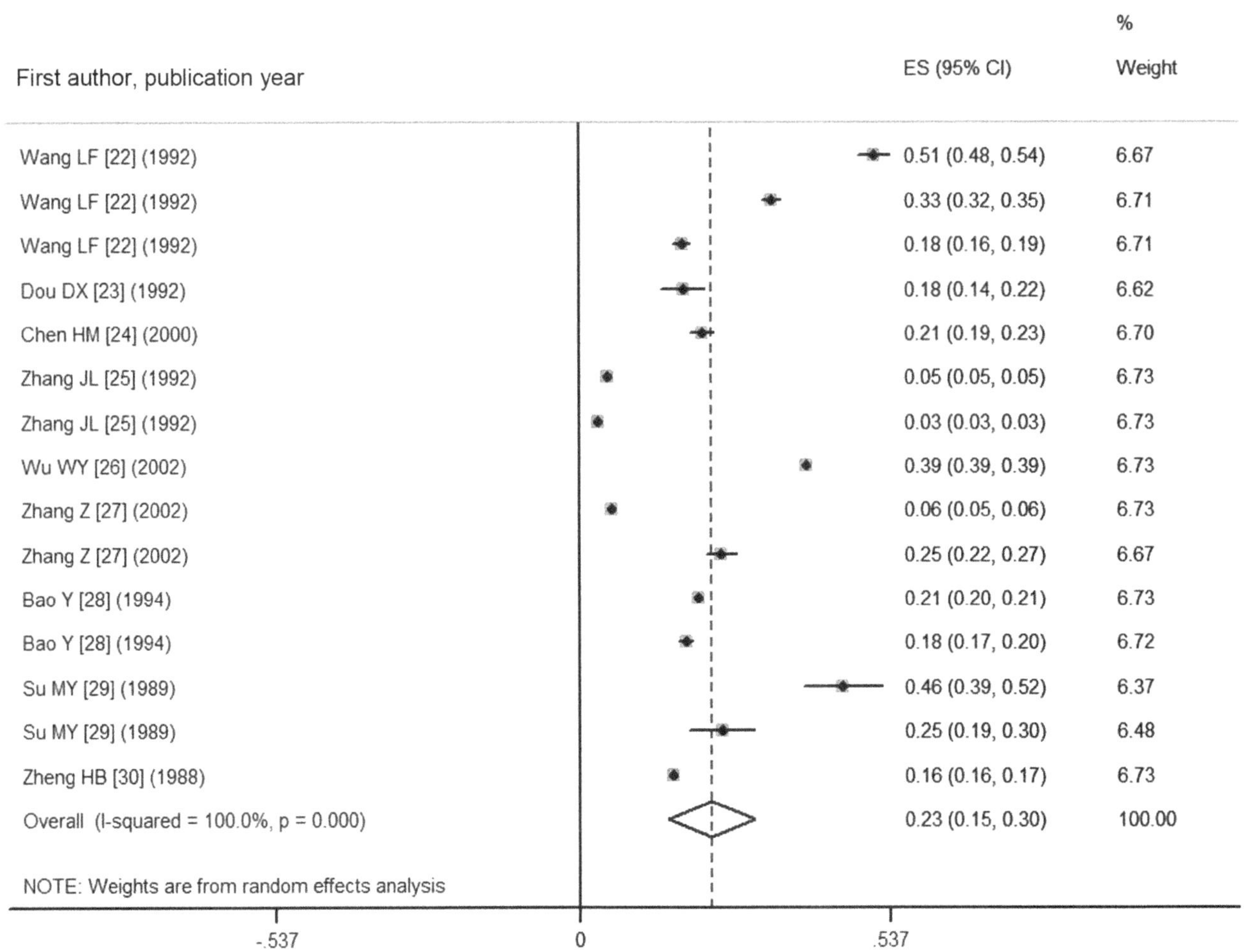

Figure 2. Forest plot displaying the pooled goiter prevalence in mainland China before 1996.

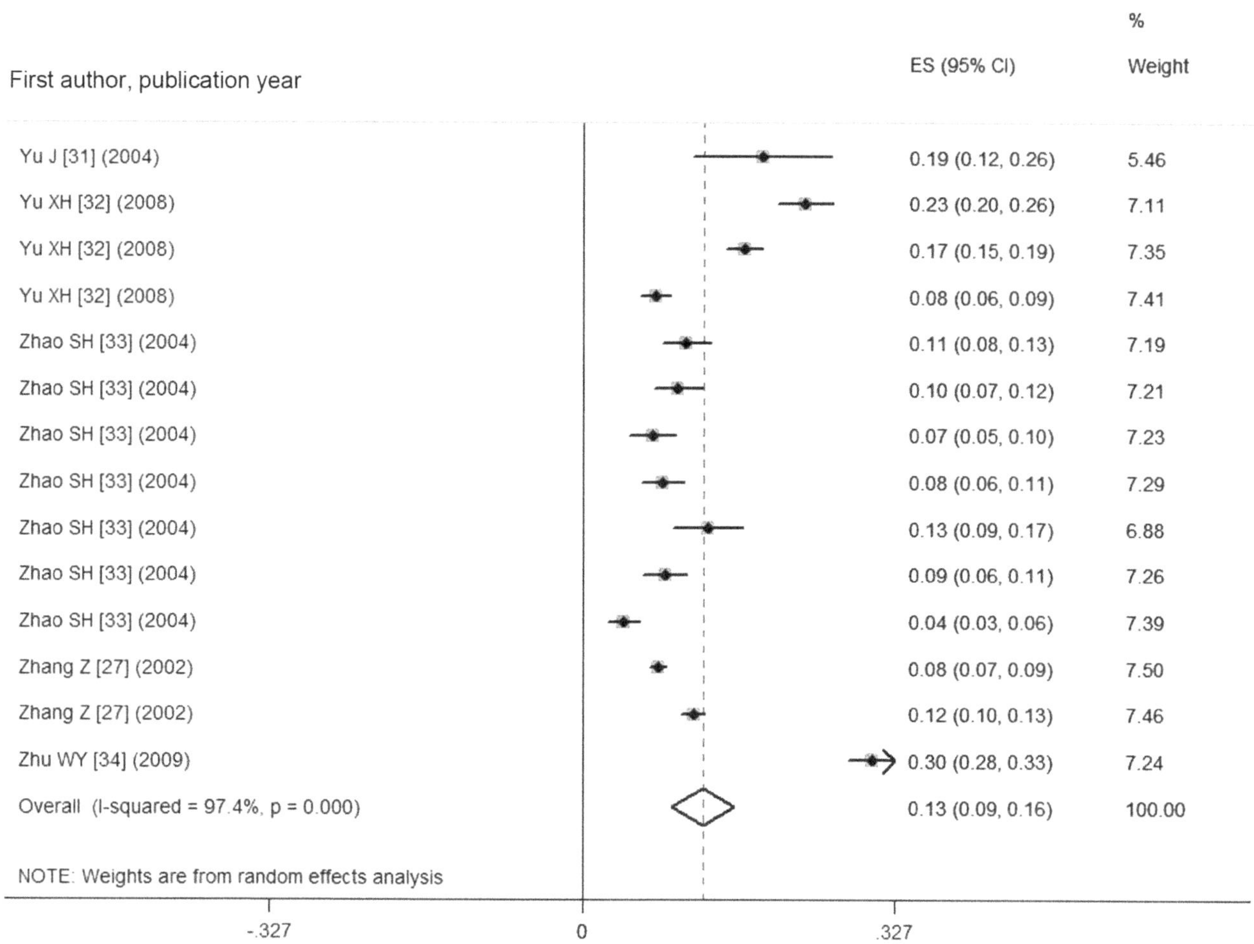

Figure 3. Forest plot displaying the pooled goiter prevalence in mainland China after 1996.

language reports of population-based studies on the prevalence of goiter and TNs using PubMed and Google Scholar, and searched all Chinese reports manually and on-line using the CNKI (Chinese National Knowledge Infrastructure), Chinese Wanfang and Chongqing VIP databases, from Jan 1985 to Feb 2014. Search key words were "goiter," "thyroid nodule(s)," "thyroid disorder(s)," "epidemiology" and "prevalence(s)". We also scanned relevant reference lists and reviews to find additional studies. Attempts were made to contact authors of the identified papers for necessary details not given in the original texts. The PRISMA guideline for systematic reviews and meta-analyses was followed closely [26], see Checklist S1.

Inclusion and Exclusion Criteria

The following inclusion criteria were adopted for paper selection: (1) Data were acquired through population-based studies instead of hospital-based studies; (2) study participants were recruited from a random community-based sample, rather than from volunteers or those receiving routine-health examinations, and the subjects had to be living in mainland China; (3) the studies contained sufficient information to conduct pooled analysis of the prevalence; (4) if the same study data were reported in both English and Chinese, the English publication was included.

Studies were excluded if: (1) they were reviews or case reports; (2) the participants suffered from any related diseases or took medicines known to affect thyroid structure or function; (3) the study focused on participants with one underlying condition (such as pregnant women and smokers) or a certain occupation; (4) they were duplicate publications.

Data Extraction

The literature was searched independently by two reviewers. Any discrepancies between the extracted data of the two reviewers were reconciled through discussion. The literature-search process is shown in Figure 1. For all included studies, the first author's name, publication date, study year, age, location, sample size, events data and prevalence were recorded.

Iodine Status

Median UIC is recognized as the most practical biochemical marker for iodine nutrition [27]. Using the criteria from WHO/UNICEF/ICCIDD [1], the iodine status was identified based on

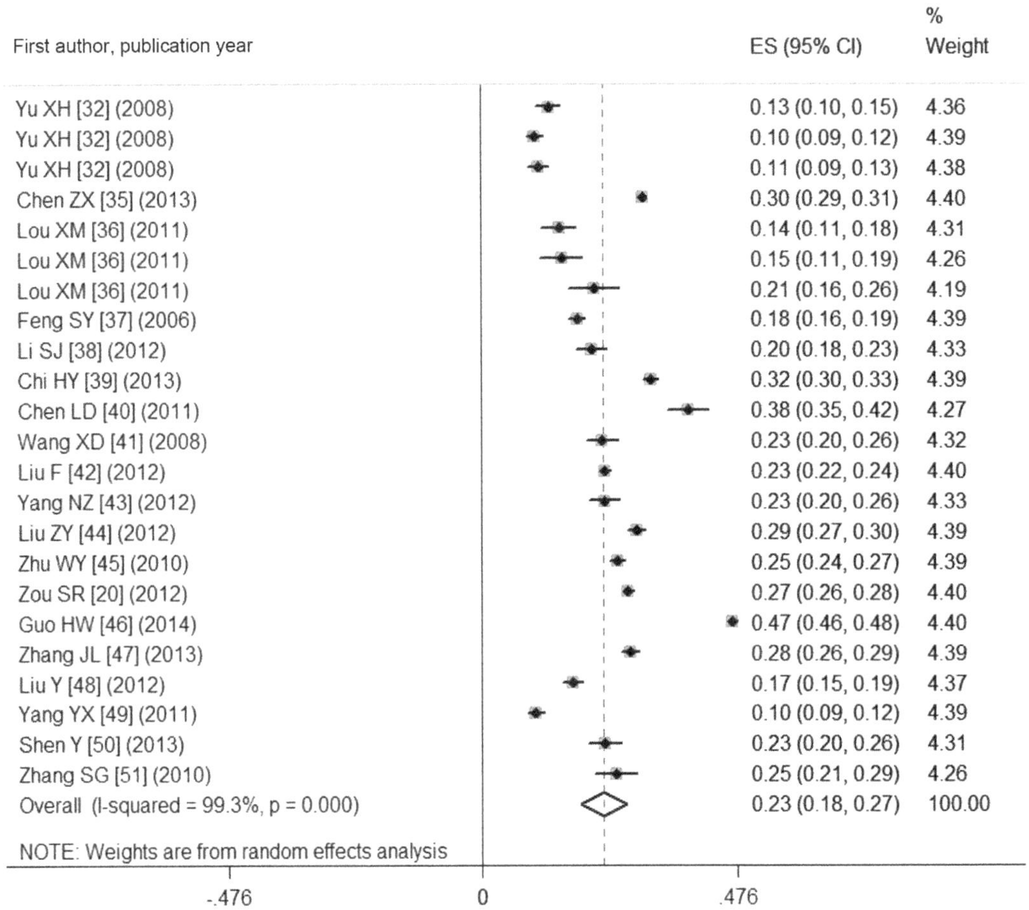

Figure 4. Forest plot of the pooled prevalence of TNs in mainland China.

the median UIC, where the median UIC ≤99 μg/L is insufficient, 100–199 μg/L is adequate, 200–299 μg/L is more than adequate and a median UIC ≥300 μg/L is considered to be excessive.

Statistical Analysis

The pooled prevalence and 95% confidence intervals (CIs) were used to estimate the prevalence of goiter and TNs in mainland China. All meta-analyses were calculated for heterogeneity using the Chi-square based Q test and the I^2 test (25, 50 and 75% were considered low, moderate and high levels of heterogeneity, respectively) [28]. For a moderate or high level of heterogeneity we adopted a random-effects meta-analysis rather than using a fixed-effects model. Addressing heterogeneity and performing a secondary analysis required subgroup analysis. Publication bias was estimated through Egger's test. A *p*-value less than 0.05 indicated statistical significance. Meta-analyses were carried out in Stata Version 11.0 (Stata Corp LP, TX). Differences in prevalence among different groups were analyzed using the Chi-square test with SPSS Version 17.0 (SPSS Software, Chicago, IL).

Results

Characteristics of Papers

Figure 1 provides a schematic representation of the process for identifying, screening, and including studies in the review. The search strategy resulted in 31 articles (4 published in English and 27 in Chinese), reporting 52 studies—29 studies reporting goiter prevalence estimates (15 before 1996 and 14 after) and 23 on TNs. Table 1 provides a descriptive summary of these studies.

All studies were based on general population samples. Before 1996, 436,182 people met the inclusion criteria for goiter; the criteria for diagnosis were in line with those of WHO, which was based on palpations. Another 14,359 people met the criteria for goiter after 1996. Goiter diagnosis after 1996 was based on palpation or ultrasound. After a diagnose with ultrasound, 59,098 people met the inclusion criteria for TNs.

Pooled Prevalence of Goiter and TNs

As shown in Figs 2 and 3, the pooled prevalence of goiter before 1996 was 22.8% (95% CI: 15.3%, 30.3%), with the actual numbers ranging from 3.11 to 50.89%; after 1996, the pooled prevalence, 12.6% (95% CI: 9.4%, 15.8%) in the range of 4.27–

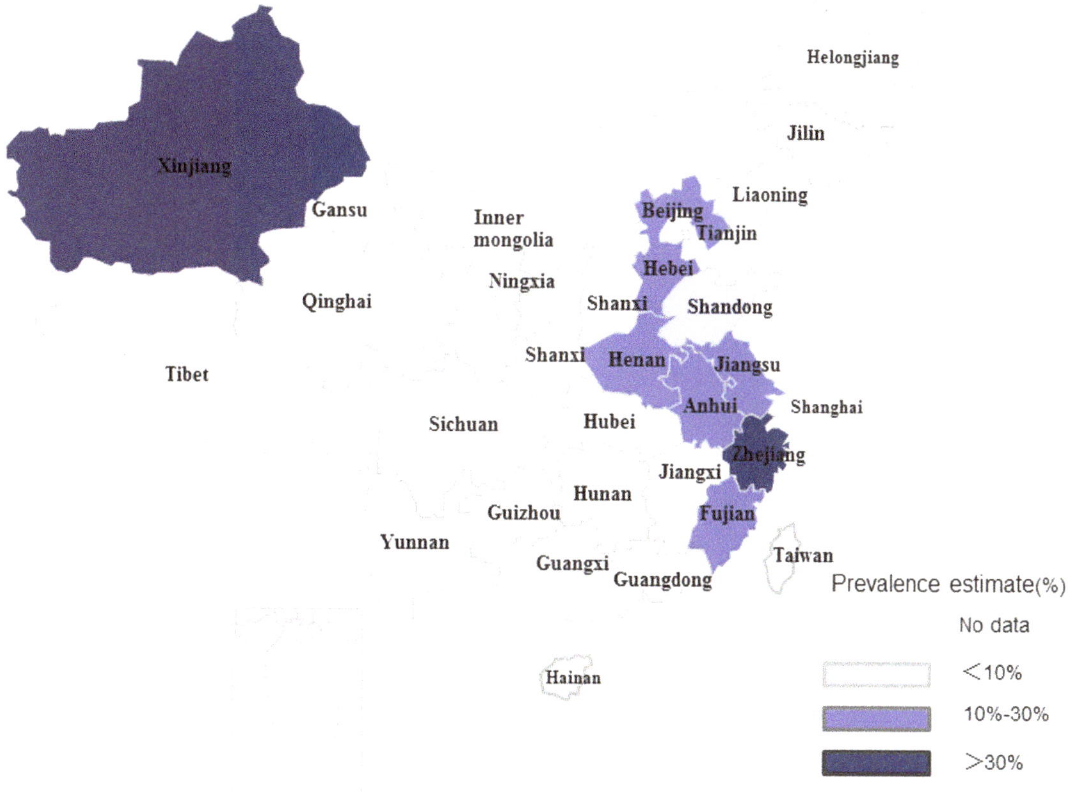

Figure 5. Regional distribution of pooled goiter prevalence in mainland China before 1996.

30.31%, was significantly lower compared with the prevalence prior to 1996 ($\chi^2 = 532.56$, $p<0.001$). Figure 4 shows a pooled prevalence of 22.7% (95%CI: 18.3%, 27.0%) for TNs with individual studies ranging from 10.12–46.56%. Individual disease conditions of the provinces and municipalities are shown in the maps in Figs 5–7.

Subgroup Analysis

Goiter prevalences before and after 1996 and TNs were analyzed in subgroups, divided by location (North, South, East, West and Central China) and the type of area (rural, urban and mixed), as shown in Tables 2–4.

As shown in Table 2, before 1996, rural area ($\chi^2 = 48054.05$, $p<0.001$), inland area ($\chi^2 = 1479.00$, $p<0.001$), high altitude ($\chi^2 = 52150.24$, $p<0.001$), small study sample size ($\chi^2 = 255.52$, $p<0.001$), location in West China ($\chi^2 = 2023.41$, $p<0.001$), and both low and high levels of iodine intake ($\chi^2 = 8809.32$, $p<0.001$) might indicate a high prevalence of goiter.

As shown in Table 3, after 1996, subgroups including rural area ($\chi^2 = 448.82$, $p<0.001$), diagnosis using ultrasound ($\chi^2 = 101.98$, $p<0.001$) and study year 2002–2014 ($\chi^2 = 421.05$, $p<0.001$) had a greater prevalence of goiter. Of note, iodine nutrition may also be associated with this greater prevalence. Among the four iodine intake categories, the prevalence of goiter was lowest in the subgroup with adequate iodine, 4.3% (95% CI: 2.6%, 5.9%), and prevalence data for the insufficient subgroup was 23.2% (95% CI: 20.3%, 26.1%) and for excess iodine subgroup was 14.5% (95% CI: 8.8%, 20.1%), both of which were higher ($\chi^2 = 190.17$, $p< 0.001$).

For TNs, prevalence among subgroups of location and study year was very different (Table 4). Prevalence rates for North, East and West China were 11.0% (95% CI: 9.7%, 12.3%), 25.5% (95% CI: 21.2%, 29.8%) and 18.3% (95% CI: 7.6%, 28.9%) ($\chi^2 = 800.56$, $p<0.001$), respectively. In terms of the study year, 11.0% (95% CI: 9.7%, 12.3%) of people investigated between 1999 and 2001 were diagnosed with TNs and this increased to 24.4% (95% CI: 20.2%, 28.7%) after 2002 ($\chi^2 = 538.27$, $p< 0.001$).

Analysis of Heterogeneity and Publication Bias

We noted a significant overall heterogeneity within the studies ($p<0.001$, $I^2 = 97.4$–100.0%), which decreased through subgroup analyses. Egger's test for the three independent research categories revealed no evidence of publication bias ($p = 0.101$, 0.148 and 0.113, respectively).

Discussion

We examined 52 epidemiological research studies covering 14 provinces, municipalities and autonomous regions in China. We systematically analyzed the prevalence of goiter and TNs prior to and after 1996, when China implemented the USI program. To our knowledge this is one of the first studies of this kind.

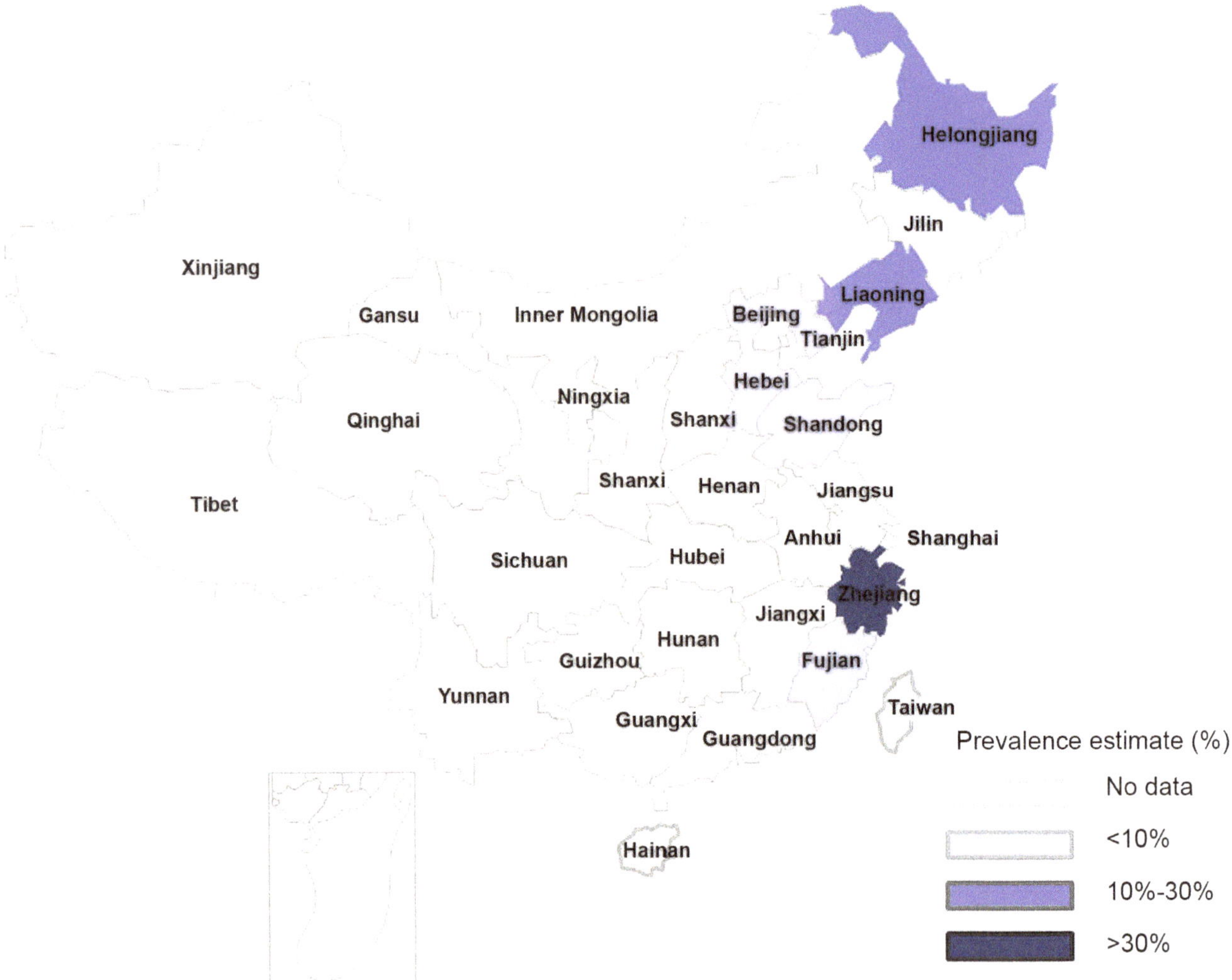

Figure 6. Regional distribution of pooled goiter prevalence in mainland China after 1996.

Research indicates that the prevalence of goiter in children 8–10 years-of-age is an indicator of local iodine consumption [1]. Our analysis, however, focused on the general population, to provide epidemiological information concerning the disease itself. Iodine nutrition is certainly an important factor for goiter, and the association between iodine intake and goiter prevalence has been investigated extensively.

Indian researchers reported that the prevalence of goiter was 65.9% in an iodine-deficient area [59], which decreased to 27.7% two decades after the USI program [60]. In Denmark, the goiter prevalence was 13.4% in an area with mild iodine deficiency and 19.7% in an area with moderate iodine deficiency, indicating that even a modest increase in iodine intake might significantly reduce IDDs [61]. In China, the USI program was launched in 1996 to prevent IDDs, establishing an important time boundary for our study. We observed a trend similar to the study in India. The overall goiter prevalence was 22.8% prior to 1996 and this was halved (declined to 12.6%). Thus, the USI program might be beneficial in China.

Also, iodine excess may increase thyroid volume [1]. In our subgroup analyses, both before and after 1996, the prevalence of goiter significantly changed with iodine status, with data suggesting hormesis—emphasizing that overdoses of iodine, as well as deficiencies may be associated with high prevalence of goiter. Meanwhile, previous studies suggest a goitrogenic effect of excess iodine in school-age children and adults [62–67]. In areas with high iodine content in the drinking water, school-age children had elevated median UIC and endemic goiter, suggesting that, in addition to adjusting the iodine content of salt, improving water quality is also necessary [62,63]. In a prospective study, 10 normal men accepted daily oral intake of excess iodine for 1 month. At the end of this treatment, their mean thyroid volume increased, which eventually returned to

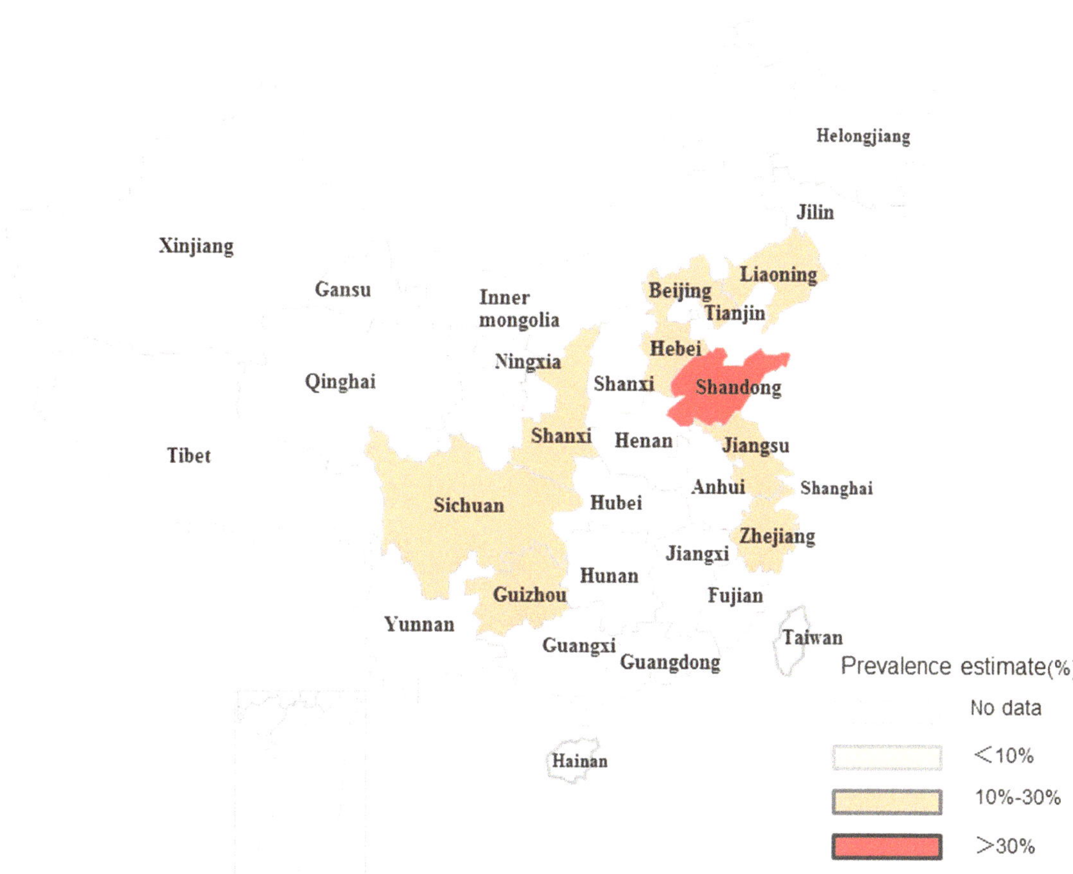

Figure 7. Regional distribution of pooled prevalence of TNs in mainland China.

baseline within 4 weeks after iodine withdrawal [64]. LeMar reported that excess iodine from tetraglycine hydroperiodide tablets caused a reversible thyroid stimulating hormone (TSH)-dependent thyroid enlargement [65]. For Peace Corps volunteers, after the removal of excess iodine from water, the mean serum iodine declined sharply, and the goiter rate fell from 44 to 30% [66]. In animal models, excessive iodine intake has been shown to lead to thyroid enlargement [67]. Thus, iodine excess should be scrutinized. In agreement with this concern, we observed that after 1996, the pooled goiter prevalence increased from 10.7% before 2002 to 25.1% afterwards, indicating an impending problem.

We also observed that altitude correlated with goiter: the plateau environment was associated with higher goiter frequency than residence in the plains and hills, a finding similar to trends in previous surveys that may be explained by deficiencies in natural iodine at high altitudes and limited educational and economic support for the people who reside there [68–70].

There is a longstanding controversy regarding the relationship between the prevalence of TNs and iodine nutrition because of the varied epidemiological situation across the globe. Among a Swedish population with adequate iodine, the rate of TNs was only 2.6% [71]. German data from a previously iodine deficient area revealed a 20.2% prevalence of TNs, with a smaller rate for men [72]. Mexico, which formerly was mildly iodine deficient, now consumes more than normal iodine intake and here the locally-identified TNs frequency was 19.6% [73]. Overall, the prevalence of TNs in mainland China was similar to that of other countries and regions of historic iodine deficiency and present states of iodine sufficiency. In addition, our data indicate that the prevalence of TNs after 2002 was higher than the rate prior to 2002—11.0% of those investigated from 1999–2001 were diagnosed with TNs, and this increased to 24.4% between 2002 and 2014.

Unlike goiter, which has a strong etiological relationship with iodine nutrition, the prevalence of TNs also depends on sex, age and head-and-neck radiation exposure history [74,75]. According to the present information, TNs are more common in cities than in the country, which may be explained by lifestyle choices [76,77]. Furthermore, females were at greater risk for TNs and this difference was not changed when females were further divided into rural, mixed and urban groups.

In conclusion, we report that the USI program in China successfully reduced the prevalence of goiter after 1996. However, the program might cause excesses iodine intake that

Table 2. Prevalence of goiter before 1996 in mainland China by different stratification factors.

Subgroups	Prevalence % (95%CI)	No of studies	Heterogeneity		Case/Total
			I^2%	*p* Value	
Area					
Rural	28.6 (20.7-36.5)	10	99.9	<0.001	82605/262005
Mixed	4.0 (2.3-5.7)	2	99.6	<0.001	5769/158692
Urban	16.1 (5.0-27.2)	3	99.6	<0.001	1569/15485
Coastal/Inland					
Coastal	5.6 (5.1-6.0)	1	-	-	584/10454
Inland	24.0 (16.0-32.1)	14	100.0	<0.001	89359/425728
Altitude					
<200	13.4 (8.3-18.5)	8	100.0	<0.001	26843/273004
200-500	31.9 (17.6-46.2)	2	99.2	<0.001	60687/155483
500-1000	-	0	-	-	-
>1000	34.3 (21.9-46.6)	5	99.2	<0.001	2413/7695
Iodine Status					
Insufficient	25.5 (12.0-39.1)	10	100.0	<0.001	67878/288418
Adequate	14.5 (−4.8-33.8)	2	97.8	<0.001	2378/48303
More than Adequate	-	0	-	-	-
Excess	19.2 (15.8-22.6)	3	98.9	<0.001	19687/99461
Method					
Palpation	22.8 (15.3-30.3)	15	100.0	<0.001	89943/436182
Ultrasound	-	0	-	-	-
Sample Size					
<5000	28.0 (21.3-34.8)	9	98.9	<0.001	3805/14713
>5000	14.9 (3.1-26.7)	6	100.0	<0.001	86138/421469
Location					
North China	16.1 (15.6-16.7)	1	-	-	2631/16324
South China	15.0 (−3.5-33.6)	2	99.5	<0.001	837/11486
East China	17.3 (4.8-29.8)	6	100.0	<0.001	83726/399088
West China	34.3 (21.9-46.6)	5	99.2	<0.001	2413/7695
Central China	21.1 (19.1-23.2)	1	-	-	336/1589
Total	**22.8 (15.3-30.3)**	**15**	**100.0**	**<0.001**	**89943/436182**

may be associated with a high prevalence of goiter. The prevalence of TNs also increased over time. Also, 5% of TNs may be malignant [14], so an increased prevalence of TNs might predict more thyroid carcinoma patients. In view of this information, in 2012, China adjusted the iodized salt concentration to 20–30 mg/kg (previously 35 mg/kg) and provincial governments and health administrative departments were allowed to formulate local standards within ±30% of recommended concentrations based on data for their area [78,79].

Our study has several limitations. First, variations in the quality of the selected papers exist. Uncertain data will confound investigations into potential influences on heterogeneity. Secondly, primary TNs articles did not use a completely unified diagnostic criterion, but they did diagnose with ultrasound. Third, data from qualified articles failed to cover most of mainland China provinces. Still, we included all available information about goiter and TNs from the past three decades and this report is the first to document the epidemiological status of both diseases before and after the USI program in mainland China. In addition, our work underscores the need for additional population-based studies in areas excluded from this analysis.

Our data show that the implementation of USI program is beneficial but may pose iodine risks; therefore, salt iodization standards should be set according to local conditions. Also, some epidemiology studies remain to be undertaken, and these are essential for comprehensive original data on the

Table 3. Prevalence of goiter after 1996 in mainland China by different stratification factors.

Subgroups	Prevalence % (95%CI)	No of studies	Heterogeneity		Case/Total
			I^2%	*p* Value	
Area					
Rural	11.5 (8.3–14.6)	11	95.0	<0.001	859/7103
Mixed	30.3 (27.9–32.7)	1	-	-	421/1389
Urban	9.7 (6.0–13.3)	2	95.5	<0.001	549/5867
Coastal/Inland					
Coastal	12.0 (7.1–16.9)	8	97.7	<0.001	982/7906
Inland	13.4 (8.5–18.4)	6	97.4	<0.001	847/6453
Altitude					
<200	13.4 (9.6–17.3)	12	97.5	<0.001	1528/11403
200–500	7.9 (0.8–15.1)	2	97.8	<0.001	301/2956
500–1000	-	0	-	-	-
>1000	-	0	-	-	-
Iodine Status					
Insufficient	23.2 (20.3–26.1)	1	-	-	189/815
Adequate	4.3 (2.6–5.9)	1	-	-	24/562
More than Adequate	9.8 (6.3–13.3)	5	94.7	<0.001	660/6604
Excess	14.5 (8.8–20.1)	7	97.7	<0.001	956/6378
Method					
Palpation	9.7 (6.0–13.3)	2	95.5	<0.001	549/5867
Ultrasound	13.2 (8.8–17.5)	12	97.6	<0.001	1280/8492
Sample Size					
<5000	12.6 (9.4–15.8)	14	97.4	<0.001	1829/14359
>5000	-	0	-	-	-
Location					
North China	16.5 (8.9–24.0)	4	97.3	<0.001	546/3497
South China	9.7 (6.0–13.3)	2	95.5	<0.001	549/5867
East China	11.6 (5.9–17.3)	8	97.9	<0.001	734/4995
West China	-	0	-	-	-
Central China	-	0	-	-	-
Study Year					
1996–2001	10.7 (8.3–13.1)	12	95.0	<0.001	1387/12858
2002–2014	25.1 (13.8–36.3)	2	88.7	0.003	442/1501
Total	**12.6 (9.4–15.8)**	**14**	**97.4**	**<0.001**	**1829/14359**

epidemiology and distribution of thyroid diseases. Our future work will include a national baseline study on thyroid diseases which will be implemented from 2014 to 2016 and these data will provide broad and accurate information for other researchers.

Acknowledgments

We are grateful to Jianming Zhang (Department of Clinical Epidemiology and Evidence-based Medicine, the First Affiliated Hospital of China Medical University), Yongze Li (Key Laboratory of AIDS Immunology of Ministry of Health, Department of Laboratory Medicine, the First Affiliated Hospital of China Medical University) and Guangcong Liu (School of Public Health, China Medical University) for methodological support. We also thank the authors of the included studies.

Table 4. Prevalence of TNs in mainland China by different stratification factors.

Subgroups	Prevalence % (95%CI)	No of studies	Heterogeneity		Case/Total
			I^2%	*p* Value	
Area					
Rural	19.1 (13.7–24.6)	7	97.7	<0.001	1300/7552
Mixed	24.0 (21.6–26.4)	10	94.5	<0.001	7926/28786
Urban	25.1 (13.2–37.1)	6	99.8	<0.001	7572/22760
Coastal/Inland					
Coastal	23.3 (20.2–26.4)	9	95.5	<0.001	5650/20797
Inland	22.5 (15.7–29.2)	14	99.6	<0.001	11148/38301
Altitude					
<200	23.4 (18.7–28.0)	20	99.3	<0.001	15568/53116
200–500	17.0 (15.1–18.9)	1	-	-	255/1500
500–1000	-	0	-	-	-
>1000	18.9 (1.7–36.1)	2	99.6	-	975/4482
Sample Size					
<5000	20.7 (17.0–24.5)	19	98.4	<0.001	6360/27724
>5000	31.7 (21.8–41.7)	4	99.7	<0.001	10438/31374
Location					
North China	11.0 (9.7–12.3)	3	35.9	0.210	371/3385
South China	-	0	-	-	-
East China	25.5 (21.2–29.8)	17	99.1	<0.001	15197/49731
West China	18.3 (7.6–28.9)	3	99.2	<0.001	1230/5982
Central China	-	0	-	-	-
Gender					
Male	16.6 (12.1–21.2)	23	99.0	<0.001	5420/24469
Rural	11.1 (5.9–16.3)	7	97.3	<0.001	302/2708
Mixed	19.2 (16.6–21.7)	10	90.4	<0.001	2854/12865
Urban	19.2 (9.1–29.2)	6	99.3	<0.001	2264/8896
Female	26.9 (22.2–31.6)	23	99.0	<0.001	11378/34629
Rural	23.3 (17.5–29.0)	7	96.1	<0.001	998/4844
Mixed	28.5 (25.9–31.1)	10	90.1	<0.001	5072/15921
Urban	29.4 (16.6–42.2)	6	99.6	<0.001	5308/13864
Study Year					
1999–2001	11.0 (9.7–12.3)	3	35.9	0.210	371/3385
2002–2014	24.4 (20.2–28.7)	20	99.2	<0.001	16427/55713
Total	**22.7 (18.3–27.0)**	**23**	**99.3**	**<0.001**	**16798/59098**

Author Contributions

Conceived and designed the experiments: WPT ZYS. Performed the experiments: WZ CH XGS. Analyzed the data: WZ CH CHX JS. Contributed reagents/materials/analysis tools: WPT. Wrote the paper: WZ CH. Revised the language/article: WPT WZ CH XGS.

References

1. World Health Organization, United Nations Children's Fund, International Council for the Control of Iodine Deficiency Disorders (2007) Assessment of iodine deficiency disorders and monitoring their elimination: A guide for program managers. Geneva, Switzerland: World Health Organization.
2. FAO/WHO (2005) Vitamin and mineral requirements in human nutrition, 2nd ed. Geneva: World Health Organization. Available: http://whqlibdoc.who.int/publications/2004/9241546123.pdf
3. Zimmermann MB (2009) Iodine deficiency. Endocr Rev 30: 376–408.
4. Ozpinar A, Kelestimur F, Songur Y, Can O, Valentin L, et al. (2014) Iodine status in Turkish populations and exposure to iodide uptake inhibitors. PLoS One 9: e88206.
5. Delange F, Bürgi H, Chen ZP, Dunn JT (2002) World status of monitoring iodine deficiency disorders control programs. Thyroid 12: 915–924.
6. Polyzos SA, Kita M, Avramidis A (2007) Thyroid nodules-Stepwose diagnosis and management. Hormones (Athens) 6: 101–119.
7. Singer PA, Cooper DS, Daniels GH, Ladenson PW, Greenspan FS, et al. (1996) Treatment guidelines for patients with thyroid nodules and well-differentiated thyroid cancer. Arch Intern Med 156: 2165–2172.
8. Mazzaferri EL (1992) Thyroid cancer in thyroid nodules: finding a needle in the haystack. Am J Med 93: 359–362.
9. Tan GH, Gharib H (1997) Thyroid incidentalomas: management approaches to nonpalpable nodules discovered incidentally on thyroid imaging. Ann Intern Med 126: 226–231.

10. Hull OH (1955) Critical analysis of two hundred twenty-one thyroid glands: study of thyroid glands obtained at necropsy in Colorado. AMA Arch Pathol 59: 291–311.
11. Mortensen JD, Woolner LB, Bennett WA (1955) Gross and microscopic findings in clinically normal thyroid glands. J Clin Endocrinol Metab 15: 1270–1280.
12. Oertel JE, Klinck GH (1965) Structural changes in the thyroid glands of healthy young men. The Med Ann Dist Columbia 34: 75–77.
13. Gharib H, Papini E, Paschke R, Duick DS, Hegedus L, et al. (2010) American Association of Clinical Endocrinologists, Associazione Medicie Endocrinologi, and European Thyroid Association medical guidelines for clinical practice for the diagnosis and management of thyroid nodules: executive summary of recommendations. J Endocrinol Invest 33: 51–56.
14. American Thyroid Association (ATA) Guidelines Taskforce on Thyroid Nodules and Differentiated Thyroid Cancer, Cooper DS, Doherty GM, Haugen BR, Kloos RT, et al. (2009) Revised American Thyroid Association management guidelines for patients with thyroid nodules and differentiated thyroid cancer. Thyroid 19: 1167–1214.
15. Endemic Disease Control Department in Ministry of Public Health (1989) China national programme 1989–1995 for the control of iodine deficiency disorders (Article in Chinese). Chin J Endemiol 8: 252–254.
16. Luton D, Alberti C, Vuillard E, Ducarme G, Oury JF, et al. (2011) Iodine deficiency in northern Paris area: impact on fetal thyroid mensuration. PLoS One 6: e14707.
17. Ministry of Health of the People's Republic of China, Ministry of Light Industry of the People's Republic of China (1994) Outline of eliminating iodine deficient disorders in China in 2000 (Article in Chinese). Beijing.
18. Zimmermann MB, Andersson M (2012) Update on iodine status worldwide. Curr Opin Endocrinol Diabetes Obes 19: 382–387.
19. Zhou RH, Zhu HM, Du YG, Dong XJ (2000) Investigation on residents' iodine-nutritional status after supplementation of iodine salt in Shijiazhuang City (Article in Chinese). Chin J Endemiol 19: 191–193.
20. Tan J, Fang PH, Lu TZ, Chen BZ, Gao S, et al. (2001) Investigation on iodine nutritional status and thyroid goiter prevalence of residents in Tianjin after salt iodination (Article in Chinese). Chin J Endocrinol Metab 17: 75–78.
21. Jin Y, Teng WP, Yuan B, Zhang YG, Yin CC (2001) Thyroid autoimmunity in members from multiplex families with Grave's disease and effect of iodine intake on its incidence (Article in Chinese). Chin J Endocrinol Metab 17: 79–82.
22. Yang F, Teng WP, Shan ZY, Wang ZY, Jin Y, et al. (2001) A comparative epidemiologic survey of hyperthyroidism in areas with different iodine intake (Article in Chinese). Chin J Endocrinol Metab 17: 197–201.
23. hang KZ, Lin YC, Fang ZP, Luo CR, Liu XY, et al. (2002) The effect of salt iodization for 10 years on the prevalence of endemic goiter and hyperthyroidism (Article in Chinese). Chin J Endocrinol Metab 18: 342–344.
24. Hou X, Wang J, Qi Q, Zhu LX, Xue XF, et al. (2003) Epidemiologic comparative study of hyperthyroidism before and after salt iodization in different iodine intake regions of Jilin Province (Article in Chinese). Chin J Endocrinol Metab 19: 104–105.
25. Wu MY, Zhang JW, Zhao JK, Zhang QL, Xie YQ, et al. (2004) Retrospective study on thyroid diseases after universal salt iodization in mild iodine deficiency area (Article in Chinese). Chin J Endocrinol Metab 20: 104–106.
26. Liberati A, Altman DG, Tetzlaff J, Mulrow C, Gøtzsche PC, et al. (2009) The PRISMA statement for reporting systematic reviews and meta-analyses of studies that evaluate health care interventions: explanation and elaboration. PLoS Medicine 6: e1000100.
27. Zou SR, Wu F, Guo CY, Song J, Huang CH, et al. (2012) Iodine nutrition and the prevalence of thyroid disease after salt iodization: a cross-sectional survey in Shanghai, a coastal area in China. PLoS One 7: e40718.
28. Higgins JP, Thompson SG, Deeks JJ, Altman DG (2003) Measuring inconsistency in meta-analyses. BMJ 327: 557–560.
29. Wang LF, Wang SL, Aihaidi, Wang XZ, Lin FF, et al. (1992) Iodine deficiency disorders and geographical environment: an investigation in the diluvia-alluvial plain in front of the Kunlun Mountains (Article in Chinese). Endemic Diseases Bulletin 7: 56–64.
30. Dou DX, Li ZP, Zhu HF, Lv XC (1992) Control of endemic goiter with iodine bricks (Article in Chinese). Mil Med Sci 16: 256–259.
31. Chen HM, Ke GY, Li DL, Zheng XX, Cui SL, et al. (2000) An observational study on the control of endemic goiter by water improvement to reduce iodine level (Article in Chinese).Chin J Endemiol 19: 275–276.
32. Zhang JL, Kang XP, Li QM, Ma LJ, Ping F, et al. (1992) A report on the effect of the prevention and treatment of endemic goiter at the basic control stage in Linyi area (Article in Chinese). J Linyi Med School 14: 327–331.
33. Wu WY, Wang XL, Wu LP (2002) The epidemiology, control and elimination of endemic goiter in Qingyuan County (Article in Chinese). Occupation and Health 18: 94–95.
34. Zhang Z, Lin YC, Fang ZP, Luo CR, Liu XY, et al. (2002) The effect of salt iodization for 10 years on the prevalence of endemic goiter and hyperthyroidism (Article in Chinese). Chin J Endocrinol Metab 18: 342–344.
35. Bao Y, Shu HS, Yu MJ, Chen T, Liu RJ, et al. (1994) An epidemiological investigation of endemic goiter in Xuzhou areas (Article in Chinese). Endemic Diseases Bulletin 9: 58–61.
36. Su MY, Yilixiati, Tang PC, Jiang XM, Kelimu, et al. (1989) A preliminary study on the difference of the incidence of endemic goiter between the agricultural areas and pasture-lands of Tekesi County, Xinjiang (Article in Chinese). Chin J Endemiol 8: 375–406.
37. Zheng HB, Feng JL, Li GQ, Qin ZQ (1988) An investigation on goiter caused by high concentration of water iodine in Cangzhou areas (Article in Chinese). Endemic Diseases Bulletin 3: 61–65.
38. Yu J, Liu SJ, Su M, Zhang SB, Ye YX, et al. (2004) A Survey of IDDs surveillance in Jixian Village of Huangchuan County, Heilongjiang Province in 2003 (Article in Chinese). Chin J Ctrl Endem Dis 19: 114–116.
39. Yu XH, Fan CL, Shan ZY, Teng XC, Guan HX, et al. (2008) A five-year follow-up study of goiter and thyroid nodules in three regions with different iodine intakes in China. J Endocrinol Invest 31: 243–250.
40. Zhao SH, Wang YG, Yan SL, Wang YH, Han L, et al. (2004) A survey of present status of thyroid goiter and urine iodine status of residents in the coastal regions of Shandong Province (Article in Chinese). Med J Qilu 19: 221–223.
41. Zhu WY, Hu XF, Zhou SQ, Wang HK, Zheng XJ, et al. (2009) An epidemiological investigation on goiter in the town residents of Zhoushan Archipelago (Article in Chinese). Zhejiang Prev Med 21: 1–3.
42. Chen ZX, Xu WM, Huang YM, Jin XY, Deng J, et al. (2013) Associations of noniodized salt and thyroid nodule among the Chinese population: a large cross-sectional study. Am J Clin Nutr 98: 684–692.
43. Lou XM, Mo Z, Zhu WM, Zhou JS, Mao GM, et al. (2011) An epidemiological analysis of thyroid nodules among population with different levels of iodine nutrition (Article in Chinese). Chin J Public Health 27: 1564–1565.
44. Feng SY, Liu C, Liu XY, Duan Y, Liu CP (2006) An epidemiological study of thyroid nodules among a community-based population in Gaochun and Chuzhou of Jiangsu (Article in Chinese). Acta Universitais Medicinalis Nanjing (Natural Science) 26: 717–720.
45. Li SJ, Cao YS, Sun S, Wang XM (2012) An analysis of the prevalence of thyroid nodules and the risk factors among population (Article in Chinese). Zhejiang Prev Med 24: 4–10.
46. Chi HY, Zhou YP, Li YB, Wang Y, Zhang HR (2013) The age distribution and thyroid function of thyroid nodules patients (Article in Chinese). Chin J Prac Med 40: 24–25.
47. Chen LD, Chen P, Lei JM (2011) An analysis on thyroid ultrasonography results of residents in Lishui, Zhejiang Province (Article in Chinese). Chin Rural Health Service Administration 31: 981–982.
48. Wang XD, Bu RF, Peng W, Duan Y, Liu XY, et al. (2008) An epidemiological study of thyroid nodules among population in Wuxi of Jiangsu Province (Article in Chinese). Chin J Prac Int Med 28: 860–862.
49. Liu F, Chen HB, Ye TY (2012) An epidemiological survey of thyroid nodules in Ruian, Zhejiang Province (Article in Chinese). Chin J Prim Med Pharm 19: 3400–3401.
50. Yang NZ, Chen Y, Yang WY, Bao XJ, Hao W, et al. (2012) A survey on iodine nutrition condition of residents in Jiaojiang District, Taizhou City, Zhejiang Province (Article in Chinese). J Environ Occup Med 29: 148–153.
51. Liu ZY, Zhou JS, Lin Q, Zhang YL (2012) An analysis on thyroid ultrasonography results of residents in Zhoushan islands (Article in Chinese). Chin J Ctrl Endem Dis 27: 57–59.
52. Zhu WY, Zhou SQ, Wang HK, Hu XF, Zheng XJ, et al. (2010) An investigation of iodine nutrition and prevalence of thyroid nodules in Zhoushan Archipelago (Article in Chinese). Chin Prev Med 11: 113–116.
53. Guo HW, Sun M, He W, Chen HH, Li W, et al. (2014) The prevalence of thyroid nodules and its relationship with metabolic parameters in a Chinese community-based population aged over 40 years. Endocrine 45: 230–235.
54. Zhang JL, Tuo SJ, Song HP, Zhou XD, Liu XY, et al. (2013) An epidemiological survey of thyroid diseases in Yan'an City (Article in Chinese). Chin J Clin Med 20: 548–550.
55. Liu Y, Yan Z, Tong NW, Lv GQ (2012) An epidemiological survey of thyroid diseases in a community-based population in Chengdu (Article in Chinese). Proceedings of the 11th Annual Meeting of Chinese Society of Endocrinology pp. 114.
56. Yang YX, Shi LX (2011) A survey of the prevalence of thyroid nodules in a community-based population in Guiyang (Article in Chinese). Proceedings of the 10th Annual Meeting of Chinese Society of Endocrinology pp. 162–163.
57. Shen Y, Zhang YY, Yuan H, Sun SF, Tao MY, et al. (2013) A survey of iodine nutritional status of the residents in Jiading District of Shanghai (Article in Chinese). Chin Tropical Med 13: 307–309.
58. Zhang SG, Jiao L, Gong Y, Cai KY, Lu MQ, et al. (2010) The epidemiological characteristics and analysis of subclinical thyroid diseases in Xuzhou coalmine areas (Article in Chinese). Acta Academiae Med Xuzhou 30: 65–67.
59. Pandav CS, Kochupillai N (1982) Endemic goitre in India: prevalence, etiology, attendant disabilities and control measures. Indian J Pediatr 49: 259–271.
60. Yadav S, Gupta SK, Godbole MM, Jain M, Singh U, et al. (2010) Persistence of severe iodine-deficiency disorders despite universal salt iodization in an iodine-deficient area in northern India. Public Health Nutr 13: 424–429.
61. Knudsen N, Bülow I, Jorgensen T, Laurberg P, Ovesen L, et al. (2000) Goitre prevalence and thyroid abnormalities at ultrasonography: a comparative epidemiological study in two regions with slightly different iodine status. Clin Endocrinol (Oxf) 53: 479–485.
62. Zhao J, Wang P, Shang L, Sullivan KM, van der Haar F, et al. (2000) Endemic goiter associated with high iodine intake. Am J Public Health 90: 1633–1635.
63. Liu P, Liu L, Shen H, Jia Q, Wang J, et al. (2014) The standard, intervention measures and health risk for high water iodine areas. PLoS One 9: e89608.
64. Namba H, Yamashita S, Kimura H, Yokoyama N, Usa T, et al. (1993) Evidence of thyroid volume increase in normal subjects receiving excess iodide. J Clin Endocrinol Metab 76: 605–608.

65. LeMar HJ, Georgitis WJ, McDermott MT (1995) Thyroid adaptation to chronic tetraglycine hydroperiodide water purification tablet use. J Clin Endocrinol Metab 80: 220–223.
66. Pearce EN, Gerber AR, Gootnick DB, Khan LK, Li R, et al. (2002) Effects of chronic iodine excess in a cohort of long-term American workers in West Africa. J Clin Endocrinol Metab 87: 5499–5502.
67. Yu JS, Shan ZY, Chong W, Mao JY, Geng YX, et al. (2011) Vitamin E ameliorates iodine-induced cytotoxicity in thyroid. J Endocrinol 209: 299–306.
68. Harris NS, Crawford PB, Yangzom Y, Pinzo L, Gyaltsen P, et al. (2001) Nutritional and health status of Tibetan children living at high altitudes. N Engl J Med 344: 341–347.
69. Abuye C, Berhane Y, Ersumo T (2008) The role of changing diet and altitude on goitre prevalence in five regional states in Ethiopia. East Afr J Public Health 5: 163–168.
70. Abu-Eshy SA, Abolfotouh MA, Al-Naggar YM (2001) Endemic goiter in schoolchildren in high and low altitude areas of Asir region, Saudi Arabia. Saudi Med J 22: 146–149.
71. Takahashi T, Fujimori K, Simon SL, Bechtner G, Edwards R, et al. (1999) Thyroid nodules, thyroid function and dietary iodine in the Marshall islands. Int J Epidemiol 28: 742–749.
72. Völzke H, Lüdemann J, Robinson DM, Spieker KW, Schwahn C, et al. (2003) The prevalence of undiagnosed thyroid disorders in a previously iodine-deficient area. Thyroid 13: 803–810.
73. Hurtado-Lopez LM, Basurto-Kuba E, Montes de Oca-Duran ER, Pulido-Cejudo A, Vazquez-Ortega R, et al. (2011) Prevalence of thyroid nodules in the Valley of Mexico. Cir Cir 79: 114–117.
74. Rojeski MT, Gharib H (1985) Nodular thyroid disease: evaluation and management. N Engl J Med 313: 428–436.
75. Gharib H (1997) Changing concepts in the diagnosis and management of thyroid nodules. Endocrinol Metab Clin North Am 26: 777–800.
76. Leng S, Liu Y, Liu HX, Zhao H, Sun GH, et al. (2011) Epidemiology of thyroid nodules in health examination participants in Dalian (Article in Chinese). Medicine and Philosophy 32: 22–24.
77. Wang CY, Mi GL, Si RH, Tao L, Wang X, et al. (2012) Epidemiology of thyroid nodules in teachers of distinction in Shijiazhuang (Article in Chinese). Hebei Med J 34: 1402–1403.
78. Ministry of Health of the People's Republic of China (2011) National Guideline for food safety: iodine concentration in table salt (Article in Chinese). Available: http://wenku.baidu.com/view/7db4f3de6f1aff00bed51eae.html. Accessed 8 August 2013.
79. Meng F, Zhao R, Liu P, Liu L, Liu S (2013) Assessment of iodine status in children, adults, pregnant women and lactating women in iodine-replete areas of China. PLoS One 8: e81294.

AltitudeOmics: Rapid Hemoglobin Mass Alterations with Early Acclimatization to and De-Acclimatization from 5260 m in Healthy Humans

Benjamin J. Ryan[1]*, Nadine B. Wachsmuth[2], Walter F. Schmidt[2], William C. Byrnes[1], Colleen G. Julian[3], Andrew T. Lovering[4], Andrew W. Subudhi[3,5], Robert C. Roach[3]

1 Department of Integrative Physiology, University of Colorado Boulder, Boulder, Colorado, United States of America, **2** Department of Sports Medicine/Sports Physiology, University of Bayreuth, Bayreuth, Germany, **3** Altitude Research Center, Department of Emergency Medicine, University of Colorado Anschutz Medical Campus, Aurora, Colorado, United States of America, **4** Department of Human Physiology, University of Oregon, Eugene, Oregon, United States of America, **5** Department of Biology, University of Colorado Colorado Springs, Colorado Springs, Colorado, United States of America

Abstract

It is classically thought that increases in hemoglobin mass (Hbmass) take several weeks to develop upon ascent to high altitude and are lost gradually following descent. However, the early time course of these erythropoietic adaptations has not been thoroughly investigated and data are lacking at elevations greater than 5000 m, where the hypoxic stimulus is dramatically increased. As part of the AltitudeOmics project, we examined Hbmass in healthy men and women at sea level (SL) and 5260 m following 1, 7, and 16 days of high altitude exposure (ALT1/ALT7/ALT16). Subjects were also studied upon return to 5260 m following descent to 1525 m for either 7 or 21 days. Compared to SL, absolute Hbmass was not different at ALT1 but increased by 3.7±5.8% (mean ± SD; $n = 20$; $p < 0.01$) at ALT7 and 7.6±6.6% ($n = 21$; $p < 0.001$) at ALT16. Following descent to 1525 m, Hbmass was reduced compared to ALT16 (−6.0±3.7%; $n = 20$; $p = 0.001$) and not different compared to SL, with no difference in the loss in Hbmass between groups that descended for 7 (−6.3±3.0%; $n = 13$) versus 21 days (−5.7±5.0; $n = 7$). The loss in Hbmass following 7 days at 1525 m was correlated with an increase in serum ferritin ($r = -0.64$; $n = 13$; $p < 0.05$), suggesting increased red blood cell destruction. Our novel findings demonstrate that Hbmass increases within 7 days of ascent to 5260 m but that the altitude-induced Hbmass adaptation is lost within 7 days of descent to 1525 m. The rapid time course of these adaptations contrasts with the classical dogma, suggesting the need to further examine mechanisms responsible for Hbmass adaptations in response to severe hypoxia.

Editor: Raghavan Raju, Georgia Regents University, United States of America

Funding: The overall AltitudeOmics study was funded, in part, by grants from the U.S. Department of Defense (W81XWH-11-2-0040 TATRC to RCR, and W81XWH-10-2-0114 to ATL); the Cardiopulmonary & Respiratory Physiology Laboratory, University of Oregon; the Altitude Research Center and the Charles S. Houston Endowed Professorship, Department of Emergency Medicine, School of Medicine, University of Colorado Denver. The funders had no role in study design, data collection and analysis, decision to publish, or preparation of the manuscript.

Competing Interests: The authors have declared that no conflicts of interest exist.

* Email: benjamin.ryan@colorado.edu

Introduction

Precise regulation of erythropoiesis is critical, as both anemia and excessive polycythemia have detrimental effects on physiological function. Hypoxia is a potent stimulator of erythropoiesis and erythropoietin (EPO) increases within hours of hypobaric hypoxia [1]. However, it is classically thought that elevations in total hemoglobin mass (Hbmass) and red cell volume (RCV) during high altitude acclimatization require several weeks to occur [2,3]. This delayed increase fits with patterns observed with exogenous EPO administration in healthy humans, where Hbmass/RCV have been consistently reported to remain unchanged within the first 12 days of treatment [4,5,6]. Although previous studies examining erythropoeitic adaptations in lowlanders adapting to altitudes greater than 4000 m for periods longer than 4 weeks have consistently reported increases in Hbmass/RCV [7,8], the time course of erythropoietic adaptation during early (i.e., first 1–3 weeks) high altitude acclimatization is less clear. For example, whereas some studies have found unchanged RCV following 2–3 weeks at 4300 m [9,10], others have found moderate increases at this same elevation over a similar time course [11,12]. More recently, studies examining the early time course of changes in Hbmass at lower altitudes (2000 m–3600 m) have reported small (2–3%) but significant increases in Hbmass following 11–13 days [13,14,15]. Data from these studies conflict with the classical dogma that at least 3–4 weeks are required for increases in Hbmass to be observed, but this remains a matter of considerable debate [16,17]. Further investigation of early erythropoietic adaptations to high altitude is warranted and, importantly, data are lacking at elevations greater than 5000 m where the hypoxic stimulus for erythropoiesis is dramatically increased [18,19].

Gains in Hbmass/RCV obtained during high altitude acclimatization are eventually lost following descent to low altitude, but the time course of this de-acclimatization also remains unclear. Based upon the traditional kinetics of red blood cell production and destruction, large reductions in Hbmass/RCV are expected to take multiple weeks to occur. Recent altitude training studies conducted at elevations between 2000 m–3600 m have reported full or partial retention of altitude-induced gains in Hbmass for 2–3 weeks following descent to sea level [14,15,17], with Hbmass eventually returning to baseline sea level values [14,17]. Hbmass/RCV have also been reported to remain elevated for several weeks following cessation of EPO treatment [5,6,20]. These studies suggest that elevations in Hbmass induced with short-term environmental or pharmacologic perturbation decay gradually over several weeks. In contrast, a study of polycythemic high altitude natives from 4380 m reported a rapid loss in RCV of ~7% within the first week of descent to sea level; this rapid loss in RCV was coupled with increases in several markers of red blood cell destruction [21]. Although this study suggested that an increased rate of red blood cell destruction may cause a rapid reduction in Hbmass following high altitude descent, the high altitude natives studied were severely polycythemic and therefore these results may not extend to subjects with less marked polycythemia. As with studies examining changes in Hbmass during the early phase of acclimatization to altitudes greater than 5000 m, we are unaware of any studies examining the early time course of loss in Hbmass following descent from altitudes greater than 5000 m.

AltitudeOmics was designed as a large collaborative research project examining early high altitude acclimatization/de-acclimatization in multiple physiological systems [22]. As a result of this overall project design, we had the unique opportunity to examine the early time course of erythropoietic adaptations with ascent to and descent from 5260 m in healthy humans. Because rapid changes in plasma volume (PV) occur within the first days of high altitude ascent (i.e., [23,24,25,26,27] and descent [26,27], early alterations in hemoglobin concentration ([Hb]) or hematocrit (Hct) do not necessarily reflect changes in Hbmass/RCV. Therefore, we measured Hbmass and blood volume compartments in lowlanders at sea level, on 3 occasions at 5260 m during 16 days of high altitude exposure, and upon initial return to 5260 m following descent to low altitude (1525 m) for either 7 or 21 days.

Methods

Study Design

A detailed description of the overall AltitudeOmics study design and subject characteristics is reported elsewhere [22]. The study was approved by the Institutional Review Boards of the Universities of Colorado and Oregon, and by the Human Research Protection Office of the U.S. Department of Defense. Subjects were informed about the possible risks and discomforts involved before giving written and verbal consent to participate.

The data reported here are novel with the exception of the basic characteristics of the 21 AltitudeOmics subjects (12 males, 9 females; age: 21±1 years; height: 176±8 cm; body mass: 70±9 kg) that have been reported previously [22]. Subjects were studied near sea level (130 m; Eugene, OR, USA) and on 4 occasions at 5260 m (Mt. Chacaltaya, Bolivia). Hbmass/BV compartments were measured in duplicate at sea level (SL) during baseline testing, with the mean of 2 tests used as the SL value. Nine to ten weeks after SL testing, subjects were flown via commercial aircraft to El Alto, Bolivia (4050 m) and then immediately driven to 1525 m (Coroico, Bolivia), where they stayed for 2 days. Subjects were then driven to 5260 m on ALT1 and Hbmass/BV parameters were assessed after 9–13 hours at this elevation. Subjects spent days ALT2-ALT4 at 3800 m (La Paz, Bolivia), with a short visit to 5260 m on ALT4, before returning to 5260 m on ALT5. Subjects remained at 5260 m from ALT5 to ALT17, and Hbmass and BV compartments were assessed on ALT7 and ALT16. On ALT17, subjects descended to 1525 m for either 7 (POST7; n = 14) or 21 days (POST21; n = 7). Subjects were transported back to 5260 m on POST7/POST21 and Hbmass/BV measurements were taken following 9–13 hours at this elevation.

Serum ferritin was assessed in all subjects 2–3 weeks prior to baseline testing. All male subjects had initial ferritin levels greater than 20 ng mL^{-1} and none received iron supplementation during the study. Women with initial ferritin levels less than 20 ng mL^{-1} (n = 7) were directed to take oral iron supplements (325 mg ferrous sulfate, 2–3 times daily) for 2–3 weeks prior to baseline testing and until departure to high altitude. One subject ceased supplementation prior to departure to high altitude due to gastrointestinal complaints. No subjects received iron supplementation following departure from SL. The decision not to provide iron supplementation during high altitude acclimatization/de-acclimatization was made based on potential confounding influences [28,29] of iron supplementation on other physiological responses that were assessed as part of the overall AltitudeOmics project.

Subjects participated in many studies as part of the AltitudeOmics project and some involved blood sampling. At SL, Hbmass/BV assessments were performed prior to any other blood sampling. At high altitude, Hbmass/BV parameters were measured following other blood sampling. The estimated volume of blood withdrawn for sampling at each altitude time point was as follows–ALT1: 212±81 mL; ALT7: 64±26 mL; ALT16: 191±10 mL; POST7/21: 147±46 mL. To examine the effect of blood sampling on Hbmass measured at ALT1, we compared our measured Hbmass values at ALT1 and SL and found that the mean values were not significantly different (see Results). Additionally, when we examined Hbmass across all time points using measured or adjusted (for estimated Hbmass withdrawn due to blood sampling), the statistical significance of our findings remained unaltered. Therefore, we have chosen to report the measured Hbmass values without adjusting for blood withdrawn for sampling but address the magnitude of Hbmass lost due to sampling in the discussion.

Analytical Methods

Hbmass and BV Parameters. Hbmass was measured using the optimized carbon monoxide (CO) rebreathing method [30,31] with minor modifications. Following at least 20 minutes of seated rest, a venous (v) blood sample (~2 mL) was obtained from an antecubital vein and used for determination of v[Hb] (OSM3 hemoximeter, Radiometer, Denmark) and vHct (microcentrifugation). The OSM3 was calibrated for [Hb] at regular intervals according to the manufacturers' recommendations. v[Hb] and vHct were analyzed in triplicate. Arterialized capillary blood samples (200 μL) were obtained from a hyperemic earlobe and measured for baseline carboxyhemoglobin (HbCO%) in sextuplicate on the OSM3. End-tidal [CO] was measured using a portable CO detector (Draeger Pac 7000, Draeger, Germany). Subsequently, a bolus of 99.9% CO was administered to subjects from a calibrated syringe into a custom-built spirometer (Spico-CO Respirations-Applikator, Blood Tec, Germany) and rebreathed for 2 minutes along with 3 to 5 L of 100% oxygen.

The volume of CO administered to subjects was chosen to induce a ~5–6% increase in HbCO%. The volume of CO administered was increased at high altitude based on the reduced barometric pressure to obtain similar ΔHbCO% in tests at sea level and high altitude. However, the largest volume of CO administered was 135 mL (maximal volume of calibrated syringe). The mean ΔHbCO% following the rebreathing procedure was 5.4±0.8%.

Potential CO leaks from the subject or rebreathing apparatus were monitored throughout the rebreathing procedure using 2 portable CO detectors. Due to the effects of CO leaks on measurement error of Hbmass [32], any test in which a CO leak was detected was excluded (total of 6 tests). End-tidal [CO] was measured 4 minutes following initial CO inhalation. Arterialized capillary blood samples (100 μL) were obtained at minutes 6 and 8 following CO inhalation and analyzed in triplicate, with the mean of minute 6 and 8 taken as post-rebreathing HbCO%. The amount of CO remaining in the spirometer was measured using a calibrated syringe and a portable CO detector (Draeger Pac 7000, Draeger, Germany). All data were compiled and used to calculate Hbmass according to previously published formulas [30,31].

The altitude in the present study was higher than any previous studies employing the optimized CO rebreathing method. To address a potential issue due to differences in oxygen saturation [33] between sea level and high altitude testing conditions, the following minor modification was made. For tests at sea level, subjects breathed a hyperoxic gas mixture (50.5% O_2, balance nitrogen, $P_IO_2 \approx 360$) for 10 minutes prior to baseline blood sampling and throughout the rest of the procedures, with the exception of the 2-minute CO rebreathing procedure, where 100% O_2 was rebreathed along with CO. At high altitude ($P_B = 408$ mmHg), subjects breathed 100% O_2 ($P_IO_2 \approx 360$) for 10 minutes prior to the baseline blood sampling and throughout the rest of the procedures. Hyperoxia was provided at both sea level and high altitude to establish similarly high oxygen saturation levels during the Hbmass procedure in both environments in order to eliminate the influence of oxygen saturation differences on the analytical determination of HbCO% on the OSM3 hemoximeter [33].

A single OSM3 unit was used for all HbCO% measurements during the study. To determine any potential confounding effects of the international transport on the OSM3 hemoximeter or high altitude *per se* on the measurement of HbCO%, we performed a quality control analysis using in-house arterial blood samples that we had obtained prior to this study at 2 levels of HbCO% (high and low HbCO%). These control samples were run in sextuplicate on 5 days during sea level testing and the mean ΔHbCO% between days was 6.84±0.05%; control samples were kept frozen at −80°C until transport–they remained stored on ice during transport and were analyzed in sextuplicate on 2 days within the first week at high altitude. The mean ΔHbCO% between these days was 6.80±0.07%. Thus, the difference in ΔHbCO% between sea level and high altitude was well within the intra-analyzer variability of ΔHbCO% using OSM3 hemoximeters [34], indicating that neither high altitude nor the international transport of the OSM3 had any confounding effects on the measurement of ΔHbCO% that is critical to Hbmass determination.

Measurement errors of Hbmass and BV parameters were calculated from duplicate baseline measurements (n = 19) according to Hopkins [35]. Measurement error for Hbmass was 1.5% (95%CI: 1.1–2.3%)–with duplicate Hbmass tests within a 1-week period, measurement error reflects primarily analytical error as the biological variation over this time frame has been shown to be minimal [36,37].

RCV, BV, and PV were derived from Hbmass, v[Hb], and vHct as follows:

1) $RCV = Hbmass \times MCHC^{-1} \times 100^{-1}$

2) $BV = RCV \times 100 \times Hct^{-1} \times 0.91^{-1}$

3) $PV = BV - RCV$

Hct was multiplied by 0.96 to account for trapped plasma; the constant of 0.91 was included in the BV calculation to correct for the ratio of body hematocrit to peripheral hematocrit [38]. Measurement errors for RCV, PV, and BV were 2.2% (95%CI: 1.6–3.2%), 4.9% (95%CI: 3.6–7.3%), and 3.4% (95%CI: 2.5–5.0%), respectively. For BV compartments, the measurement error is influenced by analytical error of Hbmass, [Hb], and Hct as well as biological variation in PV and total BV.

Serum Ferritin and EPO. Whole blood samples were collected following 30 min of rest from a catheter placed in an antecubital vein [22]. The ALT1 ferritin sample was taken after ~2 hours at 5260 m whereas the ALT1 EPO sample was taken after ~10 hours at 5260 m. Samples were drawn into 10 mL syringes and immediately transferred into serum collection vacutainers (BD, Franklin Lakes, NJ, USA). These vacutainers were inverted 5 times and then allowed to sit for 30–60 minutes at room temperature to allow for proper clotting. Tubes were spun for 20 minutes at 800 relative centrifugal force at room temperature. Once separated, serum was stored on ice for 10 minutes before being stored in either a −80°C freezer (Eugene), or in a charged nitrogen vapor shipper (Bolivia). Frozen serum samples were transported in charged nitrogen vapor shippers, and then stored at −80°C until analysis. Serum ferritin was assessed via nephelometry (within-run coefficient of variation (CV): 7%; between-run CV: 5%; Siemens BNII Nephelometer, Erlangen, Germany). Serum EPO was assessed in duplicate using a Quantikine IVD Human Epo ELISA kit (intra-assay CV: 4%; inter-assay CV: 6%; R&D Systems, Minneapolis, MN, USA).

Missing Data. As mentioned above, 6 Hbmass tests were excluded due to CO leaks. We also missed Hbmass tests due to logistical difficulties (6 tests) and subject discomfort prior to Hbmass testing (1 test). Some v[Hb] or vHct samples (total of 16 tests) were missed for logistical reasons and difficulties with obtaining or processing venous samples; in the case of missing v[Hb] or vHct, data were also excluded from the analysis of changes in BV parameters. The majority of missing tests for Hbmass and BV occurred at ALT1. Ferritin values were missing from 3 tests and EPO values were missing from 8 tests.

Statistics. Statistical analyses were performed using Statistical Package for the Social Sciences (version 20, SPSS Inc., Chicago, IL, USA) and Microsoft Excel 2008 (Redmond, WA, USA). We performed linear mixed model statistical analyses to examine our outcome variables across acclimatization using the Mixed procedure in SPSS. A major advantage of linear mixed model statistical analyses is that missing values do not result in casewise deletion of other longitudinal measurements, as is required with repeated-measures analysis of variance. Time (SL, ALT1, ALT7, ALT16), sex, and a time × sex interaction were included in the linear mixed models as fixed factors. Time comparisons were made with SL as the reference. Separate paired-tests were performed to compare ALT7 and ALT16. No adjustments were made for multiple testing. Due to largely reduced subject numbers at ALT1 for Hbmass/BV parameters, we could not be certain that the missing data at ALT1 met the missing-at-random requirement of the linear mixed model. Therefore, we performed paired t-tests to examine changes between SL and ALT1. To examine differences at POST7/POST21 compared to SL and ALT16, we used linear mixed models with time (SL, ALT16, POST), group (POST7, POST21), and a time × group interaction included as fixed factors. The POST timepoint includes POST7 and POST21 measurements, with differences between the groups descending for 7 versus 21 days assessed by comparing the effect of group. Time comparisons were made with POST as the reference–therefore, data from SL and ALT16 were excluded from these analyses for subjects missing the POST7/POST21 time point. Due to the reduced number of female subjects included at POST21 (n = 2), sex was not included in these models. We performed simple linear regressions to examine relationships between variables. For all analyses, statistical significance was accepted when $p \leq 0.05$. Data are presented throughout the paper as mean ± SD unless otherwise noted. A complete list of individual data for Hbmass and serum ferritin is provided in Table S1.

Results

Subject characteristics and ferritin status during high altitude acclimatization and de-acclimatization

A detailed description of subject characteristics is presented elsewhere [22] –briefly, body mass was reduced by 2.6±1.6 kg after 16 days of high altitude exposure. Serum ferritin levels are presented in Table 1. Ferritin levels were lower in women compared to men. At ALT1, all men had ferritin above 20 ng mL^{-1}, whereas 4 of 8 women had ferritin levels below this value. Ferritin levels decreased from ALT1 to ALT16 in both men (−68±16%) and women (−65±26%) and increased following descent from high altitude in both men (+189±196%) and women (+184±283%).

Hematological adaptations during 16 days of high altitude acclimatization

EPO increased from a baseline level of 8.3±5.0 IU L^{-1} by 4.9±2.8 fold at ALT1 (n = 16), 8.3±8.7 fold at ALT7 (n = 18), and 2.5±1.6 fold at ALT16 (n = 21; all $p<0.05$ compared to SL). There were no significant correlations between the increases in EPO at ALT1, ALT7, or ALT16 and changes in Hbmass. Data comparing SL and ALT1 for subjects with Hbmass/BV measurements at both time points are presented separately in Table 2 so that the effect of acute altitude on Hbmass and BV parameters can be distinguished from inter-individual variation. We found a non-significant 11 g loss in absolute Hbmass at ALT1 compared to SL (p = 0.206); there was also a trend for relative Hbmass to be slightly (0.3 g kg^{-1}) reduced at ALT1 compared to SL (p = 0.056). A small decrease in Hbmass was expected, as Hbmass was assessed after the required blood sampling for other protocol procedures on ALT1. v[Hb], vHct, and BV compartments were not significantly different at ALT1 compared to SL.

Table 3 presents data on hematological parameters at SL, ALT7, and ALT16. Compared to SL, absolute Hbmass was increased at ALT7 (+3.7±5.8%; n = 20; $p<0.01$) and ALT16 (+7.6±6.6%; n = 21; $p<0.001$), with the gain larger at ALT16 compared to ALT7. The increase in absolute Hbmass was larger in men compared to women at ALT16. Relative Hbmass was increased compared to SL at ALT7 and ALT16; relative Hbmass was greater at ALT16 compared to ALT7 and the increases were greater in men than women at both ALT7 and ALT16. Due to the lower absolute and relative Hbmass levels in women compared to men, we also examined the percent change in absolute Hbmass from SL and found no significant difference between men and women (Figure 1A). At ALT16, Hbmass was elevated compared to SL in all 12 men and 7 out of 9 women. There was no significant correlation between ferritin level upon initial exposure to altitude and the percent change in absolute Hbmass at ALT16 (Figure 1B).

Table 1. Serum ferritin during high altitude acclimatization and de-acclimatization.

Serum Ferritin (ng ml^{-1})	Time				Significant Effects	
	SL	ALT1	ALT16	POST	Sex	Time
M	63.2±29.0 (12)	66.8±42.2 (11)	25.8±24.0 (12)	52.3±44.0 (11)	M>W	ALT16 <SL; ALT16<ALT1; ALT16<POST
W	28.9±15.5 (9)	19.7±10.9 (8)	7.5±5.2 (9)	19.6±21.3 (9)		

Data are presented as mean ± SD (ng ml^{-1}) with the number of subjects indicated in parentheses. The POST measurement took place upon initial return to 5260 m following descent to 1525 m for 7 days (7W, 7M) or 21 days (2W, 4M) duration. Linear mixed model statistical analyses were performed to examine the effects of sex and time with SL as the reference. Paired t-tests were performed to compare ALT16 with ALT1 and POST. Effects were accepted as significant when $p \leq 0.05$.

Table 2. Hematological parameters at sea level and the first day of exposure to 5260 m.

	SL	ALT1	Percent Change
Hbmass (g)	723±175 (6,6)	711±173 (6,6)	−1.6±4.4%
Rel Hbmass (g kg^{-1})	10.1±1.4 (6,6)	9.8±1.4 (6,6)	−2.7±4.4%
v[Hb] (g dL^{-1})	13.9±1.0 (8,4)	14.3±1.5 (8,4)	2.5±6.7%
vHct (%)	42.6±2.6 (8,4)	42.6±4.5 (8,4)	−0.3±6.5%
BV (ml)	6224±848 (5,3)	6130±517 (5,3)	−0.8±7.5%
Rel BV (ml kg^{-1})	83.2±6.6 (5,3)	81.9±7.3 (5,3)	−1.4±7.0%
PV (ml)	3907±416 (5,3)	3866±276 (5,3)	−0.2±11.5%
Rel PV (ml kg^{-1})	52.4±4.7 (5,3)	51.9±7.3 (5,3)	−0.9±10.9%
RCV (ml)	2317±442 (5,3)	2264±417 (5,3)	−2.1±5.0%
Rel RCV (ml kg^{-1})	30.8±3.0 (5,3)	29.9±3.3 (5,3)	−2.6±5.6%

Data are presented as mean ± SD with the number of subjects (M,W) indicated in parentheses. This table only includes data for subjects with measures at both time points so that the effect of acute altitude on Hbmass and BV parameters can be distinguished from the inter-individual variation. Paired t-tests were performed for each parameter and none of the differences were statistically significant (all p>0.05).

v[Hb] and vHct were increased at ALT7 and ALT16 compared to SL, with no significant differences between ALT7 and ALT16. Men had larger increases in v[Hb] and vHct at ALT16 compared to women. Absolute and relative PV were reduced at ALT7 and ALT16 compared to SL, with no significant difference between ALT7 and ALT16. The reduction in absolute PV at ALT16 was greater in men compared to women, but no significant difference was detected in the change in relative PV. Absolute BV was reduced at ALT7 and ALT16 compared to SL, with no significant difference between ALT7 and ALT16 or in the change in BV between men and women. Relative BV was not significantly different from SL at ALT7 or ALT16, but there was a trend (p = 0.057) for women to have a greater reduction in relative BV compared to men at ALT7. Relative BV was greater at ALT16 compared to ALT7. Changes in absolute and relative RCV mirrored changes in Hbmass.

Hematological adaptations following descent to low altitude

Table 4 presents hematological parameters for subjects with complete measurements at SL, ALT16, and POST7/POST21. For all hematological parameters, there were no significant differences in responses between POST7 and POST21 groups or any significant group × time interactions. Absolute (−6.0±3.7%) and relative (−6.8±4.3%) Hbmass declined following high altitude descent–absolute Hbmass at the POST7/POST21 measurement was not significantly different from SL (+0.8±4.5%), but relative Hbmass was slightly elevated compared to SL (+3.2±5.5%). Figure 2A shows the percent changes in absolute Hbmass from SL at ALT16 and POST7/POST21. A similar pattern was observed for RCV, with absolute and relative RCV values reduced at POST7/POST21 compared to ALT16. Absolute and relative PV were increased at POST7/POST21 compared to ALT16 and not significantly different from SL. Absolute and relative BV at POST7/POST21 were not significantly different from ALT16 or SL. v[Hb] and vHct were reduced at POST7/POST21 compared to ALT16 and not significantly different compared to SL.

The gain in Hbmass from SL to ALT16 was correlated with the reduction in Hbmass from ALT16 to POST7/POST21 (Figure 2B; r = −0.77; n = 20; p = 0.00006). The reduction in Hbmass from ALT16 to POST7 was correlated with an increase in serum ferritin (Figure 2C; r = −0.64; n = 13; p = 0.02).

Discussion

This study provides the first data on early Hbmass alterations in healthy humans with ascent to and descent from altitudes greater than 5000 m. We found an increase in Hbmass at ALT7 and a further augmentation by ALT16. However, the altitude-induced gain in Hbmass was remarkably short-lived, as descent to low altitude resulted in a reduction in Hbmass to baseline values within 7 days. The correlation between the loss in Hbmass and increase in serum ferritin following descent to low altitude suggests that this rapid reduction in Hbmass was mediated by increased red blood cell destruction. Overall, this study demonstrates the capacity for rapid alterations in Hbmass with ascent to and descent from high altitude and suggests the need to further examine mechanisms of erythropoietic adaptations to severe hypoxia.

Increase in Hbmass during high altitude acclimatization

The veracity of our finding of swift alterations in Hbmass is predicated on the validity and sensitivity of our methodological approach for measuring Hbmass. We have several reasons to believe our measurements were robust and that our findings were not the result of analytical error or artifact. First, CO rebreathing methods have been shown to have low measurement error compared to other methodological approaches for assessing the red cell compartment [39] and we achieved a measurement error of 1.5% from duplicate baseline tests in the present study. At ALT7 and ALT16, the mean increases in Hbmass we observed were 2–5 times greater than our measurement error. Second, we performed quality-control analysis for ΔHbCO% both at SL and high altitude and found near-identical results [34]. Third, the ALT7 and ALT16 measures, at which Hbmass was elevated compared to SL, took place at the same location and with the same equipment and personnel as the POST7 and POST21 measures, at which Hbmass had returned to SL values following a 7 or 21 day de-acclimatization period. Therefore, a spurious inflation of Hbmass only at ALT7 and ALT16 seems unlikely. Taken together, we are confident that our findings reflect true physiological alterations in Hbmass with early ascent to and

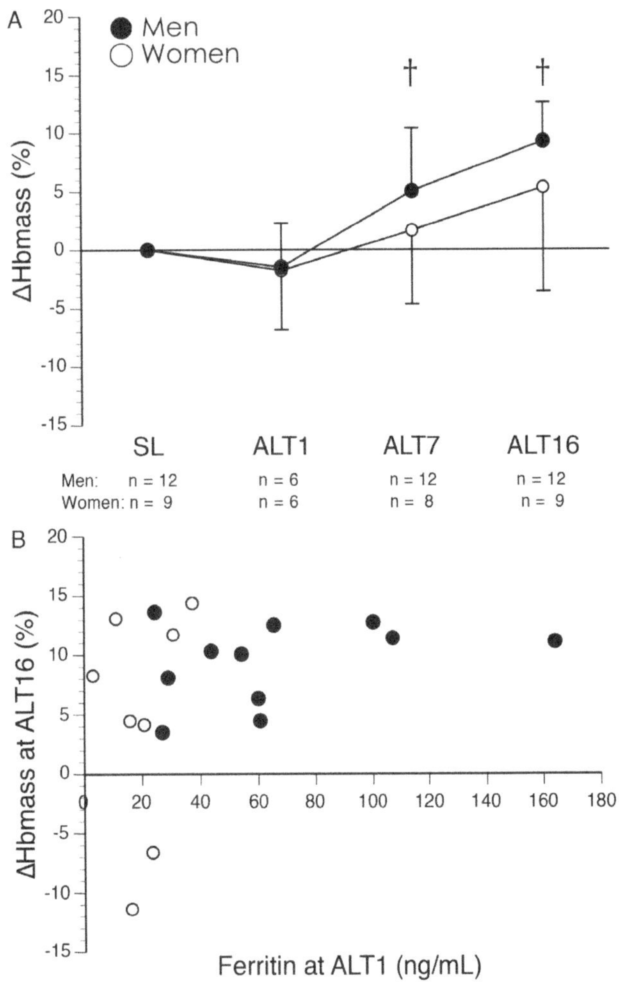

Figure 1. Hemoglobin mass in men and women during 16 days high altitude acclimatization. A) Time course of changes in absolute Hbmass. Data are presented as mean ± SD, with the number of men and women tested at each time indicated below the x-axis. †Significantly different from sea level ($p<0.05$; main effect of time). The percent changes were not significantly different between men and women ($p>0.05$). B) Relationship between serum ferritin level upon arrival at high altitude and the percent change in absolute Hbmass following 16 days at high altitude. Two subjects had missing ferritin data at ALT1 and their Hbmass data were excluded from this graph. There was no correlation between initial ferritin level upon arrival at altitude and the percent change in absolute Hbmass during high altitude acclimatization ($r = 0.33$; $n = 19$; $p = 0.16$).

descent from high altitude and were not caused by normal biological variation or analytical error.

The speed of change in Hbmass observed in our study conflicts with the classical dogma that increases in Hbmass during high altitude acclimatization take at least 3–4 weeks to develop [2,3]. Recent studies at moderate altitude (2000–3600 m) suggested that erythropoietic adaptations may be swifter than previously thought [13,14,15,17], but the speed and magnitude of increase in Hbmass we observed at ALT7 and ALT16 exceed previous findings. The magnitude of change we observed is particularly striking given that some Hbmass was lost due to sampling (estimated loss of 29±12 g at ALT1, 10±4 g at ALT7, and 30±4 g at ALT16). We report the Hbmass values that we measured without adjusting for the blood lost due to sampling–this underestimates the total increase in the amount of hemoglobin produced at high altitude (estimate presented in Figure 3), which includes the Hbmass change we measured above our SL baseline values plus the Hbmass lost due to blood sampling on ALT1, ALT7 and ALT16 combined (calculated as 69±16 g; n = 21). Our findings raise the intriguing question of what mechanism enables this rapid and robust increase in Hbmass in response to severe hypoxia.

The regulation of red cell production is known to be largely influenced by EPO [42]. EPO peaks within the first 2–3 days of altitude exposure before beginning to fall towards baseline [40,41] and it has been suggested that the rapid return of EPO to baseline levels with continued altitude exposure should reduce the magnitude of the erythropoeitic stimulus compared to exogenous EPO treatment [2]. However, single measurements of circulating EPO do not adequately reflect the complex kinetics of EPO secretion over days and weeks, and it is unclear if the fall in circulating EPO with continued altitude exposure results from a decrease in EPO expression or is related to an increased rate of clearance from circulation [42]. It is noteworthy that much of the RCV expansion in lowlanders ascending to 4540 m for a 12-month period occurred after 1–2 months [7], a time at which EPO would be expected to have returned to baseline [40,41]. Importantly, our finding of an increase in Hbmass within 7 days of ascent to high altitude is in stark contrast to studies involving exogenous EPO administration, where Hbmass has been consistently reported to remain unchanged within the first 12 days of treatment [4,5,6] despite continuous elevation of circulating EPO above baseline [4]. In comparing high altitude ascent with EPO treatment, it is important to consider that the distinct stimuli of high altitude residence *versus* pharmacological EPO administration are markedly different. Whereas the elevation in EPO with severe hypoxia is secondary to hypoxia-inducible factor (HIF) signaling [43], the provision of exogenous EPO bypasses broad HIF activation. Differences between these conditions are reflected in divergent responses in other pathways affected by HIF signaling that influence erythopoietic adaptations such as iron mobilization [4,43,44]. Ultimately, we cannot provide mechanistic data from our study explaining the swifter increase in Hbmass in our subjects compared to previous studies at lower elevations or involving exogenous EPO administration, and we are not suggesting that EPO is not a key player in augmenting erythropoiesis in response to severe hypoxia. Rather, the more rapid increase in Hbmass in severe hypoxia compared to exogenous EPO treatment suggests that mechanisms in addition to augmentation of EPO may play an important role in the rapid erythropoietic response.

To our knowledge, we are the first to compare changes in Hbmass/RCV in men and women at identical time points and under similar experimental conditions at altitudes greater than 4000 m. We found that the percent increase in absolute Hbmass following 16 days at high altitude was not significantly different between men and women. Some previous cross-sectional studies of moderate altitude residents have suggested that erythropoietic responses may be lower in females compared to males [45,46], and it has been suggested that the ventilatory-stimulating effects of the female sex hormones play a key role [47]. However, Reeves et al. found no effect of menstrual phase on ventilatory or erythropoietic adaptations in healthy women acclimatizing to 4300 m despite large differences in sex hormone levels between subjects in the luteal versus follicular phases [12]. Arterial oxygen pressure and saturation did not differ between men and women at ALT1 and therefore the impact of ventilatory effects on potential sex differences in erythropoietic responses to high altitude would be minimal in our study.

Table 3. Hematological adaptations during 16 days high altitude acclimatization in healthy men and women.

		Time			Significant Effects		
		SL	ALT7	ALT16	Sex	Time	Interaction
Hbmass (g)					M>W	ALT7>SL; ALT16>SL; ALT16>ALT7	ΔM>ΔW ALT16
	M	905±95 (12)	950±110 (12)	989±110 (12)			
	W	559±62 (9)	567±76 (8)	590±91 (9)			
Rel Hbmass (g kg^{-1})					M>W	ALT7>SL; ALT16>SL; ALT16>ALT7	ΔM>ΔW ALT7; ΔM>ΔW ALT16
	M	11.9±1.4 (12)	13.0±1.7 (12)	13.8±1.6 (12)			
	W	9.1±0.8 (9)	9.2±1.0 (8)	9.7±1.2 (9)			
v[Hb] (g dL^{-1})					M>W	ALT7>SL; ALT16>SL	ΔM>ΔW ALT16
	M	14.6±0.6 (12)	16.2±1.1 (12)	16.9±0.6 (12)			
	W	12.4±0.8 (9)	13.7±1.1 (8)	13.4±1.0 (8)			
vHct (%)					M>W	ALT7>SL; ALT16>SL	ΔM>ΔW ALT16
	M	44.2±1.4 (12)	48.5±3.0 (12)	50.6±2.2 (12)			
	W	39.1±2.3 (9)	42.4±2.8 (8)	42.1±3.3 (8)			
BV (ml)					M>W	ALT7<SL; ALT16<SL	
	M	6813±667 (12)	6434±687 (12)	6420±588 (12)			
	W	4974±565 (9)	4592±730 (7)	4821±756 (8)			
Rel BV (ml kg^{-1})					M>W	ALT16>ALT7	
	M	89.9±9.3 (12)	88.0±8.9 (12)	89.5±8.0 (12)			
	W	80.9±7.1 (9)	74.2±7.8 (7)	78.7±9.8 (8)			
PV (ml)					M>W	ALT7<SL; ALT16<SL	ΔM>ΔW ALT16
	M	4190±412 (12)	3713±473 (12)	3580±304 (12)			
	W	3287±417 (9)	2921±502 (7)	3047±499 (8)			
Rel PV (ml kg^{-1})						ALT7<SL; ALT16<SL	
	M	55.3±5.5 (12)	50.7±5.5 (12)	49.9±3.8 (12)			
	W	53.4±5.6 (9)	47.2±5.5 (7)	49.8±6.9 (8)			
RCV (ml)					M>W	ALT7>SL; ALT16>SL; ALT16>ALT7	
	M	2623±279 (12)	2721±298 (12)	2839±331 (12)			
	W	1687±188 (9)	1671±247 (7)	1773±300 (8)			
Rel RCV (ml kg^{-1})					M>W	ALT7>SL; ALT16>SL; ALT16>ALT7	ΔM>ΔW ALT7; ΔM>ΔW ALT16
	M	34.6±4.0 (12)	37.3±4.6 (12)	39.6±4.8 (12)			
	W	27.4±2.3 (9)	27.1±2.8 (7)	28.9±4.0 (8)			

Data are presented as mean ± SD with the number of subjects indicated in parentheses. Linear mixed model statistical analyses were performed to examine the effects of sex, time (with SL as the reference) and a sex × time interaction. Paired t-tests were performed to compare ALT7 with ALT16. Effects were accepted as significant when $p \leq 0.05$.

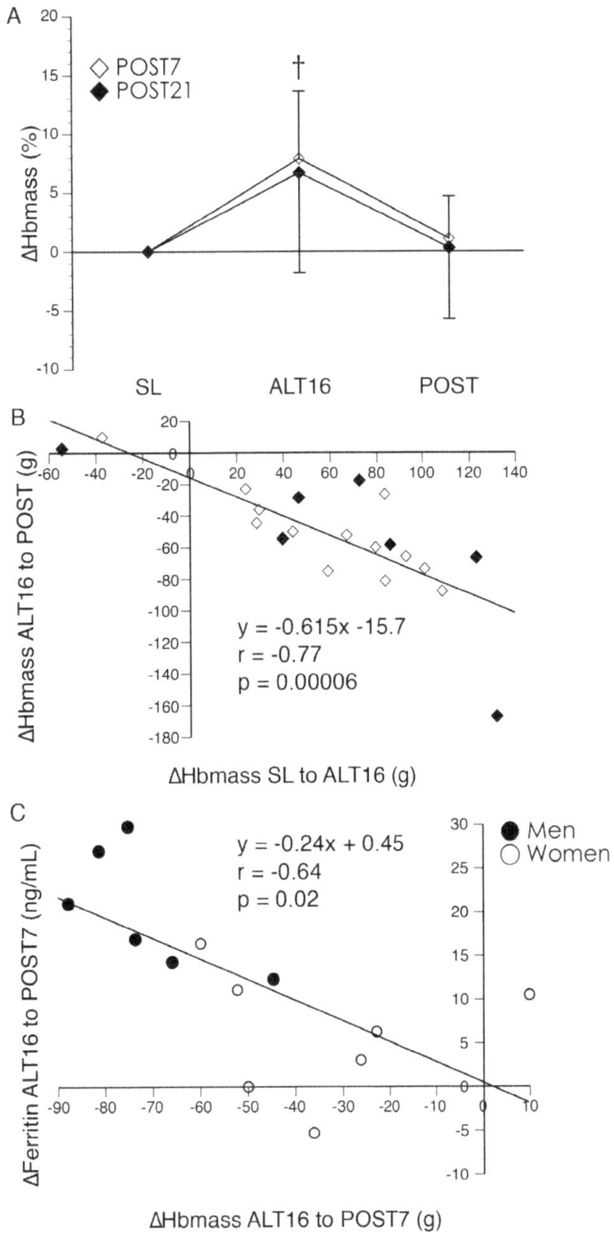

Figure 2. Change in hemoglobin mass following descent from high altitude to low altitude. Subjects were tested at high altitude at the end of a 16 day acclimatization period and upon return to high altitude after descent to low altitude (1525 m) for either 7 (POST7; n = 13) or 21 days (POST21; n = 7). Data are presented as mean ± SD. A) Changes in Hbmass. † Significantly different from POST ($p<0.05$; main effect of time). There were no significant differences between the POST7 and POST21 groups or between POST and SL ($p>0.05$). B) Relationship between changes in Hbmass following 16 days high altitude acclimatization and changes in Hbmass following descent to low altitude. C) Relationship between changes in Hbmass and changes in serum ferritin following descent to low altitude for 7 days.

Our finding that the percent change in absolute Hbmass did not differ between men and women is particularly striking given the low ferritin levels of our female subjects upon arrival at high altitude. Although subjects with low ferritin during baseline testing were directed to take oral iron supplements up until departure for high altitude, several women arrived at high altitude with low ferritin levels, and based on previous work at moderate altitude [48], one might expect that the low iron stores would prevent an increase in Hbmass. In contrast, most (7 out of 9) of the women increased Hbmass in response to high altitude exposure. However, while all 12 men had increases in Hbmass following 16 days high altitude acclimatization, 2 women failed to increase Hbmass; indeed, these 2 women had reductions in Hbmass that were similar to the calculated amount of Hbmass withdrawn from these subjects for blood sampling at altitude. We examined the EPO response of these 2 individual subjects and found that their increases in EPO with high altitude exposure were above the group median at ALT1, ALT7, and ALT16, suggesting that the failure to increase Hbmass was not caused by a lack of EPO upregulation. As can be observed in Figure 1B, these 2 women were not distinguished by particularly low iron stores upon arrival at high altitude. Indeed, our individual data demonstrate the capability to increase Hbmass despite low ferritin levels upon initial arrival at high altitude. The subject with the lowest ferritin (3 ng mL^{-1}) upon initial high altitude exposure had a relatively large (8.3%) increase in Hbmass.

It might be questioned whether the level of storage iron indicated by these low ferritin values would be sufficient to enable a large increase in Hbmass. However, previous work has demonstrated increases in intestinal iron absorption at high altitude [7,49,50] and it is possible that dietary iron intake (not measured in the current study) provided sufficient iron for increasing hemoglobin production. Additionally, recent data suggest that a decrease in skeletal muscle iron content during the first week at high altitude may increase iron available for erythropoiesis [44]. Admittedly, because we did not measure dietary iron intake or iron-related proteins in skeletal muscle, the role of these mechanisms in allowing increased erythropoiesis in our subjects with low ferritin is purely speculative. However, these other studies highlight the complexity of iron homeostasis at high altitude and suggest that the iron required for increasing erythropoiesis may have been obtained from increased intestinal absorption or mobilization of iron from skeletal muscle stores. Further studies involving Hbmass assessments coupled with more comprehensive assessments of iron homeostasis are needed to more robustly determine the relationship between iron availability and erythropoiesis at high altitude. Our data suggest that low initial iron stores do not requisitely prevent high altitude-induced erythropoiesis; however, we stress that we cannot determine from our data whether low iron stores limited the magnitude of increase in Hbmass in some subjects.

Decrease in Hbmass following descent from high altitude to low altitude

We found that the Hbmass gained during high altitude acclimatization was quickly lost following descent to 1525 m. Hbmass had returned to SL baseline in our subjects who descended to low altitude for 7 days, and there was no further decrement in the group who descended for 21 days. To our knowledge, we are the first to report a complete loss of altitude-induced Hbmass adaptation within 7 days; the speed of this de-acclimatization response contrasts with previous studies, in which Hbmass has been reported to remain elevated above baseline for multiple weeks following descent to SL [14,15,17,51]. Although a rapid loss in RCV following high altitude descent has been previously reported by Rice et al. [21], there are several aspects of our study that make our findings unique. We studied lowlanders following just 16 days of high altitude acclimatization whereas Rice et al. [21] studied polycythemic high altitude natives. This was reflected by dramatic differences in the degree of polycythe-

Table 4. Hematological adaptations following descent from high altitude to low altitude.

		Time			Significant Effects
		SL	**ALT16**	**POST**	**Time**
Hbmass (g)					**POST<ALT16**
	POST7	726±172 (6,7)	785±194 (6,7)	734±173 (6,7)	
	POST21	802±245 (5,2)	865±296 (5,2)	810±266 (5,2)	
Rel Hbmass (g kg^{-1})					**POST<ALT16; POST>SL**
	POST7	10.2±1.4 (6,7)	11.3±1.9 (6,7)	10.5±1.6 (6,7)	
	POST21	11.7±2.4 (5,2)	13.3±3.3 (5,2)	12.3±2.9 (5,2)	
v[Hb] (g dL^{-1})					**POST<ALT16**
	POST7	13.6±1.2 (5,4)	15.4±1.6 (5,4)	13.8±1.5 (5,4)	
	POST21	14.2±1.1 (5,2)	16.0±2.1 (5,2)	14.7±1.8 (5,2)	
vHct (%)					**POST<ALT16**
	POST7	42.3±2.9 (5,4)	47.0±4.3 (5,4)	42.0±4.1 (5,4)	
	POST21	43.1±2.9 (5,2)	48.5±6.1 (5,2)	44.4±4.1 (5,2)	
BV (ml)					
	POST7	6017±907 (4,4)	5694±926 (4,4)	5965±825 (4,4)	
	POST21	6125±1569 (5,2)	5820±1476 (5,2)	5914±1445 (5,2)	
Rel BV (ml kg^{-1})					
	POST7	83.6±5.2 (4,4)	81.4±7.1 (4,4)	85.0±6.0 (4,4)	
	POST21	90.1±13.2 (5,2)	90.2±12.5 (5,2)	90.9±12.0 (5,2)	
PV (ml)					**POST>ALT16**
	POST7	3813±435 (4,4)	3363±403 (4,4)	3775±423 (4,4)	
	POST21	3799±885 (5,2)	3300±664 (5,2)	3587±749 (5,2)	
Rel PV (ml kg^{-1})					**POST>ALT16**
	POST7	53.2±3.1 (4,4)	48.3±3.0 (4,4)	54.0±4.4 (4,4)	
	POST21	56.1±6.9 (5,2)	51.5±4.0 (5,2)	55.4±5.3 (5,2)	
RCV (ml)					**POST<ALT16**
	POST7	2204±485 (4,4)	2331±556 (4,4)	2190±480 (4,4)	
	POST21	2326±695 (5,2)	2520±847 (5,2)	2326±711 (5,2)	
Rel RCV (ml kg^{-1})					**POST<ALT16**
	POST7	30.4±3.6 (4,4)	33.2±5.3 (4,4)	31.0±4.2 (4,4)	
	POST21	34.0±6.7 (5,2)	38.7±9.4 (5,2)	35.5±7.3 (5,2)	

Data are presented as mean ± SD with the number of subjects (M,W) indicated in parentheses. Subjects were studied at sea level, at 5260 m after 16 days high altitude acclimatization, and upon initial return to 5260 m after descent to 1525 m for 7 (POST7) or 21 (POST21) days. Linear mixed model statistical analyses were performed to examine the effects of time (with POST as the reference), group (POST7 versus POST21) and a time × group interaction. Effects were accepted as significant when $p \leq 0.05$. There were no significant effects of group or any significant group × time interactions (all $p > 0.05$).

mia obtained at high altitude (mean [Hb] of 23.4 g dL^{-1} in the high altitude natives versus 15.5 g dL^{-1} at ALT16 in our subjects). Indeed, the majority of subjects in the study of Rice et al. [21] met the criteria for excessive erythrocytosis ([Hb]≥21 in men or ≥19 in women; [52]) whereas none of our subjects came within 2 g dL^{-1} of this criterion at ALT16. Therefore, our results show that the development of excessive polycythemia is not required for high altitude descent to induce a rapid loss in Hbmass.

Based on the kinetics of red blood cell turnover (~0.83% of circulating cells destroyed per day [53]) and the delayed influence of changes in EPO on red blood cell production [21,42], the large reduction in Hbmass we observed within 7 days is unlikely to be explained by a reduction in red blood cell production. The correlation between the loss in Hbmass and increase in serum ferritin from ALT16 to POST7 suggests an increase in red blood cell destruction, as the iron contained in destroyed red blood cells is transferred to iron stores [21]. It is possible that neocytolysis, the selective destruction of a population of young red blood cells [54,55,56], may have been the mechanism of this rapid loss in Hbmass. However, the strength of the evidence for neocytolysis has recently been questioned [57]. We did not measure markers of red blood cell production or examine red blood cell age distributions during high altitude acclimatization and de-acclimatization and therefore cannot provide direct evidence in support of, or against a role for, neocytolysis.

Our finding of a rapid loss in Hbmass following descent from high altitude contrasts with patterns observed following cessation of exogenous EPO administration [5,6,20], despite the fact that these studies induced similar or larger elevations in Hbmass and [Hb]/Hct compared to our observations. Although it was hypothesized that cessation of exogenous EPO therapy would induce neocytolysis and lead to a rapid reduction in Hbmass

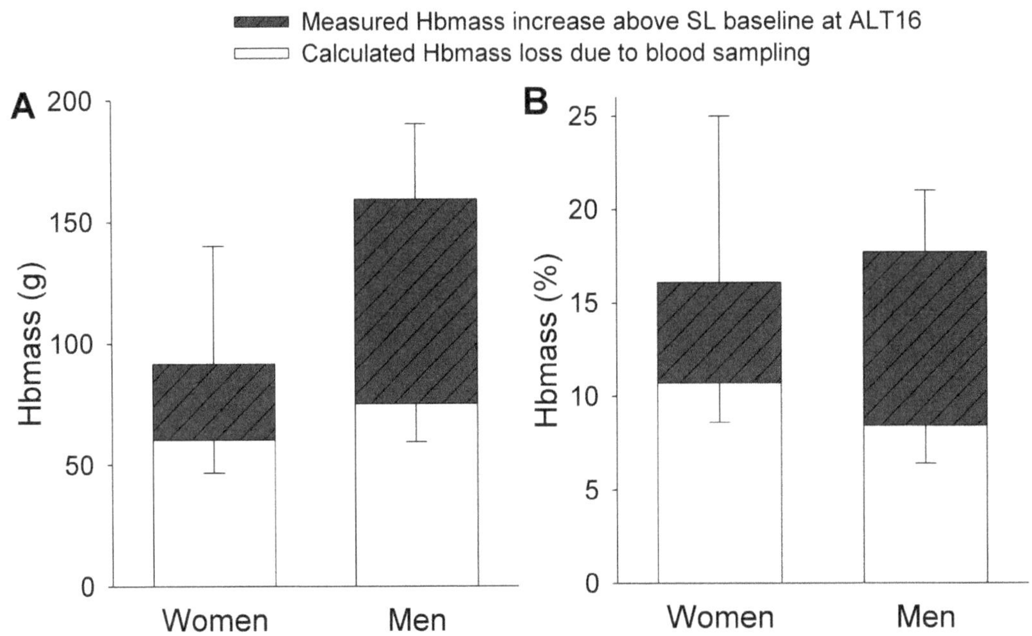

Figure 3. Estimate of the increase in hemoglobin mass produced during 16 days high altitude acclimatization determined from the measured Hbmass increase above sea level baseline plus the calculated Hbmass loss due to blood sampling. Panel A represents the absolute increase in Hbmass (g) produced. Panel B represents the percent increase in Hbmass produced. Data are presented as mean ± SD. Upward SD bars represent the SD of the increase in Hbmass measured above baseline and the downward SD bars represent the SD of calculated Hbmass loss due to blood sampling.

[21,56], recent studies provide compelling evidence that this is not the case, with Hbmass/RCV consistently reported to remain unchanged for 2 weeks following treatment cessation before beginning to fall gradually back to baseline [5,6,20]. The stimulus for increased red blood cell production with high altitude acclimatization is hypobaric hypoxia, whereas EPO treatment elevates Hbmass in the absence of systemic hypoxia. Although this suggests that the production of red blood cells under conditions of hypoxia may influence the retention of Hbmass adaptations, it is important to note that rapid reductions in Hbmass have also been reported with spaceflight [54] and dehydration-induced rapid weight loss [58] and neither of these situations involve systemic hypoxia. Further work is required to clearly establish the mechanism(s) of rapid loss of Hbmass in healthy humans.

What are the implications of the rapid loss in Hbmass following descent to low altitude on acclimatization status upon return to high altitude? The reduction in oxygen carrying capacity might be expected to impair submaximal endurance performance upon return to 5260 m; however, despite large reductions in absolute and relative Hbmass from ALT16 to POST7, the improvement in 3.2 km run time-trial performance from ALT1 to ALT16 with acclimatization was fully maintained at POST7 [22]. This calls into question the importance of the altitude-induced Hbmass adaptation for submaximal endurance performance at high altitude. Previous studies examining the effects of artificial Hbmass alterations with erythrocyte infusion [59,60], recombinant EPO treatment [61], and isovolemic hemodilution [62] have failed to observe alterations in maximal oxygen uptake or endurance performance at altitudes greater than 4300 m. Our results extend these findings by showing that the loss in Hbmass accompanying descent to low altitude does not result in impaired submaximal endurance performance upon return to high altitude. However, previous work suggests that there may be a threshold altitude above which alterations in Hbmass have minimal effects on maximal oxygen uptake [61], and we stress that our finding of maintained endurance performance despite significant loss of Hbmass may not apply to performances at less severe altitudes.

Changes in blood volume compartments during high altitude acclimatization and de-acclimatization

In support of previous high altitude studies (Reviewed in [2]), we observed large reductions in absolute and relative PV at ALT7 and ALT16. However, we did not detect a significant reduction in PV in the first 9–13 hours of initial exposure to 5260 m and the PV measured 9–13 hours after return to 5260 m following descent to low altitude was not different from SL. Some studies have found reductions in PV within the first hours of high altitude exposure [9,10] but other studies have failed to detect changes within this time window [23,24]. Differences between studies are likely influenced by several factors including hydration status, exercise prior to PV assessments, acute mountain sickness, and the methodology used to assess PV. PV returned to SL values following descent to low altitude. Previous work has indicated that the recovery of PV following high altitude descent occurs within 2 days and is influenced by changes in fluid-regulating hormones including renin, aldosterone, and vasopressin [26,27], so our finding of a recovered PV following 1 and 3 weeks at low altitude is not surprising. As expected, changes in RCV paralleled the changes we observed in Hbmass. Compared to SL, relative BV was unchanged by high altitude acclimatization and de-acclimatization, at least at the time points we assessed–relative BV was influenced both by alterations in the absolute sizes of the BV compartments and small changes in body mass [22] during high altitude acclimatization and de-acclimatization. In our subjects, reductions in relative PV during high altitude acclimatization were offset by an augmentation of relative RCV. The opposite response occurred following descent to low altitude, with the diminution in relative RCV offset by an enlargement of relative PV.

Limitations

There are some potential limitations to the current study that should be considered. The overall experimental design lacked a separate lowlander control group that was studied over time in the absence of altitude exposure. However, Hbmass has been consistently shown to be stable over time in subjects at SL [36,37] and we took several steps to ensure that the SL and high altitude measurements were comparable, as detailed above. Additionally, because examining responses to acute hypoxia on ALT1 was a key component of the overall AltitudeOmics study design, many steps were taken to minimize the subjects' exposure to hypoxia prior to ALT1 [22]. During the travel period prior to ALT1 (including flight time), subjects spent less than 20 hours exposed to hypoxia equivalent to 2000 m or greater. A recent meta-analysis of changes in Hbmass with hypoxia reported gains in Hbmass of ~1% per 100 hours spent above 2000 m [17]. Therefore, the effect of hypoxic exposure prior to ALT1 on the Hbmass response is estimated as less than 0.2%, dramatically lower than the increases we observed at ALT7 and ALT16.

As described previously, subjects were unable to maintain their normal physical activity habits at high altitude and some detraining may have occurred during acclimatization, with some fitness restoration during the period spent at low altitude [22]. Eastwood et al. found a 3.1% reduction in Hbmass after 30 days of detraining (~90% reduction in training volume) in triathletes at SL, but reported unchanged Hbmass at 10 and 20 days following training reduction [63]. A potential interaction between hypoxia and detraining on changes in Hbmass with ascent to high altitude has not been previously examined. There is a very strong cross-sectional relationship between lean body mass and Hbmass at sea level [64] and it could be speculated that the mean loss of ~1.5 kg lean body mass between ALT1 and ALT16 [22] may have reduced the erythropoietic stimulus. However, data examining a potential interaction between changes in lean body mass and Hbmass during altitude sojourn are currently lacking. Next, although subjects with low ferritin prior to baseline testing were directed to take oral iron supplements, supplementation was not directly monitored and the efficacy of supplementation in increasing serum ferritin was not determined prior to arrival at high altitude. Some subjects arrived at high altitude with low ferritin levels and it is possible that this may have limited the increase in Hbmass. However, as noted above, several subjects had robust increases in Hbmass despite low ferritin levels upon arrival.

Finally, the potential influence of blood loss due to sampling should be considered. Blood loss due to sampling occurs in many studies but its potential influence on hematological and other physiological outcomes is often ignored. The amount of blood removed due to sampling at ALT1 is of a magnitude that may induce a small EPO response at SL [65]. It is important to consider that it takes ~5 weeks to recover Hbmass lost from a 550 mL blood donation at SL [66], whereas our subjects were able to increase Hbmass above SL baseline within 7 days despite the loss of blood due to sampling. While we cannot rule out a potential interaction between blood loss due to sampling and the hypoxic stimulus on the magnitude of the erythropoietic response, it is clear that the hypoxic stimulus drives the rapid gain in Hbmass observed at 5260 m.

Conclusions

We documented the early time course of Hbmass adaptations at 5260 m and found rapid increases following just 7 and 16 days of high altitude acclimatization. The altitude-induced gain in Hbmass was remarkably short-lived, as descent to low altitude resulted in a dramatic loss in Hbmass within 7 days. The loss in Hbmass was correlated with an increase in serum ferritin, suggesting an increase in red blood cell destruction. Overall, this study demonstrates the capacity for rapid alterations in Hbmass with high altitude acclimatization and de-acclimatization in healthy men and women and suggests the need to further examine mechanisms of erythropoietic adaptations to severe hypoxia.

Acknowledgments

This paper is part of a series titled "AltitudeOmics" that together represent a group of studies that explored the basic mechanisms controlling human acclimatization to hypoxia and its subsequent retention. Many people and organizations invested enormous amounts of time and resources to make AltitudeOmics a success. Foremost, the study was made possible by the tireless support, generosity and tenacity of our research subjects. AltitudeOmics principal investigators were Colleen G. Julian, Andrew T. Lovering, Andrew W. Subudhi and Robert C. Roach. A complete list of other investigators on this multinational, collaborative effort involved in development, subject management and data collection, supporting industry partners, and people and organizations in Bolivia that made AltitudeOmics possible is available elsewhere [22].

Author Contributions

Conceived and designed the experiments: BJR NBW WFS WCB CGJ ATL AWS RCR. Performed the experiments: BJR NBW. Analyzed the data: BJR NBW WFS WCB CGJ ATL AWS RCR. Wrote the paper: BJR NBW WFS WCB CGJ ATL AWS RCR.

References

1. Eckardt K-U, Boutellier U, Kurtz A, Schopen M, Koller EA, et al. (1989) Rate of erythropoietin formation in humans in response to acute hypobaric hypoxia. J Appl Physiol 66: 1785–1788.
2. Sawka MN, Convertino VA, Eichner ER, Schnieder SM, Young AJ (2000) Blood volume: importance and adaptations to exercise training, environmental stresses, and trauma/sickness. Med Sci Sports Exerc 32: 332–348.
3. Grover RF, Bärtsch P (2001) Blood. In: High Altitude: An Exploration of Human Adaptation, edited by Hornbein TF, Schoene RB. New York & Basel: M. Dekker, Inc.
4. Robach P, Recalcati S, Girelli D, Gelfi C, Aachmann-Andersen NJ, et al. (2009) Alterations of systemic and muscle iron metabolism in human subjects treated with low-dose recombinant erythropoietin. Blood 113: 6707–6715.
5. Olsen NV, Aachmann-Andersen N-J, Oturai P, Munch-Andersen T, Bornø A, et al. (2011) Erythropoietin down-regulates proximal renal tubular reabsorption and causes a fall in glomerular filtration rate in humans. J Physiol 589: 1273–1281.
6. Durussel J, Daskalaki E, Anderson M, Chatterji T, Wondimu DH, et al. (2013) Haemoglobin mass and running time trial performance after recombinant human erythropoietin administration in trained men. PLoS ONE 8(2): e56151.
7. Reynafarje C, Lozano R, Valdivieso J (1959) The polycythemia of high altitudes: iron metabolism and related aspects. Blood 14: 433–455.
8. Pugh LGCE (1964) Blood volume and haemoglobin concentration at altitudes above 18,000 ft (5500 m). J Physiol 170: 344–354.
9. Sawka MN, Young AJ, Rock PB, Lyons TP, Boushel R, et al. (1996) Altitude acclimatization and blood volume: effects of exogenous erythrocyte volume expansion. J Appl Physiol 81: 636–642.
10. Grover RF, Selland MA, McCullough RG, Dahms TE, Wolfel EE, et al. (1998) ß-Adrenergic blockade does not prevent polycythemia or decrease in plasma volume in men at 4300 m altitude. Eur J Appl Physiol 77: 264–270.

11. Wolfel EE, Groves BM, Brooks GA, Butterfield GE, Mazzeo RS, et al. (1991) Oxygen transport during steady-state submaximal exercise in chronic hypoxia. J Appl Physiol 70: 1129–1136.
12. Reeves JT, Zamudio S, Dahms TE, Asmus I, Braun B, et al. (2001) Erythropoiesis in women during 11 days at 4,300 m is not affected by menstrual cycle phase. J Appl Physiol 91: 2579–2586.
13. Garvican L, Martin D, Quod M, Stephens B, Sassi A, et al. (2012) Time course of the hemoglobin mass response to natural altitude training in elite endurance cyclists. Scand J Med Sci Sports 22: 95–103.
14. Wachsmuth NB, Völzke C, Prommer N, Schmidt-Trucksäss A, Frese F, et al. (2013) The effects of classic altitude training on hemoglobin mass in swimmers. Eur J Appl Physiol 113: 1199–1211.
15. Wachsmuth NB, Kley M, Spielvogel H, Aughey RJ, Gore CJ, et al. (2013) Changes in blood gas transport of altitude native soccer players near sea-level and sea-level native soccer players at altitude (ISA3600). Br J Sports Med 47, i93–i99.
16. Rasmussen P, Siebenmann C, Díaz V, Lundby C (2013) Red cell volume expansion at altitude: a meta-analysis and Monte Carlo simulation. Med Sci Sports Exerc 45: 1767–1772.
17. Gore CJ, Sharpe K, Garvican-Lewis LA, Saunders PU, Humberstone CE, et al. (2013) Altitude training and haemoglobin mass from the optimised carbon monoxide rebreathing method determined by a meta-analysis. Br J Sports Med 47: i31–i39.
18. Milledge JS, Cotes PM (1985) Serum erythropoietin in humans at high altitude and its relation to plasma renin. J Appl Physiol 59: 360–364.
19. Richalet J-P, Souberbielle J-C, Antezana A-M, Déchaux M, Le Trong J-L, et al. (1994) Control of erythropoiesis in humans during prolonged exposure to the altitude of 6,542 m. Am J Physiol Regul Integr Comp Physiol 266: R756–R764.
20. Lundby C, Achman-Andersen NJ, Thomsen JJ, Norgaard AM, Robach P (2008) Testing for recombinant human erythropoietin in urine: problems associated with current anti-doping testing. J Appl Physiol 105: 417–419.
21. Rice L, Ruiz W, Driscoll T, Whitley CE, Tapia R, et al. (2001) Neocytolysis on descent from altitude: a newly recognized mechanism for the control of red cell mass. Ann Intern Med 134: 652–656.
22. Subudhi AW, Bourdillon N, Bucher J, Davis C, Elliott JE, et al. (2014) AltitudeOmics: the integrative physiology of human acclimatization to hypobaric hypoxia and its retention upon reascent. PLoS ONE 9(3): e92191.
23. Imoberdorf R, Garlick PJ, McNurlan MA, Casella GA, Peheim E, et al. (2001) Enhanced synthesis of albumin and fibrinogen at high altitude. J Appl Physiol 90: 528–537.
24. Loeppky JA, Roach RC, Maes D, Hinghofer-Szalkay H, Roessler A, et al. (2004) Role of hypobaria in fluid balance response to hypoxia. High Alt Med Biol 6: 60–71.
25. Poulsen TD, Klausen T, Richalet J-P, Kanstrup I-L, Fogh-Andersen N, et al. (1998) Plasma volume in acute hypoxia: comparison of a carbon monoxide rebreathing method and dye dilution with Evans' blue. Eur J Appl Physiol 77: 457–461.
26. Robach P, Dechaux M, Jarrot S, Vaysse J, Schneider J-C, et al. (2000) Operation Everest III: role of plasma volume expansion on $\dot{V}O_2$ max during prolonged high-altitude exposure. J Appl Physiol 89: 29–37.
27. Robach P, Lafforgue E, Olsen NV, Déchaux M, Fouqueray B, et al. (2002) Recovery of plasma volume after 1 week of exposure at 4,350 m. Pflugers Arch-Eur J Physiol 444: 821–828.
28. Smith TG, Robbins PA, Ratcliffe PJ (2008) The human side of hypoxia-inducible factor. Br J Haematology 141: 325–334.
29. Talbot NP, Smith TG, Privat C, Nickol AH, Rivera-Ch M, et al. (2011) Intravenous iron supplementation may protect against acute mountain sickness: a randomized, double-blinded, placebo-controlled trial. High Alt Med Biol 12: 265–269.
30. Schmidt W, Prommer N (2005) The optimised CO-rebreathing method: a new tool to determine total haemoglobin mass routinely. Eur J Appl Physiol 95: 486–495.
31. Prommer N, Schmidt W (2007) Loss of CO from the intravascular bed and its impact on the optimised CO-rebreathing method. Eur J Appl Physiol 100: 383–391.
32. Ryan BJ, Brothers MD, Nelson JL, Doan BK, Zupan MF, et al. (2011) Influence of carbon monoxide leaks on the measurement error of total haemoglobin mass. Scand J Clin Lab Invest 71: 523–528.
33. Hütler M, Beneke R, Littschwager A, Böning D (2001) Fraction of carboxyhaemoglobin depends on oxygen saturation of haemoglobin. Scand J - Clin Lab Invest 61: 83–88.
34. Gough CE, Sharpe K, Ashenden MJ, Anson JM, Saunders PU, et al. (2011) Quality control technique to reduce the variability of longitudinal measurement of hemoglobin mass. Scand J Med Sci Sports 21: e365–e371.
35. Hopkins WG (2000) Measures of reliability in sports medicine and science. Sports Med 30: 1–15.
36. Eastwood A, Hopkins WG, Bourdon PC, Withers RT, Gore CJ (2008) Stability of hemoglobin mass over 100 days in active men. J Appl Physiol 104: 982–985.
37. Prommer N, Sottas P-E, Schoch C, Schumacher YO, Schmidt W (2008) Total hemoglobin mass–a new parameter to detect blood doping? Med Sci Sports Exerc 40: 2112–2118.
38. Chaplin H, Mollison PL, Vetter H (1953) The body/venous hematocrit ratio: its constancy over a wide hematocrit range. J Clin Invest 32: 1309–1316.
39. Gore CJ, Hopkins WG, Burge CM (2005) Errors of measurement for blood volume parameters: a meta-analysis. J Appl Physiol 99: 1745–58.
40. Abbrecht PH, Littell JK (1972) Plasma erythropoietin in men and mice during acclimatization to different altitudes. J Appl Physiol 32: 54–58.
41. Robach P, Fulla Y, Westerterp KR, Richalet J-P (2004) Comparative response of EPO and soluble transferring receptor at high altitude. Med Sci Sports Exerc 36: 1493–1498.
42. Jelkmann W (2011) Regulation of erythropoietin production. J Physiol 589: 1251–1258.
43. Haase VH (2013) Regulation of erythropoiesis by hypoxia-inducible factors. Blood Reviews 27: 41–53.
44. Robach P, Cairo G, Gelfi C, Bernuzzi F, Pilegaard H, et al. (2007) Strong iron demand during hypoxia-induced erythropoiesis is associated with down-regulation of iron-related proteins and myoglobin in human skeletal muscle. Blood 109: 4724–4731.
45. Böning D, Rojas J, Serrato M, Ulloa C, Coy L, et al. (2001) Hemoglobin mass and peak oxygen uptake in untrained and trained residents of moderate altitude. Int J Sports Med 22: 572–578.
46. Böning D, Cristancho E, Serrato M, Reyes O, Mora M, et al. (2004) Hemoglobin mass and peak oxygen uptake in untrained and trained female altitude residents. Int J Sports Med 25: 561–568.
47. Christancho E, Reyes O, Serrato M, Mora MM, Rojas JA, et al. (2007) Arterial oxygen saturation and hemoglobin mass in postmenopausal untrained and trained altitude residents. High Alt Med Biol 8: 296–306.
48. Stray-Gundersen J, Alexander C, Hochstein A, deLemos D, Levine BD (1992) Failure of red cell volume to increase to altitude exposure in iron deficient runners (Abstract). Med Sci Sports Exerc 24: S90.
49. Mairbäurl H, Schobersberger W, Oelz O, Bärtsch P, Eckardt KU, et al. (1990) Unchanged in vivo P50 at high altitude despite decreased erythrocyte age and elevated 2,3,-diphosphoglycerate. J Appl Physiol 68: 1186–1194.
50. Goetze O, Schmitt J, Spliethoff K, Theurl I, Weiss G, et al. (2013) Adaptation of iron transport and metabolism to acute high-altitude hypoxia in mountaineers. Hepatology 58: 2153–2162.
51. Böning D, Maassen N, Jochum J, Steinacker J, Halder A, et al. (1997) After-effects of a high altitude expedition on blood. Int J Sports Med. 18: 179–185.
52. León-Velarde F, Maggiorini M, Reeves JT, Aldashev A, Asmus I, et al. (2005) Consensus statement on chronic and subacute mountain sickness. High Alt Med Biol 6: 147–157.
53. Finch CA, Harker LA, Cook JD (1977) Kinetics of the formed elements of human blood. Blood 50: 699–707.
54. Alfrey CP, Udden MM, Leach-Huntoon C, Driscoll T, Pickett MH (1996) Control of red blood cell mass in spaceflight. J Appl Physiol 81: 98–104.
55. Alfrey CP, Rice L, Udden MM, Driscoll TB (1997) Neocytolysis: physiological down-regulator of red-cell mass. Lancet 349: 1389–1390.
56. Rice L, Alfrey CP (2005) The negative regulation of red cell mass by neocytolysis: physiologic and pathophysiologic manifestations. Cell Physiol Biochem 15: 245–250.
57. Risso A, Cianna A, Achilli C, Antonutto G, Minetti G (2014) Neocytolysis: none, one or many? A reappraisal and future perspectives. Front Physiol 5: 54.
58. Reljic D, Hässler E, Jost J, Friedmann-Bette B (2013) Rapid weight loss and the body fluid balance and hemoglobin mass of elite amateur boxers. J Athletic Training 48: 109–117.
59. Young AJ, Sawka MN, Muza SR, Boushel R, Lyons T, et al. (1996) Effects of erythrocyte infusion on $\dot{V}O_2$ max at high altitude. J Appl Physiol 81: 252–259.
60. Pandolf KB, Young AJ, Sawka MN, Kenney JL, Sharp MW, et al. (1998) Does erythrocyte infusion improve 3.2 km run performance at high altitude? Eur J Appl Physiol 79: 1–6.
61. Robach P, Calbet JAL, Thomsen JJ, Boushel R, Mollard P, et al. (2008) The ergogenic effect of recombinant human erythropoietin on $\dot{V}O_2$ max depends on the severity of arterial hypoxemia. PLoS ONE 3(8): e2996.
62. Calbet JAL, Radegran G, Boushel R, Sondengaard H, Saltin B, et al. (2002) Effect of blood haemoglobin concentration on $\dot{V}O_2$ max and cardiovascular function in lowlanders acclimatised to 5260 m. J Physiol 545: 715–728.
63. Eastwood A, Bourdon PC, Snowden KR, Gore CJ (2012) Detraining decreases Hbmass of triathletes. Int J Sports Med 33: 253–257.
64. Schumacher YO, Ahlgrim C, Pottgiesser T (2008) Evaluation of anthropometrical reference parameters for hemoglobin mass in endurance athletes. J Sports Med Phys Fitness 48: 509–514.
65. Miller ME, Cronkite EP, Garcia JF (1982) Plasma levels of immunoreactive erythropoietin after acute blood loss in man. Br J Haematol 52: 545–549.
66. Pottgiesser T, Specker W, Umhau M, Dickhuth H-H, Roecker K, et al. (2009) Recovery of hemoglobin mass after blood donation. Transfusion 48: 1390–1397.

11

Haemolysis and Perturbations in the Systemic Iron Metabolism of Suckling, Copper-Deficient *Mosaic* Mutant Mice – An Animal Model of Menkes Disease

Małgorzata Lenartowicz[1]*, Rafał R. Starzyński[2], Wojciech Krzeptowski[3], Paweł Grzmil[1], Aleksandra Bednarz[1], Mateusz Ogórek[1], Olga Pierzchała[1], Robert Staroń[2], Anna Gajowiak[2], Paweł Lipiński[2]*

1 Department of Genetics and Evolution, Institute of Zoology, Jagiellonian University, Kraków, Poland, **2** Department of Molecular Biology, Institute of Genetics and Animal Breeding, Polish Academy of Sciences, Magdalenka, Poland, **3** Department of Cell Biology and Imaging, Institute of Zoology, Jagiellonian University, Kraków, Poland

Abstract

The biological interaction between copper and iron is best exemplified by the decreased activity of multicopper ferroxidases under conditions of copper deficiency that limits the availability of iron for erythropoiesis. However, little is known about how copper deficiency affects iron homeostasis through alteration of the activity of other copper-containing proteins, not directly connected with iron metabolism, such as superoxide dismutase 1 (SOD1). This antioxidant enzyme scavenges the superoxide anion, a reactive oxygen species contributing to the toxicity of iron *via* the Fenton reaction. Here, we analyzed changes in the systemic iron metabolism using an animal model of Menkes disease: copper-deficient *mosaic* mutant mice with dysfunction of the ATP7A copper transporter. We found that the erythrocytes of these mutants are copper-deficient, display decreased SOD1 activity/expression and have cell membrane abnormalities. In consequence, the *mosaic* mice show evidence of haemolysis accompanied by haptoglobin-dependent elimination of haemoglobin (Hb) from the circulation, as well as the induction of haem oxygenase 1 (HO1) in the liver and kidney. Moreover, the hepcidin-ferroportin regulatory axis is strongly affected in *mosaic* mice. These findings indicate that haemolysis is an additional pathogenic factor in a mouse model of Menkes diseases and provides evidence of a new indirect connection between copper deficiency and iron metabolism.

Editor: James F. Collins, University of Florida, United States of America

Funding: This work was supported by grant no. K/PBO/000142 from the National Science Center of Poland. This work was supported by The National Science Centre grant 2012/05/B/NZ4/02423 and partially by funding from the Jagiellonian University within the SET project, which is cofinanced by the European Union. The funders had no role in study design, data collection and analysis, decision to publish, or preparation of the manuscript.

Competing Interests: The authors have declared that no competing interests exist.

* Email: malgorzata.lenartowicz@uj.edu.pl (ML); p.lipinski@ighz.pl (PL)

Introduction

Copper and iron are essential biometals, both existing in two main oxidation states, i.e. Cu(I)/Cu(II) and Fe(II)/Fe(III). The extensive range of redox potential available to both metals by varying their interactions with coordinating ligands, as well as their capacity to participate in one-electron transfer reactions, are the reasons why copper and iron are essential for almost all living organisms. Both metals serve as cofactors for enzymes that catalyze diverse redox reactions underlying fundamental metabolic processes, including respiratory oxidation, DNA, microRNA and neurotransmitter synthesis, oxygen radical scavenging and connective tissue formation [1,2].

In mammals, iron is much more abundant than copper [3], mainly because it is an essential component of haem in the oxygen-carrying molecules haemoglobin and myoglobin. On the other hand, the biological activities of copper and iron also have a toxic aspect, since both cuprous [Cu(I)] and ferrous [Fe(II)] ions are able to react with hydrogen peroxide in the Fenton cycle, yielding the highly destructive hydroxyl radical, the most reactive free radical species known. It is therefore vital that copper and iron are carefully sequestered and transported to their intracellular destinations. Regulatory systems have evolved to maintain iron [1] and copper [2] homeostasis. Interestingly, some pathways of iron homeostasis largely depend on the activity of copper-containing ferroxidases such as caeruloplasmin (Cp) and hephaestin. The former is mainly synthesized in hepatocytes in the form of apo-Cp. Incorporation of copper into apo-Cp results in the formation of the redox-active holoenzyme and is mediated by the P-type ATPase, ATP7B during transit through the trans-Golgi network. Cp is then secreted to the circulation where it functions to deliver copper to other tissues. Although Cp-bound copper accounts for about 90% of the total serum copper, it is not indispensable for efficient copper distribution in the body [3,4,5]. It has been shown that an alternative spliced glycosylphosphatidylinositol (GPI) variant of Cp (Cp-GPI) originally characterized in the brain [6] is of particular importance for iron metabolism [3,5]. Cp-GPI cooperates with ferroportin (Fpn), the sole cellular iron exporter known in mammals [7], to facilitate the movement of iron out of cells. First, ferrous ions transported into the circulation by ferroportin are oxidized by Cp-GPI and ferric ions are then bound by transferrin. Second, Cp-GPI is required for the stability of cell surface ferroportin [8].

Copper deficiency has not been reported to significantly and directly influence ferroportin gene expression [9,10], but on the other hand, treatment of J774 macrophage cells with copper has been shown to induce ferroportin and to increase iron efflux from these cells [11]. The cooperation Cp-GPI and ferroportin is crucial for iron recycling by reticuloendothelial cells and iron release by hepatocytes [3]. The role of Cp in iron metabolism has been reported in the congenital human disease acaeruloplasminemia, in which mutations in the caeruloplasmin gene lead to hypoferraemia and iron loading in the liver [12,13]. Hepatic iron overload also occurs in acquired copper deficiency and is likely mediated by hypocaeruloplasminemia [14]. Furthermore, iron overload was reported in Wilson disease, a genetic disorder caused by the mutation in *ATP7B* gene. The lack of ATP7B activity in patients with Wilson disease results in impaired copper loading to apo-Cp and in consequence in decreased Cp ferroxidase activity [15].

Hephaestin shares 50% homology with Cp and is a ferroxidase required for the egress of iron from intestinal enterocytes into the circulation. Sex-linked anaemia (sla) mice, carrying mutations in the gene encoding hephaeastin develop moderate to severe microcytic hypochromic anaemia [16]. Systemic iron deficiency has been also reported in copper-deficient mice displaying decreased hephaestin ferroxidase activity in the intestine [17]. Evidence of the nutritional requirement for copper in maintaining iron homeostasis dates back to the study of Hart et al. in 1928, in which copper was found to be necessary for haemoglobin formation in rats fed on a copper-deficient milk-based diet [18]. Numerous examples of the correlation between copper deficiency and poor iron status have been provided by studies on rapidly growing suckling piglets [19,20].

In mammals, dietary copper is transferred across the apical membrane into enterocytes in its reduced (cuprous) form by copper transporter 1. Transport through the enterocyte basolateral membrane is mediated by ATP7A, a P-type ATPase copper transporter. In the blood copper is bound to albumin or α2-macroglobulin and is delivered to the liver *via* the portal circulation [21,22]. Copper deficiency is associated with Menkes disease, a life-threatening pathology in man, which is due to mutations in the *ATP7A* gene, resulting in defective functioning of ATP7A [21,23]. The general pattern of copper content in the organs of patients with Menkes disease indicates that copper is scarce in the brain, liver and heart, while it accumulates in the small intestine and kidneys [23]. This is consistent with the role of ATP7A as a membrane protein transporting copper out of duodenal enterocytes [21]. In other cells, under physiological conditions, this protein is primarily localized to the trans-Golgi network, but it is also detected in some other post Golgi compartments [21]. However, when cells are exposed to increased copper concentrations, ATP7A is trafficked to the plasma membrane and its main role is to prevent toxic intracellular accumulation of copper by expelling copper ions from the cell's interior [24,25].

Mouse *Atp7a* mutants closely mimicking patients with Menkes disease serve as animal models of this inherited disorder and have recently been extensively used to explore metabolic copper-iron interactions [26,27]. The *mosaic* mutation ($Atp7a^{mo-ms}$) belongs to the group of *mottled* mutations, which severely affect copper metabolism, and is caused by mutation of the X-linked *Atp7a* gene. In *mosaic* mutants, a G to C nucleotide exchange in exon 15 of the *Atp7a* gene results in an arginine to proline substitution in the highly conserved 6th transmembrane domain of the ATP7A protein. The mutated protein is mislocalized and is not translocated to the plasma membrane [28]. Hemizygous mutant males exhibit a severe phenotype including defects in pigmentation and hair structure, decreased body weight, and neurological problems such as ataxia, tremor and progressive paresis of the hind limbs. The *mosaic* mutation is usually lethal by day 17 of life [28].

Here, we analyzed potential changes in iron metabolism in copper-deficient 14-day old male *mosaic* mutant mice. The conception of our study was based on the assumption that copper deficiency may decrease the activity of Cu,Zn-superoxide dismutase (SOD1), an enzyme playing a crucial role in erythrocyte antioxidant defense, and thus may sensitize these cells to haemolysis, a pathological condition in which systemic iron metabolism is seriously affected [29]. Accordingly, we and others have previously demonstrated that mice with a disrupted *Sod1* gene are prone to haemolytic insult [30,31]. Our results show that *mosaic* mutant mice exhibit some perturbations in systemic iron metabolism that are characteristic of moderate haemolysis.

Materials and Methods

Animals

Mice used in these experiments were bred in the Department of Genetics and Evolution, Jagiellonian University, and derived from a closed outbred colony. The animals were obtained by mating heterozygous *ms*/+ females with normal (+/−) males. The experimental material consisted of two groups of 14-day-old control (+/−) and mosaic mutant (*ms*/−) males. All mice were housed at constant temperature (22°C) under artificial light (12-hour photoperiod) and fed a standard Murigran diet (Motycz, Poland). Experiments were performed in accordance with Polish legal requirements under the licence of the First Local Ethical Committee on Animal Testing at the Jagiellonian University in Krakow (permission number: 85/2012). The animals were sacrificed by cervical dislocation.

Blood and tissue collection

Blood samples were collected from a neck vein to EDTA-coated tubes. The EDTA-treated whole blood was used for the immediate preparation of smears. Blood samples were incubated at 4°C for 2 hours, and then serum and erythrocyte fractions were obtained by centrifugation at 2000×g for 10 min. The liver and kidneys were excised from mice following laparotomy. Tissue, serum and red blood cell (RBC) samples were immediately frozen in liquid nitrogen and stored at −80°C prior to molecular analysis.

Measurement of erythrocyte copper content

The level of copper in erythrocytes from *ms*/− and +/− male mice was measured by atomic absorption spectrophotometry. Erythrocyte samples were weighed and digested in 2 ml of boiling Suprapur-grade nitric acid (Merck). After cooling to room temperature (RT), each sample was suspended in 10 ml of deionized water. Reference material samples were prepared in a similar manner. The copper concentration was measured using the graphite furnace AAS technique (AAnalyst 800, Perkin-Elmer). Three samples of nitric acid were used as blanks. In addition, three samples of a standard reference material, Cu = 189±4 mg/kg, were analyzed for normalization of the obtained data.

Measurement of superoxide dismutase activity

SOD activity in erythrocyte total extracts was measured by gel electrophoresis using the Nitroblue Tetrazolium (NBT)/riboflavin method as described previously [32]. Briefly, 15 μg samples of the erythrocyte extracts were resolved by electrophoresis on 12% polyacrylamide gels under non-denaturing and non-reducing conditions. After electrophoresis, the activity of SOD was visualized by immersion of the gels in staining buffer [50 mM potassium phosphate (pH 7.8), 0.1 mM EDTA, 28 mM TEMED, 3 μM riboflavin, 0.25 mM NBT] for 30 min in the dark at RT. Gels were then exposed to light until the SOD activity bands became visible as bright bands on a dark blue background. The reaction was stopped by rinsing the gels with water and they were scanned and quantified immediately using a Molecular Imager with Quantity One software (Bio-Rad). The activities of Cu,Zn-SOD and Mn-SOD were distinguished by selective inhibition of the former activity by incubation of the gels in a buffer containing 3 mM KCN prior to staining, as described by Salin and Bridges [33].

Immunoblot analysis

SOD1 was detected in total extracts (15 μg) obtained from peripheral erythrocytes using rabbit polyclonal anti-superoxide dismutase 1 antibody (Abcam; ab16831). To determine plasma haptoglobin (Hp) levels, 7 μl samples of 20-fold diluted mouse serum were used. Hp was detected with a chicken antibody raised against human Hp (US Biological). Its cross-reactivity with the mouse protein was demonstrated previously [31]. Ferritin levels in cytosolic extracts (20 μg) of mouse liver were analyzed using purified rabbit mouse liver ferritin antiserum (kindly provided by Dr. J. Brock, Glasgow University, Glasgow, UK) [34]. Haem oxygenase 1 (HO1) was detected in hepatic and renal crude membrane extracts (80 μg) using a rabbit polyclonal antibody raised against rat liver HO1 (StressGen). Actin, the loading control for serum and tissue extracts, was detected using an anti-human goat polyclonal antibody (Sigma; sc1615). Immunoreactive bands were disclosed using the ECL Plus Western blotting detection system (Amersham Life Sciences). Reactive bands were quantified relative to actin using a Molecular Imager with Quantity One software (Bio-Rad).

Real-time Quantitative RT-PCR

HO1 and hepcidin (Hepc) hepatic mRNAs were measured by real-time quantitative RT-PCR as described previously [31]. Specific cDNA fragments were amplified using the following pairs of oligonucleotide primers: HO1, 5′-GTCGTGGTCAGTCAA-CATGG-3′ (forward) and 5′-TCTTGCCTGGCTCTCTTCTC-3′ (reverse); Hepc, 5′-CAATGTCTGCCCTGCTTTCT-3′ (forward) and 5′-TCTCCTGCTTCTCCTTG-3′ (reverse). The reactions were performed in a Light Cycler (Roche Diagnostics) and Light Cycler 3.5 Software was used for data analysis. Expression was quantified relative to that of a control transcript encoding glyceraldehyde-3-phosphate dehydrogenase [GAPDH; 5′-GACCACAGTCCATGCCATCAC-3′ (forward) and 5′-TCCACCACCCTGTTGCTGTAG-3′ (reverse)].

Quantitative hepatic non-haem iron measurement

The non-haem iron content of liver fragments (100 mg) was determined by acid digestion of the samples at 100°C for 10 h, followed by colorimetric measurement of the absorbance of the iron-ferrozine complex at 560 nm as described previously [35].

Immunofluorescence (IF) and confocal analysis of liver and kidney sections

After the sacrifice of mice, the liver and kidneys were immediately excised and fixed in 4% paraformaldehyde (Sigma) in phosphate-buffered saline (PBS) (Sigma) at 4°C for 24 h. After washing 3 times for 30 min in PBS, both tissues were successively soaked in 12.5 and 25% sucrose (Merck) for 1.5 and 12 h, respectively at 4°C. The tissues were then embedded in Tissue-Tek compound, frozen in liquid nitrogen and sectioned into 20-μm slices using a cryostat (Leica). The sections were washed in PBS and permeabilized by bathing in PBS/0.1% Triton X-100 (Sigma) for 10 min. Non-specific antibody binding was blocked by incubation of the tissue sections in PBS/3% BSA (Merck) for 1.5 h. For ferroportin (Fpn) detection in the liver, sections were incubated at RT with primary rabbit polyclonal anti-Fpn antibody (Alpha Diagnostic) diluted 1:250 in PBS/3% BSA. The sections were then washed 3 times with PBS and incubated with Cy3 (indocarbocyanine)-conjugated goat anti-rabbit antibody (Jackson Immunoresearch) diluted 1:500 in PBS/3% BSA. For haem oxygenase 1 (HO1) detection, liver and kidney sections were prepared as described above and incubated overnight at RT with primary rabbit polyclonal anti-HO1 antibody (StressGen) diluted 1:250 in PBS/3% BSA. The sections were washed 3 times with PBS and then incubated with Cy3-conjugated goat anti-rabbit antibody diluted 1:500 in PBS/3% BSA. In the liver we also performed co-labeling of HO1 and Fpn with F4/80, a membrane macrophage marker [36]. Liver sections were incubated overnight with either anti-Fpn or with anti-HO-1 antibody and rat anti-mouse F4/80 monoclonal antibody (Serotec) diluted 1:500 in PBS/3% BSA. The sections were then incubated with a mixture of Cy3-conjugated goat anti-rabbit antibody and Alexa 488 goat anti-rat antibody (Jackson Immunoresearch) in PBS/3% BSA for 1 h. Finally, the sections were washed 3 times for 10 min in PBS at RT and mounted using Vectashield with 4′,6-diamidine-2-phenylindole (DAPI; Vector Labs). As a negative control, some sections were prepared without incubating with primary antibody. IF was analyzed with a Zeiss LSM 510 Meta confocal microscope (Carl Zeiss, Jena, Germany) using the 60x objective.

Statistical Analysis

Statistical analysis was performed using a two-tailed Student's t test, with p values of <0.05 and <0.01 being considered statistically significant and highly significant, respectively.

Results

Copper deficiency and decreased SOD1 activity and expression in erythrocytes of mutant *ms/−* mice

14-day-old *mosaic* mutant mouse males exhibit a tissue copper concentration pattern typical of Menkes disease, i.e. reduced levels in both liver and brain and increased levels in both kidney and duodenum [37,38]. Here, we analyzed for the first time the copper content in circulating RBCs of such mutants and found that it was nearly 60% lower compared to wild-type animals (Figure 1A). Bearing in mind that the bioavailability of copper is crucial for maintaining SOD1 activity at the required level [39], we then assessed the activity of this key antioxidant enzyme in erythrocytes of both mutant and wild-type males. Similarly to the copper concentration, SOD1 activity in erythrocytes measured by the NBT/riboflavin method [32] was substantially reduced in *ms/−* mice as shown by densitometry of SOD1 bands (Figure 1B). Moreover, we found that this decrease was at least partly due to the reduced SOD1 protein level in *mosaic* erythrocytes, detected by western immunoblotting (Figure 1C).

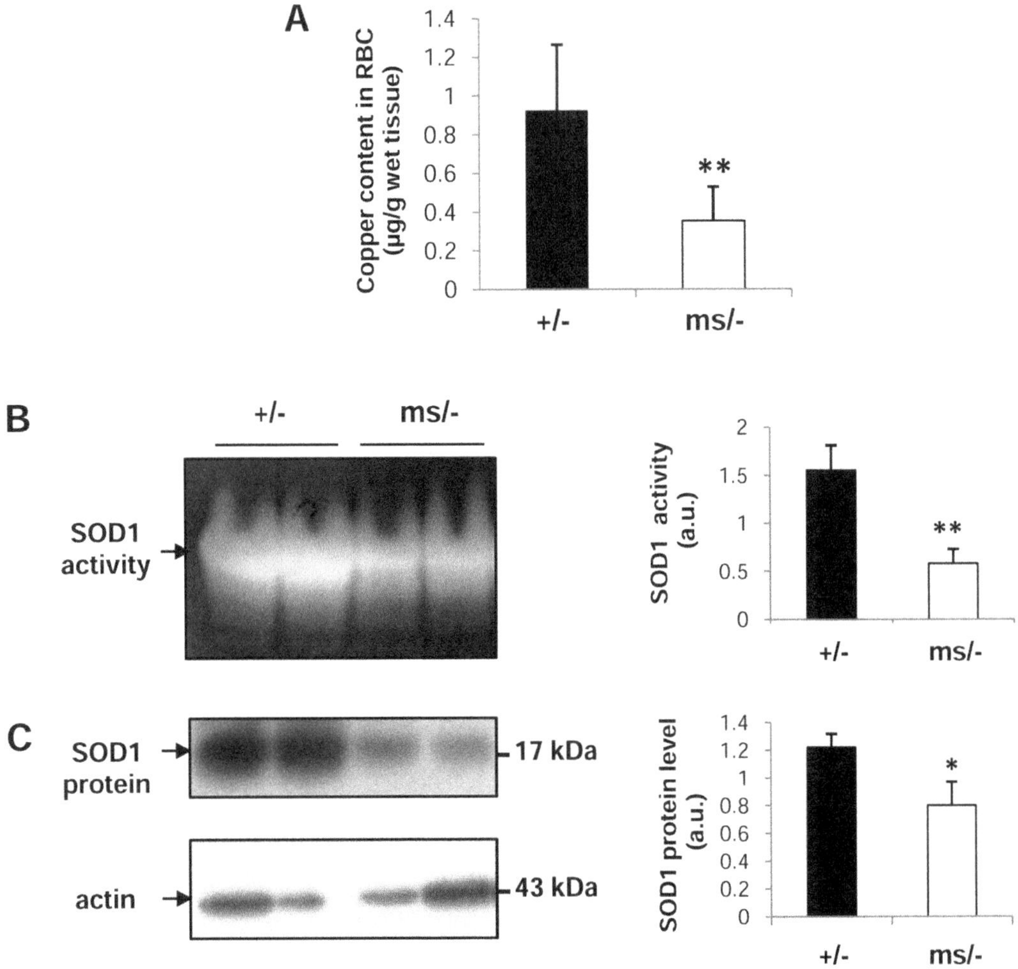

Figure 1. Decreased copper content and activity/expression of SOD1 in circulating erythrocytes from *ms/−* mice. (**A**) Decreased copper content in erythrocytes of *ms/−* mice. Values are expressed as the means ± S.D. for erythrocyte samples obtained from 15 control (+/−) and 15 mutant (*ms/−*) males. (**B**) *left-hand panel*, the activity of SOD was measured after resolution by gel electrophoresis using the Nitroblue Tetrazolium (NBT)/riboflavin method as described in the Experimental section. The analyses were performed using erythrocyte total extracts obtained from *ms/−* and +/− males and representative results are shown. (**C**) *left-hand panel*, SOD1 levels in erythrocytes were analyzed by western blotting as described in the Experimental section. The analyses were performed using erythrocyte total extracts obtained from *ms/−* and control (+/−) males, and representative results are shown. The blot was reprobed with monoclonal anti-actin antibody as a loading control. (**B,C**) *right-hand panels*, the intensity of the SOD bands was quantified with a molecular Imager using Quantity One software (Bio-Rad) and is plotted in arbitrary units to present activity (**B**) and protein level (**C**). Results are expressed as the mean ± S.D. for 5 mice of both the *ms/−* and +/− genotypes. Significant differences are indicated (* - $P<0.05$; ** - $P<0.01$).

Haemolysis and haemoglobin (Hb)-scavenging systems in mutant *ms/−* mice

We and others have shown that in SOD1 knock-out (KO) mice, erythrocytes become sensitive to rupture due to oxidative stress and, in consequence, KO SOD1 mice display clear signs of haemolysis [30,31]. Therefore, in the present study we attempted to identify hallmarks of intravascular haemolysis in *ms/−* mice. It was immediately noticeable that serum obtained from the blood of *ms/−* mice, centrifuged immediately after neck vein puncture, was a reddish color (Figure 2A). Wright staining of blood smears from *ms/−* mice revealed a large percentage of irregularly-shaped RBCs, the morphology of which strongly resembled that of acanthocytes (Figure 2B). We then examined the serum level of haptoglobin (Hp), an acute phase protein that traps free Hb released from ruptured erythrocytes and eliminates it from the circulation [40,41]. In contrast to free Hp, the stable Hp-Hb complex binds the CD163 receptor with high affinity and is rapidly delivered mainly to the reticulo-endothelial system by endocytosis [40,41]. Therefore, a decrease in the Hp concentration in the serum is generally considered a marker of accelerated haemolysis [40,41]. Western blot analysis showed that Hp was completely depleted in the plasma of *ms/−* mice (Figure 2C), suggesting intensive plasma clearance of free Hb.

Increase in hepatic and renal haem oxygenase 1 (HO1) expression in mutant *ms/−* mice

Hb produced by haemolysis is recovered from the circulation by the liver in a process that entails the transcriptional induction of HO1 expression [42], which represents the most important protective system against haem toxicity. A comprehensive assessment of HO1 expression and localization in the liver clearly showed significant induction of the *Hmox1* gene (coding HO1) at both the mRNA (Figure 3A) and protein levels (Figure 3B, 3C and 3D) in *mosaic* mutants. Co-localization studies demonstrated that

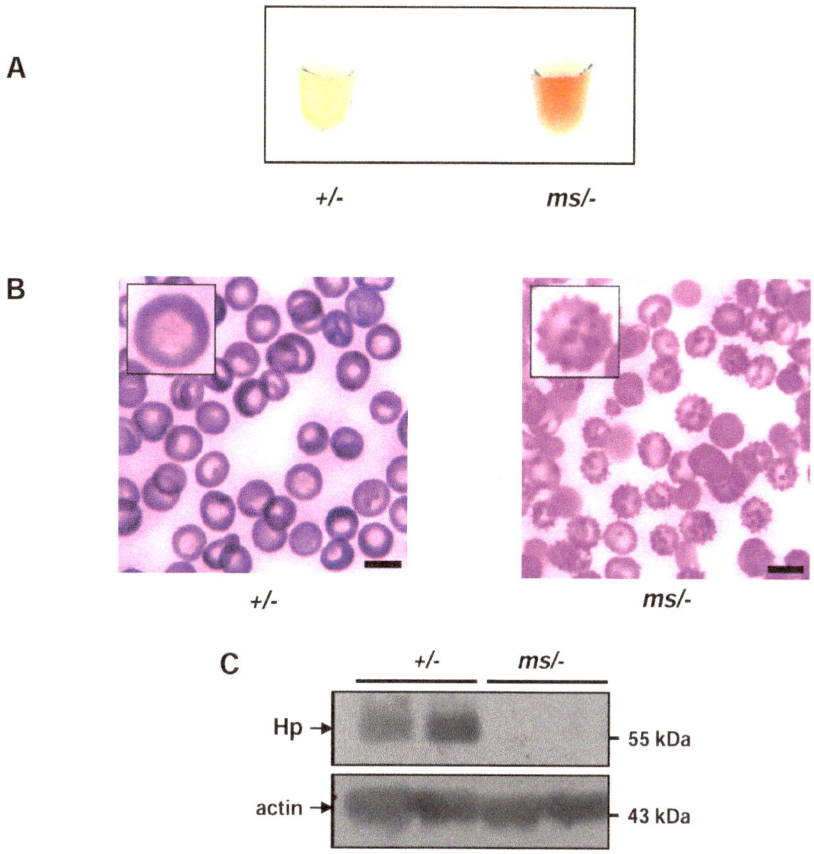

Figure 2. Haemolysis and acanthocytosis in *ms/−* mice. (**A**) Serum of control (+/−) and mutant (*ms/−*) males obtained by centrifugation. (**B**) Peripheral blood smears of *ms/−* mice showing increased numbers of acanthocytes. High magnification images of a normal and an abnormally-shaped erythrocyte are shown (insets). Six animals from both the control and *ms/−* male groups were examined and one typical sample of each is shown. Bars correspond to 5 μm. (**C**) Plasma levels of haptoglobin (Hp) were assessed by western blotting as described in the Experimental section. The blot was reprobed with monoclonal anti-actin antibody as a loading control.

HO1 was mainly located in Kupffer cells in both control and mutant males (identified by staining with the anti-F4/80 antibody specific for a macrophage membrane marker [36]) (Figure 3D). Quantitative RT-PCR (Figure 4A) and western blotting (Figure 4B) analyses showed that HO1 expression was also increased in the kidney of *ms/−* mice. Microscopic analysis of immunofluorescent (IF) staining and transmitted light images indicated that expression of HO1 in the renal cortex of control males expression of HO1 occurred mainly in the renal glomeruli (Figure 4 C, upper panel), whereas in the mutant males, HO1 expression was strongly up-regulated in the cells of renal tubules (Figure 4C, bottom panel).

Decreased ferroportin (Fpn) and increased hepcidin (Hepc) expression in the liver of *ms/−* mice

Assessment of the functioning of the Hepc-Fpn axis is an indispensable element in the analysis of iron metabolism. It has been reported that Fpn, the sole cellular iron exporter known in mammalian cells [7], is up-regulated in the liver in various mouse models of haemolysis [29,31]. Using IF detection we found substantial hepatic Fpn down-regulation in *ms/−* males compared with control animals (Figure 5A). Confocal analysis of dual staining with antibodies specific for Fpn and the plasma membrane macrophage marker F4/80, indicated strong co-localization, suggesting that Fpn is located in liver macrophages (Kupffer cells) in both wild-type and *mosaic* mutant males (Figure 5B). Detailed analysis of the microscopic images revealed strong cell membrane localization of Fpn in control animals (Fpn staining precisely overlaps that of F4/80), whereas membrane expression of Fpn on Kupffer cells appeared much weaker in the mutants (Figure 5B, bottom panel). Quantitative RT-PCR analysis showed an increase in the Hepc mRNA level of about 10-fold in the livers of *ms/−* mice compared with those of +/− animals. Assuming that systemic inflammation may be responsible for the transcriptional induction of *Hamp* gene expression, it is noteworthy that the kidneys of *ms/−* males showed clear signs of inflammation including cellular vacuolization, necrosis of the renal tubule epithelial cells, lymphocyte infiltration, and damage to renal glomeruli structures [43,44].

Hepatic and renal iron status in *ms/−* mice

In the context of accelerated Hb clearance and the enhanced capacity to degrade excess haem in the liver and kidneys of *ms/−* males, we investigated the consequences of these activities on the iron status in both organs. Although our data showed a tendency for hepatic and renal iron accumulation in *ms/−* males compared with +/− animals (Figure 6A and 6C), the differences in non-haem iron content between these mice were not significant (P values $>$ 0.05). In general, the ferritin level serves as a marker of iron loading in cells and tissues [45]. Moreover, it is usually elevated in

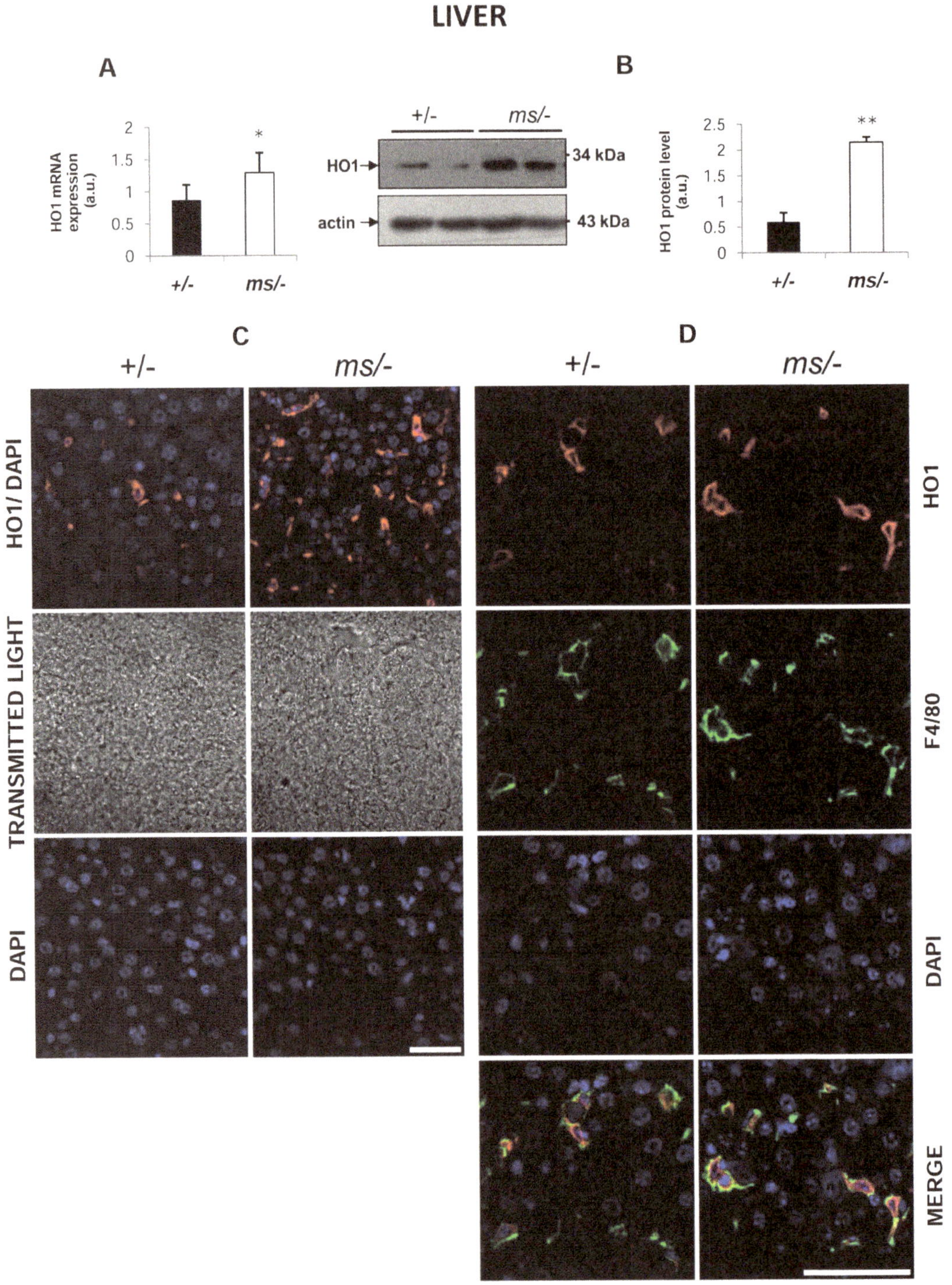

Figure 3. Increased expression of haem oxygenase 1 (HO1) in Kupffer cells of *ms/−* mice. (**A**) Real-time quantitative PCR analysis of hepatic HO1 mRNA expression. The histogram displays HO1 mRNA levels in arbitrary units (means ± S.D., n = 6). (**B**) *left-hand panel* Western blot analysis of HO1 protein levels in hepatic membrane fractions prepared from +/− and *ms/−* males. The blot was reprobed with polyclonal anti-human actin antibody as a loading control. *right-hand panel* Immunolabelled HO1 bands from six mice were quantified using a Molecular Imager and HO1 protein levels (means ± S.D.) are plotted in arbitrary units. * - $P<0.05$. (**C**) *top panel* Immunofluorescent staining of HO1 in +/− and *ms/−* livers analyzed by confocal microscopy. *middle panel* Tissue morphology observed in transmitted light. *bottom panel* To confirm the specificity of Fpn detection, liver sections of +/− and *ms/−* males were incubated with only the secondary antibody. No HO1 staining was detected in these negative controls. Nuclei were counterstained with DAPI. Bars correspond to 50 μm. (**D**) Colocalization (*bottom panel*) of HO1 (red channel) and F4/80, a macrophage marker (green channel) in the livers of +/− and *ms/−* males analyzed by confocal microscopy. Nuclei were counterstained with DAPI. Bars correspond to 50 μm.

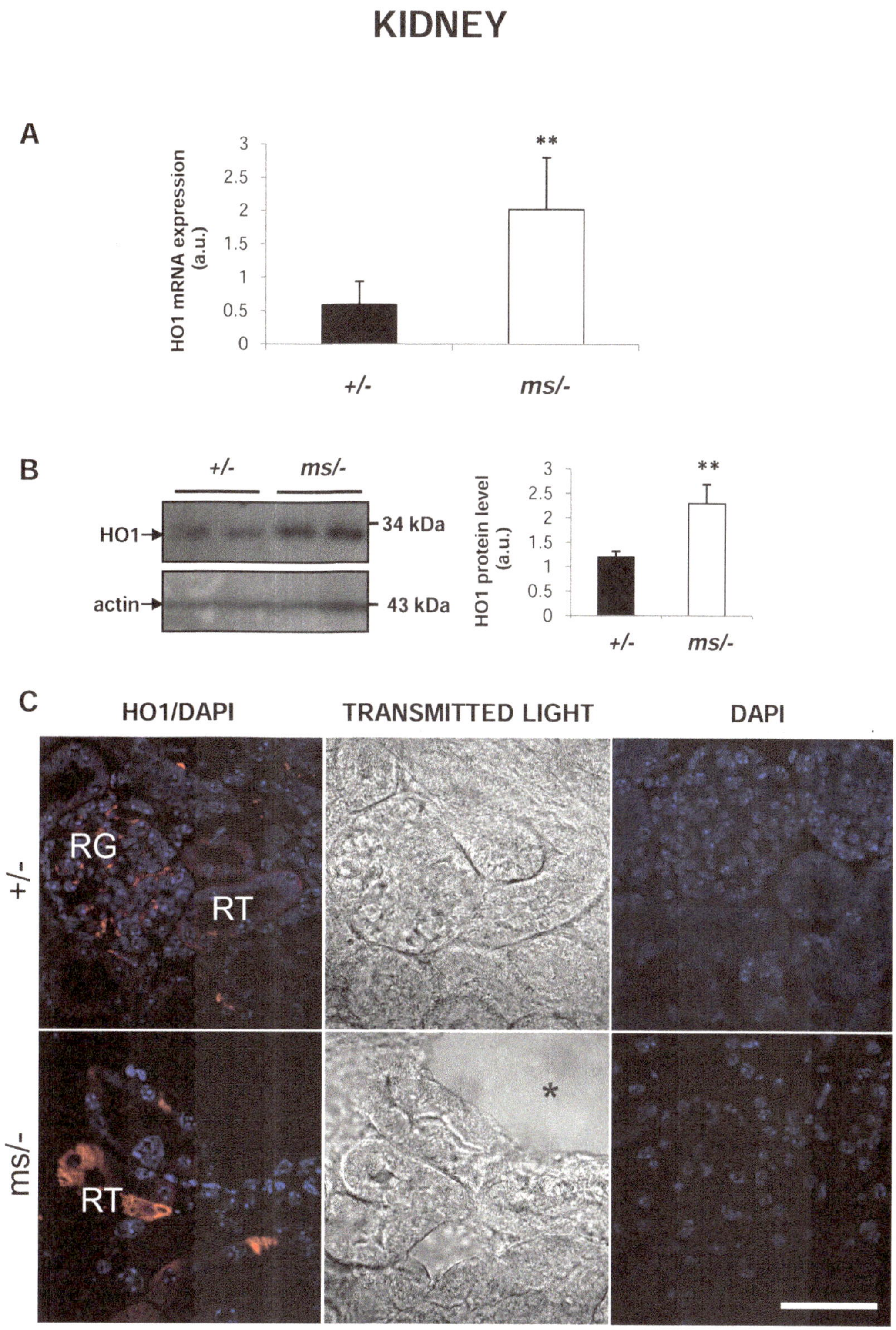

Figure 4. Increased expression of haem oxygenase 1 (HO1) in kidneys of *ms/−* mice. (**A**) Real-time quantitative PCR analysis of renal HO1 mRNA expression. The histogram displays HO1 mRNA levels in arbitrary units (means ± S.D., n = 6). (**B**) *left-hand panel* Western blot analysis of HO1 protein levels in hepatic membrane fractions prepared from +/− and *ms/−* males. The blot was reprobed with polyclonal anti-human actin antibody as a loading control. *right-hand panel* Immunolabelled HO1 bands from six mice were quantified using a Molecular Imager and HO1 protein levels (means ± S.D.) are plotted in arbitrary units. ** – $P<0.01$. (**C**) *left-hand panel* Immunofluorescent staining of HO1 in +/− and *ms/−* kidneys analyzed by confocal microscopy. RN – renal tubules; RG – renal glomeruli. *middle panel* Transmitted light image shows the structure of glomeruli and tubules as well as the presence of a large lesion (asterisk) in the kidney of a mutant. *right-hand panel* To confirm the specificity of HO1 detection, kidney sections of +/− and *ms/−* males were incubated with only the secondary antibody. No HO1 staining was detected in these negative controls. Nuclei were counterstained with DAPI. Bars correspond to 50 μm.

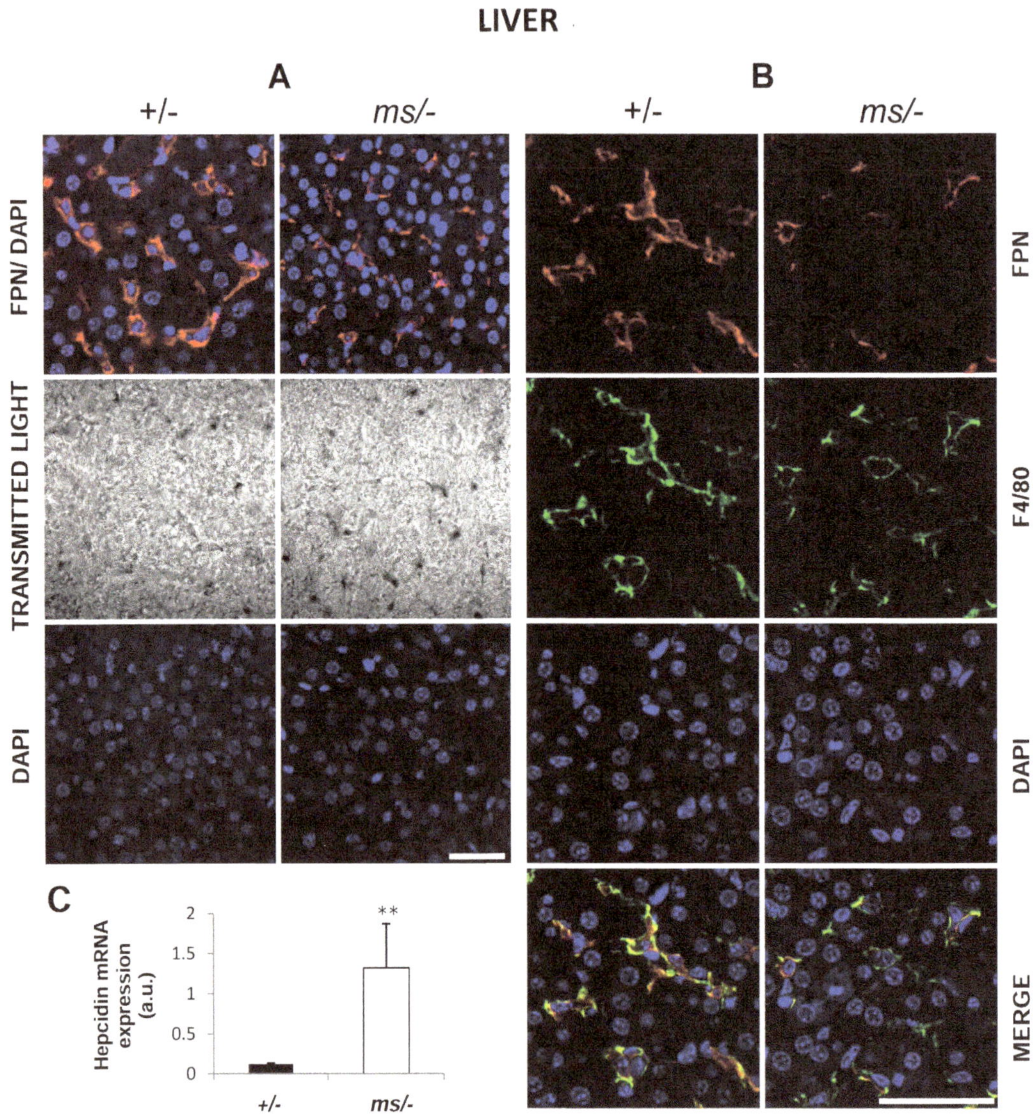

Figure 5. Correlation between decreased ferroportin (Fpn) protein level and increased hepcidin (Hepc) mRNA expression in the liver of *ms/−* males. (**A**) Immunofluorescent staining of Fpn in +/− and *ms/−* males. *top panel* Livers analyzed by confocal microscopy. *middle panel* Tissue morphology observed in transmitted light. *bottom panel* To confirm the specificity of Fpn detection, liver sections of +/− and *ms/−* males were incubated with only the secondary antibody. No Fpn staining was detected in these negative controls. Nuclei were counterstained with DAPI. Bars correspond to 50 μm. (**B**) Colocalization (*bottom panel*) of Fpn (red channel) and F4/80, a macrophage marker (green channel) in liver from +/− and *ms/−* males analyzed by confocal microscopy. Nuclei were counterstained with DAPI. Bars correspond to 50 μm. (**C**) Real-time quantitative PCR analysis of hepatic Hepc mRNA expression in +/− and *ms/−* males. The histogram displays Hepc mRNA levels in arbitrary units (means ± S.D., n = 6). Significant difference is indicated (** - P<0.01).

the kidneys and liver under conditions of haemolysis [29,46]. Analysis of liver and kidney cytosolic extracts by western blotting revealed significantly higher ferritin expression in *ms/−* males compared with the control animals (Figure 6B and 6D).

Discussion

The interaction between the multi-copper ferroxidases caeruloplasmin and hepheastin, and ferroportin in the egress of iron from cells is a major biological link between copper and iron, and the best characterized at the molecular level [3]. It is assumed that mutation of genes encoding caeruloplasmin and hephaestin as well as copper deficiency, which decreases the ferroxidase activity of both enzymes, reduces the amount of iron available for erythropoiesis and contributes to the accumulation of iron in the liver, intestine and brain [3]. Another important interaction between these two biometals is copper-dependent iron utilization for haemoglobin synthesis by erythroid cells [18], but the molecular nature of this process is poorly understood [47]. Recently, an additional copper-iron relationship was identified in mice under conditions of nutritional copper deficiency [48]. This involves a series of consecutive events such as iron-deficiency anaemia, hypoxia, stabilization of HIF2-α in duodenal enterocytes and subsequent transcriptional up-regulation of genes responsible for enhanced iron absorption [48].

In the present study, we examined the adaptive response of systemic iron regulation to copper deficiency, which causes altered activity of the first-line defence antioxidant cuproenzyme, super-

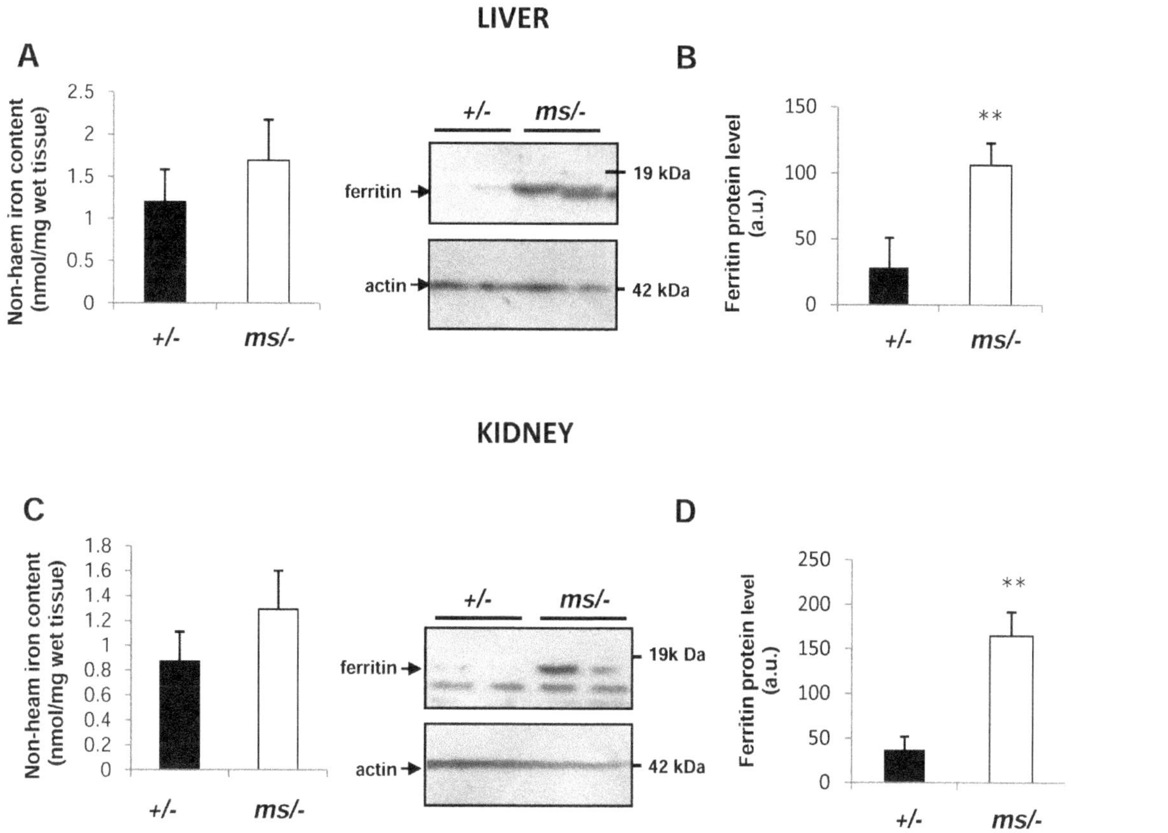

Figure 6. Hepatic and renal iron status in control (+/−) and mutant (*ms/−*) mice. Non-haem hepatic (**A**) and renal (**C**) iron content was measured as described in the Experimental section. Values are expressed as the means ± S.D. for both liver and kidney samples obtained from 15 mice of each genotype. L-ferritin levels in hepatic (**B**) and renal (**D**) cytosolic protein extracts (50 µg/lane) were assessed by western blot analysis *left-hand panels*. The blots were reprobed with polyclonal anti-human actin antibody as a loading control. (**B**) and (**D**) *right-hand panels* Immunolabelled ferritin bands from four mice were quantified using a Molecular Imager and ferritin protein levels (means ± S.D.) are plotted in arbitrary units. ** – P< 0.01.

oxide dismutase 1 (SOD1, Cu,Zn-SOD), a scavenger of the superoxide anion radical ($O_2^{\bullet -}$) [49]. Previous study performed on 10 and 11-day-old mice showed that both dietary copper deficiency in wild-type mice and copper insufficiency in *brindled* mutant mice (*Atp7a*$^{mo-br}$) lead to the decrease in SOD1 activity in many organs such as liver, spleen, brain, heart, thymus and bone marrow [50]. Decrease in SOD1 activity was also described in organs of 13-day old *brindled* and *blotchy* (*Atp7a*$^{mo-blo}$) mutant males [51]. This study was designed to test whether copper deficiency is responsible for decreased SOD1 activity in erythrocytes, resulting in membrane damage, haemolysis and subsequent changes in systemic iron metabolism. This hypothesis was formulated in the light of the following information: 1) SOD1-associated copper accounts for more than half of the total copper content in circulating erythrocytes [52]; 2) nutritional copper deficiency has been shown to decrease both the expression and activity of SOD1 in erythrocytes [39]; 3) we [31] and others [30] have demonstrated the occurrence of haemolysis in mice lacking Cu,Zn-SOD; and 4) haemolysis entails substantial changes in iron metabolism [29].

In our experiments we used a well characterized *mosaic* mouse line, representing a model of Menkes disease, which carries a mutation in the *Atp7a* gene and therefore lacks the ATP7A copper-transporting P-type ATPase [28]. When untreated with copper, *mosaic* mutant hemizygous males die by day 17 of life [28] and so we used 14-day-old animals in our study. Their pattern of body copper content and distribution is typical for Menkes disease, i.e. increased copper accumulation in the small intestine and kidneys, and severe copper deficiency in the brain, liver and heart [37,38]. To our knowledge, erythrocyte copper content has never been described in patients with Menkes disease or in mouse models of this condition. Considering that the duodenal ATP7A transporter plays a crucial role in copper uptake to the organism [21], it is plausible that its dysfunction in *ms/−* male mice may result in impaired copper delivery to erythroid precursors and in consequence, low copper levels in peripheral erythrocytes. Indeed, measurement of the copper concentration in circulating *ms/−* erythrocytes showed a decrease of about 60% compared with that of healthy controls. This decrease correlated strongly with the down-regulation of both SOD1 expression (30%) and activity (70%). A reduction in erythrocyte SOD1 activity in response to dietary copper deficiency has been described in various mammalian species [53–55] including mice [39]. Obviously, altered functioning of Cu,Zn-SOD increases the risk of oxidative stress. With regard to erythrocytes, this phenomenon is well documented in SOD1 null mice, in which the lack of Cu,Zn-SOD activity is responsible for increased oxidative stress in circulating erythrocytes [30,56] and the production of autoantibodies against erythrocytes [30]. These events were found to be causally connected with the increased sensitivity of erythrocytes to oxidative injury and haemolysis [30,31]. Although *ms/−* erythrocytes still display about 30% of normal SOD1 activity, the serum obtained from these animals clearly has a haemolytic appearance. The threshold level of SOD1 activity required to protect erythrocytes against oxidative stress is unknown, although it was previously shown that a decrease in SOD1 activity in $Sod1^{+/-}$ erythrocytes to half of the value in $Sod1^{+/+}$ cells is still sufficient to ensure the protective activity of the enzyme [56]. Interestingly, *ms/−* male mice have a large number of acanthocytes (about 40%) in the peripheral blood. Acanthocytosis may occur due to alteration of the lipid composition and fluidity of the red cell membrane, but can also be caused by dehydration in a subpopulation of acanthocytic erythrocytes. Indeed, *mosaic* suckling males show macroscopic signs of dehydration such as low body weight, loss of liquids due to diarrhea, and increased density of the plasma. It is worth noting that mild to moderate haemolysis was reported to be associated with acanthocytosis [57]. One of the valuable hallmarks of intravascular haemolysis is the disappearance of haptoglobin (Hp) from the serum [40,41]. Hp is an acute-phase protein involved in the clearance of haemoglobin (Hb) from the bloodstream to prevent its toxicity [40,41]. When Hb is released from ruptured erythrocytes, it is instantly bound by Hp and forms a stable Hp-Hb complex [40,41], which is then rapidly removed from the circulation by binding to the CD163 receptor, present mainly on tissue macrophages including Kupffer cells [58]. Since free Hp does not bind to CD163, specific recognition of the Hp-Hb complex by this receptor explains the decrease in Hp concentration in the plasma during accelerated haemolysis [40,41]. However, in contrast to humans, the mouse CD163 may also directly bind Hb that is not complexed with Hp [59]. Nevertheless, we found that the serum of *ms/−* mice was completely depleted of Hp, suggesting that the Hb scavenging mechanism functions very efficiently in these mutant males. The next steps of Hb inactivation are its lysosomal degradation followed by haem breakdown catalyzed by haem oxygenase 1 (HO1) [reviewed in 42]. Besides functioning as a substrate of HO1, haem is known to be the most potent transcriptional inducer of the *Hmox1* gene [60]. Unsurprisingly, increases in the level of both the HO1 transcript and protein were detected in the liver of *ms/−* mutants. Significantly, we previously found that the expression of HO1 was also strongly induced in the liver of $Sod1^{-/-}$ mice displaying moderate haemolytic anaemia [31]. Furthermore, transcriptional induction of hepatic HO1 was observed under conditions of intravascular haemolysis in β-thalassemic and sickle mice [29] as well as during malaria [61]. The identification of Kupffer cells as a site of hepatic HO1 expression in *ms/−* mice strongly suggests that these cells are mostly charged with the detoxification of haem derived from Hb taken up from the bloodstream. HO1 also appears to be largely responsible for haem catabolism during erythrophagocytosis [62]. Therefore, it is noteworthy that in agreement with the subcellular localization of HO1 found in mouse bone marrow-derived macrophages during erythrophagocytosis [62], immunostaining of this enzyme was predominantly intracytosolic in the Kupffer cells of *ms/−* mice.

Studies on Hp-null mice showed that even under conditions of physiological haemolysis, Hb is filtered by the kidneys [63]. Renal filtration of Hb also occurs in normal subjects (mice and humans) when the buffering capacity of Hp is overwhelmed in acute haemolysis [40,41]. Studies in disease models demonstrated that the kidney can adapt to increased amounts of Hb by inducing HO1 [63]. Such a situation seems to occur in *ms/−* mice. Indeed, in the kidneys of these animals we showed a marked induction of HO1 in cells of the renal tubules, very possibly as a consequence of glomerular filtration of Hb. However, it is also possible that the *Hmox1* gene is induced in *ms/−* mouse kidney in response to an inflammatory reaction, the occurrence of which has been well documented in the kidneys of 14-day-old *mosaic* males [43,44]. It has recently been claimed that the protective antioxidant effect of HO1 depends, at least in part, on co-induction of ferritin, a cytosolic protein that binds, stores and thus detoxifies reactive iron released by haem breakdown [64]. Accordingly, in both the liver and kidneys of *ms/−* males, ferritin was elevated at the protein level compared to their healthy littermates. However, the *Hmox1* gene might also be induced in the kidneys of *ms/−* mice in response to the inflammatory reaction caused by excessive copper accumulation. Available data suggest a likely mechanism for this copper overload. In the kidneys of healthy animals, copper reabsorption from the urine occurs via the proximal renal tubules [65,66]. Most of copper ions are then transferred back to the circulation *via* ATP7A located in the basolateral membranes of epithelial cells of these tubules [67]. This explains why dysfunction of ATP7A protein in *Atp7a* mutants results in toxic copper accumulation at the renal-proximal epithelium, a phenomenon detected in various mouse models of Menkes disease [65,66], including *mosaic* mice [43,44].

Apart from the induction of the Hp-CD163-HO1 pathway [42], the adaptive changes in the iron metabolism under haemolytic conditions also involve the redistribution of iron from macrophages back to the circulation. This process is mediated by ferroportin (Fpn), the sole cellular exporter of ionic iron known in mammalian cells [7]. We previously demonstrated that enhanced expression of hepatic Fpn in haemolytic anemia in KO SOD1 mice ensures the iron supply required for erythropoiesis [31]. Surprisingly, in *ms/−* mice, Fpn was down-regulated in Kupffer cells, the principal cell type expressing Fpn in the liver. According to the consensus of the hepcidin-ferroportin regulatory axis [7], such down-regulation of Fpn expression strongly suggested the concomitant up-regulation of hepatic hepcidin. Indeed, hepcidin was elevated at the mRNA level by more than 10-fold in *ms/−* mutants compared with control males. We hypothesize that the renal inflammation induced in *mosaic* mice by heavy copper overload [38,43,44] diffuses throughout the organism of *ms/−* mice and mediates transcriptional activation of the *Hamp* gene in the liver. Accordingly, it is well established that plasma hepcidin levels remain persistently high in patients with chronic kidney disease [68]. Furthermore, inflammatory mediators such as interleukin-6 and -1 participate in the iron-independent induction of the *Hamp* gene [69]. Despite increased and decreased expression of HO1 and Fpn, respectively, we observed only a tendency in both liver and kidney of *ms/−* mice to accumulate non-haem iron, although the elevated level of ferritin in both organs seems to support some retention of iron in these tissues. It is possible that the extent of iron loading in the two examined organs is quite limited. A similar lack of global hepatic iron loading has also been reported in haemolytic mice lacking Cu,Zn-SOD1 [31].

In summary, we have identified a new indirect relationship between copper deficiency in the mouse model of Menkes disease and systemic iron metabolism. The key point in this interconnection is decreased activity of the erythrocyte antioxidant cuproenzyme Cu,Zn-SOD, resulting in oxidative stress, increased permeability of erythrocyte membranes and haemolysis. Hb released from damaged erythrocytes causes the mobilization of a protective system neutralizing Hb toxicity, including Hp-dependent elimination of Hb from the circulation as well as the degradation of haem derived from Hb by HO1 in the liver and kidneys. Importantly, our results show for the first time that suckling mice adapt their iron metabolism to haemolytic insult in a similar manner to adult animals. Finally, haemolysis has been identified as an additional pathological symptom in a mouse model of Menkes diseases.

It is largely known that similarly to *mosaic* mutants [44], Menkes patients suffer from kidney and urinary tract dysfunctions and develop chronic renal inflammation [70]. Increased hepcidin synthesis under these pathological conditions may reduce availability of iron for erythropoiesis and in combination with haemolysis may contribute for the development of anemia. Taking together, our results point out a need to monitor iron status in Menkes patients.

Acknowledgments

We would like to thank the Confocal Microscopy Laboratory (Institute of Zoology, Jagiellonian University) for access and assistance with the confocal microscope - LSM 510 META Axiovert 200 M, ConfoCor 3 (Carl Zeiss MicroImaging GmbH, Jena, Germany). We thank John Gittins for critically reading the manuscript prior to submission.

Author Contributions

Conceived and designed the experiments: ML PL. Performed the experiments: RRS WK PG AB OP MO AG RS. Analyzed the data: RRS WK PG. Contributed reagents/materials/analysis tools: ML RRS. Wrote the paper: PL ML.

References

1. Hentze MW, Muckenthaler MU, Galy B, Camaschella C (2010) Two to tango: regulation of mammalian ironmetabolism. Cell 142: 24–38.
2. Lutsenko S (2010) Human copper homeostasis: a network of interconnected pathways. Curr Opin Chem Biol 14: 211–217.
3. Collins JF, Prohaska JR, Knutson M (2010) Metabolic crossroads of iron and copper. Nutr Rev 68: 133–147.
4. Hellman NE, Gitlin JD (2002) Ceruloplasmin metabolism and function. Annu Rev Nutr 22: 439–58.
5. Prohaska JR (2011) Impact of copper limitation on expression and function of multicopper oxidases (ferroxidases). Adv Nutr 2: 89–95.
6. Patel BN, David S (1997) A novel glycosylphosphatidylinositol-anchored form of ceruloplasmin is expressed by mammalian astrocytes. J Biol Chem. 272: 20185–90.
7. Ganz T (2005) Cellular iron: ferroportin is the only way out. Cell Metab 1: 155–157.
8. De Domenico I, Ward DM, di Patti MC, Jeong SY, David S, et al. (2007) Ferroxidase activity is required for the stability of cell surface ferroportin in cells expressing GPI-ceruloplasmin. EMBO J 26: 2823–31.
9. Chung J, Prohaska JR, Wessling-Resnick M (2004) Ferroportin-1 is not upregulated in copper-deficient mice. J Nutr 134: 517–21.
10. Prohaska JR, Broderius M (2012) Copper deficiency has minimal impact on ferroportin expression or function. Biometals 25: 633–42.
11. Chung J, Haile DJ, Wessling-Resnick M (2004) Copper-induced ferroportin-1 expression in J774 macrophages is associated with increased iron efflux. Proc Natl Acad Sci U S A 101: 2700–5.
12. Harris ZL, Takahashi Y, Miyajim H, Serizawa M, MacGillivray RT, et al. (1995) Aceruloplasminemia: molecular characterization of this disorder of iron metabolism. Proc Natl Acad Sci U S A 92: 2539–2543.
13. Yoshida K, Furihata K, Takeda S, Nakamura A, Yamamoto K, et al. (1995) A mutation in the ceruloplasmin gene is associated with systemic hemosiderosis in humans. Nat Genet 9: 267–272.
14. Thackeray EW, Sanderson SO, Fox JC, Kumar N (2011) Hepatic iron overload or cirrhosis may occur in acquired copper deficiency and is likely mediated by hypoceruloplasminemia. J Clin Gastroenterol 45: 153–58.
15. Hayashi H, Hattori A, Tatsumi Y, Hayashi K, Katano Y, et al. (2013) Various copper and iron overload patterns in the livers of patients with Wilson disease and idiopathic copper toxicosis. Med Mol Morphol 46: 133–40
16. Vulpe CD, Kuo YM, Murphy TL, Cowley L, Askwith C, et al. (1999) Hephaestin, a ceruloplasmin homologue implicated in intestinal iron transport, is defective in the sla mouse. Nat Genet 21: 195–199.
17. Chen H, Huang G, Su T, Gao H, Attieh ZK, et al. (2006) Decreased hephaestin activity in the intestine of copper-deficient mice causes systemic iron deficiency. J Nutr 136: 1236–41.
18. Hart EB, Steenbock H, Waddell J, Elvehjem CA (1928) Iron in nutrition: VII. Copper as a supplement to iron for hemoglobin building in the rat. J Biol Chem 77: 797–812.
19. Cartwright GE, Gubler CJ, Bush JA, Wintrobe MM (1956) Studies of copper metabolism. XVII. Further observations on the anemia of copper deficiency in swine. Blood 11: 143–153.
20. Lee GR, Nacht S, Lukens JN, Cartwright GE (1968) Iron metabolism in copper-deficient swine. J Clin Invest 47: 2058–2069.
21. Lutsenko S, Barnes NL, Bartee MY, Dimitriev OY (2007) Function and regulation of human copper-transporting ATPases. Physiol Rev 87: 1011–1046.
22. Van den Berghe PV, Folmer DE, Malingré HE, van Beurden E, Klomp AE, et al. (2007) Human copper transporter 2 is localized in late endosomes and lysosomes and facilitates cellular copper uptake. Biochem J 407: 49–59.
23. Møller LB, Mogensen M, Horn N (2009) Molecular diagnosis of Menkes disease: genotype-phenotype correlation. Biochimie 91: 1273–1277.
24. Mercer JF, Barnes N, Stevenson J, Strausak D, Llanos RM (2003) Copper-induced trafficking of the Cu-ATPases: a key mechanism for copper homeostasis. Biometals 16: 175–184.
25. La Fontaine S, Mercer JFB (2007) Trafficking of the copper-ATPases, ATP7A and TP7B: Role in copper homeostasis. Arch Biochem Biophys 463: 149–167.
26. Gulec S, Collins JF (2013) Investigation of iron metabolism in mice expressing a mutant Menke's copper transporting ATPase (Atp7a) protein with diminished activity (Brindled; Mo (Br) (/y)). PLoS One 8: e66010.
27. Gulec S, Collins JF (2014) Silencing the Menkes copper-transporting ATPase (Atp7a) gene in rat intestinal epithelial (IEC-6) cells increases iron flux via transcriptional induction of ferroportin 1 (Fpn1). J Nutr 144: 12–19.
28. Lenartowicz M, Grzmil P, Shoukier M, Starzyński R, Marciniak M, et al. (2012) Mutation in the CPC motif-containing 6th transmembrane domain affects intracellular localization, trafficking and copper transport efficiency of ATP7A protein in mosaic mutant mice-an animal model of Menkes disease. Metallomics 4: 197–204.
29. Vinchi F, De Franceschi L, Ghigo A, Townes T, Cimino J, et al. (2013) Hemopexin therapy improves cardiovascular function by preventing heme-induced endothelial toxicity in mouse models of hemolytic diseases. Circulation 127: 1317–1329.
30. Iuchi Y, Okada F, Onuma K, Onoda T, Asao H, et al. (2007) Elevated oxidative stress in erythrocytes due to an SOD1 deficiency causes and triggers autoantibody production. Biochem J 402: 219–227.
31. Starzyński RR, Canonne-Hergaux F, Willemetz A, Gralak MA, Woliński J, et al. (2009) Haemolytic anaemia and alterations in hepatic iron metabolism in aged mice lacking Cu,Zn-superoxide dismutase. Biochem J 420: 383–390.
32. Beauchamp C, Fridovich I (1971) Superoxide dismutase: improved assays and an assay applicable to acrylamide gels. Anal Biochem 44: 276–287.
33. Salin ML, Bridges SM (1981) Absence of the iron-containing superoxide dismutase in mitochondria from mustard (Brassica campestris). Biochem J 195: 229–233.
34. Bouton C, Chauveau MJ, Lazereg S, Drapier JC (2002) Recycling of RNA binding iron regulatory protein 1 into an aconitase after nitric oxide removal depends on mitochondrial ATP. J Biol Chem 277: 31220–31227.
35. Torrance JD, Bothwell TH (1980) Iron stores. Methods Hematol 1, 90–115.
36. van den Berg TK, Kraal G (2005) A function for the macrophage F4/80 molecule in tolerance induction. Trends Immunol 26, 506–509.
37. Lenartowicz M, Starzyński R, Wieczerzak K, Krzeptowski W, Lipiński P, et al. (2011) Alterations in the expression of the Atp7a gene in the early postnatal development of the mosaic mutant mice (Atp7a mo-ms) - an animal model for Menkes disease. Gene Expr Patterns 11: 1–7.
38. Lenartowicz M, Sasuła K (2000) Altered copper metabolism in the Mosaic mutant mice. Nutr Res 10: 1519–1529.
39. West EC, Prohaska JR (2004) Cu,Zn-superoxide dismutase is lower and copper chaperone CCS is higher in erythrocytes of copper-deficient rats and mice. Exp Biol Med (Maywood) 229: 756–764.
40. Ascenzi P, Bocedi A, Visca P, Altruda F, Tolosano E, et al. (2005) Hemoglobin and heme scavenging. IUBMB Life 57: 749–759.
41. Nielsen MJ, Møller HJ, Moestrup SK (2010) Hemoglobin and heme scavenger receptors. Antioxid Redox Signal 12: 261–273.
42. Thomsen JH, Etzerodt A, Svendsen P, Moestrup SK (2013) The haptoglobin-CD163-heme oxygenase-1 pathway for hemoglobin scavenging. Oxid Med Cell Longev 2013: 523652.
43. Lenartowicz M, Sasuła K, Zawadowska B (2001) Alterations in kidney morphology in mice with mosaic mutation. Folia Histochem Cytobiol 39: 275–281.
44. Lenartowicz M, Windak R, Tylko G, Kowal M, Styrna J (2010) Effects of copper supplementation on the structure and content of elements in kidneys of mosaic mutant mice. Biol Trace Elem Res 136: 204–220.
45. Batts KP (2007) Iron overload syndromes and the liver. Mod Pathol. 20 Suppl 1: S31–S39.
46. Starzyński RR, Canonne-Hergaux F, Lenartowicz M, Krzeptowski W, Willemetz A, et al. (2013) Ferroportin expression in haem oxygenase 1-deficient mice. Biochem J 449: 69–78.
47. Gulec S, Collins JF (2014) Silencing the Menkes copper-transporting ATPase (Atp7a) gene in rat intestinal epithelial (IEC-6) cells increases iron flux via transcriptional induction of ferroportin 1 (Fpn1). Annu Rev Nutr 144: 12–9.
48. Matak P, Zumerle S, Mastrogiannaki M, El Balkhi S, Delga S, et al. (2013) Copper deficiency leads to anemia, duodenal hypoxia, upregulation of HIF-2α and altered expression of iron absorption genes in mice. PLoS One 8: e59538.

49. Zelko IN, Mariani TJ, Folz RJ (2002) Superoxide dismutase multigene family: a comparison of the CuZn-SOD (SOD1), Mn-SOD (SOD2), and EC-SOD (SOD3) gene structures, evolution, and expression. Free Radic Biol Med 33: 337–49.
50. Prohaska JR (1983) Changes in tissue growth, concentrations of copper, iron, cytochrome oxidase and superoxide dismutase subsequent to dietary or genetic copper deficiency in mice. J Nutr 113: 2048–58.
51. Phillips M, Camakaris J, Danks DM (1986) Comparisons of copper deficiency states in the murine mutants blotchy and brindled. Changes in copper-dependent enzyme activity in 13-day-old mice. Biochem J 238: 177–83.
52. Evans GW (1973) Copper homeostasis in the mammalian system. Physiol Rev 53: 535–70.
53. Williams DM, Lynch RE, Lee GR, Cartwright GE (1975) Superoxide dismutase activity in copper-deficient swine. Proc Soc Exp Biol Med 149: 534–536.
54. Andrewartha KA, Caple IW (1980) Effects of changes in nutritional copper on erythrocyte superoxide dismutase activity in sheep. Res Vet Sci 28: 101–104.
55. Okahata S, Nishi Y, Hatano S, Kobayashi Y, Usui T (1980) Changes in erythrocyte superoxide dismutase in a patient with copper deficiency. Eur J Pediatr 134: 121–124.
56. Grzelak A, Kruszewski M, Macierzyńska E, Piotrowski Ł, Pułaski Ł, et al. (2009) The effects of superoxide dismutase knockout on the oxidative stress parameters and survival of mouse erythrocytes. Cell Mol Biol Lett 14: 23–34.
57. Palek J, Jarolim P (1995) Red cell membrane disorders. In: Hoffman R, et al., eds. Hematology. 2nd ed. New York, NY: Churchill LivingstoneInc; 1995: 690–694.
58. Kristiansen M, Graversen JH, Jacobsen C, Sonne O, Hoffman HJ, et al. (2001) Identification of the hemoglobin receptor. Nature 409: 198–201.
59. Etzerodt A, Kjolby M, Nielsen MJ, Maniecki M, Svendsen P, et al. (2013) Plasma clearance of hemoglobin and haptoglobin in mice and effect of CD163 gene targeting disruption. Antioxid Redox Signal 18: 2254–2263.
60. Maines MD (2005) The heme oxygenase system: update. Antioxid Redox Signaling 7: 1761–1766.
61. Dey S, Bindu S, Goyal M, Pal C, Alam A, et al. (2012) Impact of intravascular hemolysis in malaria on liver dysfunction: involvement of hepatic free heme overload, NF-κB activation, and neutrophil infiltration. J Biol Chem 287: 26630–26646.
62. Delaby C, Rondeau C, Pouzet C, Willemetz A, Pilard N, et al. (2012) Subcellular localization of iron and heme metabolism related proteins at early stages of erythrophagocytosis. PLoS One 7: e42199.
63. Fagoonee S, Gburek J, Hirsch E, Marro S, Moestrup SK, et al. (2005) Plasma protein haptoglobin modulates renal iron loading. Am J Pathol 166: 973–83.
64. Gozzelino R, Soares MP (2014) Coupling heme and iron metabolism via ferritin H chain. Antioxid Redox Signal 20: 1754–1769.
65. Kirby BJ, Danks DM, Legge GJ, Mercer JF (1998) Analysis of the distribution of Cu, Fe and Zn and other elements in brindled mouse kidney using a scanning proton microprobe. J Inorg Biochem 71: 189–197.
66. Suzuki-Kurasaki M, Okabe M, Kurasaki M (1997) Copper-metallothionein in the kidney of macular mice: a model for Menkes disease. J Histochem Cytochem 45: 1493–14501.
67. Linz R, Barnes NL, Zimnicka AM, Kaplan JH, Eipper B, et al. (2008) Intracellular targeting of copper-transporting ATPase ATP7A in a normal and Atp7b-/- kidney. Am J Physiol Renal Physiol 294: F53–61.
68. Małyszko J, Myśliwiec M (2007) Hepcidin in anemia and inflammation in chronic kidney disease. Kidney Blood Press Res 30: 15–30.
69. Lee P, Peng H, Gelbart T, Wang L, Beutler E (2005) Regulation of hepcidin transcription by interleukin-1 and interleukin-6. Proc Natl Acad Sci U S A 102: 1906–1910.
70. Zaffanello M, Maffeis C, Fanos V, Franchini M, Zamboni G (2006) Urological complication and copper replacement in childhood Menkes syndrome. Acta Pediatr 95: 785–790.

12

Effect of Vitamin D Supplementation on Cardiometabolic Risks and Health-Related Quality of Life among Urban Premenopausal Women in a Tropical Country – A Randomized Controlled Trial

Mazliza Ramly[1]*, Moy Foong Ming[2], Karuthan Chinna[1], Suhaili Suboh[1], Rokiah Pendek[3]

1 Department of Social and Preventive Medicine, Faculty of Medicine, University of Malaya, Kuala Lumpur, Malaysia, **2** Julius Centre University of Malaya, Department of Social and Preventive Medicine, Faculty of Medicine, University of Malaya, Kuala Lumpur, Malaysia, **3** Department of Medicine, Faculty of Medicine, University of Malaya, Kuala Lumpur, Malaysia

Abstract

Background: Many observational studies linked vitamin D to cardiometabolic risks besides its pivotal role in musculoskeletal diseases, but evidence from trials is lacking and inconsistent.

Aim: To determine whether Vitamin D supplementation in urban premenopausal women with vitamin D deficiency can improve cardiometabolic risks and health-related quality of life (HRQOL).

Design: A double-blind randomized controlled trial was conducted in Kuala Lumpur, Malaysia. A total of 192 vitamin D deficient (<50 nmol/l) premenopausal women were randomized to receive either vitamin D 50,000 IU or placebo once a week for 2 months and then monthly for 10 months. Primary outcomes were serum 25(OH)D, serum lipid profiles, blood pressure and HOMA-IR measured at baseline, 6 months and 12 months. HRQOL was assessed with SF-36 at baseline and 12 months.

Results: Ninety three and ninety-nine women were randomised into intervention and placebo groups respectively. After 12 months, there were significant differences in the serum 25(OH)D concentration (mean difference: 49.54; 95% CI: 43.94 to 55.14) nmol/l) and PTH levels (mean difference: −1.02; 95% CI: −1.67 to −0.38 pmol/l) in the intervention group compared to placebo group. There was significant difference between treatment group in both serum 25(OH)D and PTH. There was no effect of supplementation on HOMA-IR, serum lipid profiles and blood pressure (all $p>0.05$) between two groups. There was a small but significant improvement in HRQOL in the components of vitality (mean difference: 5.041; 95% CI: 0.709 to 9.374) and mental component score (mean difference: 2.951; 95% CI: 0.573 to 5.329) in the intervention group compared to placebo group.

Conclusion: Large and less frequent dosage vitamin D supplementation was safe and effective in the achievement of vitamin D sufficiency. However, there was no improvement in measured cardiometabolic risk factors in premenopausal women. Conversely vitamin D supplementation improves some components of HRQOL.

Trial Registration: Australian New Zealand Clinical Trial Registry ACTRN12612000452897

Editor: D. W. Cameron, University of Ottawa, Canada

Funding: The study was funded by the University Malaya (Post Graduate Research Grant, PV080/2012A) and the Ministry of Education High Impact Research Grant (MOE HIR No. E 2000069-20001). The funders had no role in study design, data collection and analysis, decision to publish or preparation of the manuscript.

Competing Interests: The authors have declared that no competing interests exist.

* Email: drmazliza@siswa.um.edu.my

Introduction

Vitamin D is well known for its fundamental role in bone mechanism and calcium homeostasis [1,2]. More recently, many studies found that vitamin D may play an important role in the prevention of cardiovascular diseases and metabolic syndrome risk factors [2–6]. The mechanisms in which vitamin D may protect against these diseases include activation of the renin-angiotensin-aldosterone systems, increase arterial intimae thickness, enhancement in insulin secretion and insulin sensitivity and inflammatory cytokines [2]. Many observational studies have shown that vitamin D deficiency, defined as serum 25(OH)D<50 nmol/l or 20 ng/ml [7] is associated with cardiometabolic diseases [4,8–10]. A meta-analysis of prospective studies by Khan et al [5] evaluated association between vitamin D levels and metabolic outcomes in healthy adults, demonstrated a significant inverse association of vitamin D status with metabolic syndrome. However, findings from this review were not able to establish causality, which required robust evidence from clinical trials. Clinical trials on the other hand produced inconsistent results [11–17]. These trials had marked study design variation in terms of samples size, study duration, participants' characteristics, primary outcomes, intervention dosage and formulation. Furthermore, existing randomized controlled trials were generally short duration (less than one year), insufficient dosage or underpowered.

Vitamin D deficiency is established risk factors for osteoporosis, falls and fractures and all these may impair HRQOL. Vitamin D deficiency can occur to any individuals regardless of age or health condition. Yet, assessment of HRQOL in vitamin D deficiency was only performed in elderly population. These observational studies found vitamin D deficiency to be inversely associated with mental and physical HRQOL [18–24]. Furthermore, most studies were restricted to disease-specific populations such as the postmenopausal osteoporotic women [18,19,22,23], elderly with heart failure [25] and elderly on dialysis [20]. Nevertheless, one observational study was found to examine the association between vitamin D and HRQOL among healthy premenopausal women [26] and another assessed the association between vitamin D and HRQOL among elderly in community setting [24]. Both studies observed inverse association between vitamin D and HRQOL. To our best knowledge, so far there are no other clinical trials evaluating the effect of vitamin D supplements on HRQOL in a healthy population.

Therefore, we designed this double-blind randomized placebo-controlled trial to determine whether vitamin D supplement can improve cardiometabolic risk factors such as blood pressure (BP), homeostasis model assessment insulin resistance (HOMA-IR), triglycerides (TG) and high-density lipoprotein cholesterol (HDL) as well as HRQOL in urban pre-menopausal women who were vitamin D deficient.

Method

The protocol for this trial is reported in full details in the published protocol [27]. The CONSORT checklist and Table S1 and Table S2 are available as supporting information; see Checklist S1, Table S1 and Table S2.

This was a randomized placebo-controlled, doubled-blind parallel trial. All premenopausal women aged 30 years old and above, working in a public university in Kuala Lumpur, Malaysia ($n = 389$) were screened for vitamin D deficiency (serum 25(OH)D≤20 ng/ml or ≤50 nmol/l). Exclusion criteria included abnormal serum PTH level (reference range for healthy adult was 1.1–7.3 pmol/l) and serum calcium (>2.7 nmol/l), known to have illnesses such as granuloma forming disorder, lymphoma, sarcoidosis or any types of cancer and taking daily vitamin D supplementation >1000 IU/day as well as pregnant women. Finally, 192 subjects were recruited in this trial (Figure 1).

The study was divided into two phases. Recruitment and screening including baseline clinical and anthropometry measurements were obtained in Phase one. All selected participants who meet the inclusion criteria in Phase one was ultimately invited to participate in this trial and proceed to Phase two. Written informed consent was obtained from these selected participants at this phase. The randomization and intervention of the first cohort ($n = 110$) commenced in October 2012 while the second cohort ($n = 82$) commenced in January 2013 (Phase two) (Figure 1). Intervention consisted of 50,000 IU (0.5 gram) of cholecalciferol (25(OH)D3) powder or placebo (0.5 gram) taken orally by diluting the powder into warm water before consumption. The consumption frequency was once a week for 8 weeks (equivalent to 7142 IU/day) and then once a month for 10 months (equivalent to 1667 IU/day) [7]. The consumption of 50,000 IU of vitamin D per week or per month is considered to be safe as the tolerable upper intake level for vitamin D is 10,000 IU per day [28]. We provided treatment for participants in the placebo group for 4 months after the trial completed, as it was unethical to withhold treatment. To ensure compliance with the intervention, participants were required to consume the active supplements or placebo in front of researcher during every follow-up. For those who did not attend the appointment, the researcher visited them at their workplace to give them the active supplements or placebo personally.

The randomization sequence was created using GraphPad Software with a 1:1 allocation by a staff (AC) with no involvement in the trial. The participant's names were matched with the random number sequence. The names of participants from intervention and placebo were printed and pasted on to the tubes filled with either vitamin D powder or placebo. The contents were not labelled on the bottles to maintain the allocation concealment. The tubes used were identical for both active intervention and placebo. Allocation sequence data was kept by AC in a secure place so that it could not be accessed or influenced by anyone, including the researchers. Outcomes measurements, randomization and allocation were fully concealed from the researchers, staffs involved in the trial and participants until the completion of data collection.

The primary outcome measures were serum 25(OH)D, systolic blood pressure, diastolic blood pressure, fasting blood insulin, fasting blood glucose, HOMA-IR, triglycerides, high-density lipoprotein cholesterol, low-density lipoprotein cholesterol and HRQOL using the SF-36 questionnaire.

Participants were recalled for clinical and anthropometry measurements at 6 months and 12 months. Serum calcium results at 6 months were checked for abnormality to detect any adverse reaction due to high dose of vitamin D supplementation. Participants were also advised to contact the researchers immediately if they suspected a reaction to supplements. Participants who were found to be pregnant at some point in the trial were also excluded in view of ethical consideration.

Methods for all measurements, questionnaires and laboratory analysis are reported in full details in the published protocol [27]. Homeostasis model assessment of insulin resistance (HOMA-IR) was used to establish a measure for insulin resistance. It can be calculated from a simple linear equation based on pairing FBS and Fasting Blood Insulin to establish a measure for insulin resistance: HOMA-IR = FBS(mmol/L)×Fasting Blood Insulin/22.5 [21]. Vitamin D concentration was analyzed using electrochemiluminescence immunoassay (ECLIA) vitamin D3 (25-OH) method on the Cobas E-411 analyzer. All tests and analyses were carried out by the Clinical Diagnostic Laboratory, University Malaya Medical Centre.

Statistical methods

A minimum of 88 subjects was required for each arm of the trial to demonstrate a significant difference at 80% power and a two-sided 5% significance. The calculations were based on the results by Zittermann et al. [29] which achieved a reduction in triglycerides of 0.19±0.54 mmol/L in vitamin D group while there is an increment of 0.03±0.50 in placebo group. Assuming a drop-out rate of 10%, 97 subjects would need to be recruited per arm. Sample size calculation was conducted using the OpenEpi Software version 2.3.1.

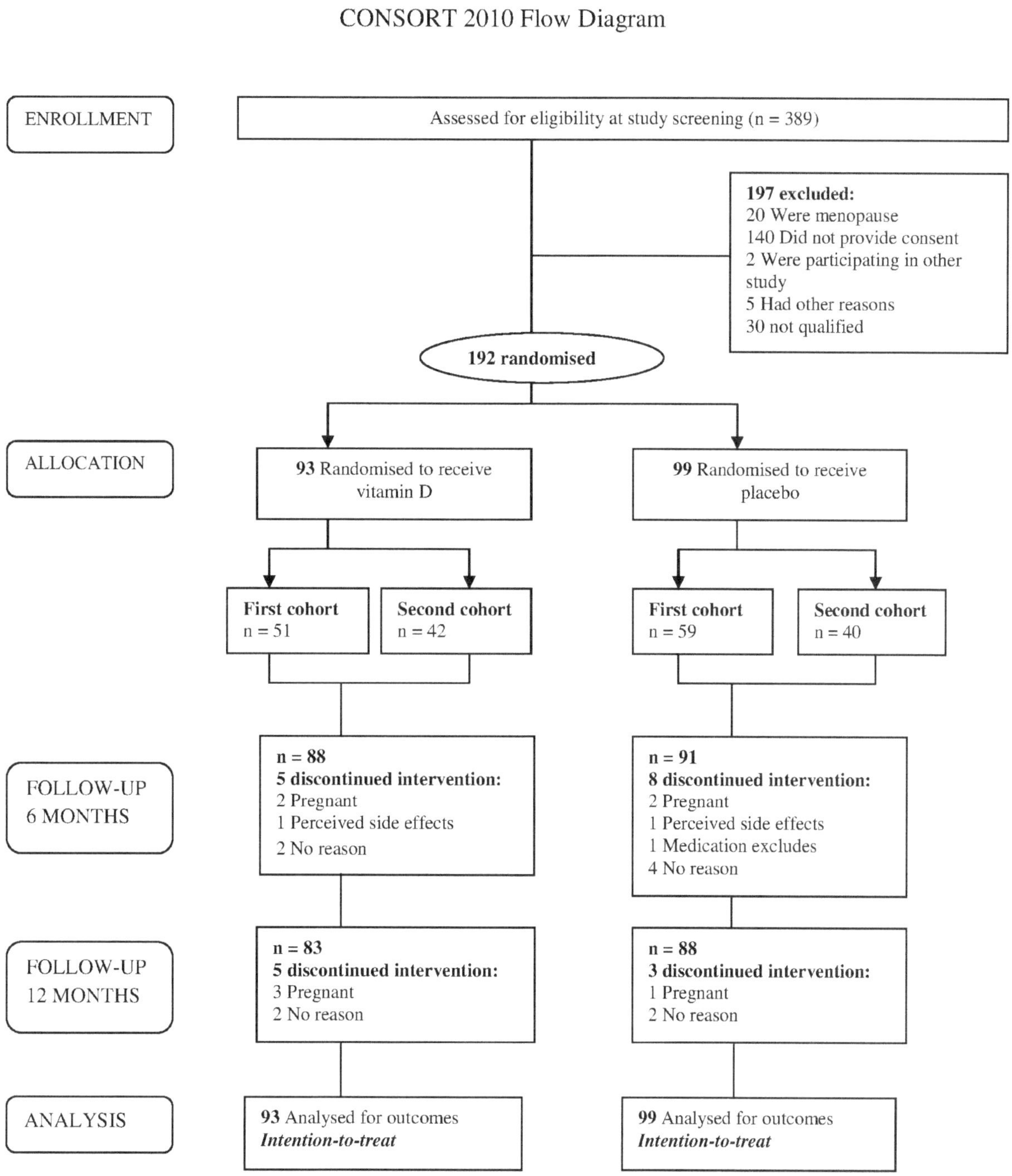

Figure 1. Flow diagram of the study, showing numbers of participants who were randomly assigned, received the intended treatment and were analyzed for the primary outcomes.

For baseline characteristics, descriptive statistics were used. Categorical data was described using count and percentages. All numerical data was checked for normality. Normally distributed variables were presented as mean ± standard deviation while abnormally distributed variables were presented as median ± interquartile range. Statistical comparisons were performed with independent *t-test*, Mann-Whitney U test or Chi-square test as appropriate. P-value was preset at 0.05. Some of the cases were loss to follow-up, therefore linear mixed effects procedure was used to test the differences in primary outcomes from baseline to follow-up at 6 months and 12 months. Data were analyzed according to the intention-to-treat principle. We also performed a linear mixed effects sensitivity analysis using complete cases. All statistical analysis was performed using the SPSS software version 16.0 (SPSS Inc, 2009, Chicago, Illinois).

Ethical approval

This trial was approved by the Medical Ethics Committee of University Malaya Medical Centre (reference number 907.22).

Trial registration no: ACTRN12612000452897. Written informed consent was obtained from all participants.

Results

Figure 1 shows the flow of participants in the trial. Three hundred eighty-nine potentially suitable participants were identified and invited for screening. Of these, a total of 192 women were randomly assigned to either intervention or placebo group. In total 21 women withdrew from the trial due to pregnancy, perceived side effects (amenorrhea) or no particular reasons. There were no reports of vitamin D intoxication or adverse reaction. A total of 171 participants completed the follow-up of 12 months.

Baseline data

Baseline characteristics of the participants are shown in Table 1. Both groups were similar in all the reported measures ($P>0.05$). Their mean age was 42±5 years, majority were Malays (>89%) and had at least secondary education (92%). A total of 15.6% of the participants had high cholesterol, 8.9% had hypertension and only 1% had diabetes mellitus. The mean scores for the HRQOL components were in the range of 60 to 70.

Effects of vitamin D supplements on cardiometabolic risk factors

Primary outcomes for both groups at baseline, 6 months and 12 months are presented (Table 2). Mean serum 25(OH)D concentrations in the intervention group increased drastically in the first 6 months (mean difference: 53.72; 95% CI: 49.23 to 58.18 nmol/l) followed with a small increment after that (mean difference: 1.83; 95% CI: −0.94 to 4.61 nmol/l). There was also significant increase in the mean serum 25(OH)D in the placebo group after 6 months (mean difference: 7.17; 95% CI: 1.46 to 12.85 nmol/l), however the level was still in the deficient category (<50 nmol/l). A total of 91.6% of the intervention group achieved 25(OH)D more than 50 nmol/l (20 ng/ml) and 63.4% achieved a level of 75 nmol/l (30 ng/ml) or higher. In contrast, 13.1% of the placebo group had 25(OH)D above 50 nmol/l and only 1% had a value of 75 nmol/l or higher. Mean PTH concentration remained suppressed in the intervention group as the mean serum 25(OH)D increased, however the change in PTH was not statistically significant. In the placebo group, the mean PTH concentration increased from baseline to 6 months (mean difference: 1.04; 95% CI: 0.49 to 1.60 pmol/l) but declined slightly at 12 months (mean difference: −0.58, 95% CI: −1.12 to −0.05 pmol/l). There were significant differences in mean concentrations of total 25(OH)D and PTH between treatment groups after 12 months of treatment.

BMI did not declined in the intervention group between baseline to 6 months (mean difference: 0.85, 95% CI: −1.07 to 2.77 kg/m^2), however these changes were not clinically significant and did not differ between treatment groups. There were significant differences in the change in serum calcium, systolic blood pressure and LDL within the intervention group ($p<0.05$). Serum calcium and LDL were significantly different over time within the placebo group ($p<0.05$). However, these changes did not differ between treatment groups and were not clinically significant. An increase in serum 25(OH)D in the intervention group induced a reduction in HOMA-IR whereas the reverse was observed in the placebo group. However, these changes were not statistically significant between treatment groups. Sensitivity analysis using complete cases showed similar results (Table S1).

There was a reduction in proportion of metabolic syndrome from 28% to 25.8% in the intervention group, while in placebo group, the proportion increased from 22.2% to 23.2%. There was no difference between groups ($p = 0.762$). Among participants with metabolic risks at baseline ($n = 26$ for intervention group and $n = 22$ for placebo group), there was a small but significant improvement ($p = 0.021$) in the proportion of low HDL in the intervention group at the end of the trial. Similar improvement was also noted in the proportions of high blood pressure, abdominal obesity and elevated glucose, however all these were not statistically significant (data not shown).

Effects of vitamin D supplements on health-related quality of life

The health-related quality of life (HRQOL) of the intervention and placebo groups is presented in Table 3. At baseline, the mean scores of HRQOL components in the SF-36 were in between 60 to 70. Vitamin D supplement improved general health of the intervention group (mean difference: 3.65; 95% CI: 0.57 to 7.73). However, there was no significant difference when compared to the placebo group. Apparently there was a small but significant improvement in vitality (mean difference: 5.041; 95% CI: 0.709 to 9.374) and mental component score (mean difference: 2.951; 95% CI: 0.573 to 5.329) in the intervention group compared to placebo group. Sensitivity analysis using complete cases were also performed for HRQOL and it also showed similar results (Table S2).

Discussion

Our participants were urban, premenopausal women working in a public university in the capital city of Malaysia. Although they were vitamin D deficient, the proportion of them having non-communicable diseases (NCD) such as hypertension and diabetes was relatively low compared to the general population [30]. However, more than 20% of them had metabolic syndrome. Their mean BMI was in the overweight category. This reflected that our participants were at risks for CVD in the future. As expected, the participants' scores for some of the HRQOL components, namely the physical functioning, role physical and social functioning were found to be lower than the general population [31].

In the present study, we demonstrated 12 months of vitamin D supplementation at a dosage of 50,000 IU per week for the first 2 months and 50,000 IU per month for the next 10 months increased serum 25(OH)D to sufficient level among our participants. However, correction of vitamin D deficiency did not improve HOMA-IR, HDL, LDL or triglycerides. Nevertheless, among participants with metabolic syndrome, vitamin D supplementation improved HDL level, offering a promising non-pharmacologic intervention in the prevention of metabolic syndrome. We also found that vitamin D supplements improved the HRQOL among the participants particularly in vitality and mental component scores.

Our results also showed the dosage and frequency of Vitamin D supplementation was safe and effective. More than 80% of participants from the intervention group achieved serum 25(OH)D above 50 nmol/l compared to only 13% from placebo group. These results were comparable with other studies which used daily dosage of vitamin D3 [16,17]. Although all women in the intervention group received the same dosage of vitamin D, a small proportion did not achieve a sufficient level of circulating vitamin D. This could be due to heterogeneity among women such as obesity. On further exploration of data, 6 out of 7 of these women were obese (>25 kg/m^2). This is probably because of a decreased in bioavailability of vitamin D that is sequestered in the fat of individuals with excess adipose tissue. Monthly dosage had

Table 1. Baseline socio-demographic characteristics of the intervention and placebo groups.

Characteristics	Intervention (n = 93)	Placebo (n = 99)	P-value[a]
	N (%)	N (%)	N (%)
Ethnicity			
Malay	83 (89.3%)	89 (89.9%)	0.777
Chinese	3 (3.2%)	3 (3.0%)	
Indian	7 (7.5%)	6 (6.1%)	
Others	0 (0%)	1 (1.0%)	
Level of education			
Primary	6 (6.5%)	8 (8.1%)	0.496
Secondary	43 (46.2%)	38 (38.4%)	
Tertiary	44 (47.3%)	53 (53.5%)	
History of CVD			
Diabetes mellitus	1 (1.1%)	1 (1.0%)	0.965
Hypertension	9 (9.7%)	8 (8.1%)	0.697
High cholesterol	15 (16.1%)	15 (15.2%)	0.852
Metabolic syndrome	26 (28%)	22 (22.2%)	0.359
	Mean ± SD	**Mean ± SD**	
Age (years)	42.58±5.35	42.88±4.99	0.69
BMI (kg/m^2)	27.23±5.49	27.23±5.09	0.99
Blood pressure			
Systolic (mmHg)	121.61±16.19	118.90±14.85	0.23
Diastolic (mmHg)	77.77±10.64	76.80±10.99	0.53
Serum 25(OH)D (nmol/l)	30.19±8.71	29.99±9.70	0.88
Serum calcium (mmol/l)	2.18±0.07	2.19±0.08	0.246
Serum PTH (pmol/l)	4.60±2.19	4.76±2.05	0.611
Lipid values (mmol/l)			
Total cholesterol	5.17±0.99	5.28±0.83	0.425
HDL – Cholesterol	1.45±0.49	1.44±0.35	0.846
LDL – Cholesterol	3.26±0.76	3.34±0.71	0.457
Triglycerides	1.15±0.53	1.17±0.62	0.770
HRQOL (SF-36)			
Physical functioning	74.68±20.23	70.96±24.24	0.252
Role physical	74.35±22.98	72.27±24.40	0.544
Bodily pain	73.13±19.64	71.13±18.31	0.467
General health	66.77±16.87	66.12±17.13	0.791
Vitality	65.27±11.98	61.76±13.88	0.063
Social functioning	78.77±19.50	74.26±21.85	0.134
Role emotional	78.92±22.37	76.26±23.99	0.428
Mental health	73.12±12.11	71.06±16.62	0.331
PCS	49.57±6.78	48.80±7.41	0.453
MCS	50.09±6.69	48.65±9.17	0.218
	Median; IQR	**Median, IQR**	
Insulin resistance			
Serum glucose (mmol/l)	4.80; 0.65	4.80; 0.70	0.871
Serum insulin (mU/L)	9.30; 9.95	9.20; 8.80	0.874
HOMA-IR	2.00; 2.28	2.00; 2.00	0.908

HOMA-IR, homeostasis model assessment insulin resistance; CVD, cardiovascular disease; PTH, parathyroid hormone; 25(OH)D, 25-hydroxyvitamin D; IQR, Interquartile range; PCS, Physical component score; MCS, Mental component score; BMI was calculated as weight (kilogram) divided by height (m^2).
[a]Determined with independent t-test or Mann-Whitney test for continuous variables as appropriate and with χ^2 test for categorical data.

Table 2. Summary of the outcome measurements overtime (baseline, 6 months and 12 months) – Intention-to-treat analysis.

	Intervention (n = 93)	Placebo (n = 99)	Mean difference (95% CI) between treatment group[a]
	Mean (95% CI)	Mean (95% CI)	
Se 25(OH)D (nmol/l)			
Baseline	30.19 (28.56 to 31.82)	29.98 (27.20 to 32.78)	0.19 (−2.43 to 2.82
6 month	83.91 (79.84 to 87.97)	37.15 (34.39 to 39.90)	**46.92 (42.42 to 51.43)**
12 months	85.74 (81.25 to 90.22)	36.09 (33.63 to 38.55)	**49.54 (43.94 to 55.14)***
Se PTH (pmol/l)			
Baseline	4.60 (4.18 to 5.03)	4.76 (4.34 to 5.18)	−0.16 (−0.76 to 0.45)
6 month	4.58 (4.05 to 5.10)	5.86 (5.34 to 6.38)	**−1.28 (−2.02 to −0.55)***
12 months	4.19 (3.74 to 4.66)	5.22 (4.77 to 5.67)	**−1.02 (−1.67 to −0.38)***
Se calcium (mmol/l)			
Baseline	2.18 (2.17 to 2.19)	2.19 (2.18 to 2.21)	−0.01 (−0.03 to 0.009)
6 month	2.23 (2.21 to 2.26)	2.24 (2.21 to 2.26)	−0.005 (−0.04 to 0.03)
12 months	2.24 (2.22 to 2.26)	2.22 (2.20 to 2.24)	0.02 (−0.01 to 0.05)
BMI			
Baseline	27.22 (26.14 to 28.31)	27.23 (26.18 to 28.28)	−0.005 (−1.511 to 1.500)
6 month	28.08 (26.96 to 29.19)	27.76 (26.67 to 28.86)	0.313 (−1.251 to 1.877)
12 months	27.63 (26.45 to 28.78)	27.84 (26.73 to 28.95)	−0.209 (−1.807 to 1.389)
Systolic BP			
Baseline	121.6 (118.4 to 124.8)	118.9 (115.8 to 121.9)	2.71 (−1.71 to 7.13)
6 month	126.3 (122.9 to 129.6)	123.9 (120.7 to 127.2)	2.38 (−2.27 to 7.04)
12 months	125.8 (122.6 to 128.9)	123.9 (120.8 to 126.9)	1.89 (−2.56 to 6.35)
Diastolic BP			
Baseline	77.77 (75.56 to 79.99)	76.79 (74.65 to 78.94)	0.976 (−2.107 to 4.059)
6 month	79.74 (77.38 to 82.10)	79.23 (76.97 to 81.55)	0.508 (−2.805 to 3.820)
12 months	77.52 (75.22 to 79.81)	76.76 (74.53 to 78.99)	0.757 (−2.441 to 3.954)
Se Glucose (mmol/l)			
Baseline	5.07 (4.88 to 5.25)	4.93 (4.75 to 5.12)	0.13 (−0.13 to 0.39)
6 month	5.14 (4.97 to 5.32)	5.07 (4.89 to 5.24)	0.07 (−0.17 to 0.32)
12 months	5.04 (4.83 to 5.26)	5.11 (4.90 to 5.32)	−0.07 (−0.37 to 0.23)
Se insulin (mU/L			
Baseline	13.81 (10.38 to 17.24)	11.07 (7.74 to 14.39)	2.74 (−2.04 to 7.51)
6 month	13.11 (11.18 to 15.04)	12.17 (10.27 to 14.06)	0.943 (−1.75 to 3.65)
12 months	13.93 (11.47 to 16.38)	12.74 (10.36 to 15.12)	1.19 (−2.23 to 4.61)
HOMA-IR			
Baseline	3.72 (2.25 to 5.19)	2.47 (1.04 to 3.91)	1.25 (−0.81 to 3.31)
6 month	3.12 (2.57 to 3.67)	2.84 (2.29 to 3.38)	0.28 (−0.49 to 1.05)
12 months	3.19 (2.61 to 3.78)	2.99 (2.42 to 3.56)	0.21 (−0.61 to 1.03)
TG (mmol/l)			
Baseline	1.15 (1.03 to 1.26)	1.17 (1.06 to 1.29)	−0.03 (−0.19 to 0.14)
6 month	1.38 (1.25 to 1.51)	1.19 (1.07 to 1.32)	**0.19 (0.01 to 0.37)***
12 months	1.36 (1.23 to 1.49)	1.22 (1.09 to 1.35)	0.14 (−0.33 to 0.33)
HDL-C (mmol/l)			
Baseline	1.45 (1.36 to 1.54)	1.44 (1.35 to 1.52)	0.01 (−0.11 to 0.13)
6 month	1.43 (1.36 to 1.49)	1.50 (1.44 to 1.57)	−0.08 (−0.18 to 0.02)
12 months	1.52 (1.44 to 1.59)	1.53 1.50 (1.43 to 1.58)	0.02 (−0.09 to 0.13)
LDL-C (mmol/l)			
Baseline	3.26 (3.11 to 3.41)	3.34 (3.19 to 3.48)	−0.08 (−0.29 to 0.13)
6 month	3.25 (3.09 to 3.39)	3.31 (3.17 to 3.46)	−0.07 (−0.28 to 0.15)

Table 2. Cont.

	Intervention (n = 93)	Placebo (n = 99)	Mean difference (95% CI) between treatment group[a]
	Mean (95% CI)	Mean (95% CI)	
12 months	3.62 (3.44 to 3.79)	3.63 (3.46 to 3.80)	-0.01 (-0.26 to 0.23)

*Significant at $p<0.05$.
[a]Determined with linear mixed effect.

advantage in terms of compliance. Von Hurst et al [16] reported that their participants found it difficult to comply with daily dosage of vitamin D. None of our participants reported any adverse effects of vitamin D clinically or biochemically.

Evidences from epidemiologic studies showed vitamin D deficiency was linked with cardiometabolic risks [9,10,32–40].

Table 3. Summary of the health-related quality of life parameters overtime (baseline and 12 months) – Intention-to-treat analysis.

	Intervention (n = 93)	Placebo (n = 99)	Mean difference (95% CI) between treatment group[a]
	Mean (95% CI)	Mean (95% CI)	
Physical functioning			
Baseline	74.68 (70.81 to 78.84)	70.96 (66.13 to 75.79)	3.718 (-2.624 to 10.06)
12 months	71.81 (66.53 to 77.09)	71.48 (66.62 to 76.33)	0.330 (-6.792 to 7.452)
Role physical			
Baseline	74.36 (69.62 to 79.09)	72.27 (67.41 to 77.14)	2.082 (-4.662 to 8.826)
12 months	73.45 (67.94 to 78.95)	72.84 (67.78 to 77.90)	0.605 (-6.820–8.029)
Bodily pain			
Baseline	73.13 (69.09 to 77.17)	71.13 (67.48 to 74.78)	1.998 (-3.416 to 7.411)
12 months	72.93 (67.76 to 77.09)	69.31 (65.64 to 72.97)	3.621 (-1.891 to 9.132)
General health			
Baseline	66.77 (63.29 to 70.25)	66.12 (62.71 to 69.54)	0.653 (-4.188 to 5.494)
12 months	70.42 (66.85 to 73.99)	68.66 (65.57 to 71.75)	1.763 (-2.924 to 6.449)
Vitality			
Baseline	65.27 (62.80 to 67.74)	61.76 (58.99 to 64.53)	3.511 (-0.173 to 7.196)
12 months	65.53 (62.45 to 68.61)	60.49 (57.39 to 63.58)	**5.041 (0.709 to 9.374)***
Social functioning			
Baseline	78.77 (74.76 to 82.79)	74.26 (69.91 to 78.62)	4.512 (-1.377 to 10.401)
12 months	80.27 (76.24 to 84.29)	75.11 (70.66 to 79.56)	5.151 (-0.804 to 11.107)
Role emotional			
Baseline	78.93 (74.32 to 85.53)	76.26 (71.48 to 79.62)	2.662 (-3.938 to 9.262)
12 months	80.52 (75.45 to 85.58)	74.52 (69.43 to 79.62)	5.995 (-1.138 to 13.129)
Mental health			
Baseline	73.12 (70.63 to 75.61)	71.06 (67.74 to 74.37)	2.058 (-2.065 to 6.180)
12 months	75.12 (72.16 to 78.08)	71.53 (68.25 to 74.82)	3.586 (-0.806 to 7.979)
Physical component score			
Baseline	49.57 (48.17 to 50.97)	48.80 (47.32 to 50.28)	0.772 (-1.249 to 2.793)
12 months	48.99 (47.51 to 50.47)	49.06 (47.79 to 50.32)	-0.069 (-1.997 to 1.860)
Mental component score			
Baseline	50.09 (48.71 to 51.46)	48.65 (46.82 to 50.48)	1.440 (-0.835 to 3.715)
12 months	51.34 (49.81 to 52.86)	48.39 (46.54 to 50.23)	**2.951 (0.573 to 5.329)***

*Significant at $p<0.05$.
[a]Determined with linear mixed effect.

Vitamin D insufficiency induced alterations in the calcium flux of pancreatic b-cells thus reduced insulin secretion [41,42] and this might influence on insulin resistance (IR). In addition, vitamin D insufficiency also induced elevations in PTH, which could adversely affect glucose metabolism. As expected, PTH levels decreased within the intervention group. On the other hand, the PTH levels also decreased within the placebo group. This could possibly due to unintentional increased consumption of dietary calcium in the placebo group because of Hawthorne effect. This could be the reason for no significant differences in insulin resistance or glucose levels between groups.

They were many clinical trials trying to establish the role of vitamin D deficiency in the pathogenesis of type 2 diabetes mellitus [11,12,14–17,33,34,43]. However, the results had been inconsistent. Most of these trials failed to detect any improvement in the glucose levels and insulin resistance. Our findings were consistent with results of many other published studies, in which the vitamin D supplements appeared to have no effect on fasting glucose and HOMA-IR [11,12,14,15,17]. Reasons for these negative results could be due to the studies were short duration, had small sample size and different dosage used in vitamin D formulations. On the contrary, data from two clinical trials showed that vitamin D supplementation improved plasma glucose and insulin resistance [16,43].

Systematic reviews and observational studies found associations between vitamin D deficiency and triglycerides, HDL and LDL [44–47]. However, results from trials had been inconsistent. Clinical trials by Brevlasky et al [11] and Wood et al [17] found an absence of improvement in lipid profiles, similar with our findings. On the other hand, two other clinical trials [13,29] found significant decrease in lipid in the treatment group. Major et al [13] reported that total cholesterol:HDL and LDL:HDL ratio in the treatment group were significantly decreased. Whereas, in study by Zitterman et al [29] the serum triglycerides and LDL ($p < 0.001$) were reduced after one year of treatment with 3320 IU of vitamin D daily among healthy overweight individuals with inadequate vitamin D levels. These inconsistent results could be due to variations in sample size, dosage and formulation of vitamin D supplement, characteristics of participants and duration of trials.

Our participants were generally healthy premenopausal women with vitamin D deficiency. Although 26% of them had history of CVD, majority had normal glucose and lipid values, which may be difficult to improve further with vitamin D supplement. However, individuals with higher baseline metabolic risks may benefit from vitamin D supplementation. Analysis on a subset of our participants with metabolic risks at baseline demonstrated an improvement in HDL among the intervention group. However, the null effect of vitamin D supplementation on other metabolic risk factors may be due to the small sample size of our participants with metabolic risks. Therefore, there might be inadequate power to detect the effectiveness of vitamin D on these components. Future studies should recruit women with vitamin D deficiency and at risks for metabolic syndrome or CVD.

The increase levels in some of the clinical indicators (systolic blood pressure, triglycerides, LDL-cholesterol) within both intervention and placebo groups was probably due to the advancing age that affected the pathogenesis of these indicators [48]. Twelve months of treatment with vitamin D may not be sufficient to produce a significant reduction in the cardiometabolic risk factors as more time may be needed for the vitamin D to correct the metabolic risks back to normal.

The optimal dose for vitamin D supplementation on cardiometabolic risk could also influence our results. Expert opinions for daily vitamin D dosage ranged from 600 to 2000 IU for prevention of cardiovascular or metabolic risk [28,49,50]. The Institute of Medicine Report [28] concluded that due to lack of evidence, they could not make any recommendation for non-skeletal outcomes. The method of vitamin D supplementation in our study (50,000 IU weekly for 2 months and once a month after that) differed from the daily doses (400–4000 IU) used in majority of other studies [12,15–17,43,51]. We used the recommendation by Holick [7] which stated that for an effective vitamin D deficiency treatment, higher dosage was needed at initial stage to correct the vitamin D deficient status. However, this recommendation only corrected the vitamin D deficiency. There is no current recommendation on the optimum dosage needed for improvement of cardiometabolic outcomes. There are few other studies using similar dosage [52] or larger dose of vitamin D supplementation [14,25,53] but in shorter duration (less than 6 months). Although we did not find any effect of vitamin D supplementation on cardiometabolic risks, we cannot exclude the possibility that higher dosage of supplementation for a longer duration might help in the prevention of cardiometabolic risks among individuals with existing co-morbidities or cardiometabolic events such as myocardial infarct or stroke. However, a review article has indicate that negative outcomes could be predicted due to failure to maintain circulating vitamin D over time as with monthly, quarterly or yearly bolus vitamin D dosing [54]. It appears that for the optimal benefits of vitamin D supplementation, sufficient amount of vitamin D should be provided on a daily basis to ensure that stable circulating concentrations are maintained over time as vitamin D has short circulating half-life of vitamin D. These particular reasons might explain the varying results of clinical trials. Therefore, a large-scale prospective clinical trial is needed to examine large dosage of daily versus weekly and monthly vitamin D with the same primary outcome measures.

On the other hand, we found vitamin D supplements improved the HRQOL of participants particularly in vitality and mental component score. These improvements were statistically significant but clinically insignificant. However, it has some clinical relevance as vitality assessed energy and fatigue; and women with vitamin D deficiency usually feel tired, low energy and worn out. Vitamin D is a nuclear steroid hormone which thought to be involved in brain health and function as well as neuromuscular functions. Vitamin D receptors in the cell's nucleus regulate the expression of target genes when bound to 1,25(OH)D. These receptors are expressed in areas of the brain important to behavioural regulation [55]. An observational study by Ecemis et al [26] found physical component score, mental component score, physical functioning score and vitality score were impaired in vitamin D deficient and insufficient healthy premenopausal women. Other studies did relate vitamin D status with depression [56–59] and mental component score [19]. Another observational study also concluded that women who were on daily vitamin D supplementation had higher mental HRQOL scores [19].

At baseline, our study showed slightly higher scores in bodily pain components compared to the general population [20]. Although muscle and bone pain was a common symptom of vitamin D deficiency, we did not find any significant improvement for physical components score. This may be due to non-specific definition of pain was used in the SF-36 questionnaire which we administered. For example, Huang et al [21] used VR-36 (Veteran Rand 36 items) questionnaire as well as VAS (visual analog scale) to evaluate bodily pain and found that vitamin D supplementation was effective to alleviate pain and improve other components of HRQOL. Similarly, Sakalli et al [60] used VAS and SF-36 questionnaire to detect the level of pain and they reported that single megadose of vitamin D was effective to increase QOL particularly physical functioning, role physical, bodily pain, general health, social functioning and also decrease non-specific musculoskeletal pain. On the contrary, another study that used a disease-specific tool (Minnesota Living with Heart Failure questionnaire) did not find any improvement in physical function or HRQOL in older patients with heart failure [25].

To date, very few studies examined the relationship of vitamin D and HRQOL among healthy premenopausal women without osteoporosis as the study population. So far, we only found study by Ecemis et al [26] on Vitamin D and HRQOL among the healthy premenopausal women. They reported significant association between vitamin D and HRQOL.

It is difficult to recommend sunlight exposure to improve vitamin D levels due to interpersonal variations in sunlight exposure as well as the risks of skin cancer due to excessive UV radiation. However, skin cancer is a rare disease in Asia as compared to Caucasians [61]. A study by Nurbazlin et al. [62] has found that urban women in Malaysia had significantly lower sunlight exposure and vitamin D status compared to rural women. This study shown that sun index were the major factors influencing vitamin D status in Malaysian women. A trial study on the effect of nutrition education and sun exposure on vitamin D status among postmenopausal Malay women also found serum vitamin D level was increased through nutrition education and sunlight exposure [63]. Therefore it is sensible to recommend additional sunlight exposure for Malaysian women especially those living in the urban. Besides that, the best way of preventing vitamin D deficiency is by food fortification. Food fortification has the dual advantage of being able to deliver nutrients to large segments of the population without requiring radical changes in food consumption patterns. A recent review study found vitamin D fortification using vegetable oil can be the efficacious way to increase intake of daily vitamin D in Southeast Asian countries [64]. In addition to fortification, supplementation can be the alternative solution with high and less frequent doses are advisable especially to high risk population such as elderly. Nevertheless, we need to learn more about the long term safety and efficacy of the high dosage, less frequent vitamin D supplementation.

Limitations and Strength

Although all of our participants were vitamin D deficient, only small proportion of them was at risk for CVD as our study was conducted in a non-clinical setting. From the National Health and Morbidity Survey IV (NHMS IV) conducted in 2011, only 14.5% of women age more than 18 years old were diabetic while 31.6% were hypertensive [65]. Therefore, we had difficulty recruiting women with vitamin D deficiency as those with CVD risk. So, our study was not powered to detect the effect of vitamin D supplementation on cardiometabolic risks. We were also not able to examine the incidence of cardiovascular events due to the short duration. A larger sample size of high risk population for CVD with longer follow-up and higher intakes of vitamin D supplementation may be needed to establish whether steady normalization of vitamin D levels will translate to decrease in cardiovascular event incidence. An article by Heaney [66] has indicated that inadequate intakes of vitamin D may produce more than one disease by more than one mechanisms and may require several years for the consequent morbidity to be sufficiently evident to be clinically recognizable as "disease". Similarly more established evident are needed to prove that higher intakes of vitamin D are required for its prevention. For example, preventing the osteoporosis requires almost 4 times the amount of vitamin D needed to prevent rickets and this knowledge takes years to be established.

Nevertheless, our study has several strengths that worth mention. One of them is its high quality of randomisation where there was concealment of allocation, double-blinding among the participant and researchers and placebo controlled design. This reduced bias in term of selection and information bias as self-reported HRQOL was subjective. Larger but less frequent dosage of vitamin D may be advantageous from a compliance perspective compared to daily doses. There was also no problem with seasonal confounders as Malaysia is blessed with sufficient sunshine all year round necessary for cutaneous synthesis of vitamin D. Both groups were comparable in outdoor physical activity, sunlight exposure activity and diet at baseline and there were no changes pre and post intervention. In addition, our participants' retention rate was good with only 11% drop-out from the study.

Conclusion

This trial showed that Vitamin D supplementation over one year to premenopausal vitamin D deficient women living in an urban tropical country had no meaningful effect on measured cardiometabolic risk factors, but it did improve some components of HRQOL. Our findings provided evidence for the larger dosage but lower frequency to be effective in improving serum vitamin D levels. Further long term trials of this intervention versus daily and weekly vitamin D dosing especially among the high risk individuals with existing co-morbidities are needed.

Supporting Information

Table S1 Sensitivity analysis using complete cases of the outcome measurements overtime (baseline, 6 months and 12 months).

Table S2 Sensitivity analysis using complete cases of the health-related quality of life parameters overtime (baseline and 12 months).

Checklist S1 CONSORT Checklist. CONSORT 2010 checklist of information to include when reporting a randomized trial.

Acknowledgments

The authors would like to acknowledge all participants of the trial and the management of the University of Malaya for supporting this study.

Author Contributions

Conceived and designed the experiments: MR MFM RP. Performed the experiments: MR SS. Analyzed the data: MR MFM. Contributed to the writing of the manuscript: MR MFM.

References

1. Wacker M, Holick MF (2013) Vitamin D - effects on skeletal and extraskeletal health and the need for supplementation. Nutrients 5: 111–148.
2. Holick MF (2011) Vitamin D: A D-Lightful Solution for Health. Journal of Investigative Medicine 59: 9.
3. Holick MF (2004) Vitamin D: importance in the prevention of cancers, type 1 diabetes, heart disease, and osteoporosis. Am J Clin Nutr 79: 362–371.
4. Hosseinpanah F, Yarjanli M, Sheikholeslami F, Heibatollahi M, Eskandary PS, et al. (2011) Associations between vitamin D and cardiovascular outcomes; Tehran Lipid and Glucose Study. Atherosclerosis 218: 238–242.

5. Khan H, Kunutsor S, Franco OH, Chowdhury R (2013) Vitamin D, type 2 diabetes and other metabolic outcomes: a systematic review and meta-analysis of prospective studies. Proc Nutr Soc 72: 89–97.
6. Lee JH, O'Keefe JH, Bell D, Hensrud DD, Holick MF (2008) Vitamin D Deficiency: An Important, Common, and Easily Treatable Cardiovascular Risk Factor? Journal of the American College of Cardiology 52: 1949–1956.
7. Holick MF (2009) Vitamin D Status: Measurement, Interpretation, and Clinical Application. Annals of Epidemiology 19: 73–78.
8. Anderson JL, May HT, Horne BD, Bair TL, Hall NL, et al. (2010) Relation of Vitamin D Deficiency to Cardiovascular Risk Factors, Disease Status, and Incident Events in a General Healthcare Population. The American Journal of Cardiology 106: 963–968.
9. Chacko SA, Song Y, Manson JE, Van Horn L, Eaton C, et al. (2011) Serum 25-hydroxyvitamin D concentrations in relation to cardiometabolic risk factors and metabolic syndrome in postmenopausal women. American Journal of Clinical Nutrition 94: 209–217.
10. El-Menyar A, Rahil A, Dousa K, Ibrahim W, Ibrahim T, et al. (2012) Low vitamin D and cardiovascular risk factors in males and females from a sunny, rich country. Open Cardiovascular Medicine Journal 6: 76–80.
11. Breslavsky A, Frand J, Matas Z, Boaz M, Barnea Z, et al. (2013) Effect of high doses of vitamin D on arterial properties, adiponectin, leptin and glucose homeostasis in type 2 diabetic patients. Clin Nutr 32: 970–975.
12. Harris SS, Pittas AG, Palermo NJ (2012) A randomized, placebo-controlled trial of vitamin D supplementation to improve glycaemia in overweight and obese African Americans. Diabetes Obes Metab 14: 789–794.
13. Major GC, Alarie F, Dore J, Phouttama S, Tremblay A (2007) Supplementation with calcium + vitamin D enhances the beneficial effect of weight loss on plasma lipid and lipoprotein concentrations. Am J Clin Nutr 85: 54–59.
14. Nagpal J, Pande JN, Bhartia A (2009) A double-blind, randomized, placebo-controlled trial of the short-term effect of vitamin D3 supplementation on insulin sensitivity in apparently healthy, middle-aged, centrally obese men. Diabet Med 26: 19–27.
15. Ryu OH, Lee S, Yu J, Choi MG, Yoo HJ, et al. (2013) A prospective randomized controlled trial of the effects of vitamin D supplementation on long-term glycemic control in type 2 diabetes mellitus of Korea. Endocr J.
16. von Hurst PR, Stonehouse W, Coad J (2010) Vitamin D supplementation reduces insulin resistance in South Asian women living in New Zealand who are insulin resistant and vitamin D deficient - a randomised, placebo-controlled trial. Br J Nutr 103: 549–555.
17. Wood AD, Secombes KR, Thies F, Aucott L, Black AJ, et al. (2012) Vitamin D3 supplementation has no effect on conventional cardiovascular risk factors: a parallel-group, double-blind, placebo-controlled RCT. J Clin Endocrinol Metab 97: 3557–3568.
18. Basaran S, Guzel R, Coskun-Benlidayi I, Guler-Uysal F (2007) Vitamin D status: effects on quality of life in osteoporosis among Turkish women. Quality of Life Research 16: 1491–1499.
19. Motsinger S, Lazovich D, MacLehose RF, Torkelson CJ, Robien K (2012) Vitamin D intake and mental health-related quality of life in older women: the Iowa Women's Health Study. Maturitas 71: 267–273.
20. Anand S, Kaysen GA, Chertow GM, Johansen KL, Grimes B, et al. (2011) Vitamin D deficiency, self-reported physical activity and health-related quality of life: the Comprehensive Dialysis Study. Nephrol Dial Transplant 26: 3683–3688.
21. Huang W, Shah S, Long Q, Crankshaw AK, Tangpricha V (2013) Improvement of pain, sleep, and quality of life in chronic pain patients with vitamin D supplementation. Clin J Pain 29: 341–347.
22. Michael YL, Smit E, Seguin R, Curb JD, Phillips LS, et al. (2011) Serum 25-hydroxyvitamin D and physical performance in postmenopausal women. J Womens Health (Larchmt) 20: 1603–1608.
23. Ohta H, Uemura Y, Nakamura T, Fukunaga M, Ohashi Y, et al. (2014) Serum 25-hydroxyvitamin D level as an independent determinant of quality of life in osteoporosis with a high risk for fracture. Clinical Therapeutics 36: 225–235.
24. Chao YS, Ekwaru JP, Ohinmaa A, Griener G, Veugelers PJ (2014) Vitamin D and health-related quality of life in a community sample of older Canadians. Qual Life Res.
25. Witham MD, Crighton LJ, Gillespie ND, Struthers AD, McMurdo MET (2010) The Effects of Vitamin D Supplementation on Physical Function and Quality of Life in Older Patients With Heart Failure: A Randomized Controlled Trial. Circulation: Heart Failure 3: 195–201.
26. Ecemis GC, Atmaca A (2013) Quality of life is impaired not only in vitamin D deficient but also in vitamin D-insufficient pre-menopausal women. J Endocrinol Invest 36: 622–627.
27. Ramly M, Moy FM, Pendek R, Suboh S, Tan Tong Boon A (2013) Study protocol: the effect of vitamin D supplements on cardiometabolic risk factors among urban premenopausal women in a tropical country – a randomized controlled trial. BMC Public Health 13: 416.
28. Ross AC, Manson JE, Abrams SA, Aloia JF, Brannon PM, et al. (2011) The 2011 report on dietary reference intakes for calcium and vitamin D from the Institute of Medicine: what clinicians need to know. J Clin Endocrinol Metab 96: 53–58.
29. Zittermann A, Frisch S, Berthold HK, Gotting C, Kuhn J, et al. (2009) Vitamin D supplementation enhances the beneficial effects of weight loss on cardiovascular disease risk markers. Am J Clin Nutr 89: 1321–1327.
30. Begg GA, Cleland JG, Witte KK (2010) Letter by Begg, et al regarding article, "The effects of vitamin d supplementation on physical function and quality of life in older heart failure patients: a randomized controlled trial". Circ Heart Fail 3: e24; author reply e25.
31. Azman AB, Sararaks S, Rugayah B, Low LL, Azian AA, et al. (2003) Quality of life of the Malaysian general population: results from a postal survey using the SF-36. Med J Malaysia 58: 694–711.
32. Alam U, Najam O, Al-Himdani S, Benoliel S, Jinadev P, et al. (2012) Marked vitamin D deficiency in patients with diabetes in the UK: ethnic and seasonal differences and an association with dyslipidaemia. Diabet Med 29: 1343–1345.
33. Al-Daghri N (2010) Serum 25-hydroxy-vitamin D is associated with insulin resistance and adiponectin levels in diabetic Saudi adults. Osteoporosis International 21: S726.
34. Al-Daghri NM, Alkharfy KM, Al-Saleh Y, Al-Attas OS, Alokail MS, et al. (2012) Modest reversal of metabolic syndrome manifestations with vitamin D status correction: A 12-month prospective study. Metabolism: Clinical and Experimental 61: 661–666.
35. Botella-Carretero JI, Alvarez-Blasco F, Villafruela JJ, Balsa JA, Vázquez C, et al. (2007) Vitamin D deficiency is associated with the metabolic syndrome in morbid obesity. Clinical Nutrition 26: 573–580.
36. Chailurkit LO, Aekplakorn W, Ongphiphadhanakul B (2012) The association between vitamin D status and type 2 diabetes in a Thai population, a cross-sectional study. Clin Endocrinol (Oxf) 77: 658–664.
37. Moy FM, Bulgiba A (2011) High prevalence of vitamin D insufficiency and its association with obesity and metabolic syndrome among Malay adults in Kuala Lumpur, Malaysia. BMC Public Health 11: 735.
38. Kayaniyil S, Vieth R, Harris SB, Retnakaran R, Knight JA, et al. (2011) Association of 25(OH)D and PTH with metabolic syndrome and its traditional and nontraditional components. Journal of Clinical Endocrinology and Metabolism 96: 168–175.
39. Mark F M (2009) Poor vitamin D status may contribute to high risk for insulin resistance, obesity, and cardiovascular disease in Asian Indians. Medical Hypotheses 72: 647–651.
40. Siadat ZD, Kiani K, Sadeghi M, Shariat AS, Farajzadegan Z, et al. (2012) Association of vitamin D deficiency and coronary artery disease with cardiovascular risk factors. Journal of Research in Medical Sciences 17: 1052–1055.
41. Zhou QG, Hou FF, Guo ZJ, Liang M, Wang GB, et al. (2008) 1,25-Dihydroxyvitamin D improved the free fatty-acid-induced insulin resistance in cultured C2C12 cells. Diabetes Metab Res Rev 24: 459–464.
42. Manna P, Jain SK (2012) Vitamin D up-regulates glucose transporter 4 (GLUT4) translocation and glucose utilization mediated by cystathionine-gamma-lyase (CSE) activation and H2S formation in 3T3L1 adipocytes. J Biol Chem 287: 42324–42332.
43. Pittas AG, Harris SS, Stark PC, Dawson-Hughes B (2007) The effects of calcium and vitamin D supplementation on blood glucose and markers of inflammation in nondiabetic adults. Diabetes Care 30: 980–986.
44. Maki KC, Rubin MR, Wong LG, McManus JF, Jensen CD, et al. (2009) Serum 25-hydroxyvitamin D is independently associated with high-density lipoprotein cholesterol and the metabolic syndrome in men and women. Journal of Clinical Lipidology 3: 289–296.
45. Minambres I, Sanchez-Quesada JL, Sanchez-Hernandez J, Rodriguez J, De Leiva A, et al. (2014) Vitamin D concentrations in familial combined hyperlipidemia: Effects of lipid lowering treatment. Diabetology and Metabolic Syndrome 6.
46. Rejnmark L, Vestergaard P, Heickendorff L, Mosekilde L (2010) Simvastatin does not affect vitamin d status, but low vitamin d levels are associated with dyslipidemia: results from a randomised, controlled trial. Int J Endocrinol 2010: 957174.
47. Jorde R, Grimnes G (2011) Vitamin D and metabolic health with special reference to the effect of vitamin D on serum lipids. Progress in Lipid Research 50: 303–312.
48. Ford ES, Giles WH, Dietz WH (2002) Prevalence of the metabolic syndrome among US adults: Findings from the Third National Health and Nutrition Examination Survey. Journal of the American Medical Association 287: 356–359.
49. Vacek JL, Vanga SR, Good M, Lai SM, Lakkireddy D, et al. (2012) Vitamin D Deficiency and Supplementation and Relation to Cardiovascular Health. The American Journal of Cardiology 109: 359–363.
50. Whiting S, Evans C, Foo L (2013) Recent systematic reviews indicate adults need (greater-than or equal to) 800 iu vitamin D to reduce risk of disease. Annals of Nutrition and Metabolism 63: 347.
51. Mitri J, Dawson-Hughes B, Hu FB, Pittas AG (2011) Effects of vitamin D and calcium supplementation on pancreatic beta cell function, insulin sensitivity, and glycemia in adults at high risk of diabetes: the Calcium and Vitamin D for Diabetes Mellitus (CaDDM) randomized controlled trial. Am J Clin Nutr 94: 486–494.
52. Talaei A, Mohamadi M, Adgi Z (2013) The effect of vitamin D on insulin resistance in patients with type 2 diabetes. Diabetol Metab Syndr 5: 8.
53. Tai K, Need AG, Horowitz M, Chapman IM (2008) Glucose tolerance and vitamin D: effects of treating vitamin D deficiency. Nutrition 24: 950–956.
54. Hollis BW, Wagner CL (2013) Clinical review: The role of the parent compound vitamin D with respect to metabolism and function: Why clinical dose intervals can affect clinical outcomes. J Clin Endocrinol Metab 98: 4619–4628.

55. Kalueff AV, Tuohimaa P (2007) Neurosteroid hormone vitamin D and its utility in clinical nutrition. Curr Opin Clin Nutr Metab Care 10: 12–19.
56. Ju SY, Lee YJ, Jeong SN (2013) Serum 25-hydroxyvitamin D levels and the risk of depression: a systematic review and meta-analysis. J Nutr Health Aging 17: 447–455.
57. May HT, Bair TL, Lappe DL, Anderson JL, Horne BD, et al. (2010) Association of vitamin D levels with incident depression among a general cardiovascular population. Am Heart J 159: 1037–1043.
58. Penckofer S, Kouba J, Byrn M, Estwing Ferrans C (2010) Vitamin D and depression: where is all the sunshine? Issues Ment Health Nurs 31: 385–393.
59. Shaffer JA, Edmondson D, Wasson LT, Falzon L, Homma K, et al. (2014) Vitamin D Supplementation for Depressive Symptoms: A Systematic Review and Meta-Analysis of Randomized Controlled Trials. Psychosom Med.
60. Sakalli H, Arslan D, Yucel AE (2012) The effect of oral and parenteral vitamin D supplementation in the elderly: a prospective, double-blinded, randomized, placebo-controlled study. Rheumatol Int 32: 2279–2283.
61. Lee HY, Chay WY, Tang MB, Chio MT, Tan SH (2012) Melanoma: differences between Asian and Caucasian patients. Ann Acad Med Singapore 41: 17–20.
62. Nurbazlin M, Chee WS, Rokiah P, Tan AT, Chew YY, et al. (2013) Effects of sun exposure on 25(OH) vitamin D concentration in urban and rural women in Malaysia. Asia Pac J Clin Nutr 22: 391–399.
63. Istiany A, Rahman SA, Kasim ZM, Swee WCS, Yassin Z, et al. (2012) Effect Of Nutrition Education And Sun Exposure On Vitamin D Status Among Postmenopausal Malay Women. International Journal of Science and Engineering Investigations 1: 91–97.
64. Yang Z, Laillou A, Smith G, Schofield D, Moench-Pfanner R (2013) A review of vitamin D fortification: implications for nutrition programming in Southeast Asia. Food Nutr Bull 34: S81–89.
65. Ministry of Health M (2011) National Health and Morbidity Survey (NHMS) 2011. 15th NIH Scientific Meeting incorporating NHMS 2011 and GATS conference, 2012. Holiday Villa, Subang Jaya, Selangor.
66. Heaney RP (2003) Long-latency deficiency disease: insights from calcium and vitamin D. Am J Clin Nutr 78: 912–919.

Effect of Cholecalciferol Supplementation on Inflammation and Cellular Alloimmunity in Hemodialysis Patients: Data from a Randomized Controlled Pilot Trial

Lily Li[1,2]❡, Marvin Lin[1,2]❡, Maria Krassilnikova[1,2], Katya Ostrow[1,2], Amanda Bader[1,2], Brian Radbill[1,2], Jaime Uribarri[1,2], Joji Tokita[1,2], Staci Leisman[1,2], Vijay Lapsia[1,2], Randy A. Albrecht[5,6], Adolfo García-Sastre[2,5,6], Andrea D. Branch[2,7], Peter S. Heeger[1,2,3,4]¶, Anita Mehrotra[1,2]*¶

1 Division of Nephrology, Icahn School of Medicine at Mount Sinai, New York, New York, United States of America, **2** Department of Medicine, Icahn School of Medicine at Mount Sinai, New York, New York, United States of America, **3** Recanati Miller Transplantation Institute, Icahn School of Medicine at Mount Sinai, New York, New York, United States of America, **4** Immunology Institute, Icahn School of Medicine at Mount Sinai, New York, New York, United States of America, **5** Department of Microbiology, Icahn School of Medicine at Mount Sinai, New York, New York, United States of America, **6** Global Health and Emerging Pathogens Institute, Icahn School of Medicine at Mount Sinai, New York, New York, United States of America, **7** Division of Liver Diseases, Icahn School of Medicine at Mount Sinai, New York, New York, United States of America

Abstract

Background: Memory T-cells are mediators of transplant injury, and no therapy is known to prevent the development of cross-reactive memory alloimmunity. Activated vitamin D is immunomodulatory, and vitamin D deficiency, common in hemodialysis patients awaiting transplantation, is associated with a heightened alloimmune response. Thus, we tested the hypothesis that vitamin D_3 supplementation would prevent alloreactive T-cell memory formation in vitamin D-deficient hemodialysis patients.

Methods and Findings: We performed a 12-month single-center pilot randomized, controlled trial of 50,000 IU/week of cholecalciferol (D_3) versus no supplementation in 96 hemodialysis patients with serum 25(OH)D<25 ng/mL, measuring effects on serum 25(OH)D and phenotypic and functional properties of T-cells. Participants were randomized 2:1 to active treatment versus control. D_3 supplementation increased serum 25(OH)D at 6 weeks (13.5 [11.2] ng/mL to 42.5 [18.5] ng/mL, $p<0.001$) and for the duration of the study. No episodes of sustained hypercalcemia occurred in either group. Results of IFNγ ELISPOT-based panel of reactive T-cell assays (PRT), quantifying alloreactive memory, demonstrated greater increases in the controls over 1 year compared to the treatment group (delta PRT in treatment 104.8+/−330.8 vs 252.9+/−431.3 in control), but these changes in PRT between groups did not reach statistical significance ($p=0.25$).

Conclusions: D_3 supplements are safe, effective at treating vitamin D deficiency, and may prevent time-dependent increases in T-cell alloimmunity in hemodialysis patients, but their effects on alloimmunity need to be confirmed in larger studies. These findings support the routine supplementation of vitamin D-deficient transplant candidates on hemodialysis and highlight the need for large-scale prospective studies of vitamin D supplementation in transplant candidates and recipients.

Trial Registration: Clinicaltrials.gov NCT01175798

Editor: Kathrin Eller, Medical University of Graz, Austria

Funding: This work was supported by grants from the Doris Duke Charitable Foundation (LL), National Kidney Foundation (PSH), American Heart Association (AM), and National Institute of Health: DK090317, DA0301095 (ADB), U01AI063594 (PSH), U19AI089987 (AG-S, RA), and UL1TR000067 from the National Center for Advancing Translational Sciences. The funders had no role in study design, data collection and analysis, decision to publish, or preparation of the manuscript.

Competing Interests: The authors have declared that no competing interests exist.

* Email: anita.mehrotra@mssm.edu

❡ These authors contributed equally to this work.

¶ These authors are co-senior authors on this work.

Introduction

Alloreactive memory T-cells are pathogenic mediators of transplant injury. They are among the first cells to injure vascularized allografts in animal models [1], prevent tolerance induction in mice [2], and are associated with inferior transplant outcomes both in non-human primates and in human kidney transplant recipients [3–6].

Memory T-cells can be induced by direct exposure to alloantigens through transplantation, pregnancy, or blood transfusion. Evidence also indicates that heterologous (cross-reactive) immune responses initiated by environmental pathogens and homeostatic proliferation can facilitate the induction and expansion of alloreactive memory T-cells [7,8]. Interventions to reduce graft injury caused by T-cell memory are not yet available.

The biologically active form of vitamin D, 1,25-dihydroxyvitamin D [1,25(OH)$_2$D] has immune-modulatory properties. T-cells and dendritic cells (DCs), express the vitamin D receptor (VDR) and the 1α-hydroxylase needed to convert 25-hydroxyvitamin D [25(OH)D] to 1,25(OH)$_2$D [9]. 1,25(OH)$_2$D can directly modulate the function of T-cells and DCs through a variety of mechanisms [10–13], and can enhance tolerance induction in mice [14]. Importantly, many of the immune effects of vitamin D require local, immune cell production of 1,25(OH)$_2$D from its immediate precursor, 25(OH)D, which circulates in blood [9,15,16].

Vitamin D deficiency is widespread among the general population [17], and is prevalent in patients with end-stage renal disease (ESRD) on hemodialysis (HD). The concentration of 25(OH)D is the main clinical indicator of vitamin D status and is used to define vitamin D deficiency. According to the Institute of Medicine (IOM), there is an elevation in the risk of experiencing adverse health consequences of vitamin D deficiency at 25(OH)D levels <20 ng/mL [18]. Over 80% of HD patients have serum 25(OH)D concentrations within the insufficient/deficient range despite ongoing treatment with activated vitamin D [1,25(OH)$_2$D] for prevention of uremic bone disease [19,20]. While there have been uncontrolled studies of nutritional vitamin D (D$_2$ or D$_3$) supplementation in HD patients and one short-term (3 week) randomized, controlled trial of D$_3$ supplementation [20–23], the safety, efficacy, and *immunological* impact of nutritional vitamin D repletion in HD patients, particularly in patients already receiving 1,25(OH)$_2$D, has not been tested in controlled studies.

Observational studies of kidney transplant recipients show an association between 25(OH)D deficiency and inferior graft outcomes [24,25]. Our previously published data show a strong correlation between 25(OH)D deficiency and elevated memory T-cell alloimmunity in dialysis patients, many of whom are on the transplant waiting list, independent of known sensitizing events [19]. We hypothesized that inadequate concentrations of 25(OH)D contribute to the development of alloreactive memory T-cells by reducing the local synthesis of the 1,25(OH)$_2$D that is needed to achieve optimal levels in immune cells. To test this hypothesis and to obtain preliminary data for power calculations for a larger multi-center study, we performed a pilot, single-center, randomized, controlled trial (RCT) of oral cholecalciferol (D$_3$) (versus no supplementation) to assess the impact of increased 25(OH)D on memory T-cell alloimmunity, in patients already receiving 1,25(OH)$_2$D as clinically indicated. Our data indicate that D$_3$ supplementation is safe and effective at correcting vitamin D deficiency in this setting, and may prevent the time-dependent increase of peripheral cellular alloimmunity that occurs in many dialysis patients, establishing a strong rationale for conducting a larger, multi-center RCT to confirm these findings.

Methods

Clinical Trial Design

The protocol for this trial, sample case report form, and supporting CONSORT checklist are available as supporting information; see Protocol S1, Sample Case Report Form S1, and CONSORT Checklist S1. We recruited adults (≥18 years) on hemodialysis for ≥2 months at the Icahn School of Medicine at Mount Sinai (ISMMS) and Terrence Cardinal Cooke outpatient dialysis units in New York City from August 2010 to October 2011, excluding patients with a history of acute renal failure with potential for recovery, a history of HIV/AIDS, or inability to provide informed consent. All participants gave written informed consent, and the study was conducted according to the principles expressed in the Declaration of Helsinki. The study was approved by the Icahn School of Medicine at Mount Sinai (ISMMS) Institutional Review Board (IRB #09-2275) and registered at clinicaltrials.gov (NCT01175798).

Peripheral blood was obtained during the hemodialysis procedure. All study subjects were being dialyzed using biocompatible dialysis membranes. Serum 25(OH)D concentrations were determined commercially in a CLIA-certified laboratory (Nationwide Laboratories, Ft. Lauderdale, FL) by the chemiluminescent Diasorin method (www.diasorin.com, Stillwater, MN). Subjects with serum 25(OH)D<25 ng/mL were eligible for randomization. This cut-off for randomization was pre-determined based on previous data showing the distribution of vitamin D concentrations in the population [19].

The study was an open-label pilot RCT of nutritional Vitamin D- therapy (D$_3$: cholecalciferol, purchased from BioTech Pharmacal, Inc: http://www.biotechpharmacal.com/). Participants were randomized in a 2:1 ratio using Random Allocation Software (Version 1.0.0) [26] into one of two groups: oral cholecalciferol or no treatment (currently the standard of care at the dialysis units, as routine screening for and treatment of 25(OH)D deficiency are not part of practice guidelines for this population). Randomization was stratified by baseline 25(OH)D (10–24 ng/mL and <10 ng/mL). Within each stratum, randomization occurred in permuted 12-subject blocks. Implementation of randomization was performed by a study investigator.

Those participants randomized to D$_3$ had a target 25(OH)D concentration of >35 ng/ml. The initial dose of D$_3$ was 50,000/week for 6 weeks, at which time 25(OH)D was re-measured. Subjects whose 25(OH)D remained ≤35 ng/ml continued on 50,000 IU weekly for another 6 weeks, at which point 25(OH)D concentrations were repeated. Those subjects who achieved 25(OH)D concentrations >35 ng/ml were transitioned to 10,000 IU/week. D$_3$ therapy was directly observed by a study coordinator or investigator. 25(OH)D was measured at baseline, 6 weeks, 3 months, and 6 months following randomization in both treatment and control groups, and other clinical information (routine labs, medication dosage) was collected at the same time-points.

The primary outcome was change in 25(OH)D at 6 weeks, 3 months, and 6 months. Secondary outcomes included change in clinical laboratory values (intact parathyroid hormone [PTH], serum calcium, and phosphorus), activated vitamin D requirements (mcg/treatment), and laboratory-based phenotypic and functional T-cell assays.

All study subjects continued to receive routine care at their hemodialysis unit including monthly laboratory testing of calcium, phosphorus, and intact parathyroid hormone. Dosing of hemodialysis-related intravenous medications (activated vitamin D analog) continued as per pre-specified, standardized protocols in the hemodialysis units. Nursing staff adjusting hemodialysis-related intravenous medications were blinded to treatment assignment. Study subjects undergoing kidney transplantation during the study period were not included in the final analysis (Figure 1).

Laboratory Procedures

Peripheral blood was collected during the hemodialysis procedure into BD Vacutainer tubes (BD, Franklin Lakes, NJ)

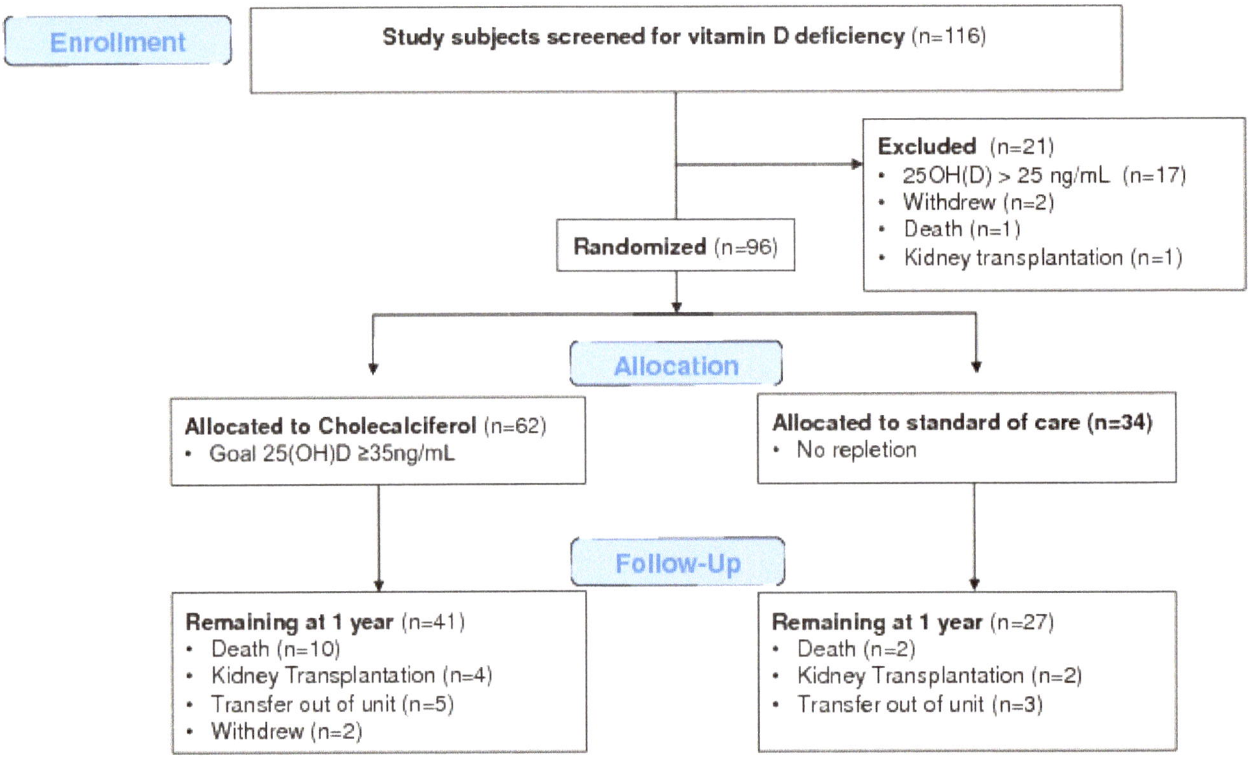

Figure 1. Study flow diagram. A total of 116 hemodialysis patients were screened, and 96 were randomized in a 2:1 ratio to receive oral cholecalciferol (n = 62) or no repletion (n = 34). There were no differences in dropout rates from transplantation (6.6% vs 5.9% at 1 year, p = .90) or death (16.4% vs 5.9% at 1 year, p = .14) between groups. A total of 68 subjects completed follow-up to 1 year. Of those 68 subjects, 51 (34 in the treatment group and 17 in the control group) had sufficient PBMC samples meeting predetermined quality-assurance criteria for immunologic assessment.

containing sodium heparin for plasma or no additive for serum. PBMCs were isolated by Ficoll gradient centrifugation, cryopreserved at a concentration of 10^7 cells/mL, and placed in a −80°C freezer for ≥24 hours prior to transfer to liquid nitrogen for long-term storage for ELISPOT assays. Serum separator tubes were left for one hour at room temperature before centrifugation at 1500 rpm for 15 minutes at 20°C, and serum was immediately divided into 0.5 mL aliquots and stored at −80°C until analysis.

10^6 PBMCs were treated overnight with Streck Cell Preservative (Streck, Omaha, Nebraska) and stained with fluorochrome-labeled antibodies the following day as per the manufacturers' recommendations for each antibody. Antibodies used for differentiation of T-cell subsets included: anti-CD4-FITC, anti-CD25-APC, anti-CD8-PE, anti-CD45RA-APC, anti-CD45RO-FITC (BD, Franklin Lakes, NJ), anti-CD4-PE-Cy7 and anti-Foxp3-PE (eBioscience, San Diego, CA). Stained cells were analyzed on a

Table 1. Baseline patient characteristics.

Characteristic	Treatment (n = 62)	Control (n = 34)	p-value
Baseline 25(OH)D, ng/mL (median, [IQR])	13.4 [9.3, 19.7]	13.1 [9.9, 18.6]	0.97
Age, years	60.2 [14.3]	58.9 [14.9]	0.66
Gender: Female	26 (41.9)	14 (41.2)	0.94
Race: Black	42 (67.7)	17 (50)	0.09
Dialysis Vintage, years (median, [IQR])	4.0 [1.3,8.0]	3.5 [1.2,7.9]	0.86
Diabetes	26 (41.9)	15 (44.1)	0.84
Current or Former Smoker	25 (40.3)	15 (44.1)	0.71
Dialysis Access: Catheter	12 (19.4)	8 (23.5)	0.45
Prior transplant	13 (21.0)	7 (20.6)	0.97
Prior blood transfusion	30 (48.4)	21 (61.8)	0.14
Prior pregnancy	20 (32.3)	13 (38.2)	0.31

Mean [SD] or count (%) unless otherwise specified.

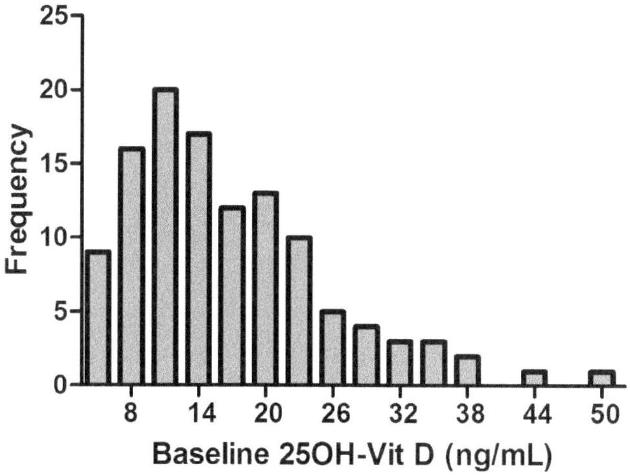

Figure 2. Baseline serum 25(OH)D concentrations in the study cohort. Distribution of serum 25(OH)D in the entire study cohort (n = 116) is shown. Median (IQR) 25(OH)D was 14.7 (10.5–21.6) ng/mL. 17 subjects with a baseline vitamin D level >25 ng/mL were excluded from randomization.

FACS Canto II flow cytometry (BD Bioscience, San Jose, CA, see Foxp3stainingeBioscience S1) and comparative results processed using FlowJo software (Tree Star, Inc, Ashland, OR).

IFNγ ELISPOT PRT assays were performed as previously described [5,19,27]. A total of 3×10^5 live responder cells were incubated with 1×10^5 of each allogeneic B cell line in duplicate or triplicate for 24 hours. Phytohemagglutinin (0.02 mg/mL) was used as a positive control. ELISPOT assays were developed according to standard operating protocol and spots quantified using an automated Immunospot Reader and CTL Immunospot Software (Cellular Technology Limited, Shaker Heights, OH). Mean numbers of IFNγ ELISPOTS from control wells (responder cells plus media only, typically <10 spots per well) were subtracted from the total number of spots in stimulated wells. Results are reported as the sum of the mean responses to each set of six stimulators [19].

Plasma anti-HLA antibody was assessed using HLA class I and class II antigen-coated microbeads (LABScreen Mixed, One Lambda Inc., Canoga Park, CA) and a flow analyzer (BioPlex 200 System with HTF, Bio-Rad, Hercules, CA) as previously described [28]. Determination of cut-off for reactivity was based on calculations as per the manufacturer's software. A new reactivity was defined by an MFI <1000 at baseline that increased to ≥5000 at one year. Results were analyzed using HLA fusion software (One Lambda Inc., Canoga Park, CA).

Statistical Analysis

Although the primary outcome was change in 25(OH)D concentrations, we attempted to power the study to detect differences in PRT results within groups over time, based on a standard deviation of 375 spots from our previous work [19], so as to provide estimates for power calculations for a larger, multi-center study. 30 subjects per group would provide 80% power to detect a difference of 200 spots in the PRT assay over time (alpha = 0.05). 30 study subjects per group would also provide 80% power to detect a difference in 25(OH)D levels *between* groups of 11 ng/mL at the 1 year time-point, based on a conservative estimate of the standard deviation of 15 ng/mL. Because we were unsure of how patients would respond to D_3 supplementation, randomization was performed in a 2:1 ratio to ensure an adequate number of patients had an increase in 25(OH)D levels over time, leading us to target an enrollment of 60 patients in the intervention group and 30 patients in the control group.

Statistical analysis was performed using SPSS version 20.0 (Chicago, IL) and GraphPad Prism 5 (GraphPad Software, Inc., La Jolla, CA). All analysis was performed on a per-protocol basis. There was no group cross-over, but, only patients reaching the 1-year time point were included in the 1-year data analysis in order to minimize the effect of missing data from patients lost to follow-up in the interim. Data are reported as medians and interquartile ranges or means and standard deviations for continuous variables, as appropriate, and as percentages of total for categorical variables. Baseline characteristics of the groups were compared using parametric (student's t-test) or non-parametric (Mann-Whitney) tests for continuous variables, as appropriate, and Chi-square or Fisher's exact tests for categorical variables, as appropriate. Changes over time were compared between groups using parametric (t-test) or non-parametric (Wilcoxon signed-rank test) tests, as appropriate. A two-tailed p-value<0.05 was considered statistically significant.

Results

Oral D_3 supplementation is safe and effective

Of 116 chronic hemodialysis patients screened, 99 (85.3%) had 25(OH)D concentrations <25 ng/mL and qualified for randomization (**Figure 1**). The median (IQR) 25(OH)D concentration of the 116 patients (**Figure 2**) was 14.7 (10.5–21.6) ng/mL. 25(OH)D concentration was independent of month (time of year)

Table 2. Laboratory parameters of bone and mineral metabolism and activated Vitamin D requirements.

	Treatment		Control		P-value*
	Baseline	12 Months	Baseline	12 Months	
25OH-D,** ng/mL (median, [IQR])	13.5 [9.8, 20.9]	40.9 [32.2, 45.5]	13.0 [10.9, 20.4]	15.8 [9.5, 19.5]	<0.001
PTH, pg/mL	465.0 (360.5)	555.9 (436.6)	434.3 (380.7)	637.4 (645.5)	0.35
Calcium, mg/dL	9.2 (0.6)	9.0 (0.7)	8.8 (1.0)	9.0 (1.0)	0.09
Phosphorus, mg/dL	5.8 (1.2)	5.3 (1.4)	5.4 (1.8)	5.1 (1.4)	0.95
Activated Vitamin D dose, mcg/treatment (median, [IQR])	4.0 [0, 9.1]	4.0 [2.5, 5.0]	3.5 [0, 5.6]	5.0 [2.3, 7.5]	0.22

Mean (SD) unless otherwise specified.
*p-values for comparison of change from baseline to 12 months between groups (treatment vs control).
**n = 41 in treatment group and 27 in control group.

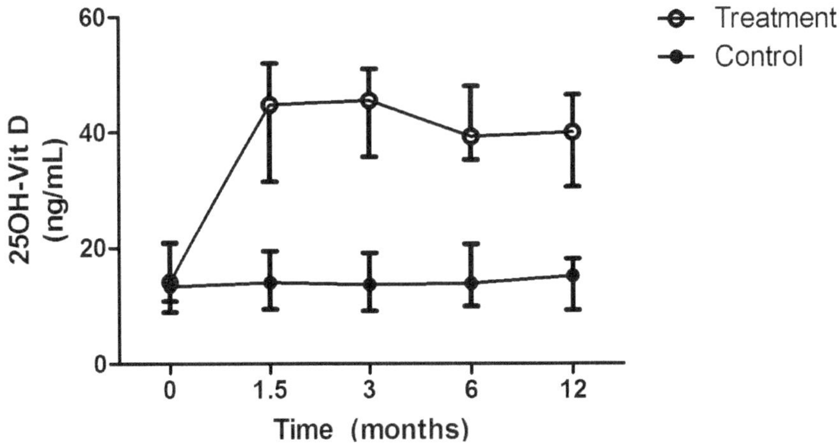

Figure 3. Effects of Vitamin D supplementation on serum 25(OH)D concentrations. Values increased by six weeks in the treatment group (13.5 [11.2] ng/mL to 42.5 [18.5] ng/mL, p<0.001), but remained low in the control group throughout the study duration. Median (IQR) are displayed on the graph.

of testing (data not shown). Reflecting the 2:1 enrollment design, 62/99 (62.6%) were randomized to treatment with cholecalciferol (D_3), and 34/99 (34.3%) were randomized to standard of care (control, no treatment); two patients withdrew, and one patient died prior to randomization (**Figure 1**). As randomization was stratified by baseline 25(OH)D concentration (10–24 ng/mL and<10 ng/mL), there were similar numbers of study subjects with baseline 25(OH)D<10 ng/mL in both groups (27.4% in the D_3 group and 23.5% in the control group, p = 0.68). Demographics of the randomized patients (**Table 1**) showed no differences between treatment and control groups in baseline 25(OH)D, age, gender, race, dialysis vintage, history of diabetes, smoking status, and dialysis access (catheter vs. arteriovenous fistula/arteriovenous graft). The majority (61.5%) of randomized patients were of self-reported African ancestry.

Therapy with oral D_3 resulted in a significant rise in serum 25(OH)D by 6 weeks (**Figure 3**), which was sustained throughout the 12 months of study. Serum 25(OH)D in the control group did not change (**Figure 3**). We did not observe any adverse events attributable to D_3 supplementation (see AdverseEventsTable S1). There were no differences in dropout rates from transplantation (6.6% vs 5.9% at 1 year, p = .90) or death (16.4% vs 5.9% at 1 year, p = .14) between groups (**Figure 1**), and importantly, the overall mortality of 11.6% at 1 year was not higher than expected for the general dialysis population based on previous reports (approximately 20%) [29]. Serum calcium, phosphorus, intact PTH, and activated vitamin D requirements (paricalcitol) were similar in the control and intervention arms through the trial (**Table 2**), and no episodes of sustained hypercalcemia occurred in either group during the study (**Table 2**, see RawData S1).

Effect of D_3 supplementation on T-cell phenotype

We used flow cytometry to analyze and quantify PBMCs collected at baseline and 1 year. Gating strategies are shown in **Figure 4** and the data are summarized in **Table 3 and Table 4**. Of 96 subjects randomized, 51 patients (34 in the treatment group and 17 in the control group) were available for 12 month follow-up, had sufficient PBMC, and were included in this analysis. None of the study subjects included in this analysis received packed red blood cell (PRBC) transfusions during the study period. At baseline, the median 25(OH)D concentration for these 51 patients was 14.1 ng/mL (IQR: 10.9–21.0 ng/mL), a value that did not differ from the parent cohort (14.7 ng/mL, IQR: 10.5–21.6 ng/mL). The baseline demographics of these subjects did not differ from those of the parent cohort (p>0.05 for each), supporting random and equal loss from the treatment and control groups, without evidence of bias.

Table 3. Effects of Vitamin D supplementation on T cell phenotypes†.

	Oral D_3 (n = 34)		**Control (n = 17)**	
	Baseline	**1 Year**	**Baseline**	**1 Year**
CD4%	37.0 [29.0,45.4]	40.6 [29.9,47.1]	34.5 [22.3,39.5]	35.7 [27.8,40.6]
Naïve CD45RA+	33.6 [20.4,44.5]	32.9 [16.8,44.8]	31.3 [19.4,49.7]	34.7 [17.3,50.1]
Memory CD45RO+	52.7 [41.0,64.9]	50.6 [39.0,66.3]	61.9 [39.9,70.4]	49.2 [41.4,72.5]
Foxp3+CD25+	7.9 [5.9,9.3]	5.9 [2.8,9.0]	7.8 [4.6,10.9]	3.9 [1.4,7.6]
CD8%	17.1 [12.8,25.8]	14.0 [9.8,22.9]	17.7 [11.6,22.8]	15.8 [13.0,18.6]
Naïve CD45RA+	64.5 [55.8,80.0]	67.7 [52.3,77.0]	68.8 [51.5,79.5]	65.8 [47.6,79.9]
Memory CD45RO+	14.6 [7.1,19.3]	14.2 [8.0,21.7]	14.6 [8.8,26.7]	20.0 [9.0,27.9]

Values are expressed as median [IQR].
†no statistically significant differences in baseline, 1 year, or change from baseline to 1 year between groups.

Table 4. Effects of Vitamin D supplementation on monocyte subsets†.

	Oral D_3 (n = 34)		Control (n = 17)	
	Baseline	**1 Year**	**Baseline**	**1 Year**
Total % Monocytes (CD19−/HLA-DR+)	6.4 [3.7,11.8]	6.2 [3.6,8.6]	5.5 [3.1,9.7]	5.9 [5.5,8.7]
Classical CD14++/CD16– % of monocytes	67.2 [53.4,78.5]	66.8 [57.2,78.2]	72.0 [64.2,79.5]	67.8 [52.5,73.4]
Nonclassical CD14lo/CD16+ % of monocytes	9.0 [4.8,16.4]	10.6 [6.6,16.7]	9.5 [6.4,13.8]	10.3 [5.3,16.4]
CCR2−/M-DC8−	2.5 [0.6,4.3]	2.1 [1.0,3.6]	1.5 [0.6,2.9]	2.0 [1.7,5.1]
CCR2−/MDC-8+	1.8 [0.6,4.5]	0.9 [0.5,1.8]	1.2 [0.5,3.3]	1.3 [0.6,2.9]

†no statistically significant differences in baseline, 1 year, or change from baseline to 1 year between groups.

We examined the percentages of CD4 and CD8 T-cells including their naïve (CD45RA+/CD45RO^{neg}) and memory (CD45RA^{neg}/CD45RO+) subsets and quantified CD4+Foxp3+ T-cells. These analyses showed no differences in memory or naïve CD4 or CD8 cell subsets between the groups at baseline and at 1 year (**Table 3**). The percentages of CD4+Foxp3+ T-cells were lower in both groups at 1 year versus baseline, but the values did not differ between groups at either time point (**Table 3**).

D_3 supplementation may prevent time-dependent increases in cellular alloimmunity

We used an IFNγ ELISPOT-based panel of reactive T-cell (PRT) assay to quantify the frequencies of alloreactive memory T-

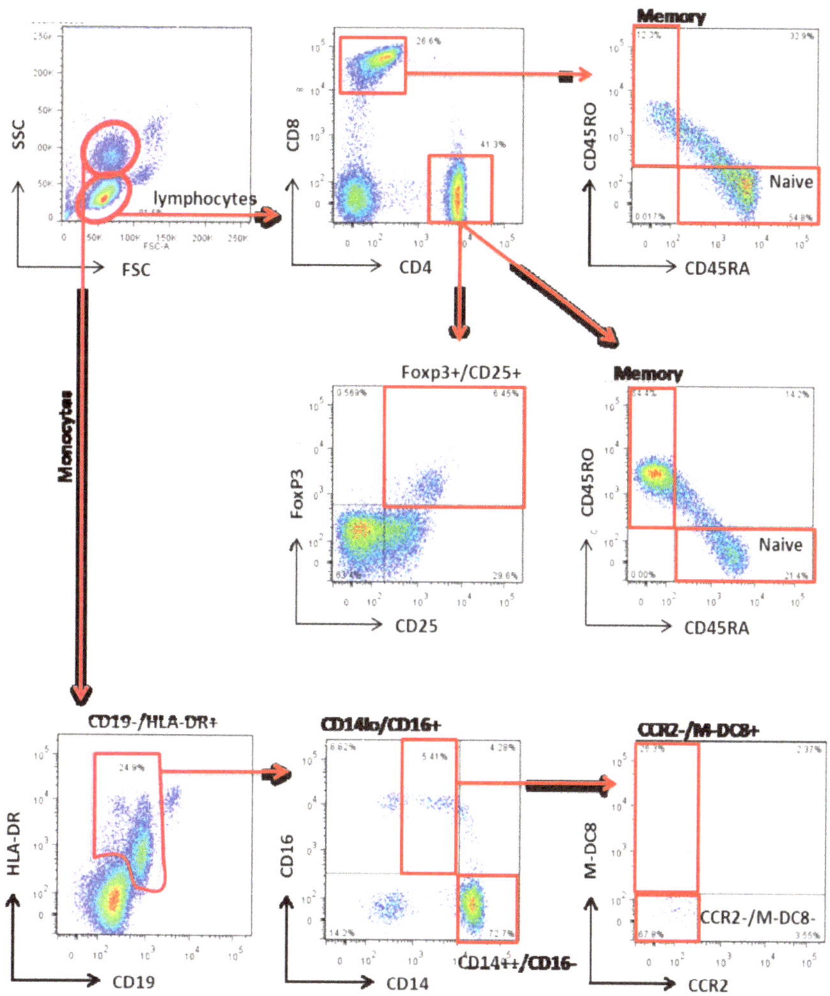

Figure 4. Gating strategy for enumeration of T cell and monocyte subsets. CD4 and CD8 memory (CD45RO+/CD45RA^{neg}) and naïve (CD45RO^{neg}/CD45RA+) T cells, and the Foxp3+/CD25+/CD4+ population containing regulatory cells were evaluated. Monocytes were identified by a CD19^{neg}/HLA-DR+ phenotype, and further characterized into the CD14++/CD16^{neg} classical subset, and the CD14^{lo}/CD16+ non-classical M-DC8+ and M-DC8^{neg} subsets.

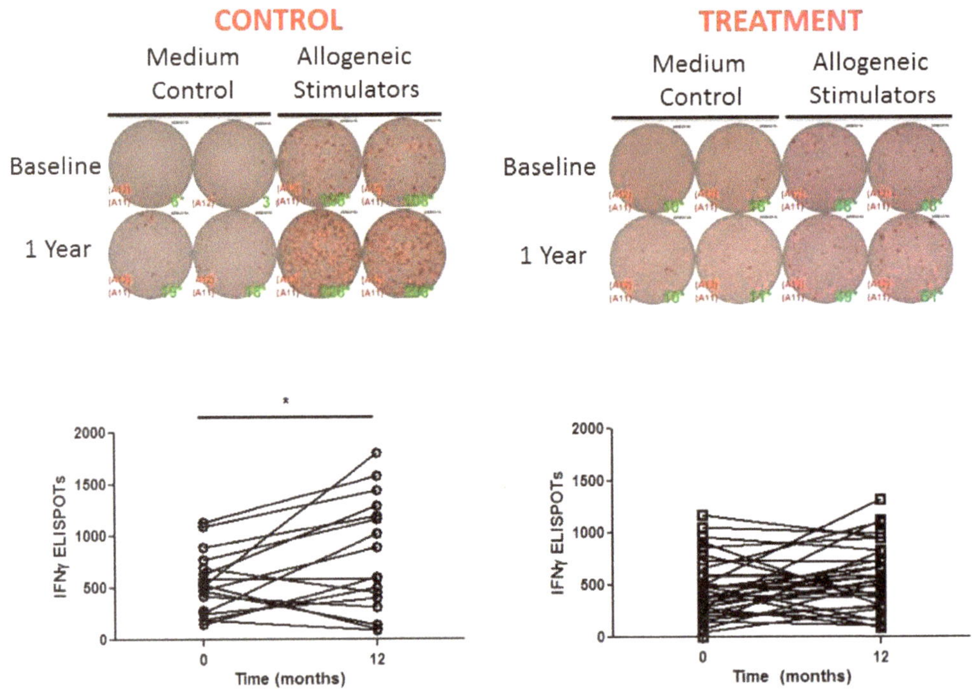

Figure 5. Vitamin D supplementation may prevent the time-dependent increase in PRT. (A) Representative ELISPOT PRT wells in duplicate at baseline and one year with no stimulation (media control) or response to allogeneic B cells. (B) Quantified results reveal a significant increase in the number of IFNγ ELISPOTs over time in the control group (517.4+/−280.8 to 797.8+/−542.3 spots, $p=0.03$), but the comparison of "delta" PRT (1 year - baseline) in the treatment vs control group did not reach statistical significance (104.8+/−330.8 in treatment vs 252.9+/−431.3 in control, $p=0.25$).

cells in each patient. In this assay, PBMC are stimulated with a panel of HLA-typed allogeneic B cell lines inducing alloreactive memory, but not naïve, T-cells to produce IFNγ [3]. Our previously published work showed that the summed responses to a randomly selected panel of 6 primary B cell lines is sufficient to provide reproducible and interpretable information [19], and that subjects with the highest PRT results were at an elevated risk for developing post-transplant acute rejection and inferior one year kidney function [5].

The PRT results were similar in the active treatment and control groups at baseline (450.9+/−301.2 vs 517.4+/−280.8 spots, $p=0.41$) (**Figure 5**). Whereas the PRT did not change over 1 year study in the patients treated with oral D_3, the PRT increased significantly in the controls (517.4+/−280.8 to 797.8+/−542.3 spots, $p=0.03$) (**Figure 5**). However, when comparing the "delta" PRT (1 year – baseline) in the treatment vs control group, this comparison did not reach statistical significance (delta PRT in treatment 104.8+/−330.8 vs 252.9+/−431.3 in control, $p=0.25$). D_3 supplementation did not alter the development of new alloantibodies (**Figure 6**).

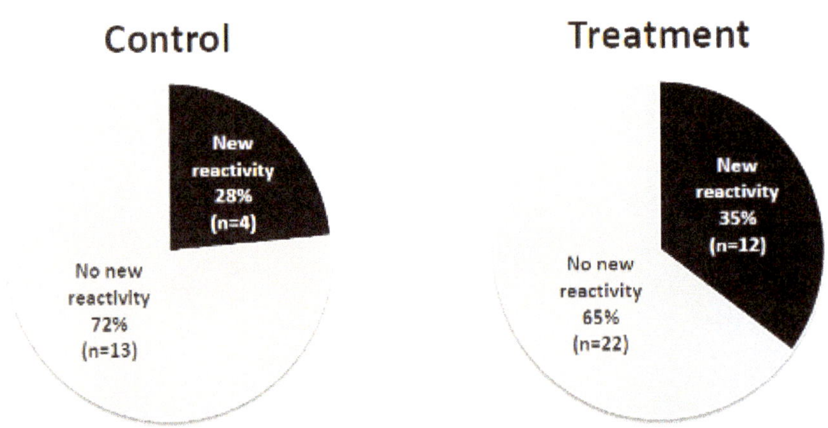

Figure 6. Vitamin D supplementation does not alter anti-HLA antibodies. Pie charts depicting the percentages of patients in each group that developed new anti-HLA antibodies between entry and 1 year ($p=0.393$). A new reactivity was defined as having a MFI <1000 at baseline and >5000 at one year using the LuminexPRA assay.

Effect of D_3 supplementation on peripheral pro-inflammatory monocytes

Peripheral blood monocytes are a heterogenous population of mononuclear cells capable of modulating inflammation and activating T cells, regulating expression of MHC, co-stimulatory molecules, and cytokines. Previous work by others showed that "non-classical" $CD14^{lo}/CD16+$ monocytes produce higher amounts of pro-inflammatory cytokines and express more cell surface HLA-DR than their classical CD14++/$CD16^{neg}$ monocyte counterparts [30]. We did not observe differences in either of these monocyte subsets, either between groups at baseline and 1 year, or between groups over time (**Table 4**).

The $CD14^{lo}/CD16+$ non-classical monocyte population is comprised of two subgroups: M-DC8+ and M-$DC8^{neg}$ cells. The M-DC8+ subset has been shown to express two-fold more HLA class I and II molecules, to produce higher amounts of IL-12, and to induce more potent Th1 immune responses for the priming of cord blood T cells versus the M-DC8- population [31]. While there appeared to be a time-dependent, 50% decrease in M-DC8+ monocytes in the treatment group (**Table 4**), this change over time was not statistically significantly different from changes in the control group over time.

Discussion

In this pilot RCT of D_3 supplementation in vitamin D-deficient hemodialysis (HD) patients, we demonstrate safety and efficacy of D_3 in the setting of concurrent therapy with activated vitamin D analogs. Subjects randomized to D_3 therapy did not experience sustained hypercalcemia or other adverse events. While our study was not powered to examine mortality, the overall mortality of the cohort did not exceed that of the dialysis population in general [29] and published data show a survival benefit from vitamin D supplementation in other populations [32].

We newly show that D_3 supplementation may inhibit the expansion of alloreactive T-cell memory over 1 year on dialysis. Although the comparison of "delta" PRT (1 year – baseline) in the treatment vs control group did not reach statistical significance, (delta PRT in treatment group: 104.8+/−330.8 vs 252.9+/−431.3 in control group, $p = 0.25$), this pilot study provides important data on standard deviation and effect size that can be used to design and power a larger clinical trial. If confirmed in a larger RCT, this would be the first demonstration of a potentially clinically relevant effect of nutritional vitamin D supplementation (D_3) that could impact standard of practice. These data expand upon our prior cross-sectional observations [19] and suggest that vitamin D supplements may prevent the induction of environmentally driven, heterologous (cross-reactive) cellular alloimmunity. The results support the therapeutic use of nutritional vitamin D (D_2 or D_3) in all hemodialysis patients, especially those on the transplant waiting list who may benefit from vitamin D's inhibitory effects on alloimmunity. We demonstrated potential effects of D_3 supplementation on cellular alloresponses in just one year; as most HD patients on the deceased-donor waiting list wait from 2–7 years for a transplant, and the risk for developing cross-reactive anti-donor T-cell immunity increases with longer HD vintage [33], the impact of vitamin D deficiency on heterologous immunity over time may be even greater, and needs to be evaluated in larger prospective multi-center longitudinal studies.

Our findings are consistent with emerging evidence in the literature that deficiency of 25(OH)D (despite exogenous $1,25(OH)_2D$ therapy) reduces local immune cell production of active vitamin D, and thereby promotes inflammation [16,34]. While hemodialysis patients are commonly treated with $1,25(OH)_2D$ analogs for the prevention of renal osteodystrophy, there are currently no recommendations for the regular surveillance or repletion of the precursor, 25(OH)D, and the prevalence of vitamin D deficiency in this population is high [20]. Vitamin D has been reported to inhibit dendritic cell (DC) differentiation and maturation and impair DC antigen presentation to attenuate the alloreactive T-cell response [10,11]. Consistent with these observations, we noted fewer proinflammatory monocytes in the treatment arm over time (**Table 4**), suggestive of an inhibitory effect on APCs, but the difference in this change between treatment and control groups was not statistically significant. Vitamin D has also been reported to promote Th2 immunity while limiting Th1 responses and to inhibit antigen-induced T-cell activation [12,13], which could prevent induction of cross-reactive alloimmunity. We acknowledge that results from this limited RCT do not reveal the mechanisms that underlie our findings; however, they suggest that vitamin D supplementation impacts alloreactive memory formation through a process that is likely to involve local production of $1,25(OH)_2D$ and provide a foundation for future detailed mechanistic studies by our group and others.

Observational studies in the kidney transplant population show an association between 25(OH)D deficiency and inferior graft outcomes [24,25,35]. In addition, a functional polymorphism in the vitamin D receptor (VDR) (*FokI*, rs10735810) leading to increased transcriptional activity has been shown to correlate with improved renal allograft survival [36]. Results of our immunological studies are consistent with these clinical observations, and highlight the need for prospective trials of vitamin D therapy in kidney transplant candidates and recipients with a focus on graft and patient outcomes, possibly stratifying by polymorphisms in the VDR and other genes involved in vitamin D metabolism and function.

Significant limitations of our study include the un-blinded nature and lack of a placebo control, thus introducing the possibility of study subject and investigator bias. However, all laboratory-based assays were performed by technicians unaware of study subject treatment assignment in an effort to minimize investigator bias. Because patients were aware of group assignment, we cannot exclude the possibility that some patients assigned to the control group obtained vitamin D supplements elsewhere. However, as 25(OH)D concentrations remained stable over time in the control group, it is unlikely that these patients were taking clinically significant doses of any vitamin D supplements.

In conclusion, the results of this pilot RCT show that nutritional vitamin D (D_3) supplementation is safe and effective in vitamin D-deficient HD patients concurrently treated with $1,25(OH)_2D$, and may prevent time-dependent increases in memory T-cell alloreactivity. Because memory T-cell alloreactivity pre-transplantation negatively affects post-transplant outcomes, and because vitamin D deficiency is associated with higher rates of acute rejection in kidney transplant recipients [35], treatment with vitamin D has the potential to improve kidney transplant outcomes and needs to be evaluated prospectively in transplant candidates/recipients. Given the apparent safety and low cost of vitamin D supplements, routine screening and correction of 25(OH)D deficiency should be considered in all dialysis units, with monitoring and reporting of the risks and benefits observed in a larger population.

Supporting Information

Adverse Events Table S1 Tabular view of adverse events.

CONSORT Checklist S1 Completed CONSORT checklist for randomized controlled trials referencing the manuscript.

Foxp3stainingeBioscience S1 Instructions for Foxp3 intracellular staining.

Protocol S1 IRB-approved study protocol detailing all study-related procedures.

Raw Data S1 Excel spreadsheet of raw data from the study.

Sample Case Report Form S1 Sample case report form from the trial used for data collection.

Acknowledgments

The authors thank the physicians, staff, and patients at the Mount Sinai 94th Street and Terrence Cardinal Cooke hemodialysis units in New York City for their participation in this study.

Author Contributions

Conceived and designed the experiments: AM PSH. Performed the experiments: LL ML MK KO AB. Analyzed the data: LL AM. Contributed reagents/materials/analysis tools: AG-S RA. Contributed to the writing of the manuscript: LL AM ADB JU PSH. Study subject recruitment: JT SL BR VL.

References

1. Schenk AD, Nozaki T, Rabant M, Valujskikh A, Fairchild RL (2008) Donor-reactive CD8 memory T cells infiltrate cardiac allografts within 24-h posttransplant in naive recipients. American journal of transplantation: official journal of the American Society of Transplantation and the American Society of Transplant Surgeons 8: 1652–1661.
2. Valujskikh A, Pantenburg B, Heeger PS (2002) Primed allospecific T cells prevent the effects of costimulatory blockade on prolonged cardiac allograft survival in mice. American journal of transplantation: official journal of the American Society of Transplantation and the American Society of Transplant Surgeons 2: 501–509.
3. Heeger PS, Greenspan NS, Kuhlenschmidt S, Dejelo C, Hricik DE, et al. (1999) Pretransplant frequency of donor-specific, IFN-gamma-producing lymphocytes is a manifestation of immunologic memory and correlates with the risk of posttransplant rejection episodes. Journal of immunology (Baltimore, Md: 1950) 163: 2267–2275.
4. Hricik DE, Rodriguez V, Riley J, Bryan K, Tary-Lehmann M, et al. (2003) Enzyme linked immunosorbent spot (ELISPOT) assay for interferon-gamma independently predicts renal function in kidney transplant recipients. American journal of transplantation: official journal of the American Society of Transplantation and the American Society of Transplant Surgeons 3: 878–884.
5. Poggio ED, Augustine JJ, Clemente M, Danzig JM, Volokh N, et al. (2007) Pretransplant cellular alloimmunity as assessed by a panel of reactive T cells assay correlates with acute renal graft rejection. Transplantation 83: 847–852.
6. Nadazdin O, Boskovic S, Murakami T, Tocco G, Smith R-N, et al. (2011) Host alloreactive memory T cells influence tolerance to kidney allografts in nonhuman primates. Science translational medicine 3.
7. Adams AB, Williams MA, Jones TR, Shirasugi N, Durham MM, et al. (2003) Heterologous immunity provides a potent barrier to transplantation tolerance. The Journal of clinical investigation 111: 1887–1895.
8. Wu Z, Bensinger SJ, Zhang J, Chen C, Yuan X, et al. (2004) Homeostatic proliferation is a barrier to transplantation tolerance. Nature medicine 10: 87–92.
9. Hewison M, Burke F, Evans KN, Lammas DA, Sansom DM, et al. (2007) Extra-renal 25-hydroxyvitamin D3-1alpha-hydroxylase in human health and disease. The Journal of steroid biochemistry and molecular biology 103: 316–321.
10. Piemonti L, Monti P, Sironi M, Fraticelli P, Leone BE, et al. (2000) Vitamin D3 affects differentiation, maturation, and function of human monocyte-derived dendritic cells. Journal of Immunology 164: 4443–4451.
11. Penna G, Adorini L (2000) 1 Alpha,25-dihydroxyvitamin D3 inhibits differentiation, maturation, activation, and survival of dendritic cells leading to impaired alloreactive T cell activation. Journal of Immunology (Baltimore, Md: 1950) 164: 2405–2411.
12. Boonstra A, Barrat FJ, Crain C, Heath VL, Savelkoul HF, et al. (2001) 1alpha,25-Dihydroxyvitamin d3 has a direct effect on naive CD4(+) T cells to enhance the development of Th2 cells. Journal of immunology (Baltimore, Md: 1950) 167: 4974–4980.
13. Bhalla AK, Amento EP, Serog B, Glimcher LH (1984) 1,25-Dihydroxyvitamin D3 inhibits antigen-induced T cell activation. J Immunol 133: 1748–1754.
14. Adorini L, Penna G, Casorati M, Davalli AM, Gregori S (2001) Induction of transplantation tolerance by 1,25-dihydroxyvitamin D(3). Transplantation proceedings 33: 58–59.
15. Liu PT, Stenger S, Li H, Wenzel L, Tan BH, et al. (2006) Toll-like receptor triggering of a vitamin D-mediated human antimicrobial response. Science (New York, NY) 311: 1770–1773.
16. Jeffery LE, Wood AM, Qureshi OS, Hou TZ, Gardner D, et al. (2012) Availability of 25-hydroxyvitamin D(3) to APCs controls the balance between regulatory and inflammatory T cell responses. Journal of immunology (Baltimore, Md: 1950) 189: 5155–5164.
17. Looker AC, Johnson CL, Lacher DA, Pfeiffer CM, Schleicher RL, et al. (2011) Vitamin D status: United States, 2001–2006. NCHS data brief: 1–8.
18. Pramyothin P, Holick MF (2012) Vitamin D supplementation: guidelines and evidence for subclinical deficiency. Curr Opin Gastroenterol 28: 139–150.
19. Sawinski D, Uribarri J, Peace D, Yao T, Wauhop P, et al. (2010) 25-OH-vitamin D deficiency and cellular alloimmunity as measured by panel of reactive T cell testing in dialysis patients. Am J Transplant 10: 2287–2295.
20. Jean G, Terrat JC, Vanel T, Hurot JM, Lorriaux C, et al. (2008) Daily oral 25-hydroxycholecalciferol supplementation for vitamin D deficiency in haemodialysis patients: effects on mineral metabolism and bone markers. Nephrology, dialysis, transplantation: official publication of the European Dialysis and Transplant Association - European Renal Association 23: 3670–3676.
21. Matias PJ, Jorge C, Ferreira C, Borges M, Aires I, et al. (2010) Cholecalciferol supplementation in hemodialysis patients: effects on mineral metabolism, inflammation, and cardiac dimension parameters. Clin J Am Soc Nephrol 5: 905–911.
22. Wasse H, Huang R, Long Q, Singapuri S, Raggi P, et al. (2012) Efficacy and safety of a short course of very-high-dose cholecalciferol in hemodialysis. The American journal of clinical nutrition 95: 522–528.
23. Saab G, Young DO, Gincherman Y, Giles K, Norwood K, et al. (2007) Prevalence of vitamin D deficiency and the safety and effectiveness of monthly ergocalciferol in hemodialysis patients. Nephron Clin Pract 105: c132–138.
24. Bienaimé F, Girard D, Anglicheau D, Canaud G, Souberbielle JC, et al. (2013) Vitamin D Status and Outcomes After Renal Transplantation. Journal of the American Society of Nephrology: JASN.
25. Kim H, Kang S-W, Yoo T-H, Kim MS, Kim SI, et al. (2012) The impact of pretransplant 25-hydroxy vitamin D deficiency on subsequent graft function: an observational study. BMC nephrology 13.
26. Saghaei M (2004) Random allocation software for parallel group randomized trials. BMC Med Res Methodol 4: 26.
27. Zand MS, Bose A, Vo T, Coppage M, Pellegrin T, et al. (2005) A renewable source of donor cells for repetitive monitoring of T- and B-cell alloreactivity. American journal of transplantation: official journal of the American Society of Transplantation and the American Society of Transplant Surgeons 5: 76–86.
28. Nair V, Sawinski D, Akalin E, Friedlander R, Ebcioglu Z, et al. (2012) Effect of high-dose intravenous immunoglobulin on anti-HLA antibodies in sensitized kidney transplant candidates. Clin Transplant 26: E261–268.
29. Goodkin DA, Bragg-Gresham JL, Koenig KG, Wolfe RA, Akiba T, et al. (2003) Association of comorbid conditions and mortality in hemodialysis patients in Europe, Japan, and the United States: the Dialysis Outcomes and Practice Patterns Study (DOPPS). Journal of the American Society of Nephrology: JASN 14: 3270–3277.
30. Ziegler-Heitbrock L (2007) The CD14+ CD16+ blood monocytes: their role in infection and inflammation. Journal of leukocyte biology 81: 584–592.
31. de Baey A, Mende I, Riethmueller G, Baeuerle PA (2001) Phenotype and function of human dendritic cells derived from M-DC8(+) monocytes. European journal of immunology 31: 1646–1655.
32. Bjelakovic G, Gluud LL, Nikolova D, Whitfield K, Wetterslev J, et al. (2011) Vitamin D supplementation for prevention of mortality in adults. Cochrane Database Syst Rev: CD007470.
33. Augustine JJ, Poggio ED, Clemente M, Aeder MI, Bodziak KA, et al. (2007) Hemodialysis vintage, black ethnicity, and pretransplantation antidonor cellular immunity in kidney transplant recipients. Journal of the American Society of Nephrology: JASN 18: 1602–1606.
34. Hewison M (2011) Vitamin D and innate and adaptive immunity. Vitamins and hormones 86: 23–62.
35. Lee JR, Dadhania D, August P, Lee JB, Suthanthiran M, et al. (2014) Circulating levels of 25-hydroxyvitamin d and acute cellular rejection in kidney allograft recipients. Transplantation 98: 292–299.
36. Lavin PJ, Laing ME, O'Kelly P, Moloney FJ, Gopinathan D, et al. (2007) Improved renal allograft survival with vitamin D receptor polymorphism. Renal failure 29: 785–789.

14

Copper-Deficiency in *Brassica napus* Induces Copper Remobilization, Molybdenum Accumulation and Modification of the Expression of Chloroplastic Proteins

Vincent Billard[1,2,3], Alain Ourry[1,2,3], Anne Maillard[1,2,3], Maria Garnica[4], Laurent Coquet[5], Thierry Jouenne[5], Florence Cruz[6], José-Maria Garcia-Mina[4], Jean-Claude Yvin[6], Philippe Etienne[1,2,3]*

1 Normandie Université, Caen, France, **2** UNICAEN, UMR 950 Ecophysiologie Végétale, Agronomie et nutritions N, C, S, Caen, France, **3** INRA, UMR 950 Ecophysiologie Végétale, Agronomie et nutritions N, C, S, Caen, France, **4** Timac Agro Spain, Poligono de Arazuri-Orcoyen, Orcoyen, Spain, **5** Plateforme de protéomique PISSARO, UMR6270 CNRS Faculté des Sciences de Rouen, Mont-Saint-Aignan, France, **6** Centre de Recherche International en Agroscience, CRIAS-TAI, Groupe Roullier, Dinard, France

Abstract

During the last 40 years, crop breeding has strongly increased yields but has had adverse effects on the content of micronutrients, such as Fe, Mg, Zn and Cu, in edible products despite their sufficient supply in most soils. This suggests that micronutrient remobilization to edible tissues has been negatively selected. As a consequence, the aim of this work was to quantify the remobilization of Cu in leaves of *Brassica napus* L. during Cu deficiency and to identify the main metabolic processes that were affected so that improvements can be achieved in the future. While Cu deficiency reduced oilseed rape growth by less than 19% compared to control plants, Cu content in old leaves decreased by 61.4%, thus demonstrating a remobilization process between leaves. Cu deficiency also triggered an increase in Cu transporter expression in roots (*COPT2*) and leaves (*HMA1*), and more surprisingly, the induction of the *MOT1* gene encoding a molybdenum transporter associated with a strong increase in molybdenum (Mo) uptake. Proteomic analysis of leaves revealed 33 proteins differentially regulated by Cu deficiency, among which more than half were located in chloroplasts. Eleven differentially expressed proteins are known to require Cu for their synthesis and/or activity. Enzymes that were located directly upstream or downstream of Cu-dependent enzymes were also differentially expressed. The overall results are then discussed in relation to remobilization of Cu, the interaction between Mo and Cu that occurs through the synthesis pathway of Mo cofactor, and finally their putative regulation within the Calvin cycle and the chloroplastic electron transport chain.

Editor: Paul A. Cobine, Auburn University, United States of America

Funding: VB's PhD grant was funded by the Regional Council of Basse-Normandie (http://www.region-basse-normandie.fr/) and Timac Agro International (http://www.timacagro.fr/). Regional Council of Basse-Normandie had no role in study design, data collection and analysis, decision to publish, or preparation of the manuscript. Timac Agro Internationnal had a role in study design and analysis.

Competing Interests: The authors have declared that no competing interests exist.

* Email: philippe.etienne@unicaen.fr

Introduction

While N, P, K and more recently S fertilizations are common practices in agriculture, the supply of micronutrients is less frequently considered. However, according to the World Health Organization [1], two billion people around the world suffer from micronutrient deficiencies (mostly Fe, Cu, Zn and Mg), causing 7.3% of disease burden. Among the micronutrients involved in human metabolism, Cu deficiency, for example, causes symptoms of diseases such as immune defects or anaemia [2]. Without stock or sufficient intake, undernourished children are the first affected [3], however Cu deficiency is also observed in developed countries [4,5]. In the human diet, Cu is mainly present in meat (especially liver and offal), fish and nuts [6]. However, these food supplies are not available to most populations suffering from micronutrients deficiencies. As a consequence, staple foods (cereals, tubers and oils) must be fortified in order to provide the minimum dose of essential micronutrients, such as Cu, for these populations [7].

Over the past 60 years, the micronutrient content (mostly Fe, Zn, Mg and Cu) has been reduced in edible products despite sufficient micronutrient availability in most cultivated soils, and this is the result of varietal selection that aimed to achieve higher yields [8,9]. Consequently, whether a genetic improvement of micronutrient uptake by roots would increase the edible plant content remains questionable. Alternatively, improving the transfer of such micronutrients in edible parts from remobilization of vegetative tissue could be an alternative for breeding if we assume that the recycling (i.e. remobilization) of such nutrients is a significant process. In addition, it has been shown that some soils can lack Cu resulting in dramatic agricultural effects [10]. Thus, Cu deficiency in plants affects human health either directly (decrease in yield) or indirectly (symptoms induced by a lack of micronutrients) [11,12].

As a transition metal [13], Cu is involved in numerous processes in plants. Most of Cu's functions in plants rely on enzymatically bound Cu (more than one hundred proteins identified so far [14]), mostly catalysing redox reactions. As a consequence, only 2% of plant Cu occurs in its free form. Chloroplasts contain about half of the total plant Cu, where it is especially associated with proteins involved in the electron transport chain such as plastocyanin [15]. Three Cu ions are also required for assembly of the active cytochrome c oxydase complex in the mitochondrial electron transport chain. Additionally, numerous proteins known to bind Cu or to be regulated by Cu are involved in the Calvin cycle or in the Tricarboxylic Acid Cycle (TCA), for example Fructose 1–6 Bis Phosphatase (FBPase), Glyceraldehyde 3 Phosphate DeHydrogenase (G3PDH) [16] and PhosphoGlycerate Kinase (PGK) [17]. Cu is also important for enzymes involved in cell detoxification, such as glutathione-S-transferase [18] or Cu-Zn superoxide dismutase [19], or in cell wall metabolism such as ascorbate and polyphenol oxidases [20].

From a genetic point of view, some studies have reported a high variation in Cu content between accessions of the same species such as spinach, pea [21] and cassava [22]. While it has been suggested that Cu management should be easily improved by breeding [4], mechanisms that could increase the Cu content in edible tissues, such as remobilization, have been poorly described in the literature.

An important agricultural crop, such as *Brassica napus*, usually requires high levels of nutrients and hence fertilization to reach an optimal yield with preserved quality. Indeed, winter oilseed rape is highly sensitive to sulphur (S) and nitrogen (N) deficiencies with negative consequences for yield and seed quality [23] and therefore, requires high doses of N and S fertilizers. These strong needs for fertilizers are partly due to the low (macro)-nutrient use efficiency (defined by the ratio of seed to plant nutrient contents) of oilseed rape. For example, it has been reported that its low N use efficiency results from a relatively inefficient endogenous N mobilization [24,25] that occurs mostly during leaf senescence [26]. In contrast, S remobilization from leaves to the seeds (linked to induction of tonoplastic sulphate transporters allowing the mobilization of sulphate previously stored in leaves [27]) is not triggered by leaf senescence but rather by S deficiency. Therefore, without S deficiency, the S content in fallen leaves remains high, up to 2% of dry weight. According to these studies, *Brassica napus* constitutes an important model of defective agro-environmental interactions in studies of nutrient remobilization from leaves. Moreover, it constitutes a relevant plant species model because its genetic proximity to *Arabidospis thaliana* provides easy access to molecular tools while maintaining an agronomic relevance.

To date, deciphering of the plant response to Cu deficiency has been performed through Fe and Zn interactions, identification and characterization of genes encoding transporters (such as *COPT* and *HMA* families), and monitoring target proteins and metabolites [28–31]. However, to our knowledge, the effect of Cu deficiency on growth and plant metabolism is currently poorly reported. Indeed, only one article [32] describes the use of a microarray approach to study modifications of the *Arabidopsis thaliana* transcriptome in response to Cu deficiency.

The first aim of this study was to quantify the effect of Cu deficiency on growth of *Brassica napus* and to assess the mobility of Cu between plant tissues (i.e. Cu remobilization). Moreover, a wider analysis of plant nutrients has been used to monitor the effect of Cu-deficiency on the uptake of some macro (Ca, K, Mg, N, P and S) and micronutrients (B, Fe, Mn, Mo, Na and Zn). Finally, a molecular approach combining proteomic and targeted transcriptomic studies has been used to identify the main metabolic pathways affected by Cu deficiency.

Materials and Methods

Growth conditions

Seeds of *Brassica napus* var. Boheme were surface-sterilized by exposure to 80% ethanol for 30 s followed by 20% sodium hypochlorite for 10 min. After 10 washes with demineralised water, seeds were germinated on perlite over demineralised water for 2 days in the dark and 1 week under natural light in a greenhouse. Just after first leaf emergence, seedlings were transferred to a 20 L tank containing the following nutrient solution: KNO_3 1.25 mM, $Ca(NO_3)_2$ 1.25 mM, KH_2PO_4 0.25 mM, $MgSO_4$ 0.5 mM, EDTA, 2 NaFe 0.2 mM, H_3BO_3 0.01 mM, $MnSO_4$ 5 μM, $ZnSO_4$ 3 μM, $(NH_4)_6Mo_7O_{24}$ 0.7 μM, $CoCl_2$ 0.1 μM, $NiCl_2$ 0.04 μM, SiO_2 0.1 mM, $CaCl_2$ 20 1.25 mM, KCl 0.25 mM. Control nutrient solution also contained NaOH 0.1 mM and $CuSO_4$ 0.7 μM while Na_2SO_4 1 μM was added to Cu-depleted nutrient solution. These nutrient solutions were renewed every two days. Plants were grown under greenhouse conditions with a thermoperiod of 20°C/17°C day/night and a photoperiod of 16 h. Natural light was supplemented with high pressure sodium lamps (Philips, MASTER GreenPower T400W) supplying an average photosynthetically active radiation of 280 μmol photons.$m^{-2}.s^{-1}$ at canopy height. After one week of growth, plants were separated into 2 sets: control plants receiving normal nutrient solution and Cu-deficient plants receiving the Cu-depleted nutrient solution (for details, see above) over 25 days. Four independent samples, each consisting of three plants, were harvested at the beginning of Cu depletion (t = 0) and after 25 days with (control) or without Cu (−Cu). Leaves and petioles present at the beginning of Cu depletion (referred as "old leaves" and "old petioles", respectively) were distinguished from leaves appearing during Cu depletion (referred as "young leaves" and "young petioles", respectively). At each date of harvest (t = 0 and t = 25 days), whole roots from control and Cu-depleted plants were collected. An aliquot of each tissue was weighed and dried in an oven (60°C) for dry weight (DW) determination and ground to fine powder for IRMS and ICP-OES analysis. Thereafter, the remaining fresh tissues were frozen in liquid nitrogen and stored at −80°C for transcriptomic and proteomic analyses.

Every five days throughout the culture period, non-destructive determination of chlorophyll content of young and old leaves was performed using a SPAD chlorophyll meter (SPAD-502 model, Minolta, Tokyo, Japan). The determination was carried using three replicates of ten measurements performed on independent leaves.

Analysis of nutrients in plant tissues

For the analysis of total N and S contents, an aliquot of around 4 mg DW of each plant organ sample was placed in tin capsules for total N and S analysis using an IRMS spectrometer (Isoprime, GV Instrument, Manchester, UK) linked to a C/N/S analyser (EA3000, Euro Vector, Milan, Italy). The total amount of N or S (N_{tot} or S_{tot}) in a tissue "i" at a given time "t" is calculated:

$$N_{tot}(\text{or } S_{tot}) = \%\ N_{i,t}(\text{or } S_{i,t}) \times DWi,t/100$$

Other nutrients (K, Ca, S, P, Mg, Fe, Na, Mn, B, Si, Zn and Cu) were analysed by Inductively Coupled Plasma Optical Emission Spectrometry (ICP-OES, Thermo Elemental Co. Iris Intrepid II XDL) with prior microwave acid sample digestion (8 mL of concentrated HNO_3 and 2 mL of H_2O_2 for 0.5 g DW), using a protocol previously described by Mora *et al.* [33].

RNA extraction

Total RNA was extracted from 200 mg of frozen samples ground to a powder with a pestle in a mortar containing liquid nitrogen. The resulting powder was suspended in 750 µl of extraction buffer [0.1 M TRIS, 0.1 M LiCl, 0.01 M EDTA, 1% SDS (w/v), pH 8] and 750 µl of hot phenol (80°C, pH 4). This mixture was vortexed for 30 s and, after addition of 750 µl of chloroform/isoamylalcohol (24:1, v/v), the homogenate was centrifuged (15 000 g, 5 min, 4°C). The supernatant was transferred into a 4 M LiCl solution and incubated overnight at 4°C. After centrifugation (15 000 g, 30 min, 4°C), the pellet was suspended in 100 µl of sterile water. RNA was then purified with an RNeasy mini kit according to the manufacturer's protocol (Qiagen, Courtaboeuf, France). Quantification of total RNA was performed by spectrophotometry at 260 nm (BioPhotometer, Eppendorf, Le Pecq, France) before Reverse Transcription (RT) and real time Quantitative Polymerase Chain Reaction (Q-PCR) analysis.

Reverse transcription (RT) and Q-PCR analysis

For RT, 1 µg of total RNA was converted to cDNA with an "iScript cDNA synthesis kit" according to the manufacturer's protocol (Bio-Rad, Marne-la-Coquette, France).

Q-PCR amplifications were performed using specific primers for each housekeeping gene (*EF1-α* and *18S rRNA*) and target genes (Table 1). Q-PCRs were performed with 4 µl of 200x diluted cDNA, 500 nM of primers, and 1x SYBR Green PCR Master Mix (Bio-Rad, Marne-la-Coquette, France) in a real-time thermocycler (CFX96 Real Time System, Bio-Rad, Marne-la-Coquette, France). A 2 step program, composed of 42 cycles of a denaturing step at 95°C for 15 s followed by an annealing and extending step at 60°C for 40 s, was used for all pairs of primers (Table 1) except for *COPT2*, for which we used a 3 step program. In this case the denaturing step was as described previously. Annealing was at 58.6°C for 10 s and was followed by an extending step at 72°C for 30 s. For each pair of primers, a threshold value and PCR efficiency were determined using a cDNA preparation diluted >10-fold. For all pairs of primers, PCR efficiency was around 100%. The specificity of PCR amplification was examined by monitoring the presence of the single peak in the melting curves after Q-PCRs and by sequencing the Q-PCR product to confirm that the correct amplicon was produced from each pair of primers (Eurofins, Ebersberg, Germany). The relative expression of the genes in each sample was compared with the control sample [corresponding to untreated plants at the same time of harvest] and was determined with the delta delta Ct (ΔΔCt) method using the following equation [34]: Relative expression = $2^{-\Delta\Delta Ct}$, with $\Delta\Delta Ct = \Delta Ct_{treated}$-$\Delta Ct_{control}$ and with $\Delta Ct = Ct_{target\ gene} - [\sqrt{(Ct_{EF1-\alpha} \times Ct_{18S\ rRNA})}]$, where Ct refers to the threshold cycle determined for each gene in the exponential phase of PCR amplification and $[\sqrt{(Ct_{EF1-\alpha} \times Ct_{18S\ rRNA})}]$ corresponds to the geometric average of Ct of the reference genes. Using this analysis method, the relative expression of the different genes in the control sample of the experiment was equal to 1 [34], and on this basis the relative expression of other treatments was then compared with the control. For *COPT2*, because no transcript was detected in control plants (*i.e.* $Ct_{control}$ is undetermined), values are not expressed relatively to control but as $2^{-\Delta Ct}$.

Extraction and determination of total proteins

Two hundred mg of fresh matter from old leaf samples were ground to a fine powder in liquid nitrogen in the presence of 50 mg of poly(vinylpolypyrrolidone) (PVPP). The addition of PVPP is used to fix plant polyphenols that might interfere with the quantification of proteins or during separation of proteins by electrophoresis. The ground material was dissolved in 1.75 mL of TCA/acetone solution (10% TCA (w/v) prepared in acetone). After centrifugation (3 min, 16 000 g, 4°C), the protein pellet was purified according to the protocol adapted from Wang *et al.* [35]. The protein pellet obtained after precipitation with TCA/acetone (10% TCA (w/v) was suspended in 1.75 mL of 0.1 M ammonium acetate dissolved in 80% methanol. After homogenization and centrifugation (16 000 g, 3 min, 4°C), the pellet was washed with 1.75 mL of 80% acetone and centrifuged again (16 000 g, 3 min, 4°C). The supernatant was removed and the pellet was dried under vacuum (Speedvac Concentrator 5301, Eppendorf, France) for 5 min at 50°C and then suspended with 0.8 mL of phenol at pH 7.9 and in 0.8 mL of dense SDS buffer (30% sucrose, 2% SDS, 0.1 M Tris-HCl, pH 8.0, 0.5% 2-mercaptoethanol). After 5 min incubation at 4°C and centrifugation (16 000 g, 3 min, 4°C), the phenol phase was transferred to a new tube and supplemented with 1.75 mL of 0.1 M ammonium acetate and stored at -20°C overnight. Afterwards, ammonium acetate was used to precipitate proteins to enable their collection by centrifugation (16 000 g, 5 min, 4°C). The protein pellet was then washed with 1.75 mL of 100% methanol and again with 1.75 mL of 80% acetone. Residual acetone was removed by vacuum evaporation over a few minutes. The pellet was resuspended in 400 µL of R2D2 rehydration buffer [5 M urea, 2 M thiourea, 2% CHAPS, 2% N-decyl-N,N-dimethyl-3-ammonio-1-propanesulfonate, 20 mM dithiothreitol, 5 mM Tris (2-carboxy- ethyl) phosphine, 0.5% IPG buffer] (GE Healthcare, Saclay, France), pH 4 to 7 [36]. The total protein concentration was determined by the method previously described by Bradford [37] using bovine serum albumin as standard.

Table 1. Q-PCR primer sets.

Gene	Accession number	Forward	Reverse	Gene Function
EF1-α	DQ312264	5′-gcctggtatggttgtgacct-3′	5′-gaagttagcagcacccttgg-3′	
18S rRNA	GQ380689	5′-cggataaccgtagtaattctag-3′	5′-gtactcattccaattaccagac-3′	
COPT2	NM_114557	5′-tgcacatgaccttcttttgg-3′	5′-gtcatcggagggtttgttga-3′	Cu uptake
HMA1	NM_119890.6	5′-gtacagctgaccgaggaagc-3′	5′tgcccataaatgggttcaat-3′	Cu allocation to chloroplast
MOT1	NM_128127	5′-ctcgccaggatttggactta-3′	5′agatccccaacacgaacaag-3′	Mo uptake

EF1α and *18S rRNA* were housekeeping genes used for relative gene expressions by Q-PCR analysis.

Two-dimensional electrophoresis (2-DE) and image analysis

2-DE was performed according to the protocol detailed by Desclos *et al.* [25]. Gels were stained using the silver-staining procedure described by Blum *et al.* [38] and scanned with a ProXPRESS 2D proteomic imaging system (Perkin-Elmer, Courtaboeuf, France). Images of the 2-DE gels were analysed using the Progenesis SameSpots software v3.0 (Nonlinear Dynamics, Newcastle upon Tyne, UK) according to the manufacturer's protocol. Gels from three independent biological replicates were used. Spot detection, warping, and matching were performed automatically by the software and manually validated. Artefacts due to non-specific silver nitrate staining or spots that could not be confidently verified as true matches were disregarded rather than manually edited, and misalignments were corrected by manual warping when appropriate. Mw and *pI* were calculated using SameSpots software calibrated with commercial molecular mass standards (prestained precision protein standards; Bio-Rad, Marne-la-Coquette, France) run in a separate marker lane on 2-DE gel.

RuBisCO relative quantification

In order to observe maximum spots, silver staining was performed on 2-DE with a saturated RuBisCO signal. The amount of RuBisCO was then measured by Experion Pro260 Analysis Kit (Bio-Rad, Marne-la-Coquette, France). The Experion automated electrophoresis system applies a combination of microfluidic separation technology and sensitive fluorescent detection of proteins [39]. The protein extracts were treated with the Experion reagents and then separated on the Experion automated electrophoresis station according to the manufacturer's instruction. Peak areas corresponding to large and small RuBisCO subunits were then compared using software given by manufacturer.

Protein Identification by ESI LC-MS/MS

Spots of interest were excised from 2D gels and washed several times with water and dried for a few minutes. Trypsin digestion was performed overnight with a dedicated automated system (MultiPROBE II, Perkin-Elmer). The gel fragments were subsequently incubated twice for 15 min in a 0.1% CH_3CN solution in water to allow extraction of peptides from the gel pieces. Peptide extracts were then dried and dissolved in starting buffer for chromatographic elution, consisting of 3% CH_3CN and 0.1% HCOOH in water. Peptides were enriched and separated using lab-on-a-chip technology (Agilent, Massy, France) and fragmented using an on-line XCT mass spectrometer (Agilent). The ESI LC-MS/MS data were converted into DTA- format files that were further searched for proteins with MASCOT Daemon (Matrix Science [40]). For protein identification, two strategies were employed to mine the maximum data. Measured peptides were searched in the NCBI nr-protein sequence database, *viridiplantae* (green plants [41]), and in the *Brassica* EST database (*Brassica* Genome Gateway 2007, [42]). Proteins with two or more unique peptides matching the protein sequence with a score >53, as defined by MASCOT, were considered as a positive identification. The spectra of each peptide were verified manually. In cases where protein identification data were lacking, BLAST analysis was performed [43].

Data and statistical analysis

Regarding the growth, ICP-OES and IRMS analyses, all experiments were conducted with 4 independent biological replicates each corresponding to 3 plants. Proteomics and Q-PCR analyses were performed on 3 independent biological replicates each corresponding to 3 plants. Data are given as mean ± SE for n = 3 or 4. For Q-PCR, SE and Student's T-test were based on ΔΔCt (or ΔCt for *COPT2*, see above for more information), when the relation between values is still linear. According to Yuan *et al.* 2006 [44], a confidence interval of each mean value (with min and max values) can be calculated and has been presented in the results section as [mean of relative expression] (Min value-Max value) with Min value = $2^{-(\Delta\Delta Ct+SE)}$ and Max value = $2^{-(\Delta\Delta Ct-SE)}$ (Min value = $2^{-(\Delta Ct+SE)}$ and Max value = $2^{-(\Delta Ct-SE)}$ for *COPT2*). Conversion of the results of an exponential process into a linear comparison of amounts leads to an asymmetric distribution [34].

All data were analysed with Student's T-test ($p<0.05$) and marked by an asterisk (*) or cross (†) when significantly different.

Results

Cu depletion affects the growth and Cu content of *B. napus*

After 25 days of culture, control whole plant DW increased from 3.23±0.24 g to 39.67±1.26 g (table 2). The total DW of Cu-depleted plants was decreased by 18.4% relative to control plants (table 2, from 39.67 to 32.37 g DW.plant^{-1}). This was the result of a significant reduction in root DW (from 4.11±0.23 in control plants to 3.73±0.06 g DW.plant^{-1} in Cu-depleted plants) and secondly, of old petioles DW (from 8.07±0.60 to 6.31±0.49 g DW.plant^{-1}). No significant differences in growth rates were found for other organs. Control plants accumulated 251.5 µg of Cu while the Cu content in Cu-depleted plants only rose from 29.0±4.0 µg to 74.8±3.0 µg. The slight increase in total Cu in Cu-depleted plants was the result of a trace of Cu found in the mineralized water used for the nutrient solution (0.47±0.00 µM, data not shown). In roots of control plants, the amount of Cu increased from 14.7±3.0 µg to 155.2±13.2 µg but only reached 43.4±1.5 µg in Cu deficient plants. In aerial tissues that developed under Cu depletion, the Cu amount was reduced from 11.8±1.9 µg to 2.6±0.7 µg and from 76.2±4.8 µg to 16.2±2.3 µg in petioles and leaves, respectively. In petioles already present at the time of the Cu depletion, the amount of Cu rose from 2.1±0.2 µg to 8.0±0.7 µg during depletion while it reached 20.3±2.4 µg in control plants at the end of the experiment. The amount of Cu in old leaves of control plants did not vary significantly during the experiment, while in Cu-depleted plants, it was reduced from 12.2±1.1 µg to 4.7±1.0 µg indicating a remobilization of 61.4±4.2% of the Cu initially present in these leaves.

No significant difference was observed for RuBisCO by *Experion* method (Figure 1.A). During the whole experiment, the leaf chlorophyll content (SPAD values, Figure 1.B) were not significantly different between control and Cu-depleted plants. At the end of the experiment, this was confirmed in old leaves (Figure 1.C). Also, N content in old leaves didn't present any difference between the two conditions (Figure 1.D).

Cu depletion increases expression of Cu transporters in *Brassica napus*

The relative expression of genes involved in Cu transport (*HMA1, COPT2*) is given in Figure 1. Expression of the *HMA1* gene encoding a chloroplastic Cu transporter was monitored in leaves, whereas *COPT2*, which encodes a transporter involved in Cu uptake, was monitored in roots. The relative number of *HMA1* transcripts increased 2.68 fold (2.23-3.24) after 25d of Cu

Table 2. Biomass and Cu content in *Brassica napus* L. at t = 0 and after 25 days of culture with (control) or without Cu (−Cu).

		t=0	Control (25d)	-Cu (25d)
Old leaves	DW (g)	2.13±0.17	4.78±0.79	4.83±0.93
	Cu amount (μg)	12.2±1.1	17.0±2.5	4.7±1.0*†
	% remobilized	NA	NA	60.36±4,15
Old petioles	DW (g)	0.63±0.04	8.07±0.60	6.31±0.49*†
	Cu amount (μg)	2.1±0.2	20.3±2.4*	8.0±0.7*†
Young leaves	DW (g)	NA	12.7±0.94	8.83±1.64
	Cu amount (μg)	NA	76.2±4.8	16.2±2.3 †
Young petioles	DW (g)	NA	10.02±0.78	8.66±0.55
	Cu amount (μg)	NA	11.8±1.9	2.6±0.7 †
Roots	DW (g)	0.48±0.03	4.11±0.23*	3.73±0.06*
	Cu amount (μg)	14.7±3.0	155.2±13.2*	43.4±1.5*†
Total	DW (g)	3.23±0.24	39.67±1.26*	32.37±1.71*†
	Cu amount (μg)	29.0±4.0	280.5±13.5*	74.8±3.0*†

* and † represent significant differences at $p<0.05$ compared to t = 0 and control, respectively. NA: Not Applicable.

depletion (Figure 2.A). Transcripts of *COPT2* were detected only in roots from Cu-depleted plants suggesting that the expression of the *COPT2* transporter was up-regulated and/or de-repressed in *Brassica napus* roots in response to Cu deficiency (Figure 2.B).

Cu depletion affects uptake of some mineral nutrients

Figure 3 shows that Cu deprivation decreased Cu uptake by 81.8±2.0%, but also affected the uptake of Na (−41.0±3.8%), B (−31.6±2.1%) and Mg (−28.5±2.8%). while plant dry weight was reduced by 18.4±2.5% (Table 2). Cu deficiency had no effect on total plant uptake for nutrients such as N, Ca, K, S, P, B, Fe, Mn and Zn, despite the difference of biomass. In contrast, uptake of Mo was increased by 121.8% despite the reduced plant growth and was associated with a very strong up-regulation of the molybdenum transporter 1 gene (*MOT1*, Figure 2.C), having an important role in efficient Mo uptake [45,46]. Indeed, in Cu-depleted plants, the number of *MOT1* transcripts was found to be 159.61 fold (127–200) higher than in control plants.

Cu depletion induces proteomic modifications

Leaves already present at the beginning of Cu depletion were the most affected tissues, not only due to their decreased Cu content and hence the mobilization of Cu (by about 60%) to other tissues, but also according to their decrease of Mg (−42.1±11.0%), Na (−42.6±13.6%), Ca (−35.8±10.0%) and Fe (−27.9±13.5%) contents. Therefore, leaves were selected for a comparative proteomic approach in order to highlight the main metabolic modifications induced by Cu depletion. Representative 2D gels corresponding to protein extracts from leaves of control and Cu-depleted plants are shown in Figure 4. On each gel, 693 proteins were identified. Their comparative analysis revealed 48 proteins significantly up- or down-regulated by Cu depletion. Because different spots correspond to different isoforms of the same protein, only 33 different proteins were identified. Among them, 25 proteins were accumulated in Cu-depleted old leaves. Transketolase-like protein (#7 to 11, Figure 4 and Table 3) was the strongest protein induced with four isoforms that were accumulated more than fourfold compared to control. On the other hand, repression was significant in only 8 of the 33 identified

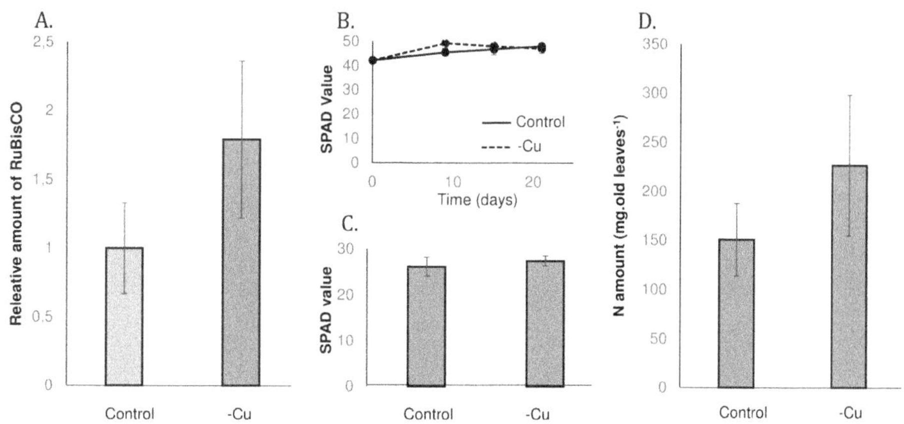

Figure 1. Parameters associated with senescence. (A.) Relative amount of RuBisCO in old leaves. Relative chlorophyll content (SPAD value) during (B.) the whole experiment at whole plant level and (C.) after 25 days of depletion in old leaves (D.) N content in old leaves.

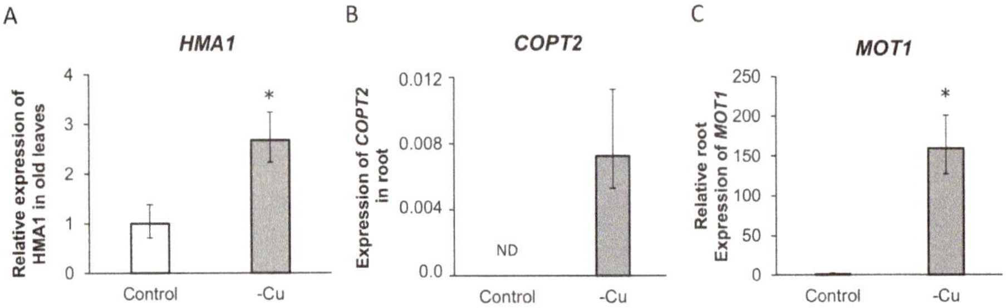

Figure 2. Relative accumulation of transcript of Cu transporters (A. *HMA1* in old leaves and B. *COPT2* in roots) and Molybdenum transporter 1 (C. *MOT1* in roots) in *Brassica napus* L after 25 days of culture with (control) or without Cu (−Cu). Control is represented by white bars and -Cu by grey bars. *MOT1* and *HMA1* values are expressed as $2^{-\Delta\Delta Ct}$ while *COPT2 value* is expressed as $2^{-\Delta Ct}$ (for details, see "Material and Methods"). * represents significant differences at $p<0.05$. ND: not detected.

proteins, with the Oxygen Evolving Enhancer (OEE, #33 to 37) having the greatest repression in our study (−2.3 to −3.93). Among all proteins (Table 3), five were involved in stress responses (disease/defence or defence/secondary metabolite), for example glutathione reductase (#18), and seventeen proteins were involved in energy processes, for example aldolase (#27) and ATP synthase (#17). Protein annotations in databases also indicated that chloroplasts were the main locations of the identified proteins with 17 references, including the most repressed, OEE (#33 to 37), and the most induced, Transketolase-like protein (#7 to 11).

Considering some of the characteristic Cu proteins reported in the literature [47], Plastocyanin was too small (around 10 kDa) to be found on our gels while Cu-Zn superoxide dismutase and Polyphenol oxidase were not differentially expressed and/or detected.

Discussion

Cu remobilization from old leaves is induced by Cu deficiency

In this study, the effectiveness of Cu deficiency can be attested by the low Cu concentration found in old and young leaves of Cu depleted plants (0.97±0.03 $\mu g.g^{-1}$ DW and 1.66±0.40 $\mu g.g^{-1}$ DW, respectively) which was lower than the usually admitted minimum concentration (5 $\mu g.g^{-1}$ DW) [48]. Using Cu deficiency we were able to demonstrate a decrease in the Cu content of leaves by 61.4±4.2% (Table 2). To our knowledge, alongside work on *Arabidopsis thaliana* [49], this is one of the few studies that shows that Cu can be recycled between leaves. However, the Cu remobilization could be underestimated in our conditions because some traces of Cu were found in the nutrient solution, as suggested by the slight increase in the overall Cu content in Cu-depleted plants (Table 2). A precise estimation of Cu remobilization would require the use of stable isotopes. This remobilization of Cu in leaves was concomitant with an increase in *COPT2* and *HMA1* expression. Despite a tendency of an increase of RuBisCO and N amounts, the RuBisCO, N amounts and chlorophyll contents in old leaves were not significantly differentially affected between control and Cu-depleted plants (Figure 1). Then we could assume that Cu remobilization was not associated with leaf senescence. This is also consistent with the down-regulation of senescence-associated proteases such as FtsH2 (#14, Table 3), a protease involved in the degradation of photosystem II [26,50]. Thus, this study suggests that Cu depletion induces a Cu mobilization independent of the distinguishing marks of senescence. This is different to what has been found for N for example, whose deficiency is known to increase leaf senescence in *Brassica napus* [25].

Effect of Cu deficiency on metabolic pathway in chloroplasts from old leaves of *B. napus*

Because the spots of our 2D-E gels correspond to the most abundant proteins in old leaves, numerous proteins (especially transporters and transcription factors) corresponding to transcripts

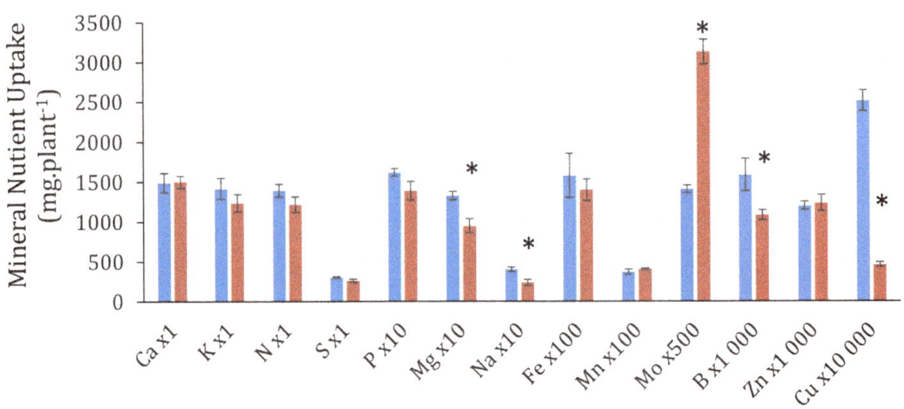

Figure 3. Mineral nutrient uptake in control plants (blue) and Cu-depleted plants over 25 Days (red). Due to large differences between nutrients, factors have been attributed to each nutrient to allow representation on the same graph. * indicates significant difference between control and Cu depleted plants at p = 0.05.

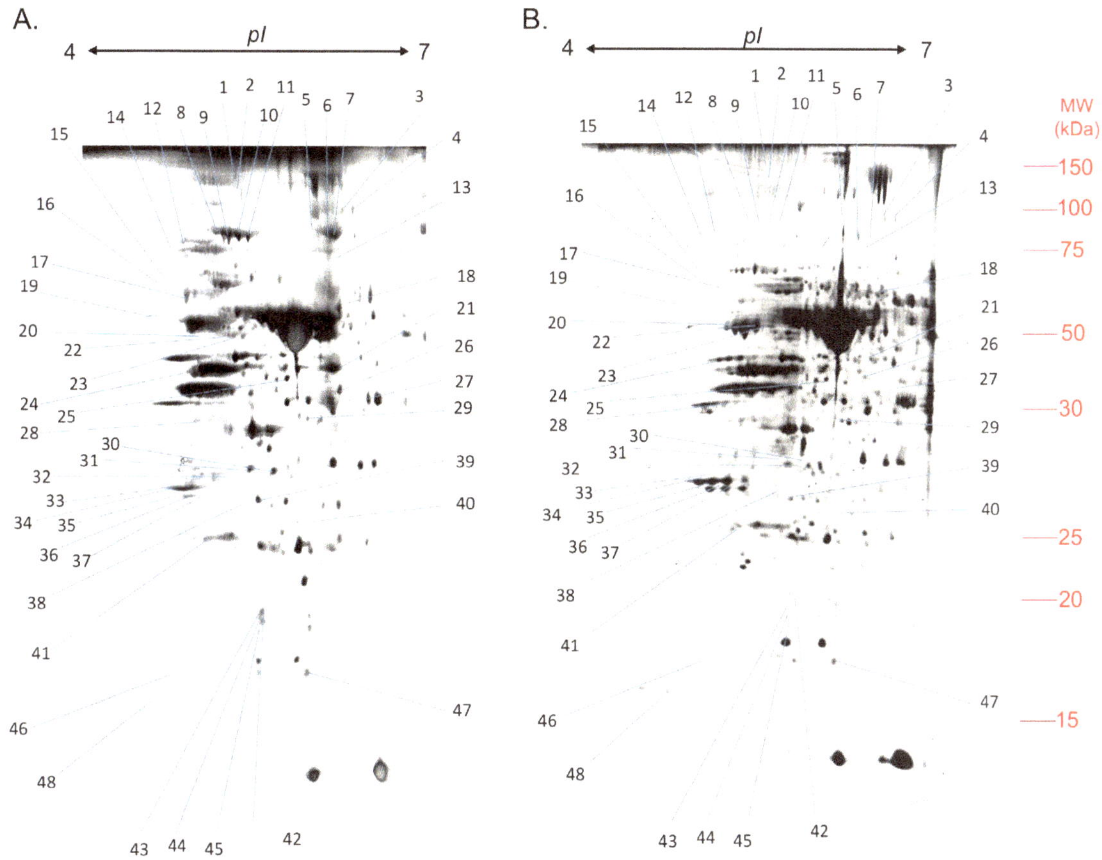

Figure 4. Representative Silver-stained 2-DE gels of proteins from old leaves of *Brassica napus* L. after 25 days of culture with (control, A) or without Cu (−Cu, B). A total of 150 µg of total proteins was loaded on an IEF strip forming an immobilized pH linear gradient from 4 to 7 (for details, see "Materials and Methods"). Numbers indicate sequenced and identified proteins presented in table 3. Molecular mass markers (MW in kDa) are listed on the right side of the gel.

identified in previous studies as regulated by Cu depletion could not be observed in the present work. Thus, this study complement previous transcriptomic data on Cu remobilisation [51,52]. This proteomic analysis of Cu-deficient old leaves showed that more than half of the up or down-regulated proteins were localised in chloroplasts (Table 3) indicating potential disturbance, despite an absence of chlorophyll content variation (Figure 1.B, C). Five of these proteins are involved in the Calvin cycle and 5 are involved in the thylakoid electron transport chain (Figure 5). From a general point of view, among the 33 proteins that were differentially expressed relatively to control plants (Table 3), 11 of them are known to rely on the presence of Cu for their synthesis and/or activity, and 9 were over expressed (#15, 16, 17, 19, 27, 29, 39 and 43). As a consequence, it could be suggested that the lack of Cu reduced their activity which may explain their up-regulation (or alternatively reduced their down-regulation). A similar regulation would also occur for enzymes that are located upstream or downstream of such copper deficiency up-regulated proteins. For example, this is the case (Figure 5) within the Calvin cycle for Transketolases (#6–11) or TPI (#41), which are located upstream and downstream of Aldolase (#27), a copper dependent protein that was up-regulated by Cu-deficiency.

Among Cu binding or regulated enzymes within the Calvin cycle (FBPase [53], GAPDH, Aldolase [16], RuBisCO [18], PGK [17]), only Aldolase (#27) and PGK (#21) were found to be over represented (Table 3 and Figure 5). However, whilst RuBisCO was not significantly affected (Figure 1), its main regulator RuBisCO activase (#24) was increased by about 3 folds (Table 3). It should be noted that PGK, Aldolase, Transketolase and TPI are also involved in glycolysis (in the cytosol or plastids [54]) and their regulation should therefore induce mitochondrial defects.

GAP is a crosspoint between numerous pathways, with B6 vitamin biosynthesis being one of them [55]. However, under an impaired Calvin cycle, more GAP would be available for this cycle (Figure 5). Vitamin B6 can also be synthesized through Pyridoxin biosynthesis protein (#32, Table 3) which is over represented in old leaves of Cu-depleted *B. napus*. The B6 dependent protein Glutamate-1-semialdehyde aminomutase (GSA, #25) [56] with a role in chlorophyll biosynthesis also accumulated (Figure 5).

Differentially expressed proteins located in thylakoids (Figure 5) could be subdivided into two groups: the first one including OEE (#33 to 37), NADPH subunit 48 (#20) and ATP synthase (#17) were down-regulated, which is consistent with previous work reporting a down-regulation of photosynthesis-related genes in response to Cu deficiency [51]. The second group corresponded to [Fe-S] cluster containing proteins such as Ferredoxin (#30 and 31) and Rieske domain protein (#47), which were over expressed in response to Cu depletion. We suggest that overall the electron transport chain was down-regulated, but an impairment of [Fe-S] cluster biosynthesis could be compensated by an up-regulation of *de novo* synthesis of [Fe-S] proteins. This stimulation of [Fe-S] cluster proteins can be linked to the accumulation of Rhodanese

Table 3. Abundance of identified proteins over (positive value) or under (negative value) accumulated in old leaves of Cu-depleted *B. napus* relative to control plants.

Spot no.	Relative Abundance	Exp. pI/ Mw	Theo. pI/Mw	PM	SC (%)	Protein name/Organism/NCBI accession no.	Functional classification/Sub-Cellular localization	Note
1	3.12	5.7/115	5.39/104.3	30	20	Myrosinase binding protein [*Brassica napus*]/gi|1711296	11. Disease/Defence	
2	2.11	6.3/99	6.59/102.2	117	40	Chaperone protein ClpC, chloroplastic-like [*Fragaria vesca* subsp. vesca]/gi|470122943	08. Intracellular traffic/Chloroplast	
3	1.75	6.64/90	6.12/84.3	58	24	Cobalamin-independent methionine synthase [*Arabidopsis lyrata* subsp. lyrata]/gi|297807807	01. Metabolism	**Zn** [73]
4	2.78	6.53/91	6.12/84.3	29	19	Cobalamin-independent methionine synthase [*Arabidopsis lyrata* subsp. lyrata]/gi|297807807	01. Metabolism	**Zn** [73]
5	4.16	6.26/80	6.16/81.2	13	13	NADH Ubiquinone oxydoreductase 75 kD subunit [*Arabidopsis thaliana*]/gi|30693102	02. Energy/Chloroplast-Mitochondria	[Fe-S] cluster
6	5.23	6.5/81	5.80/81.5	15	18	Transketolase-like protein [*Arabidopsis thaliana*]/gi|7329685	02. Energy/Chloroplast-Mitochondria	
7	2.22	6.41/80	6.12/79.9	13	10	Transketolase [*Arabidopsis thaliana*]/gi|30689983	02. Energy/Chloroplast-Mitochondria	
8	4.79	5.74/75	6.16/81.2	46	24	Transketolase-like protein [*Arabidopsis thaliana*]/gi|7329685	02. Energy/Chloroplast-Mitochondria	
9	4.17	5.78/75	6.16/81.2	61	27	Transketolase-like protein [*Arabidopsis thaliana*]/gi|7329685	02. Energy/Chloroplast-Mitochondria	
10	4.46	5.67/76	6.16/81.2	62	29	Transketolase-like protein [*Arabidopsis thaliana*]/gi|7329685	02. Energy/Chloroplast-Mitochondria	
11	4.23	5.54/74	6.16/81.2	44	26	Transketolase-like protein [*Arabidopsis thaliana*]/gi|7329685	02. Energy/Chloroplast-Mitochondria	
12	2.06	5.25/73	5.08/70.7	49	37	Heat shock cognate protein HSC70 [*Brassica napus*]/gi|2655420	08, intracellular traffic/Chloroplast	*Zn* [16]
13	−2.07	6.48/70	5.56/63.4	10	11	Phosphoglucomutase [*Arabidopsis thaliana*]/gi|15223226	02. Energy/Chloroplast	
14	−2.03	5.17/69	5.62/72.0	25	16	ATP-dependent zinc metalloprotease FTSH 2, chloroplastic-like [*Brachypodium distachyon*]/gi|357123383	06. Prot. Dest. & Storage/Chloroplast	*Zn* [74]
15	1.54	6.14/64	5.22/49.4	11	7	Thylakoid rhodanese-like protein [*Arabidopsis thaliana*]/gi|18411523	02. Energy/Chloroplast	***Cu*** and ***Zn*** [75]
16	1.4	6.08/62	5.66/47.6	5	4	Thylakoid rhodanese-like protein [*Arabidopsis thaliana*]/gi|18411523	02. Energy/Chloroplast	***Cu*** and ***Zn*** [75]
17	2.63	5.25/62	5.97/47.0	85	42	ATPase subunit I [*Arabidopsis lyrata* subsp. lyrata]/gi|297837977	02. Energy/Chloroplast-Mitochondria	*Cu* and *Zn* [16]
18	−2.67	6.52/61	8.03/60.6	15	19	Glutathione reductase [*Brassica juncea*]/gi|13448672	20. Defence & Secondary metabolism/Vacuole	*Cu* [16]
19	2.09	4.92/55	5.23/50.6	7	5	Rhodanese-like domain-containing protein 4, chloroplastic-like [*Cicer arietinum*]/gi|502179307	01. Metabolism/Chloroplast	***Cu*** [75]
20	−2.27	5.45/50	6.49/51.0	19	16	NAD(P)H dehydrogenase subunit 48 [*Arabidopsis thaliana*] gi|18394307	02. Energy/Chloroplast	
21	1.52	6.44/47	5.91/50.1	25	21	Phosphoglycerate kinase 1 [*Arabidopsis thaliana*]/gi|15230595	02. Energy/Chloroplast-Mitochondria	*Cu* [17]
22	1.92	5.58/53	6.06/54.2	19	19	Mitochondrial processing peptidase alpha subunit, putative [*Arabidopsis thaliana*] gi|21594004	06. Prot. Dest. & Storage/ Mitochondria	
23	2.81	5.53/52	6.06/54.2	7	11	Mitochondrial processing peptidase alpha subunit, putative [*Arabidopsis thaliana*] gi|21594004	06. Prot. Dest. & Storage/ Mitochondria	
24	2.97	5.11/46	6.78/47.9	61	46	Chloroplast ribulose-1,5-bisphosphate carboxylase/oxygenase activase [*Brassica oleracea*]/gi|383470439	02. Energy/Chloroplast	

Table 3. Cont.

Spot no.	Relative Abundance	Exp. pI/ Mw	Theo. pI/Mw	PM	SC (%)	Protein name/Organism/NCBI accession no.	Functional classification/Sub-Cellular localization	Note
25	1.7	6.03/44	6.43/50.2	44	32	Glutamate-1-semialdehyde 2,1-aminomutase 2 [*Arabidopsis thaliana*]/gi|15229018	01. Metabolism	B6 dependent [56]
26	1.42	6.44/42	5.91/15.1	16	45	Cinnamyl alcohol dehydrogenase [*Brassica napus*]/gi|6683959	01. Metabolism	
27	1.46	6.64/40	6.22/38.4	19	37	Fructose-bisphosphate aldolase [*Arabidopsis thaliana*]/gi|15231715	02. Energy/Chloroplast-Mitochondria	*Cu* [16] and ***Zn*** [76]
28	1.47	5.24/37	5.14/32.0	9	35	40S ribosomal protein [*Brassica napus*]/gi|15214300	05. Protein synthesis/Ribosome	
29	1.33	6.16/37	8.54/35.8	29	31	Mitochondrial NAD-dependent malate dehydrogenase [*Arabidopsis thaliana*]/gi|21592905	02. Energy/Mitochondria	*Cu* [16] and ***Zn*** [77]
30	1.72	5.7/32	8.32/40.3	49	34	Ferredoxin-NADP(+)-oxidoreductase 1 [*Arabidopsis thaliana*]/gi|15239282	02. Energy/Chloroplast	[Fe-S] cluster
31	1.56	5.8/32	8.66/40.1	34	29	Ferredoxin-NADP+ reductase [*Arabidopsis thaliana*]/gi|5730139	02. Energy/Chloroplast	[Fe-S] cluster
32	2.1	5.84/32	6.12/33.0	13	25	Pyridoxine biosynthesis protein [*Lotus japonicus*]/gi|72256517	11. Disease/Defence/Cytosol	B6 biosynthesis [55]
33	−3.93	4.88/31	5.92/35.0	5	15	Oxygen-evolving enhancer protein 1–2 [*Arabidopsis thaliana*]/gi|15230324	02. Energy/Chloroplast	***Mn*** [78]
34	−2.3	4.92/30	5.92/35.0	81	54	Oxygen-evolving enhancer protein 1–2 [*Arabidopsis thaliana*]/gi|15230324	02. Energy/Chloroplast	***Mn*** [78]
35	−2.56	4.94/30	5.93/35.1	36	48	Photosystem II subunit O-2 [*Arabidopsis lyrata* subsp. lyrata]/gi|297819782	02. Energy/Chloroplast	***Mn*** [78]
36	−2.95	5.03/30	5.93/35.1	67	52	Photosystem II subunit O-2 [*Arabidopsis lyrata* subsp. lyrata]/gi|297819782	02. Energy/Chloroplast	***Mn*** [78]
37	−2.8	5.32/30	5.92/35.0	84	55	Oxygen-evolving enhancer protein 1–2 [*Arabidopsis thaliana*]/gi|15230324	02. Energy/Chloroplast	***Mn*** [78]
38	1.69	5.61/29	8.65/33.7	13	11	Thioredoxin-like protein CDSP32 [*Arabidopsis thaliana*]/gi|15222954	11. Disease/Defence/Cytosol	
39	3.81	5.73/29	5.54/29.5	23	17	Carbonic anhydrase 1 [*Arabidopsis thaliana*]/gi|30678347	01. Metabolism/Chloroplast	***Cu*** and ***Zn*** [79]
40	−1.81	6.17/27	6.28/27.6	29	34	Mitochondrial F1F0-ATP synthase subunit Fad [*Arabidopsis thaliana*]/gi|15227104	02. Energy/Mitochondria	Cu [18] and *Zn* [16]
41	1.55	5.28/26	7.67/33.3	10	16	Triosephosphate isomerase [*Arabidopsis thaliana*]/gi|15226479	02. Energy/Chloroplast-Mitochondria	
42	2.41	5.73/20	5.37/19.9	9	26	Uncharacterized protein [*Arabidopsis thaliana*]/gi|18391006	13. Unclassified	
43	2.79	5.7/19	5.47/35.7	41	38	Chloroplast beta-carbonic anhydrase [*Brassica napus*]/gi|297787439	01. Metabolism/Chloroplast	***Cu*** and ***Zn*** [79]
44	2.6	5.75/19	6.81/21.8	6	17	Germin-like protein [*Arabidopsis thaliana*]/gi|1755154	12. Unclear Classification	
45	1.99	5.7/19	6.27/22.0	7	23	RecName: Full = Germin-like protein 1; Flags: Precursor [*Sinapis alba*]/gi|1169944	12. Unclear Classification	
46	−2.6	4.99/17	9.12/24.7	18	31	Peroxiredoxin-2E [*Arabidopsis thaliana*]/gi|15231718	11. Disease/Defence/Cytosol	
47	2.74	6.11/17	8.80/24.3	22	22	Rieske FeS protein [*Arabidopsis thaliana*]/gi|9843639	02. Energy/Chloroplast	[Fe-S] cluster
48	−1.76	4.58/16	5.24/17.9	6	15	Probable glycine cleavage system H protein 2 [*Arabidopsis thaliana*] gi|15223217	02. Energy/Chloroplast	

Experimental and theoretical pI/Mw, the number of LC–MS/MS matched peptides (PM), the SCORE and the percentage of sequence coverage (SC) obtained are also indicated. For each protein, the assigned best–matched protein is listed with the organism in which it was identified and its GenBank protein accession number is indicated. Elements given in notes correspond to ligand (in italics) or regulators (in bold) of the corresponding protein described in previous studies (indicated in brackets).

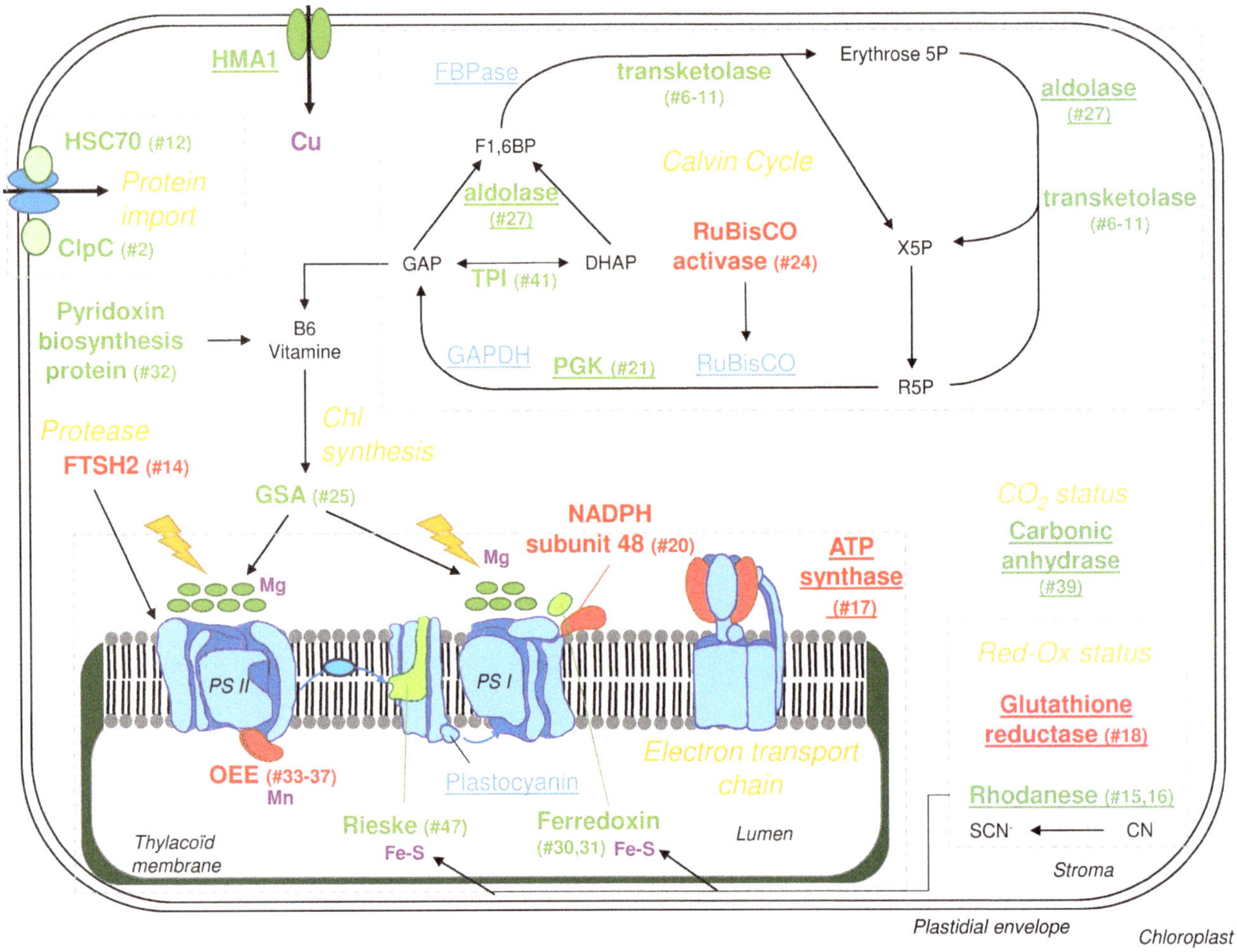

Figure 5. Effect of Cu deficiency on metabolic pathwayspathway in chloroplasts from old leaves of *B. napus*. Bold red indicates a decrease in the amount of protein while bold green indicates an increase. Spot number(s) corresponding to proteins identified in table 3 are indicated in parentheses. Intermediate metabolites are in black, proteins not identified in 2D–E analysis are in blue. Pathways are encircled by grey dashed lines and named in orange italics. Underlines indicate Cu binding and/or known Cu regulation. Other elements known to bind and/or regulate proteins are indicated in purple. PS I: Photosystem I; PS II Photosystem II; R5P: ribulose-5-phosphate; X5P: xylose-5-phosphate; F1,6BP: Fructose-1,6-bisphosphate; GAPDH: GlycerAldehyde Phosphate DeHydrogenase; PGK: PhosphoGlucoKinase; GAP: GlycerAldehyde-3-Phosphate; FBPase: Fructose-1,6-BisPhosphatase; TPI: Triose Phosphate Isomerase; GSA: Glutamate-1-Semialdehyde 2,1-Aminomutase; OEE: Oxygen Evolving Enhancer; Chl: Chlorophyll; CN: cyanate; SCN: Thiocyanate.

family members (#15 to 16), previously described as protecting [Fe-S] clusters [57] in addition to their role in cyanate detoxification.

Previous studies [52,58] highlighted the transcription factor SPL7 (SQUAMOSA-promoter binding link protein 7) which seems to coordinate the early response to Cu deficiency by targeting a Cu response element (CuRE) in the promoter of genes differentially expressed during Cu deficiency. Unfortunately, we couldn't performed an analysis on promoters of genes corresponding to the proteins presented in table 3 as *B. napus* genome sequence is not yet available. However, regulation seems to be complex as Cu deficiency induces a down-regulation at transcript level of carbonic anhydrase [52], but it was up-regulated at protein level in our study (#39). It should be noted that the Carbonic anhydrase regulation is independent from SPL7 [52] and thus its regulation should not be directly induced by Cu deficiency. Moreover, previous studies on Cu deficiency also reported a variation of microRNAs [51,52] or proteases ([59] as well as FTSH2 #14, Table 3 and Figure 5) that could impact on the translation and the proteolysis and thus lead to differences between transcriptomic and proteomic results.

Crosstalk between Cu, [Fe-S] and Mo

Surprisingly, among all quantified mineral nutrients, only Mo uptake was strongly increased in Cu-depleted plants (Figure 1) and this was further linked to strong up-regulation of *MOT1* gene in roots (Figure 2).

The relation between Mo and Cu homeostasis has been reported several times but remains poorly explained [60–63]. As an example, in lesser yam (*Dioscorea esculenta*) [63], molybdenum reached a higher concentration in Cu depleted plants than in plants submitted to any other nutrient deficiencies.

The crosstalk between Cu-Mo and Cu-[Fe-S] established from the literature and the present study are summarised in Figure 6 and can explain the up-regulation of Mo uptake (Figure 1) and expression of [Fe-S] proteins (Rieske #47 and Ferredoxin #30, 31, table 3) by Cu deficiency. Indeed, the chloroplast produces its own [Fe-S] clusters through the SUF (sulfur assimilation proteins)

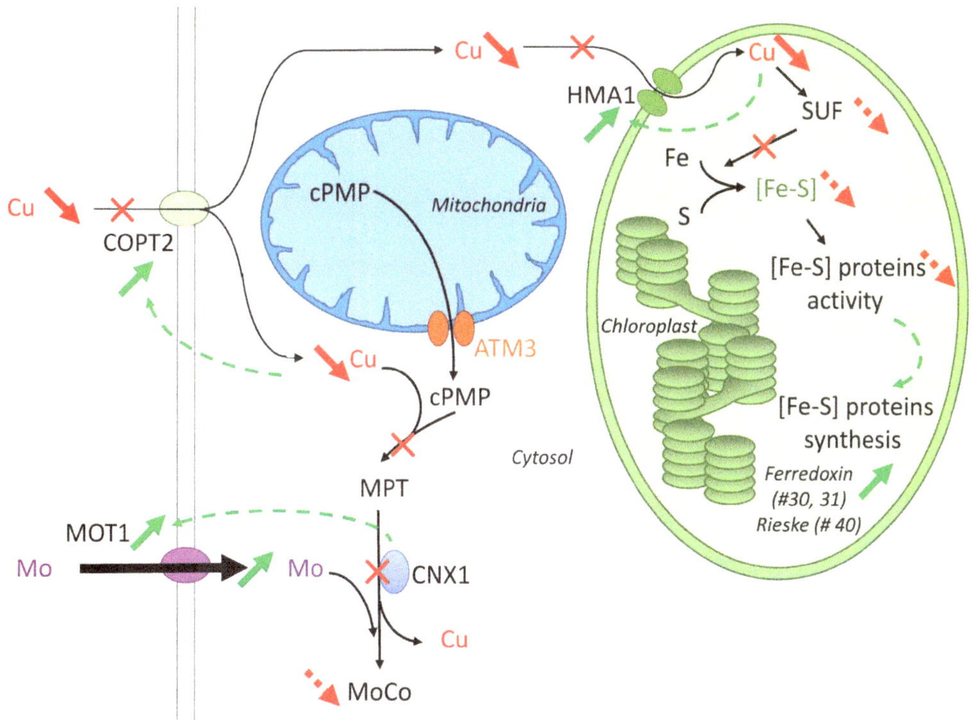

Figure 6. Crosstalk between Cu, [Fe-S] and Mo. Bold arrows indicate variation (green: increase; red: decrease). Full arrows represent observations from this study while dashed arrows have been deduced from the literature. The synthesis of chloroplastic [Fe-S] clusters is controlled by SUF (Sulphur Assimilation Protein), itself controlled by the level of Cu. On the other hand, in the mitochondria, the MoCo precursor cPMP, is exported through mitochondrial membrane by support of the ATM3 transporters. In the cytosol, the second and third steps of MoCo biosynthesis are highly dependent on Cu levels. MoCo is then incorporated into Mo proteins such as Nitrate reductase and into Mo-[Fe-S] proteins such as Xanthine dehydrogenase. The up-regulation of Copt2, HMA1 and Mot1 could be explained by feedback signals due to a low [Cu] in cell, in cytosol and an impairment of CNX1 activity respectively. cPMP: cyclic Pyranopterin MonoPhosphate; MPT: MolybdoPTerin; ATM: ATP-binding cassette Transporters of Mitochondria.

machinery [64], which may be inhibited by Cu deficiency, as previously described in *Bacillus subtilis* [65]. As previously discussed, our leaf proteomic analysis revealed two identified proteins that were over-expressed during Cu deficiency, Ferredoxin and Rieske protein which contain [Fe-S] clusters (#30, 31, 47, Table 3, Figure 6). We may hypothesized that their activity was lowered due to [Fe-S] cluster destabilization by Cu-depletion. This should lead to the observed up-regulation of both proteins to compensate for a possible loss of activity. To minimize the effect of Cu deficiency in chloroplast, the Cu transport across Chloroplast membrane is stimulated through the up regulation of *HMA1* (Figure 2.C, 5, 6).

MOT1 was previously identified as a S transporter (*SULTR5;2*) and it was identified very recently as a high affinity transporter of Mo [45]. Its localization remains unclear (mitochondrial membrane [46] or plasma membrane [45]). Its precise function has not been reported yet, but its importance for an efficient Mo uptake is acknowledged [66]. At cellular level, Mo is essentially used by the Molybdenum Cofactor (MoCo) which is essential for key enzymes such as nitrate reductase and aldehyde oxidase [66]. The first step of the MoCo biosynthesis occurs in the mitochondria and produces cPMP (Figure 6, [67]). cPMP is then exported across the mitochondria membrane by support of the ATM3 transporter [68]. In the cytosol, it must bind Cu in order to be metabolised into MPT representing a step that should be affected in Cu depleted plants. Then, the CNX1 multidomain protein releases Cu and inserts Mo from MPT to give a functional MoCo molecule [69]. It has been reported that CNX1 binds to the cytoskeleton [70] and could have a role as a Mo sensor, interacting with MOT1 transporter to regulates Mo concentration in the cell [71]. Overall, it would explain how the Cu deficiency indirectly up-regulates the Mo uptake through the increase of MOT1 expression. On the other side, a transcriptomic analysis of *Arabidopsis thaliana* WT and *mot1* mutants submitted to Mo deficiency [72] did not reveal a modification of the expression of genes involved in Cu metabolism.

The impairment of Mo metabolism could also be the cause of Ferredoxin and Rieske up-regulation. Indeed, a strong crosstalk exists between Fe and Mc metabolisms: some proteins involved in MoCo biosynethesis are Fe-S (but these Fe-S clusters assembly are independent from the SUF machinery) [66], and Ferredoxin transcripts were up-regulated during an Mo deficiency in *mot1* mutants [72].

Acknowledgments

We are most grateful to the PLATIN' (Plateau d'Isotopie de Normandie) core facility for all element analysis used in this study and the authors deeply appreciate the technical help of Josette Bonnefoy and Marie-Paule Bataillé. The authors thank Laurence Cantrill for improving the English in the manuscript. The authors deeply thank the reviewers for greatly improving the quality of this manuscript with their comments.

Author Contributions

Conceived and designed the experiments: VB AO PE JCY FC. Performed the experiments: VB AM MG JMGM TJ LC. Analyzed the data: VB AM

MG LC. Contributed reagents/materials/analysis tools: MG JMGM TJ LC. Contributed to the writing of the manuscript: VB AO PE.

References

1. Allen L, World Health Organization, Food and Agriculture Organization of the United Nations (2006) Guidelines on food fortification with micronutrients. Geneva; Rome: World Health Organization; Food and Agriculture Organization of the United Nations.
2. Collins JF, Klevay LM (2011) Copper. Adv Nutr 2: 520–522. doi:10.3945/an.111.001222.
3. Steinnes E (2009) Soils and geomedicine. Environ Geochem Health 31: 523–535. doi:10.1007/s10653-009-9257-2.
4. White PJ, Broadley MR (2005) Biofortifying crops with essential mineral elements. Trends Plant Sci 10: 586–593. doi:10.1016/j.tplants.2005.10.001.
5. Ruston D, Great Britain. Office for National Statistics. Social Survey Division, Medical Research Council. Human Nutrition Research, Great Britain. Food Standards Agency (2004) The national diet & nutrition survey: adults aged 19 to 64 years: volume 4: nutritional status (anthropometry and blood analytes), blood pressure and physical activity. London: TSO.
6. ANSES (2012) Anses Table Ciqual 2012 Composition nutritionnelle des aliments. Ciqual Fr Food Comp Table Version 2012. Available: http://www.ansespro.fr/TableCIQUAL/index.htm. Accessed 11 February 2014.
7. Bouis I (2012) Biofortification: Leveraging agriculture to reduce hidden hunger. Ed Shenggen Fan Rajul Pandya-Lorch: 83.
8. Fan M-S, Zhao F-J, Fairweather-Tait SJ, Poulton PR, Dunham SJ, et al. (2008) Evidence of decreasing mineral density in wheat grain over the last 160 years. J Trace Elem Med Biol Organ Soc Miner Trace Elem GMS 22: 315–324. doi:10.1016/j.jtemb.2008.07.002.
9. Garvin DF, Welch RM, Finley JW (2006) Historical shifts in the seed mineral micronutrient concentration of US hard red winter wheat germplasm. J Sci Food Agric 86: 2213–2220. doi:10.1002/jsfa.2601.
10. Peverill KI, Sparrow LA, Reuter DJ (1999) Soil Analysis: An Interpretation Manual. Csiro Publishing. 427 p.
11. Alloway BJ (2013) Bioavailability of Elements in Soil. In: Selinus O, editor. Essentials of Medical Geology. Springer Netherlands. 351–373. Available: http://link.springer.com/chapter/10.1007/978-94-007-4375-5_15. Accessed 11 February 2014.
12. Andersen P (2007) A Review of Micronutrient Problems in the Cultivated Soil of Nepal. Mt Res Dev 27: 331–335. doi:10.1659/mrd.0915.
13. Yruela I (2013) Transition metals in plant photosynthesis. Metallomics 5: 1090–1109. doi:10.1039/C3MT00086A.
14. Yruela I (2009) Copper in plants: acquisition, transport and interactions. Funct Plant Biol 36: 409. doi:10.1071/FP08288.
15. Hänsch R, Mendel RR (2009) Physiological functions of mineral micronutrients (Cu, Zn, Mn, Fe, Ni, Mo, B, Cl). Curr Opin Plant Biol 12: 259–266. doi:10.1016/j.pbi.2009.05.006.
16. Tan Y-F, O'Toole N, Taylor NL, Millar AH (2010) Divalent Metal Ions in Plant Mitochondria and Their Role in Interactions with Proteins and Oxidative Stress-Induced Damage to Respiratory Function. Plant Physiol 152: 747–761. doi:10.1104/pp.109.147942.
17. Bailey E, Stirpe F, Taylor CB (1968) Regulation of rat liver pyruvate kinase. The effect of preincubation, pH, copper ions, fructose 1,6-diphosphate and dietary changes on enzyme activity. Biochem J 108: 427–436.
18. Kung C-CS, Huang W-N, Huang Y-C, Yeh K-C (2006) Proteomic survey of copper-binding proteins in Arabidopsis roots by immobilized metal affinity chromatography and mass spectrometry. Proteomics 6: 2746–2758. doi:10.1002/pmic.200500108.
19. Tainer JA, Getzoff ED, Richardson JS, Richardson DC (1983) Structure and mechanism of copper, zinc superoxide dismutase. Nature 306: 284–287. doi:10.1038/306284a0.
20. Broadley M, Brown P, Cakmak I, Rengel Z, Zhao F (2012) Chapter 7 - Function of Nutrients: Micronutrients. In: Marschner P, editor. Marschner's Mineral Nutrition of Higher Plants (Third Edition). San Diego: Academic Press. 191–248. Available: http://www.sciencedirect.com/science/article/pii/B9780123849052000078. Accessed 14 April 2014.
21. Grusak MA, Cakmak I (2005) 12 Methods to improve the crop-delivery of minerals to humans and livestock. Plant Nutr Genomics: 265.
22. Chavez AL, Bedoya JM, Sánchez T, Iglesias C, Ceballos H, et al. (2000) Iron, carotene, and ascorbic acid in cassava roots and leaves. Food Nutr Bull 21: 410–413.
23. Dubousset L, Etienne P, Avice JC (2010) Is the remobilization of S and N reserves for seed filling of winter oilseed rape modulated by sulphate restrictions occurring at different growth stages? J Exp Bot 61: 4313–4324. doi:10.1093/jxb/erq233.
24. Etienne P, Desclos M, Le Gou L, Gombert J, Bonnefoy J, et al. (2007) N-protein mobilisation associated with the leaf senescence process in oilseed rape is concomitant with the disappearance of trypsin inhibitor activity. Funct Plant Biol 34: 895–906.
25. Desclos M, Dubousset L, Etienne P, Le Caherec F, Satoh H, et al. (2008) A proteomic profiling approach to reveal a novel role of Brassica napus drought 22 kD/water-soluble chlorophyll-binding protein in young leaves during nitrogen remobilization induced by stressful conditions. Plant Physiol 147: 1830–1844. doi:10.1104/pp.108.116905.
26. Avice J-C, Etienne P (2014) Leaf senescence and Nitrogen Remobilization Efficiency in oilseed rape (Brassica napus L.). J Exp Bot in press. doi:JEXBOT/2014/119172, IF: 5,54.
27. Abdallah M, Dubousset L, Meuriot F, Etienne P, Avice J-C, et al. (2010) Effect of mineral sulphur availability on nitrogen and sulphur uptake and remobilization during the vegetative growth of Brassica napus L. J Exp Bot 61: 2635–2646. doi:10.1093/jxb/erq096.
28. Waters BM, Armbrust LC (2013) Optimal copper supply is required for normal plant iron deficiency responses. Plant Signal Behav 8.
29. Garcia-Molina A, Andrés-Colás N, Perea-García A, Neumann U, Dodani SC, et al. (2013) The Arabidopsis COPT6 transport protein functions in copper distribution under copper-deficient conditions. Plant Cell Physiol 54: 1378–1390. doi:10.1093/pcp/pct088.
30. Deng F, Yamaji N, Xia J, Ma JF (2013) A member of the heavy metal P-type ATPase OsHMA5 is involved in xylem loading of copper in rice. Plant Physiol 163: 1353–1362. doi:10.1104/pp.113.226225.
31. Higashi Y, Takechi K, Takano H, Takio S (2013) Involvement of microRNA in copper deficiency-induced repression of chloroplastic CuZn-superoxide dismutase genes in the moss Physcomitrella patens. Plant Cell Physiol 54: 1345–1355. doi:10.1093/pcp/pct084.
32. Wintz H, Fox T, Wu Y-Y, Feng V, Chen W, et al. (2003) Expression Profiles of Arabidopsis thaliana in Mineral Deficiencies Reveal Novel Transporters Involved in Metal Homeostasis. J Biol Chem 278: 47644–47653. doi:10.1074/jbc.M309338200.
33. Mora V, Bacaicoa E, Zamarreño A-M, Aguirre E, Garnica M, et al. (2010) Action of humic acid on promotion of cucumber shoot growth involves nitrate-related changes associated with the root-to-shoot distribution of cytokinins, polyamines and mineral nutrients. J Plant Physiol 167: 633–642. doi:10.1016/j.jplph.2009.11.018.
34. Livak KJ, Schmittgen TD (2001) Analysis of Relative Gene Expression Data Using Real-Time Quantitative PCR and the $2-\Delta\Delta CT$ Method. Methods 25: 402–408. doi:10.1006/meth.2001.1262.
35. Wang W, Scali M, Vignani R, Spadafora A, Sensi E, et al. (2003) Protein extraction for two-dimensional electrophoresis from olive leaf, a plant tissue containing high levels of interfering compounds. ELECTROPHORESIS 24: 2369–2375. doi:10.1002/elps.200305500.
36. Méchin V, Consoli L, Le Guilloux M, Damerval C (2003) An efficient solubilization buffer for plant proteins focused in immobilized pH gradients. Proteomics 3: 1299–1302. doi:10.1002/pmic.200300450.
37. Bradford MM (1976) A rapid and sensitive method for the quantitation of microgram quantities of protein utilizing the principle of protein-dye binding. Anal Biochem 72: 248–254.
38. Blum H, Beier H, Gross HJ (1987) Improved silver staining of plant proteins, RNA and DNA in polyacrylamide gels. ELECTROPHORESIS 8: 93–99. doi:10.1002/elps.1150080203.
39. Bradová J, Matějová E (2008) Comparison of the Results of SDS PAGE and Chip Electrophoresis of Wheat Storage Proteins. Chromatographia 67: 83–88. doi:10.1365/s10337-008-0545-2.
40. Matrix science (n.d.) Mascot search engine | Protein identification software for mass spec data. Available: http://www.matrixscience.com/. Accessed 11 February 2014.
41. RefSeq: NCBI Reference Sequence Database (n.d.). Available: http://www.ncbi.nlm.nih.gov/refseq/. Accessed 22 April 2014.
42. Brassica Genome Gateway (n.d.). Available: http://brassica.nbi.ac.uk/. Accessed 11 February 2014.
43. BLAST: Basic Local Alignment Search Tool (n.d.). Available: http://blast.ncbi.nlm.nih.gov/Blast.cgi?CMD=Web&PAGE_TYPE=BlastHome. Accessed 14 February 2014.
44. Yuan JS, Reed A, Chen F, Stewart CN (2006) Statistical analysis of real-time PCR data. BMC Bioinformatics 7: 85. doi:10.1186/1471-2105-7-85.
45. Tomatsu H, Takano J, Takahashi H, Watanabe-Takahashi A, Shibagaki N, et al. (2007) An Arabidopsis thaliana high-affinity molybdate transporter required for efficient uptake of molybdate from soil. Proc Natl Acad Sci 104: 18807–18812. doi:10.1073/pnas.0706373104.
46. Baxter I, Muthukumar B, Park HC, Buchner P, Lahner B, et al. (2008) Variation in molybdenum content across broadly distributed populations of Arabidopsis thaliana is controlled by a mitochondrial molybdenum transporter (MOT1). PLoS Genet 4: e1000004.
47. Ravet K, Danford FL, Dihle A, Pittarello M, Pilon M (2011) Spatiotemporal analysis of copper homeostasis in Populus trichocarpa reveals an integrated molecular remodeling for a preferential allocation of copper to plastocyanin in the chloroplasts of developing leaves. Plant Physiol 157: 1300–1312. doi:10.1104/pp.111.183350.
48. Marschner P (2012) Marschner's Mineral Nutrition of Higher Plants. Academic Press. 668 p.

49. Del Pozo T, Cambiazo V, González M (2010) Gene expression profiling analysis of copper homeostasis in Arabidopsis thaliana. Biochem Biophys Res Commun 393: 248–252. doi:10.1016/j.bbrc.2010.01.111.
50. Burda K, Kruk J, Schmid GH, Strzalka K (2003) Inhibition of oxygen evolution in Photosystem II by Cu(II) ions is associated with oxidation of cytochrome b559. Biochem J 371: 597–601. doi:10.1042/BJ20021265.
51. Bernal M, Casero D, Singh V, Wilson GT, Grande A, et al. (2012) Transcriptome sequencing identifies SPL7-regulated copper acquisition genes FRO4/FRO5 and the copper dependence of iron homeostasis in Arabidopsis. Plant Cell Online 24: 738–761.
52. Andrés-Colás N, Perea-García A, de Andrés SM, Garcia-Molina A, Dorcey E, et al. (2013) Comparison of global responses to mild deficiency and excess copper levels in Arabidopsis seedlings. Metallomics 5: 1234–1246.
53. Slovacek RE, Monahan BC (1983) Reductive activation of fructose-1,6-bisphosphatase and the peroxide effect on chloroplast photosynthesis. Arch Biochem Biophys 224: 310–318.
54. Munoz-Bertomeu J, Cascales-Minana B, Mulet JM, Baroja-Fernandez E, Pozueta-Romero J, et al. (2009) Plastidial Glyceraldehyde-3-Phosphate Dehydrogenase Deficiency Leads to Altered Root Development and Affects the Sugar and Amino Acid Balance in Arabidopsis. Plant Physiol 151: 541–558. doi:10.1104/pp.109.143701.
55. Mooney S, Hellmann H (2010) Vitamin B6: Killing two birds with one stone? Phytochemistry 71: 495–501. doi:10.1016/j.phytochem.2009.12.015.
56. Hennig M, Grimm B, Contestabile R, John RA, Jansonius JN (1997) Crystal structure of glutamate-1-semialdehyde aminomutase: an alpha2-dimeric vitamin B6-dependent enzyme with asymmetry in structure and active site reactivity. Proc Natl Acad Sci U S A 94: 4866–4871.
57. Cereda A, Carpen A, Picariello G, Tedeschi G, Pagani S (2009) The lack of rhodanese RhdA affects the sensitivity of Azotobacter vinelandii to oxidative events. Biochem J 418: 135. doi:10.1042/BJ20081218.
58. Yamasaki H, Hayashi M, Fukazawa M, Kobayashi Y, Shikanai T (2009) SQUAMOSA promoter binding protein–like7 is a central regulator for copper homeostasis in Arabidopsis. Plant Cell Online 21: 347–361.
59. Castruita M, Casero D, Karpowicz SJ, Kropat J, Vieler A, et al. (2011) Systems Biology Approach in Chlamydomonas Reveals Connections between Copper Nutrition and Multiple Metabolic Steps. Plant Cell Online 23: 1273–1292. doi:10.1105/tpc.111.084400.
60. Lidon FC, Henriques FS (1993) Effects of copper toxicity on growth and the uptake and translocation of metals in rice plants. J Plant Nutr 16: 1449–1464. doi:10.1080/01904169309364626.
61. Wallace A, Romney EM, Alexander GV, Kinnear J (1977) Phytotoxicity and some interactions of the essential trace metals iron, manganese, molybdenum, zinc, copper, and boron. Commun Soil Sci Plant Anal 8: 741–750. doi:10.1080/00103627709366768.
62. Basak A, Mandal LN, Haldar M (1982) Interaction of phosphorus and molybdenum in relation to uptake and utilization of molybdenum, phosphorus, zinc, copper and manganese by rice. Plant Soil 68: 261–269.
63. O'Sullivan JN, Ernest J (2007) Nutrient deficiencies in lesser yam (Dioscorea esculenta) characterized using constant–water table sand culture. J Plant Nutr Soil Sci 170: 273–282. doi:10.1002/jpln.200625049.
64. Pilon M, Abdel-Ghany SE, Van Hoewyk D, Ye H, Pilon-Smits EAH (2006) Biogenesis of iron-sulfur cluster proteins in plastids. Genet Eng (N Y) 27: 101–117.
65. Chillappagari S, Seubert A, Trip H, Kuipers OP, Marahiel MA, et al. (2010) Copper Stress Affects Iron Homeostasis by Destabilizing Iron-Sulfur Cluster Formation in Bacillus subtilis. J Bacteriol 192: 2512–2524. doi:10.1128/JB.00058-10.
66. Bittner F (2014) Molybdenum metabolism in plants and crosstalk to iron. Front Plant Sci 5. Available: http://www.ncbi.nlm.nih.gov/pmc/articles/PMC3916724/. Accessed 18 August 2014.
67. Mendel RR (2013) The Molybdenum Cofactor. J Biol Chem 288: 13165–13172. doi:10.1074/jbc.R113.455311.
68. Teschner J, Lachmann N, Schulze J, Geisler M, Selbach K, et al. (2010) A Novel Role for Arabidopsis Mitochondrial ABC Transporter ATM3 in Molybdenum Cofactor Biosynthesis. Plant Cell Online 22: 468–480. doi:10.1105/tpc.109.068478.
69. Kuper J, Llamas A, Hecht H-J, Mendel RR, Schwarz G (2004) Structure of the molybdopterin-bound Cnx1G domain links molybdenum and copper metabolism. Nature 430: 803–806. doi:10.1038/nature02681.
70. Schwarz G, Schulze J, Bittner F, Eilers T, Kuper J, et al. (2000) The Molybdenum Cofactor Biosynthetic Protein Cnx1 Complements Molybdate-Repairable Mutants, Transfers Molybdenum to the Metal Binding Pterin, and Is Associated with the Cytoskeleton. Plant Cell Online 12: 2455–2471. doi:10.1105/tpc.12.12.2455.
71. Tejada-Jiménez M, Galván A, Fernández E, Llamas Á (2009) Homeostasis of the micronutrients Ni, Mo and Cl with specific biochemical functions. Curr Opin Plant Biol 12: 358–363. doi:10.1016/j.pbi.2009.04.012.
72. Ide Y, Kusano M, Oikawa A, Fukushima A, Tomatsu H, et al. (2011) Effects of molybdenum deficiency and defects in molybdate transporter MOT1 on transcript accumulation and nitrogen/sulphur metabolism in Arabidopsis thaliana. J Exp Bot 62: 1483–1497. doi:10.1093/jxb/erq345.
73. Ferrer J-L, Ravanel S, Robert M, Dumas R (2004) Crystal Structures of Cobalamin-independent Methionine Synthase Complexed with Zinc, Homocysteine, and Methyltetrahydrofolate. J Biol Chem 279: 44235–44238. doi:10.1074/jbc.C400325200.
74. Komenda J, Knoppová J, Krynická V, Nixon PJ, Tichý M (2010) Role of FtsH2 in the repair of Photosystem II in mutants of the cyanobacterium Synechocystis PCC 6803 with impaired assembly or stability of the CaMn4 cluster. Biochim Biophys Acta BBA - Bioenerg 1797: 566–575. doi:10.1016/j.bbabio.2010.02.006.
75. Volini M, Van Sweringen B, Chen F-S (1978) Effects of metal-ion binding on rhodanese activity. Arch Biochem Biophys 191: 205–215. doi:10.1016/0003-9861(78)90083-8.
76. Berry A, Marshall KE (1993) Identification of zinc-binding ligands in the class II fructose-1,6-bisphosphate aldolase of Escherichia coli. FEBS Lett 318: 11–16.
77. Mahmoud YA, el Souod SM, Niehaus WG (1995) Purification and characterization of malate dehydrogenase from Cryptococcus neoformans. Arch Biochem Biophys 322: 69–75.
78. Ikeuchi M, Inoue Y (1986) Characterization of O2 evolution by a wheat photosystem II reaction center complex isolated by a simplified method: disjunction of secondary acceptor quinone and enhanced Ca2+ demand. Arch Biochem Biophys 247: 97–107.
79. Giulia M, Caricato R, Elena M, Erroi E, Schettino T (2012) Carbonic Anhydrase and Heavy Metals. In: Ekinci D, editor. Biochemistry. InTech. Available: http://www.intechopen.com/books/biochemistry/carbonic-anhydrase-and-heavy-metals. Accessed 19 February 2014.

15

Vacuolar-Iron-Transporter1-Like Proteins Mediate Iron Homeostasis in Arabidopsis

Julia Gollhofer[1], Roman Timofeev[1], Ping Lan[2], Wolfgang Schmidt[3,4,5], Thomas J. Buckhout[1]*

1 Institute of Biology, Humboldt University Berlin, Berlin, Germany, **2** State Key Laboratory of Soil and Sustainable Agriculture, Institute of Soil Science, Chinese Academy Sciences, Nanjing, PR China, **3** Academia Sinica, Institute of Plant and Microbial Biology, Taipei, Taiwan, **4** Graduate Institute of Biotechnology, National Chung Hsing University, Taichung, Taiwan, **5** Genome and Systems Biology Degree Program, College of Life Science, National Taiwan University, Taipei, Taiwan

Abstract

Iron deficiency is a nutritional problem in plants and reduces crop productivity, quality and yield. With the goal of improving the iron (Fe) storage properties of plants, we have investigated the function of three Arabidopsis proteins with homology to Vacuolar Iron Transporter1 (AtVIT1). Heterologous expression of *Vacuolar Iron Transporter-Like1* (*AtVTL1*; At1g21140), *AtVTL2* (At1g76800) or *AtVTL5* (At3g25190) in the yeast vacuolar Fe transport mutant, *Δccc1*, restored growth in the presence of 4 mM Fe. Isolated vacuoles from yeast expressing either of the *VTL* genes in the *Δccc1* background had a three- to four-fold increase in Fe concentration compared to vacuoles isolated from the untransformed mutant. Transiently expressed GFP-tagged AtVTL1 was localized exclusively and AtVTL2 was localized primarily to the vacuolar membrane of onion epidermis cells. Seedling root growth of the Arabidopsis *nramp3/nramp4* and *vit1-1* mutants was decreased compared to the wild type when seedlings were grown under Fe deficiency. When expressed under the 35S promoter in the *nramp3/nramp4* or *vit1-1* backgrounds, *AtVTL1*, *AtVTL2* or *AtVTL5* restored root growth in both mutants. The seed Fe concentration in the *nramp3/nramp4* mutant overexpressing *AtVTL1*, *AtVTL2* or *AtVTL5* was between 50 and 60% higher than in non-transformed double mutants or wild-type plants. We conclude that the VTL proteins catalyze Fe transport into vacuoles and thus contribute to the regulation of Fe homeostasis *in planta*.

Editor: Stephan Neil Witt, Louisiana State University Health Sciences Center, United States of America

Funding: This work was supported by the Deutsche Forschungsgemeinschaft to TJB (BU 713: 4-1). The funders had no role in study design, data collection and analysis, decision to publish,or preparation of the manuscript.

Competing Interests: The authors have declared that no competing interests exist.

* Email: thomas.buckhout@rz.hu-berlin.de

Introduction

Regulation of the cellular Fe concentration poses the problem of balancing Fe deficiency against toxicity [1]. Equilibrium is maintained by strict regulation of Fe uptake and storage in the cell. Uptake of soil Fe in Arabidopsis is catalyzed by the Fe^{2+} transporter AtIRT1 [2,3]. Transcription of *AtIRT1* is greatly increased under conditions of Fe deficiency [2], and AtIRT1 is also post-translationally modified to regulate its partitioning between the trans-Golgi network and plasma membranes [4]. Prior to transport, soil Fe^{3+}-chelates are reduced by the plasma membrane ferric reductase, AtFRO2 [5]. The coupling of uptake to reduction is a hallmark of strategy I plants, and an analogous mechanism is also found in *Chlamydomonas* [6] and *Saccharomyces* [7] among other organisms. The reduction-based acquisition of Fe is aided by secretion of Fe-binding compounds and H^+-ATPase-mediated acidification of the rhizosphere [8,9,10,11].

Once in the cell, Fe^{2+} can be incorporated into proteins or stored in cellular compartments. In chloroplast and presumably mitochondria, several thousand Fe atoms are stored per ferritin molecule [12]. However, in Arabidopsis only 5% of Fe is stored in ferritin, and vacuoles appear to be the major compartment for seed Fe storage [13]. Vacuolar Fe uptake was shown to be catalyzed by the ferroportin homologue, AtFPN2 [14,15], and by the CCC1-like protein AtVIT1 (16); however, the primary substrates of AtFPN2 have been reported to be Ni and Co in addition to Fe [14,15]. AtVIT1 has a specific function in the vacuolar transport of Fe into xylem parenchyma of developing embryos, and the *vit1-1* mutant shows misdistribution of Fe in seeds; although, *vit1-1* mutant seeds have unchanged Fe concentration compared with the wild type [16]. Efflux of Fe from the vacuole is catalyzed by two NRAMP proteins, NRAMP3 and NRAMP4. The double mutant *nramp3/nramp4* shows decreased Fe mobilization from the vacuole in germinating seeds [17].

Two rice orthologs of AtVIT1, OsVIT1 and OsVIT2 [18], and one in tulip, TgVIT1 [19], have been shown to catalyze vacuolar Fe transport. TgVIT1 catalyzes the transport of Fe into the proximal perianth cell vacuole, which was shown to be essential for blue color development in tulips. Both OsVIT1 and OsVIT2 complemented the yeast *Δccc1* mutant, and vacuoles that were isolated from complemented cells had increased Fe and Mn concentrations. In addition, both rice genes complemented the Zn transport mutant, *Δzrc1*, and vacuoles isolated from these cells also had an increased Zn concentration [18]. The transcript abundance of *OsVIT2* increased within hours in roots and shoots grown under conditions of excess Fe (4 mM) but decreased in roots and shoots when rice was grown under Fe-deficient conditions. In contrast, *OsVIT1* expression responded only weakly to changes in the Fe status. *OsVIT1* and *OsVIT2* were expressed in flag leaf blades and sheaths, respectively. Consistent with the localization of expression, the *osvit1-1* and *osvit2-1* T-DNA knockout mutants had decreased Fe and Zn content in flag leaves with no change in Mn. Seeds of *osvit1-1* and *osvit2-1* had correspondingly increased Fe and Zn content. OsVIT1 and OsVIT2 were shown to regulate the partitioning of Fe and Zn in rice between source and sink tissues [18].

In an analysis of the transcriptional response of Arabidopsis roots to Fe deficiency, we and others have identified three genes whose mRNA abundance decreased in Fe-deficient roots and whose putative amino acid sequences showed significant homology to AtVIT1 and consequently also to yeast Ccc1p [20,21,22]. These genes belong to a small, five-membered family that has been annotated as nodulin or nodulin-like in databases. These genes will be subsequently referred to as *Vacuolar Iron Transporter-Like* (*VTL*). The *VTL* family was found both in mono- and dicotyledon plants, as well as *Chamydomonas* and *Physcomitrella*. Promoter-β-glucuronidase (GUS) assays showed expression of *AtVTL1* in roots, hypocotyls, and cotyledons of seedlings with the greatest activity associated with the vascular bundle and the root stele [21]. The promoter activity was greatly reduced in Fe-deficient seedlings, consistent with the transcriptional analysis. In the present report, we show that AtVTL1 (At1g21140) and AtVTL2 (At1g76800) are localized to the vacuolar membrane in plants, and that AtVTL1, AtVTL2 and AtVTL5 (At3g25190) complement the *Δccc1* mutation in *Saccharomyces*. Over-expression of *AtVTL1*, *AtVTL2* and *AtVTL5* also complemented the Fe deficiency-dependent root growth phenotype in the *nramp3/nramp4* double mutation and the *vit1-1* mutation in Arabidopsis seedlings. These results indicate that the three members of the *VTL* family are involved in regulation of cellular Fe homeostasis, likely by acting as vacuolar Fe transporters.

Materials and Methods

Arabidopsis Growth Conditions

Arabidopsis seeds were surface-sterilized, vernalized and grown hydroponically as described by Gollhofer et al. [21]. Seeds of the accession Columbia (Col-0) were obtained from the Arabidopsis Biological Resource Center (Ohio State University, Columbus, Ohio). Plants were grown hydroponically according to the method described by Buckhout et al. [20], and the hydroponic nutrient solution was composed of KNO_3 (3 mM), $MgSO_4$ (0.5 mM), $CaCl_2$ (1.5 mM), K_2SO_4 (1.5 mM), NaH_2PO_4 (1.5 mM), H_3BO_3 (25 μM), $MnCl_2$ (1 μM), $ZnSO_4$ (0.5 μM), $(NH_4)_6Mo_7O_{24}$ (0.05 μM) $CuSO_4$ (0.3 μM), Fe-EDTA (40 μM) with the pH adjusted to 6.0 with KOH. For growth on Petri dishes, the method of Santi and Schmidt [11] was used. The medium contained: KNO_3 (5 mM), $Ca(NO_3)_2$ (2 mM), $MgSO_4$ (2 mM), KH_2PO_4 (2.5 mM), $MnCl_2$ (14 μM), H_3BO_3 (70 μM), $ZnSO_4$ (1 μM), $CuSO_4$ (0.5 μM), Na_2MoO_4 (0.2 μM), $CoCl_2$ (0.01 μM), NaCl (10 μM), and Fe-EDTA (40 μM). Sucrose (44 mM) and 5 mM MES (2-[N-morpholino]ethanesulfonic acid) were included, and the pH was adjusted to 5.5. The medium was solidified with 0.8% agar (Fluka, Taufkirchen, Germany). For determination of root growth seedlings were photographed at the appropriate time, the photographs enlarged and root length measured.

Analysis of the Fe Concentration in Arabidopsis Seeds and in Yeast Vacuoles

The Fe content in seeds was determined by the BPDS method [23]. Dried and powdered samples (4–8 mg) were mixed with glass beads (~20; ø 425–600 μm) in 2 ml Eppendorf tubes and incubated at 95°C in 75 μl nitric acid (65%) for 6 h to digest the plant material. Fifty μl of H_2O_2 (30%) was added and the solution incubated at 56°C for 2 h. The volume was adjusted to 200 μl with water. Twenty μl of this solution were diluted in 980 μl of BPDS buffer (1 mM bathophenanthroline disulfonic acid, 0.6 M sodium acetate and 0.48 M hydroxylammonium chloride). The concentration of Fe-BPDS was determined photometrically at 535 nm. A standard calibration curve was prepared by dilution of a stock $FeSO_4$ solution dissolved in 0.1 N HCl. Samples were measured in triplicate and the experiments were conducted at least three times.

Yeast Growth, Complementation and Isolation of Vacuoles

The yeast strain used in this study was *Δccc1* (*ura3, leu2, his3, ade2, can1, CCC1::HIS3*) in DY150. Yeast transformation was carried out by the Li-acetate method [24]. Yeast growth was determined under selection on agar plates with 10^0–10^5 cells per dot.

Vacuoles were isolated as described by Li et al. [25]. Briefly, cells harvest at $OD_{600} = 0.4$ were suspended in 30 ml of 0.1 M Tris-HCl (pH 9.3) buffer containing 10 mM dithiothreitol and incubated for 10 min at 30°C. The cells were washed once with spheroplast buffer (1.2 M sorbitol, 20 mM K-phosphate, pH 7.4) and incubated with 20 μg/ml lyticase for 30 min at 30°C. Spheroplasts were collected by centrifugation at 3,500 *g* for 5 min., and the pellet was resuspended in 10 ml of 15% Ficoll buffer (15% Ficoll (Sigma) in 0.2 M sorbitol and 10 mM PIPES-KOH, pH 6.8). Fifty μg/ml DEAE-Dextran (Amersham Pharmacia Biotech) were added to the spheroplasts, and the sample was incubated for 3 min. on ice and for an additional 5 min. at 30°C. The lysate (10 ml) was transferred to SW28 centrifuge tubes (Beckman Instruments) and overlaid with 10 ml of 8% Ficoll, 10 ml of 4% Ficoll, and 10 ml of 0% Ficoll. The tubes were centrifuged at 110,000 *g* for 3 h. The vacuolar fraction was collected from the 0%/4% interphase. Fe concentration of yeast vacuoles was determined by the BPDS method [23].

Transformation and Transient Expression of *GFP::VTL*

Arabidopsis wild-type Col-0 was transformed using the floral dip method of Clough and Bent [26]. Transgenic plants were selected for BASTA resistance on potting soil.

Onion epidermal cells were co-bombarded with 2.5 μg of plasmids bearing free GFP or GFP-tagged *VTL* genes (35S:*GFP::AtVTL1* or 35S:*GFP::AtVTL2*) and the vacuole marker plasmid vac-rk CD3 975 [27]. Plasmids were coated on 1 μm gold particles and delivered into onion epidermal cells at a pressure of 900 psi by a PDS 1000/He particle delivery system (BioRad, U.S.A). After bombardment, onion slices (2 cm^2) were placed in a Petri dish containing Murashige and Skoog (MS) salts, 30 g/l sucrose and 1.5% agar (pH = 5.7). Following a minimum of 24 h, the epidermis cells were observed under a confocal laser scanning microscope (Zeiss LSM510 Meta) using a ×63 water objective. Vac-rk CD3 975 images were captured in the 560 to 615 nm range after excitation at 543 nm with a HeNe laser beam. The GFP images were captured in the 505 to 530 nm range after excitation at 488 nm with an argon laser beam. Image overlay was carried out by Z-stack analysis at 0.8 μm intervals and further processed with the projection function under LSM510-Expert Mode software.

qRT-PCR

Total RNA was isolated using TRIsure (Bioline) and treated with DNase using DNAse Kit (Fermentas) as suggested by the manufacturer. cDNA was synthesized using DNA-free RNA with oligo-dT(18) primer and RevertAid reverse transcriptase (Thermo scientific). The cDNA was used as a PCR template in a 10 µl reaction system using the SensiMix SYBR No-ROX Kit (Bioline) with programs recommended by the manufacturer in a CFX96 Realtime system (BioRAD). Three biological replicates were performed for each sample. The $\Delta\Delta C_T$ method was used to determine the relative transcript abundance

Results

Complementation of the yeast mutant *Δccc1* by *AtVTL1*, *AtVTL2* and *AtVTL5*

As in Arabidopsis, the yeast vacuole is the major compartment for Fe storage but also protects the cell from Fe toxicity. The yeast gene *CCC1* encodes a vacuolar Fe^{2+}/Mn^{2+} transporter that catalyzes Fe^{2+} uptake into the vacuole. The *Δccc1* mutant is hypersensitive to Fe toxicity, not growing in the presence of greater than ca. 3 mM Fe [25]. Because of the homology of the VTL family member to yeast Ccc1p and Arabidopsis AtVIT1 and because of the transcriptional repression of *AtVTL1*, *AtVTL2* and *AtVTL5* under conditions of Fe deficiency, the ability of the three *AtVTL* genes to complement the *Δccc1* yeast mutant was investigated. When expressed in yeast, the VTL proteins were effective in complementing of the *Δccc1* phenotype in the order *AtVTL1*> *AtVTL2*> *AtVTL5* (Fig. 1). These results are consistent with an AtVTL-dependent decreased the cytosolic Fe in the *Δccc1* mutant, presumably by transport of Fe into the vacuole.

To test this hypothesis, the Fe concentration in isolated yeast vacuoles was investigated. Intact yeast vacuoles were isolated by floatation through a Ficoll step gradient as described by Li et al. [25]. We confirmed the composition of the vacuolar fraction by re-centrifugation the fraction on a continuous sucrose gradient followed by marker enzyme analysis (Fig. S1). As expected, the vacuole marker, bafilomycin-sensitive ATPase, co-localized with membrane proteins and no detectable plasma membrane (vanadate-sensitive ATPase) or endoplasmic reticulum (NADPH cytochrome c reductase) activities were detected in the gradient. Vacuoles, isolated from log-phase *Δccc1* cells or from *Δccc1* cells transformed with the control vector grown in liquid SD medium containing 1 mM $FeSO_4$, had approximately 2 nmoles Fe per µg protein, whereas *Δccc1* cells expressing *AtVTL1*, *AtVTL2* or *AtVTL5* had a greater than 3-fold higher Fe content (Fig. 2A).

Localization of AtVTL1 was demonstrated by transforming *Δccc1* cells with *AtVTL1* fused to a 3′ His tag (*AtVTL1-H$_6$*). *Δccc1* cells that were transformed with *AtVTL1-H$_6$* complemented the Fe-sensitive phenotype (Fig. S2). Using a His-tag antibody, AtVTL1-H_6 protein was localized to the vacuolar fraction at the 0/4% Ficoll interface (Fig. 2B). Iron was also concentrated in this fraction compared to fractions in other regions of the Ficoll gradient. The immunological signals in the pellet and 15%/8% Ficoll interface were most like the result of vacuolar membranes from ruptured vacuoles that that did not float through the gradient. We demonstrated that AtVTL1 was localized on the yeast vacuolar membrane, where it presumably catalyzed transport of Fe into the yeast vacuole.

Localization of AtVTL1 and AtVTL2 *in planta*

The localization of AtVTL1 and AtVTL2 was investigated in onion epidermis cells. Attempts to localize AtVTL5 in onion or tobacco leaf cells have not been successful. Onion cells were transformed by particle bombardment with 35S:*GFP::VTL1* or 35S:*GFP::VTL2* reporter gene constructs. In the case of AtVTL1, the GFP fluorescence co-localized with the vacuolar marker vac-rk CD3-975 (Fig. 3A, [27]). When cells were plasmolyzed in 0.8 M mannitol, the GFP signal remained associated with the vacuole (Fig. 3B). The localization of AtVTL2 in epidermis cells was predominately associated with the vacuolar membrane (Fig. 3A); however, GFP fluorescence was also found to be associated with the plasma membrane and the cytoplasm upon plasmolysis (Fig. 3B). The localization of the two AtVTL proteins on the onion vacuolar membrane was consistent with the complementation results in *Saccharomyces* and with the increased Fe concentration in vacuoles isolated from *VTL*-expressing yeast cells.

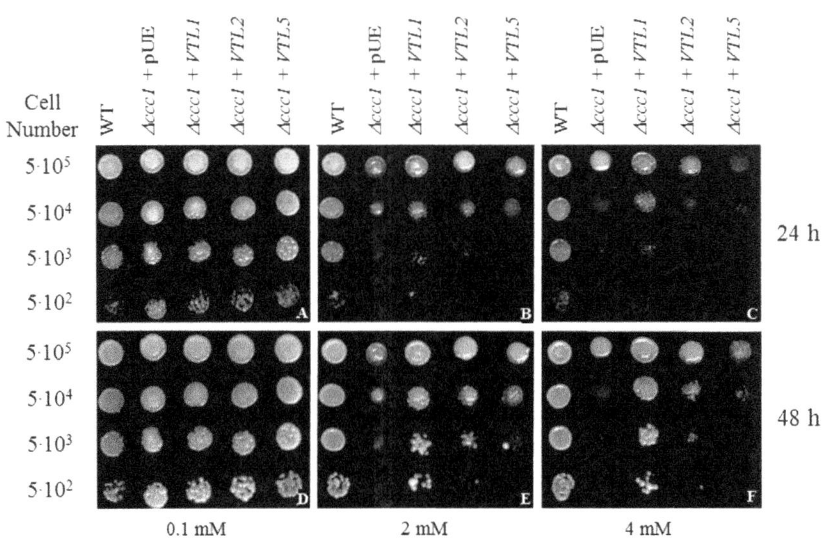

Figure 1. Complementation of the *Δccc1* by heterologous expression of the *VTL* genes. *Δccc1* (vacuolar Fe^{2+}/Mn^{2+} transporter) cells were transformed with each of the three VTL genes or the empty vector (pUE) under the control of the PGK promoter and grown on SD medium containing $FeSO_4$ at the concentrations indicated for 24 or 48 h at 30°C. Cells were plated at the densities indicated in the figure.

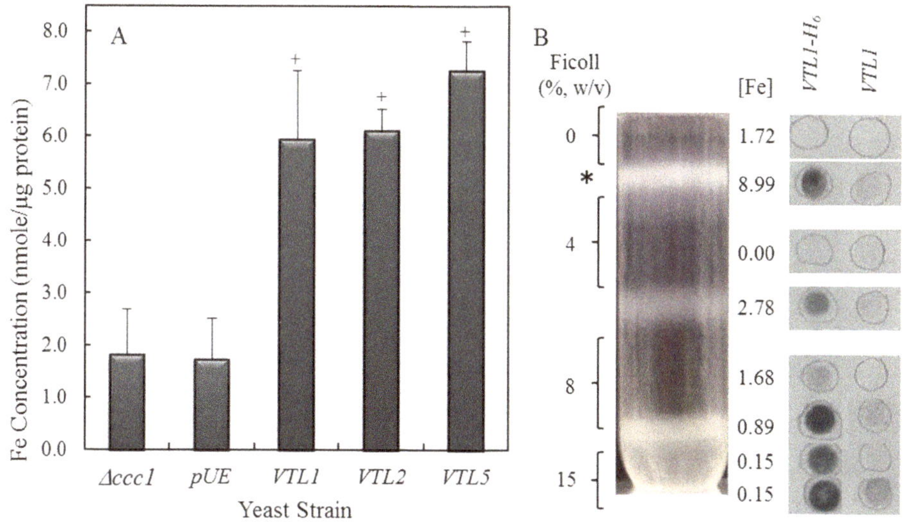

Figure 2. Determination of the Fe concentration in *Δccc1* cells transformed with *AtVTL1, AtVTL2* or *AtVTL5*. (**A**) Shown is the Fe concentration in yeast vacuoles isolated from the *Δccc1* mutant, *Δccc1* transformed with an empty plasmid (pUE), *AtVTL1, AtVTL2* or *AtVTL5*. Error bars indicate the standard error of the mean. Bar graphs labeled with "+" are significantly different for the *Δccc1* mutant ($p<0.05$). (**B**) Vacuoles were isolated from *Δccc1* yeast cells transformed with His-tagged *AtVTL1* (*VTL1-H$_6$*) or with untagged *AtVTL1* (*VTL1*) as a control. AtVTL1-H$_6$ was localized by dot-blots using an anti-His antibody. The positions of the dot-blots are approximate. The Fe concentrations (nmole/µg protein) in the fraction corresponding to the dot-blot are given.

Complementation of the *nramp3/nramp4* and the *vit1-1* mutants

Over-expression of *AtVTL1* in Arabidopsis did not greatly alter Fe content of shoots and roots [21], nor were changes observed in the kinetics of the response to Fe deficiency, as determined by the root plasma membrane Fe^{3+}-chelate reductase and chlorophyll content (Figs. S3A and B). In an attempt to characterize their functions, we have ectopically expressed the *AtVTL* genes in the Arabidopsis *nramp3/nramp4* double mutant background (17). Over-expression was confirmed by semi-quantitative RT-PCR (Fig. S4). Both NRAMP3 and NRAMP4 have been shown to be Fe vacuolar efflux carriers. The double mutant had no obvious phenotype when grown on soil; however, growth of mutant seedlings was retarded shortly after germination on an Fe-deficient substrate [17]. The phenotype was not persistent and disappeared after a few days of growth or with supplemental Fe in the media. Under Fe deficiency root growth of the *nramp3/nramp4* double mutant and of the double mutant transformed with the empty vector (GL1), was greatly inhibited compared to the wild-type control at 5 d following germination (Fig. 4 and Fig. S5; $p<0.001$) [17]. Importantly, over-expression of *AtVTL1*, *AtVTL2* or *AtVTL5* in *nramp3/nramp4* complemented this mutant growth phenotype. The early seedling root length was significantly increased (Fig. 4 and Fig. S5; $p<0.001$) compared to the double mutant; however, the roots were still significantly shorter than those of the wild type ($p<0.001$). Thus, over-expression of *AtVTL1*, *AtVTL2* or *AtVTL5* partially restored the wild-type phenotype in the *nramp3/nramp4* double mutant.

The proposed function of NRAMP3 and NRAMP4 was to mobilize Fe from the vacuole of young seedlings [17]. We hypothesized that over-expression of the AtVTLs might have increased total seed Fe, and thereby increased the Fe supply to the germinating seedling. To test this, we analyzed the Fe concentration in *nramp3/nramp4* seeds that over-expressed the *AtVTL* genes. The results of these analyses demonstrated that the *AtVTL1*, *AtVTL2* or *AtVTL5* over-expressing lines had between 40 and 60% increased Fe concentration compared to either the wild type or the *nramp3/nramp4* double mutant (Fig. 5; $p<0.01$). These results supported the concept that an increased content of Fe in the seeds could have supplied the embryo with sufficient Fe even when efflux from the vacuole through the NRAMP transporters was compromised.

As mentioned above, the CCC1-like protein, AtVIT1, is localized on the vacuolar membrane and functions in the transport of Fe into the parenchyma cell of the provascular strands in developing embryos. The *vit1-1* mutant showed misdistribution of Fe; although, *vit1-1* mutant seeds had unchanged Fe content compared to the wild type (Fig. 5) [16]. *vit1-1* had a severely chlorotic phenotype when grown on alkaline soil [16]. In addition, we observed that *vit1-1* displayed a short-root phenotype similar to the *nramp3/nramp4* mutant when grown on Fe-deficient media in the presence of the Fe^{2+} chelator Ferrozine (Fig. 6 and Fig. S6). Over-expression of *AtVTL1*, *AtVTL2* or *AtVTL5* restored root growth to greater than the wild-type length ($p>0.001$), thus complementing the *vit1-1* mutation.

Regulation of *AtVTL1*, *AtVTL2* and *AtVTL5* Gene Expression

Finally, we investigated the response of *AtVTL1*, *AtVTL2* and *AtVTL5* to nutrient supply using quantitative qRT-PCR. Previously, we reported that the transcriptional activity of these genes positively correlated with the Fe supply [20]. Quantitative RT-PCR analyses confirmed these results (Fig. 7). Compared to Fe-sufficient controls (40 µM Fe), the transcript abundance of *AtVTL1*, *AtVTL2* and *AtVTL5* was decreased under Fe deficiency and increased in plants grown on media containing 120 µM Fe. Similarly, transcript abundance also decreased under Zn deficiency for *AtVTL1*, *AtVTL2* and *AtVTL5* (Fig. 7). However, when the Zn concentration was increased to 5 µM, the transcript abundance for *AtVTL1*, *AtVTL2* and *AtVTL5* was not significantly different from that of control plants grown on standard media (Fig. 7). The *VTL* genes were unable to restore growth in the Zn sensitive *Δzrc1*

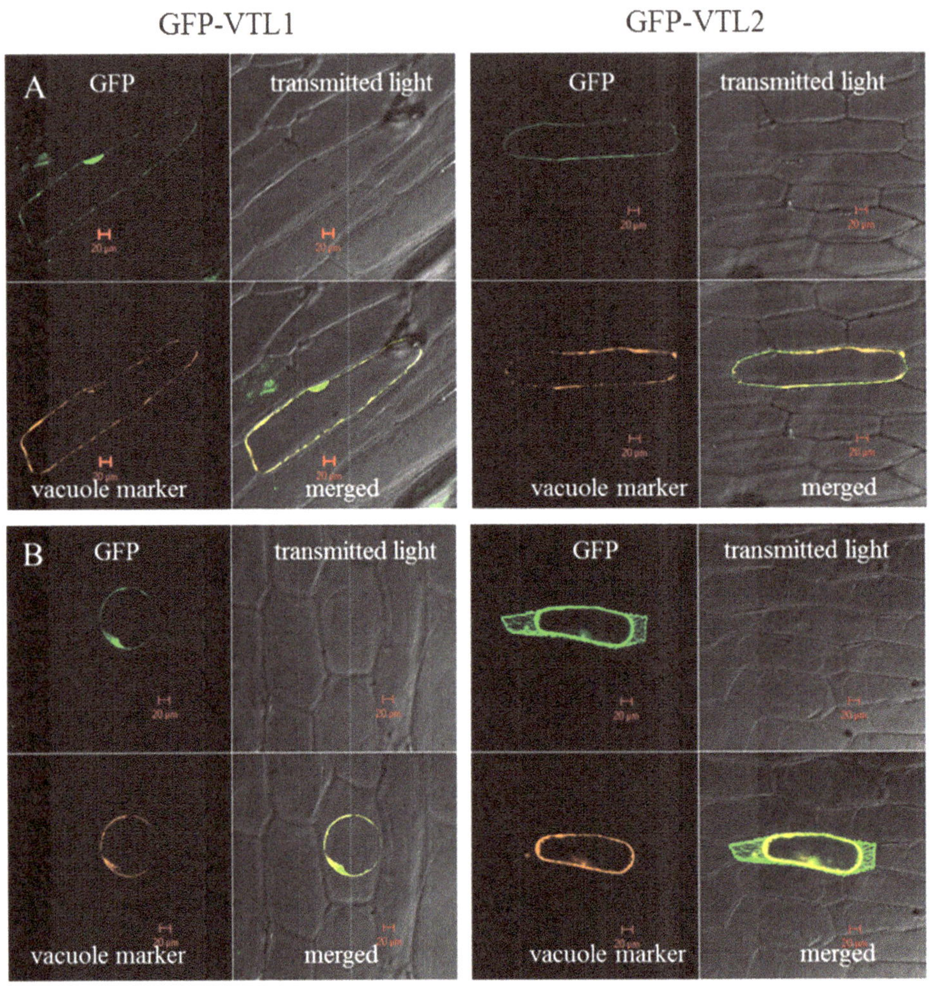

Figure 3. Transient 35S:GFP*::VTL1* and 35S:GFP*::VTL2* expression in onion epidermis cells. The GFP-VTL1 fluorescent signal co-localized with the vacuolar marker, vac-rk CD3-975, in turgescent (**A**) and plasmolyzed (**B**) cells. The GFP-VTL2 signal was also observed on the plasma membrane and cytoplasma (**B**).

mutant (Fig. S7). Thus, a function of AtVTL1, AtVTL2 or AtVTL5 in vacuolar Zn transport is unlikely. Since *AtVTL1*, *AtVTL2* and *AtVTL5* responded positively to Fe supply and since their over-expression complemented vacuolar Fe transport mutations in yeast and Arabidopsis mutants, we conclude that *VTL* genes encode protein involved in Fe homeostasis, presumably as Fe vacuolar transporters.

Discussion

Heterologous expression of *AtVIT1*, *OsVIT1*, *OsVIT2* and *TgVIT1* in the *Δccc1* mutant has been shown to complement the *Δccc1* mutation by restoring Fe uptake into the vacuole, and thus, to protect the cell from the deleterious effects of high cytosolic Fe ([6,18,19]. Vacuolar Fe transporter activity has been reported for FPN2, NRAMP3 and NRAMP4. Whereas AtVIT1 and FPN2 transported Fe into vacuoles, the two NRAMPs were shown to be efflux carriers. Previously, we have identified five genes in Arabidopsis, which encoded proteins with significant sequence homology to AtVIT1 [20]. The transcript abundance of *AtVTL1*, *AtVTL2* and *AtVTL5* was rapidly decreased in roots under conditions of Fe deficiency [21,28]. We have shown in this report, that heterologous expression of *AtVTL1*, *AtVTL2* and *AtVTL5* in yeast *Δccc1* cells restored their ability to grow in the presence of 4 mM Fe. Since the heterologous expression of these genes in yeast correlated with increased Fe in the vacuolar fraction, we proposed that these three proteins increased Fe transport into the vacuole and thereby reduced toxic Fe in the cytoplasm of *Δccc1* cells.

VTLs are Localized to the Arabidopsis Vacuolar Membrane

Transient expression of *GFP::VTL1* and *GFP::VTL2* chimeric proteins in onion epidermis cells resulted in a specific co-localization of GFP::VTL1 with the vacuolar marker vac-rk CD3-975. In the case of *GFP::VTL2* transient expression, a prominent signal was co-localized with the vacuole marker, but GFP fluorescence was also found in the cytoplasm and associated with the plasma membrane, indicating possible localization of AtVTL2 on other membranes in addition to the vacuole. Attempts at localizing AtVTL5 have not been successful.

Evidence for a function of AtVTL1, 2 and 5 in Fe homeostasis was obtained by complementation of the *nramp3/nramp4* and *vit1-1* mutations. The NRAMP3 and NRAMP4 proteins act redundantly as vacuolar Fe efflux carriers. The abundance of both

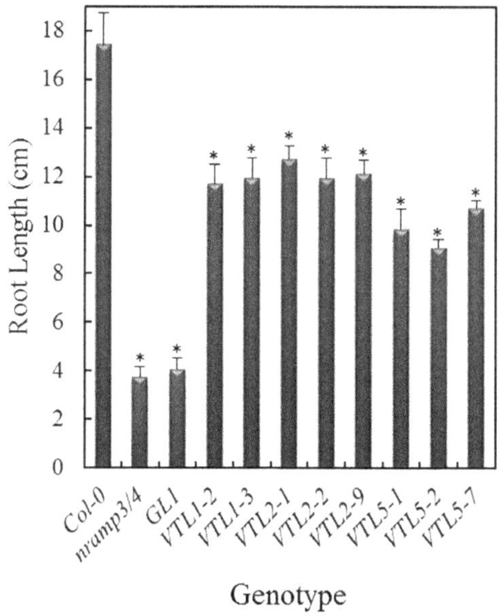

Figure 4. Complementation of the *nramp3/nramp4* double mutant by over-expression of AtVTLs. The three VTL genes were over-expressed in the *nramp3/nramp4* double mutant background under the control of the 35S promoter and root length was determined after 5 days of growth. Seedlings were grown without added Fe. Seedlings were grown on agarose Petri plates as described in the Materials and Methods. Asterisks indicate significant differences from the wild-type ($p<0.001$).

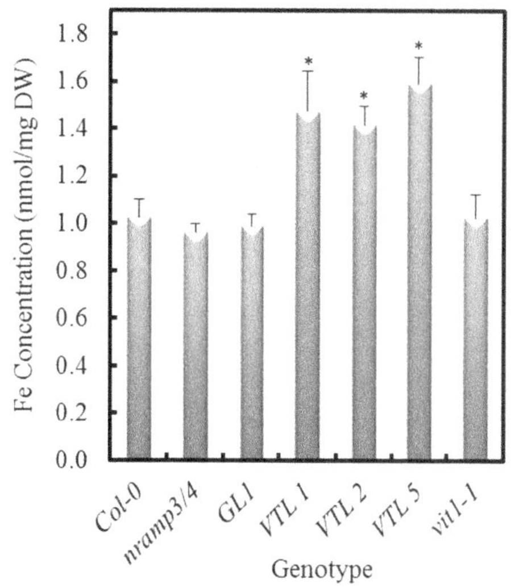

Figure 5. Fe concentration of Arabidopsis seeds. Fe was determined in the wild-type (Col-0), the *nramp3/nramp4* double mutant, the vector control (GL1), the *vit1-1* mutant and in seeds from the double mutant expressing one of the three VTL genes under the control of the 35S promoter. Asterisks indicate significant differences from the wild-type ($p<0.01$).

NRAMPs was increased during Fe deficiency, and in the double mutant, greening of cotyledons and early root growth of seedlings were delayed compared to controls when seeds were germinated under Fe deficiency [17]. This inhibition of root growth could be largely eliminated by supplying Fe to the growth medium. The root growth phenotype was complemented by over-expression of *AtVTL1, 2* or *5* in the *nramp3/nramp4* mutant. In addition the total Fe content of seeds from over-expressing *AtVTL1, 2* or *5* plants was increased compared to the wild type and the mutant. It might have seemed paradoxical that a mutation in a vacuole efflux transport system could be complemented by a putative vacuolar uptake transporter; however, an increased vacuolar Fe concentration might have been sufficient to compensate for a decreased efflux caused by the mutations in *NRAMP3* and *NRAMP4*.

The *vit1-1* mutant also displayed a Fe deficiency-dependent inhibition of seedling root growth that is likely the result of a mis-localization of Fe in the seed radicle. Over-expression of *AtVTL1, 2* or *5* might have restored the Fe supply to the growing root. In summary and based on the complementation activity in yeast, the increased vacuolar Fe concentration in yeast cells expressing AtVTL1, 2 or 5, the localization of AtVTL1 and 2 on the vacuolar membrane in onion epidermis cells and the restoration of seedling root growth in the *nramp3/nramp4* and *vit1-1* mutants, a critical role for the VTL proteins in the subcellular distribution of Fe is apparent.

AtVTLs and Metal Homeostasis

Low substrate specificity is commonly found in cation transports. For example, AtIRT1 is the predominant plasma membrane Fe^{2+} transporter and is essential for Fe uptake from the soil [3]. In the absence of Fe or in the presence of excess divalent cations, AtIRT1 can also catalyze the transport of Zn, Mn and Cd [3,29]. Both NRAMP3 and NRAMP4 have been shown also to be vacuolar Mn exporters [30]; although, transcription was correlated with the Fe and not the Mn nutrient status. Lanquar et al. [30] envision a passive function of NRAMP3 and NRAMP4 in cycling of Mn from the vacuole to the plastid in mesophyll cells. The *nramp3/nramp4* double mutant is hypersensitive to Zn and Cd, and as Sinclair and Krämer [31] suggested, the cause of the hypersensitivity appeared to be an indirect effect related to

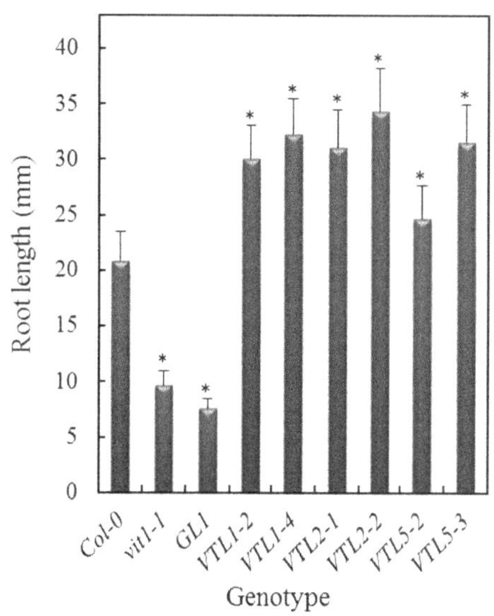

Figure 6. Complementation of the *vit1-1* mutant by over-expression of *AtVTL1*, *AtVTL2* or *AtVTL5*. The three VTL genes were over-expressed under the control of the 35S promoter in the *vit1-1* background. Root length was determined after 13 days of growth on agarose Petri plates as described in the Materials and Methods ion ES medium without added Fe and in the presence of the Fe^{2+} chelator, Ferrozine. Asterisks indicate significant differences from the wild-type ($p<0.001$). Shown are results from 2 independent transformants.

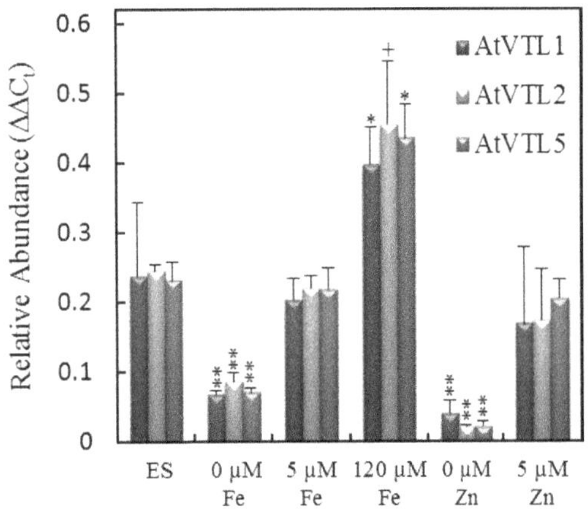

Figure 7. RT-qPCR of At*VTL1*, At*VTL2* and *AtVTL5* in response to Fe and Zn supply. Seedlings were grown on agarose petri plates as described in the Materials and Methods. Growth conditions were: ES medium (ES); "0", ES without Fe or Zn or at the concentrations indicated. RT-qPCR was standardized to the expression of the *ACTIN2*. Symbols indicate significant differences to expression in the ES medium in three biological replicates: **, $p<0.001$; *, $p<0.01$; and +, $p<0.05$.

impaired Fe and Mn transport. Although the transcript data do support a role for the VTLs in Fe homeostasis, a role in homeostasis of other divalent cations analogous to the roles of NRAMP3 and NRAMP4 cannot be excluded.

Five Zn transport genes are among the Arabidopsis genes that response to Fe deficiency [32]. Four of these genes that transport Zn into the vacuole are strongly induced under Fe deficiency. The remaining gene, *AtZIP3*, was repressed and shown to catalyzed Zn uptake into cells. Zn has been shown to accumulate in roots grown under Fe-deficient conditions, likely the result of the Zn transport activity of IRT1 [3,31]. It is noteworthy that the expression of *AtVTL1*, *AtVTL2* and *AtVTL5* was greatly decreased under Zn deficiency but unchanged when grown under Zn excess (Fig. 7). Expression of *AtVTL1*, *AtVTL2* and *AtVTL5* in the yeast *Δzrc1*, a vacuolar Zn transport mutant, did not complement this mutation (Fig. S7).

Although a direct role of the VTL proteins in Zn transport is lacking, an involvement of Zn in Fe homeostasis has been clearly demonstrated. Transcriptional regulation in strategy I plants to Fe deficiency is mediated in part by the bHLH transcription factors FIT (bHLH029) [33,34,35] and POPEYE (bHLH047, PYE) [36]. The central components of PYE regulation include PYE (At3g47640), IAA–LEUCINE-RESISTANT3 (ILR3, bHLH105, At5g54680) and BRUTUS (BTS, At3g47640). *PYE* is weakly and *BTS* is strongly induced under Fe deficiency [20,36], and PYE and BTS both interact but with ILR3 in a yeast two-hybrid assay but not with each other [36]. Either a ternary complex of PYE-ILR3-BTS or the competition between PYE and BTS for ILR3 has been proposed as the regulatory switch in the PYE network [36]. PYE directly regulated genes that were associated with the response to Fe deficiency including: *FRO3*, *NAS4* and *ZIF1*. The transcription of *AtVTL1*, *2* and *5* was increased 1.9, 16.9 and 2.9-fold, respectively, in the *pye-1* knockout mutant [36], and roots of the *pye-1* mutant had an elevated Fe content compared with controls. These observations are consistent with the positive correlation between the root Fe concentration and transcript abundance of *AtVTL1*, *2* and *5* (Fig. 7) [21].

In the *ilr3-1* gain-of-function mutant, the transcript abundance of *AtVTL1*, *2* and *5* was decreased between 3- and 4-fold; an observation that can be explained by a gain-of-function in the PYE-ILR3-BTS repression [22]. In general, BTS and the rice homologs OsHRZs negatively regulate the Fe deficiency response in Arabidopsis and rice, and thus plants with decreased expression of these genes showed tolerance to Fe deficiency [36,37]. Recombinant BTS has been shown to bind both Fe and Zn, primarily at the hemerythrin domain of the protein [36]. In a recent model, Kobayshi and Nishizawa [38] have proposed a mechanism for transcriptional regulation through the BTS/OsHRZ proteins based on binding of Zn and Fe to the hemerythrin domain of these proteins. In their model, Fe binding to BTS/OsHRZ in the absence of Zn would lead to repression PYE-regulated gene expression as seen in Fig. 7. The implications of their model are germane to the repression of *VTL* transcription under Zn deficiency observed in our experiments. Taken together, we have identified a group of putative Fe transporters that participate in the Fe homeostasis in Arabidopsis. As vacuolar Fe transporters these proteins may have importance in biofortification efforts in the future.

Supporting Information

Figure S1 Sucrose density gradient isolation of membrane in the yeast vacuolar fraction. The vacuolar fraction was isolated as described in the Materials and Methods, and the vacuoles ruptured by repeated pipetting. The membranes were layered onto a continuous, 10 to 60% sucrose gradient and centrifuged at 110,000x*g* in a swing-out rotor over-night. The gradient was fractionated into 1 ml fractions and marker enzymes for the vacuole (bafilomycin-sensitive ATPase), plasma membrane (vanadate-sensitive ATPase) and endoplasmic reticulum (cytochrome *c* reductase) were determined by the method of Luster and Buckhout (Plant Physiol. 1989; 91(3): 1014-9). The activity of the vanadate-sensitive ATPase and the cytochrome c reductase were below the limits of detection.

Figure S2 Complementation of the yeast *Δccc1* (vacuolar Fe^{2+}/Mn^{2+} transporter) mutant with his-tagged *AtVTL1* and *AtVTL2* genes. Cells were transformed with the empty vector (pUE) or the *VTL* gene containing a H_6 tag under the control of the PGK promoter and grown on YPD medium containing 7.5 mM $FeSO_4$.

Figure S3 A. Chlorophyll content in wild-type (Col-0) and wild-type plants over-expressing *AtVTL1* grown in the Fe concentrations indicated. Shown are chlorophyll a and b and the chlorophyll a/b ratio. **B. Analysis of the Fe^{3+}-chelate reductase activity in Col-0 and Col-0 plants over-expressing *AtVTL1*.** Bars are standard error of the mean.

Figure S4 Semi-quantitative PCR of of *AtVTL1*, *AtVTL2* and *AtVTL5*. Expression was determined in Col-0 (WT), the *nramp3/nramp4* double mutant and in the double mutant over-expressing each of the *VTL1*, *VTL2* or *VTL5* genes. Expression was standardized to the level of *ACTIN2* expression.

Figure S5 Root growth in the *nramp3/nramp4* double mutant transformed with *AtVTL1*, *AtVTL2* or *AtVTL5*. Seedlings were grown for 5 days on standard media lacking Fe (see Materials and Methods). Shown are results from two to three independent transformants taken from one repetition of the experiment reported in Fig. 4.

Figure S6 Root growth in the *vit1-1* mutant transformed with *AtVTL1*, *AtVTL2* or *AtVTL5*. Seedlings were grown for 13 days on standard media (see Materials and Methods) lacking Fe and in the presence of the Fe^{2+} chelator, Ferrozine. Shown are results from an experiment similar to that reported in Fig. 6.

Figure S7 Complementation of the *Δzrc1* by heterologous expression of the *VTL* genes. *Δzrc1* (vacuolar Zn^{2+} transporter) cells were transformed with each of the three VTL genes or the empty vector (pUE) under the control of the PGK promoter and grown on SD medium containing $ZnSO_4$ at the concentrations indicated for 24 or 48 h at 30°C. Cells were plated at the densities indicated in the figure.

Acknowledgments

We thank Drs. Mary-Lou Guerinot, Jerry Kaplan and Sebastian Thomine for kindly providing the *Saccharomyes* and Arabidopsis mutants used in this study and Christin Schläwicke for determination of seed Fe and leaf chlorophyll. We gratefully acknowledge the excellent technical support of Marion Dewender and Susanne Olstowski-Jacoby.

Author Contributions

Conceived and designed the experiments: JG WS TJB. Performed the experiments: JG RT PL. Analyzed the data: JG RT PL WS TJB. Contributed reagents/materials/analysis tools: JG RT PL. Wrote the paper: WS TJB.

References

1. Kosman DJ (2010) Redox cycling in iron uptake, efflux, and trafficking. J Biol Chem 285: 26729–26735. doi: 10.1074/jbc.R110.113217.
2. Eide D, Broderius M, Fett J, Guerinot ML (1996) A novel iron-regulated metal transporter from plants identified by functional expression in yeast. Proc Natl Acad Sci U S A 93: 5624–5628.
3. Vert G, Grotz N, Dedaldechamp F, Gaymard F, Guerinot ML, et al. (2002) IRT1, an Arabidopsis transporter essential for iron uptake from the soil and for plant growth. Plant Cell 14: 1223–1233.
4. Barberon M, Zelazny E, Robert S, Conéjéro G, Curie C, et al. (2011) Monoubiquitin-dependent endocytosis of the iron-regulated transporter 1 (IRT1) transporter controls iron uptake in plants. Proc Natl Acad Sci USA 108: E450–458. doi: 10.1073/pnas.1100659108.
5. Robinson NJ, Procter CM, Connolly EL, Guerinot ML (1999) A ferric-chelate reductase for iron uptake from soils. Nature 397: 694–697. doi: 10.1038/17800.
6. Eckhardt U, Buckhout TJ (1998) Iron assimilation in Chlamydomonas reinhardtii involves ferric reduction and is similar to Strategy I higher plants. Journal of Experimental Botany 49: 1219–1226.
7. Kosman DJ (2003) Molecular mechanisms of iron uptake in fungi. Mol Microbiol 47: 1185–1197.
8. Rodriguez-Celma J, Lin W-D, Fu G-M, Abadia J, Lopez-Millan A-F, et al. (2013) Mutually exclusive alterations in secondary metabolism are critical for the uptake of insoluble iron compounds by Arabidopsis and Medicago truncatula. Plant Physiol 162: 1473–1485. doi: 10.1104/pp.113.220426.
9. Fourcroy P, Siso-Terraza P, Sudre D, Saviron M, Reyt G, et al. (2014) Involvement of the ABCG37 transporter in secretion of scopoletin and derivatives by Arabidopsis roots in response to iron deficiency. New Phytol 201: 155–167. doi: 10.1111/nph.12471.
10. Schmid NB, Giehl RFH, Doll S, Mock H-P, Strehmel N, et al. (2014) Feruloyl-CoA 6′-Hydroxylase1-dependent coumarins mediate iron acquisition from alkaline substrates in arabidopsis. Plant Physiol 164: 160–172. doi: 10.1104/pp.113.228544.
11. Santi S, Schmidt W (2009) Dissecting iron deficiency-induced proton extrusion in Arabidopsis roots. New Phytol 183: 1072–1084. doi: 10.1111/j.1469-8137.2009.02908.x.
12. Briat J-F, Duc C, Ravet K, Gaymard F (2010) Ferritins and iron storage in plants. Biochim Biophys Acta 1800: 806–814. doi: 10.1016/j.bbagen.2009.12.003.
13. Ravet K, Touraine B, Boucherez J, Briat J-F, Gaymard F, et al. (2009) Ferritins control interaction between iron homeostasis and oxidative stress in Arabidopsis. Plant J 57: 400–412. doi: 10.1111/j.1365-313X.2008.03698.x.
14. Morrissey J, Baxter IR, Lee J, Li L, Lahner B, et al. (2009) The ferroportin metal efflux proteins function in iron and cobalt homeostasis in Arabidopsis. Plant Cell 21: 3326–3338. doi: 10.1105/tpc.109.069401.
15. Schaaf G, Honsbein A, Meda AR, Kirchner S, Wipf D, et al. (2006) AtIREG2 encodes a tonoplast transport protein involved in iron-dependent nickel detoxification in Arabidopsis thaliana roots. J Biol Chem 281: 25532–25540. doi: 10.1074/jbc.M601062200.
16. Kim SA, Punshon T, Lanzirotti A, Li L, Alonso JM, et al. (2006) Localization of iron in Arabidopsis seed requires the vacuolar membrane transporter VIT1. Science 314: 1295–1298. doi: 10.1126/science.1132563.
17. Lanquar V, Lelievre F, Bolte S, Hames C, Alcon C, et al. (2005) Mobilization of vacuolar iron by AtNRAMP3 and AtNRAMP4 is essential for seed germination on low iron. EMBO J 24: 4041–4051. doi: 10.1038/sj.emboj.7600864.
18. Zhang Y, Xu Y-H, Yi H-Y, Gong J-M (2012) Vacuolar membrane transporters OsVIT1 and OsVIT2 modulate iron translocation between flag leaves and seeds in rice. Plant J 72: 400–410. doi: 10.1111/j.1365-313X.2012.05088.x.
19. Momonoi K, Yoshida K, Mano S, Takahashi H, Nakamori C, et al. (2009) A vacuolar iron transporter in tulip, TgVit1, is responsible for blue coloration in petal cells through iron accumulation. Plant J 59: 437–447. doi: 10.1111/j.1365-313X.2009.03879.x.
20. Buckhout TJ, Yang TJW, Schmidt W (2009) Early iron-deficiency-induced transcriptional changes in Arabidopsis roots as revealed by microarray analyses. BMC Genomics 10. doi: 10.1186/1471-2164-10-147.
21. Gollhofer J, Schlawicke C, Jungnick N, Schmidt W, Buckhout TJ (2011) Members of a small family of nodulin-like genes are regulated under iron deficiency in roots of Arabidopsis thaliana. Plant Physiol Biochem 49: 557–564. doi: 10.1016/j.plaphy.2011.02.011.
22. Rampey RA, Woodward AW, Hobbs BN, Tierney MP, Lahner B, et al. (2006) An Arabidopsis basic helix-loop-helix leucine zipper protein modulates metal homeostasis and auxin conjugate responsiveness. Genetics 174: 1841–1857. doi: 10.1534/genetics.106.061044.
23. Blair D, Diehl H (1961) Bathophenanthrolinedisulphonic acid and bathocuproinedisulphonic acid, water soluble reagents for iron and copper. Talanta 7: 163–174.
24. Rose M, Winston F, Hieter P (1990) Methods in yeast genetics: A laboratory course manual. Cold Spring Harbor, New York: Cold Spring Harbor Press.
25. Li L, Chen OS, McVey Ward D, Kaplan J (2001) CCC1 is a transporter that mediates vacuolar iron storage in yeast. J Biol Chem 276: 29515–29519. doi: 10.1074/jbc.M103944200.
26. Clough SJ, Bent AF (1998) Floral dip: a simplified method for Agrobacterium-mediated transformation of Arabidopsis thaliana. Plant J 16: 735–743.
27. Nelson BK, Cai X, Nebenfuhr A (2007) A multicolored set of in vivo organelle markers for co-localization studies in Arabidopsis and other plants. Plant J 51: 1126–1136. doi: 10.1111/j.1365-313X.2007.03212.x.
28. Yang TJW, Lin W-D, Schmidt W (2010) Transcriptional profiling of the Arabidopsis iron deficiency response reveals conserved transition metal homeostasis networks. Plant Physiol 152: 2130–2141. doi: 10.1104/pp.109.152728.
29. Cohen CK, Fox TC, Garvin DF, Kochian LV (1998) The role of iron-deficiency stress responses in stimulating heavy-metal transport in plants. Plant Physiol 116: 1063–1072.
30. Lanquar V, Ramos MS, Lelievre F, Barbier-Brygoo H, Krieger-Liszkay A, et al. (2010) Export of vacuolar manganese by AtNRAMP3 and AtNRAMP4 is required for optimal photosynthesis and growth under manganese deficiency. Plant Physiol 152: 1986–1999. doi: 10.1104/pp.109.150946.
31. Sinclair SA, Kramer U (2012) The zinc homeostasis network of land plants. Biochim Biophys Acta 1823: 1553–1567. doi: 10.1016/j.bbamcr.2012.05.016.
32. Schmidt W, Buckhout TJ (2011) A hitchhiker's guide to the Arabidopsis ferrome. Plant Physiol Biochem 49: 462–470. doi: 10.1016/j.plaphy.2010.12.001.
33. Colangelo EP, Guerinot ML (2004) The essential basic helix-loop-helix protein FIT1 is required for the iron deficiency response. Plant Cell 16: 3400–3412. doi: 10.1105/tpc.104.024315.
34. Jakoby M, Wang H-Y, Reidt W, Weisshaar B, Bauer P (2004) FRU (BHLH029) is required for induction of iron mobilization genes in Arabidopsis thaliana. FEBS Lett 577: 528–534. doi: 10.1016/j.febslet.2004.10.062.
35. Yuan Y, Wu H, Wang N, Li J, Zhao W, et al. (2008) FIT interacts with AtbHLH38 and AtbHLH39 in regulating iron uptake gene expression for iron homeostasis in Arabidopsis. Cell Res 18: 385–397. doi: 10.1038/cr.2008.26.
36. Long TA, Tsukagoshi H, Busch W, Lahner B, Salt DE, et al. (2010) The bHLH transcription factor POPEYE regulates response to iron deficiency in Arabidopsis roots. Plant Cell 22: 2219–2236. doi: 10.1105/tpc.110.074096.
37. Kobayashi T, Nagasaka S, Senoura T, Itai RN, Nakanishi H, et al. (2013) Iron-binding Haemerythrin RING ubiquitin ligases regulate plant iron responses and accumulation. Nat Commun 4. doi: 10.1038/ncomms3792.
38. Kobayashi T, Nishizawa NK (2014) Iron sensors and signals in response to iron deficiency. Plant Sci 224C. doi: 10.1016/j.plantsci.2014.04.002.

16

Vitamin D Status among Thai School Children and the Association with 1,25-Dihydroxyvitamin D and Parathyroid Hormone Levels

Lisa A. Houghton[1]*, Andrew R. Gray[2], Michelle J. Harper[1], Pattanee Winichagoon[3], Tippawan Pongcharoen[3], Sueppong Gowachirapant[3], Rosalind S. Gibson[1]

1 Department of Human Nutrition, University of Otago, Dunedin, New Zealand, **2** Department of Preventive and Social Medicine, University of Otago, Dunedin, New Zealand, **3** Institute of Nutrition, Mahidol University, Salaya, Thailand

Abstract

In several low latitude countries, vitamin D deficiency is emerging as a public health issue. Adequate vitamin D is essential for bone health in rapidly growing children. In the Thai population, little is known about serum 25-hydroxyvitamin D [25(OH)D] status of infants and children. Moreover, the association between 25(OH)D and the biological active form of 1,25-dihydroxyvitamin D [1,25(OH)]$_2$D is not clear. The specific aims of this study were to characterize circulating serum 25(OH)D, 1,25(OH)$_2$D and their determinants including parathyroid hormone (PTH), age, sex, height and body mass index (BMI) in 529 school-aged Thai children aged 6–14 y. Adjusted linear regression analysis was performed to examine the impact of age and BMI, and its interaction with sex, on serum 25(OH)D concentrations and 1,25(OH)$_2$D concentrations. Serum 25(OH)D, 1,25(OH)$_2$D and PTH concentrations (geometric mean $\pm$ geometric SD) were 72.7$\pm$1.2 nmol/L, 199.1$\pm$1.3 pmol/L and 35.0$\pm$1.5 ng/L, respectively. Only 4% (21 of 529) participants had a serum 25(OH)D level below 50 nmol/L. There was statistically significant evidence for an interaction between sex and age with regard to 25(OH)D concentrations. Specifically, 25(OH)D concentrations were 19% higher in males. Moreover, females experienced a statistically significant 4% decline in serum 25(OH)D levels for each increasing year of age ($P = 0.001$); no decline was seen in male participants with increasing age ($P = 0.93$). When BMI, age, sex, height and serum 25(OH)D were individually regressed on 1,25(OH)$_2$D, height and sex were associated with 1,25(OH)$_2$D with females exhibiting statistically significantly higher serum 1,25(OH)$_2$D levels compared with males ($P < 0.001$). Serum 1,25(OH)$_2$D among our sample of children exhibiting fairly sufficient vitamin D status were higher than previous reports suggesting an adaptive mechanism to maximize calcium absorption.

Editor: Dominique Heymann, Faculté de médecine de Nantes, France

Funding: This study was supported by the Micronutrient Initiative Fund, Ottawa, Canada; the Institute of Nutrition, Mahidol University, Salaya, Thailand; and University of Otago Research Grants. The funders had no role in study design, data collection and analysis, decision to publish, or preparation of the manuscript.

Competing Interests: The authors have declared that no competing interests exist.

* Email: lisa.houghton@otago.ac.nz

Introduction

Vitamin D status influences the absorption of calcium and phosphate from the gut and is known mainly for its role in bone health across the lifecycle. During periods of rapid growth in childhood, health consequences of vitamin D deficiency include growth retardation, skeletal deformities and an increased fracture risk later in life [1]. Vitamin D is also associated with non-skeletal health outcomes including modulation of the immune response, reduction of inflammation, insulin production, neuromuscular function, and regulation of cell growth, differentiation and apoptosis [2,3].

The main source of vitamin D is endogenous production following exposure of 7-dehydrocholesterol in the skin to sunlight (ultraviolet-B irradiation) to produce 25-hydroxyvitamin D [25(OH)D], best known as a marker of vitamin D status. Circulating 25(OH)D is then converted to its biologically active form, 1,25-dihydroxyvitamin D [1,25(OH)$_2$D]. Natural food sources rich in vitamin D are scarce. Studies on serum 25(OH)D concentrations have shown a high prevalence (from 15% to 80%) of vitamin D deficiency and insufficiency in several pediatric and adolescents populations [4–13]. These findings have been demonstrated not only in higher latitudes, but also in lower latitude countries with ample sunshine. This is possibly due to avoidance of sunlight, indoor lifestyles, clothing coverage and sunscreen use, adiposity, and low dietary intake of vitamin D-rich foods or supplements. Another dietary factor, which may contribute to the development of vitamin D deficiency, is a low calcium diet which, by inducing secondary hyperparathyroidism and elevating 1,25(OH)$_2$D, results in increased catabolism of 25(OH)D and a depletion of vitamin D stores [14–18].

Thailand, located in the southeastern part of Asia at latitudes between 5°30′ N and 20°30′ N, is amenable to year round vitamin D synthesis. Dietary intake of vitamin D among Thais are low because foods are not fortified with vitamin D. Dietary calcium intake has also been reported to be low in children in Thailand

[19,20]. The Thai diet is predominantly based on rice, vegetables and some meats, and is often low in milk and milk products. The suboptimal calcium content of the diet may be further compromised by a high level of phytate [21]. A recent study of vitamin D status in Thai adults revealed relatively high mean serum 25(OH)D levels with the prevalence of insufficiency [serum 25(OH)D <50 nmol/L] ranging from 3% in the Northeast to 14% in the Bangkok region [22]. Data are currently lacking on the vitamin D status of Thai children. Given the emerging body of evidence on the role of vitamin D in health throughout life, we investigated the vitamin D status of a large sample of school-aged children from northeast Thailand. The specific aims of this study were to characterize circulating levels of serum 25(OH)D, 1,25(OH)$_2$D and their determinants including PTH, age, sex, height and body mass index (BMI). Moreover, we examined the impact of age and BMI, and its interaction with sex, on serum 25(OH)D concentrations in these prepubertal children ranging in age from six to 14 years.

Materials and Methods

Participants

The present study used endline data from a 31-wk randomized controlled trial (RCT; ClinicalTrials.gov ACTRN12605000341628) assessing the efficacy of a seasoning powder fortified with iron, zinc, iodine and vitamin A for reducing anemia and improving micronutrient status of northeast Thai schoolchildren [23] [24]. The original study was conducted during the school year between June 2002 and March 2003. The participants (261 males, 268 females) were aged 6.0–14.0 y and were randomly selected to participate in the trial from primary schools situated in ten poorest rural subdistricts of the Trakarn Phutphon district, Ubon Rachathani province (latitude 15°N). All of the subdistricts were of low socioeconomic status. For the RCT, children were stratified in each school into four strata: females grades 1–3; males grades 1–3; females grades 4–6; males grades 4–6. Fifteen children were selected randomly from each stratum where possible and in strata with less than fifteen children, all children were selected. To minimize clustering, only one child per household was selected. Children were eligible for the study if they were apparently healthy, and had a hemoglobin concentration greater than 80 g/L. Of the 569 children enrolled in the original study, 25(OH)D, 1,25(OH)$_2$D and PTH data were available from 529, 523 and 518 children, respectively, at study endline. Endline samples were collected during the summer season between the months of February and March 2003 (i.e., dry season). The Human Ethics Committee from the University of Otago (New Zealand) and Mahidol University (Thailand) approved the study protocol, and written informed consent was obtained from the children's parents or guardians.

Sociodemographic and anthropometric variables

A pretested sociodemographic and health status questionnaire was administered to an adult member of each participating household. Measurements of weight and standing height were taken using standardized techniques by a trained anthropometrist. Z-scores for height, weight and body mass index (BMI) were calculated using the age- and sex-specific WHO Child Growth Standards [25]. Stunted children were defined as those with height-for-age z-score less than −2, and underweight and thinness were defined as weight-for-age z-scores less than −2 and BMI-for-age z-score less than −2, respectively.

Blood sample collection and biochemical assessment

Morning, nonfasting peripheral venipuncture blood samples were drawn by trained nurses into trace element-free evacuated tubes (Becton Dickinson, Franklin Lakes, NJ), centrifuged (2500 X g, 10 min, room temperature) and serum was stored at −70°C.

Serum 25(OH)D$_2$ and 25(OH)D$_3$ were determined in-house using isotope-dilution liquid chromatography-tandem mass spectrometry (API 3200 Applied Biosystems Inc.) according to the method of Maunsell et al [26]. This method quantifies 25(OH)D$_2$ and 25(OH)D$_3$ including the 3-epimer form, which is not separated from 25(OH)D$_3$. The limit of quantification for the assay was <5 nmol/L for both metabolites. The assay's within-run (5% or less) and between-day imprecision (10% or less) was determined using the UTAK Tri-Level control material (UTAK Laboratories, Inc. CA, USA). Traceability was confirmed directly to National Institute of Standards & Technology (NIST) Standard Reference Material (SRM) 972 level 1–4. Levels of serum 1,25-dihydroxyvitamin D were measured by a ^{125}I-based radioimmunoassay (IDS Immuno-Diagnostic Systems, Boldon, UK) with a normal reference range of 48–150 pmol/L as stated by the manufacturer. Lower limit of detection was 8 pmol/L with an assay range of approximately 7–500 pmol/L. The within-run CVs ranged from 6% to 25% and between-day CV (n = 9) was 16%. Intact PTH was determined using an automated electrochemiluminescence immunoassay (Elecsys 1010, Roche Diagnostics). Manufacturer controls (Elecsys Precision Bone 1, 2 and 3) were analysed with each reagent kit. The mean (inter-assay CV, %, n = 7) for the three controls were 55 (8.1%), 197 (1.2%) and 829.1 (1.6%) ng/L, respectively, and were within the range of results provided by the manufacturer.

Statistical methods

Results for serum 25(OH)D, 1,25(OH)$_2$D and PTH were available for 529, 523 and 518 children, respectively. All available data were used for each analysis (in some cases serum samples were insufficient for assays and missing values were considered missing completely at random). Descriptive statistics were used to summarize the data. Initially, unadjusted linear regressions were performed to assess associations between age, sex, and anthropometric factors and circulating 25(OH)D, 1,25(OH)$_2$D and PTH concentrations. Adjusted linear regression analysis was subsequently performed to determine the independent contributions of demographic, biochemical and anthropometric determinants of circulating 25(OH)D and1,25(OH)$_2$D concentrations. Interactions between age and sex and between BMI and sex were investigated and where 25(OH)D or 1,25(OH)$_2$D were included in the model, interactions were also tested between these and sex. Log-transformations were investigated and used when the properties of the model residuals were improved in terms of normality, homoscedasticity, and linearity. Non-linearities were examined including a quadratic term, which was retained when statistically significant. Robust standard errors were used to account for clustering within each of the ten schools. All analyses were conducted using Stata 11.2 (StataCorp, College Station, TX, USA) with a 2-sided 0.05 level of significance used in all cases.

Results

Demographic characteristics and selected anthropometric parameters of the participants are shown in **Table 1**. Of the children with 25(OH)D available, the prevalence of stunting, underweight and thinness were 10.2% (54 of 529), 17.4% (48 of 276) and 11.6% (61 of 528), respectively. No child was taking a vitamin and mineral supplement.

Table 1. Selected characteristics of the study sample[1].

Variable	n	
Age, *y*	529	9.9±1.7
5 to 8 y, %	91	17.5
8 to 10 y, %	181	33.5
10+ y, %	257	49.0
Girls, %	268	50.5
Menarche, %	5	2.0
Weight, *kg*	536	26.3±1.3
Height, *cm*	537	131.5±10.4
BMI, kg/m	536	14.8 (2.2)
Weight-for-age *z* score[2]	279	−1.3 (1.1)
Height-for-age *z* score	537	−1.0 (1.2)
BMI-for-age *z* score	536	1.0 (1.2)
Serum 25-hydroxyvitamin D, *nmol/L*	529	72.7±1.2
Serum 1,25-dihydroxvitamin D, *pmol/L*	523	199.1±1.3
Parathyroid hormone, *ng/L*	518	35.0±1.5

[1]Values are geometric mean ± geometric SD or median (IQR) unless specified. *Note*: Geometric SD is a factor, not a quantity. *Powers* of the geometric SD can be either multiplied by (or divided into) the geometric mean to determine the set of values that lie *n* geometric SDs from the mean.
[2]WHO Reference 2007 does not provide weight-for-age charts beyond 10 years of age.

The distributions of serum 25(OH)D, 1,25(OH)$_2$D, PTH values were all positively skewed and so geometric means and standard deviations are used to describe their distributions. One implausibly low value for 1,25(OH)$_2$D was excluded from analysis (13 pmol/L). In the study sample as a whole, geometric mean (SD) serum 25(OH)D concentration was 72.7 (1.2) nmol/L, ranging from 36.1 to 127.0 nmol/L (**Table 1**). Only 21 (4%) participants had a serum 25(OH)D level below 50 nmol/L (20 ng/mL), of whom 4 (1% of the total sample) participants had circulating 25(OH)D concentrations below 40 nmol/L (16 ng/mL). The overall geometric means (SD) for serum 1,25(OH)$_2$D and PTH concentration was 199.1 (1.3) pmol/L (range 66 to 481 pmol/L) and 35.0 (1.5) ng/L (range 7.9 to 241 ng/L), respectively.

Table 2 presents the geometric mean (95% CI) serum 25(OH)D, 1,25(OH)$_2$D, and PTH for the children by sex and age groups. Regression analyses of the association between potential determinants (sex, age height and BMI) and serum 25(OH)D and 1,25(OH)$_2$D are presented in **Table 3**. Unadjusted linear regression indicated that serum 25(OH)D was statistically significantly positively associated with height and negatively associated with age, with boys having a statistically significantly higher serum 25(OH)D than females. In adjusted analyses, there was statistically significant evidence for an interaction between sex and age with regards to 25(OH)D concentrations. Specifically, serum 25(OH)D concentrations were 19% higher in males at the mean age (9.9 years). Furthermore, there was evidence of sex differences in the association with age ($P<0.001$). We did not observe a decline in 25(OH)D concentrations in male participants with increasing age ($P=0.90$), however, females experienced a statistically significant 4% decline in serum 25(OH)D levels for each increasing year of age (**Figure 1**).

Unadjusted linear regression indicated that serum 1,25(OH)$_2$D was statistically significantly positively associated with height-for-age Z-score (**Table 3**). In contrast to 25(OH)D, boys had a statistically lower serum 1,25(OH)$_2$D than females. There was also evidence of an n-shaped association with BMI, with 1,25(OH)$_2$D levels peaking around 19.9 pmol/L. All of the above relations remained statistically significant in the adjusted model. For PTH, females also appeared to have a statistically significantly higher serum PTH in the unadjusted model, although this effect was attenuated (approximately halved) in the adjusted model and was no longer statistically significant ($P=0.10$). As expected, serum 25(OH)D remained statistically significantly negatively associated with serum PTH concentrations in the adjusted model and height remained significantly positively associated with PTH. For every one unit increase in height-for-age Z score, 1,25(OH)$_2$D and PTH concentrations increased by 7% and 8%, respectively. Stunting (height-for-age Z-score<-2 SD, *n* 54 children) was not associated with either 1,25(OH)$_2$D or PTH concentrations (data not shown).

Discussion

To our knowledge, this is the first study in Thailand to evaluate differences in 25(OH)D status with age and to directly compare boys with girls in a large sample of healthy school aged children. Using cut-offs recommended by the U.S. Institute of Medicine (IOM) [serum 25(OH)D <50 nmol/L] [27], the present study results indicate that only 4% of the children were vitamin D deficient and PTH concentrations were within normal range. The low prevalence of vitamin D deficiency in our data contradicts recent findings demonstrating 30–52% prevalence of deficiency among healthy school-aged children from different regions of the country [28]. Several other studies in various clinical pediatric groups including asthmatic and thalassemia Thai patients [29,30] have also reported a high prevalence of vitamin D deficiency, although these selected patient groups are known to be predisposed to the development of vitamin D deficiency. Potential reasons for the discrepancy between our finding and the substantially higher prevalence recently reported include differences in the analytical measurement employed. In our study, serum 25(OH)D concentrations were measured using isotope dilution LC-MS/MS, which tends to have higher sensitivity and selectivity, and consequently often reports higher values over

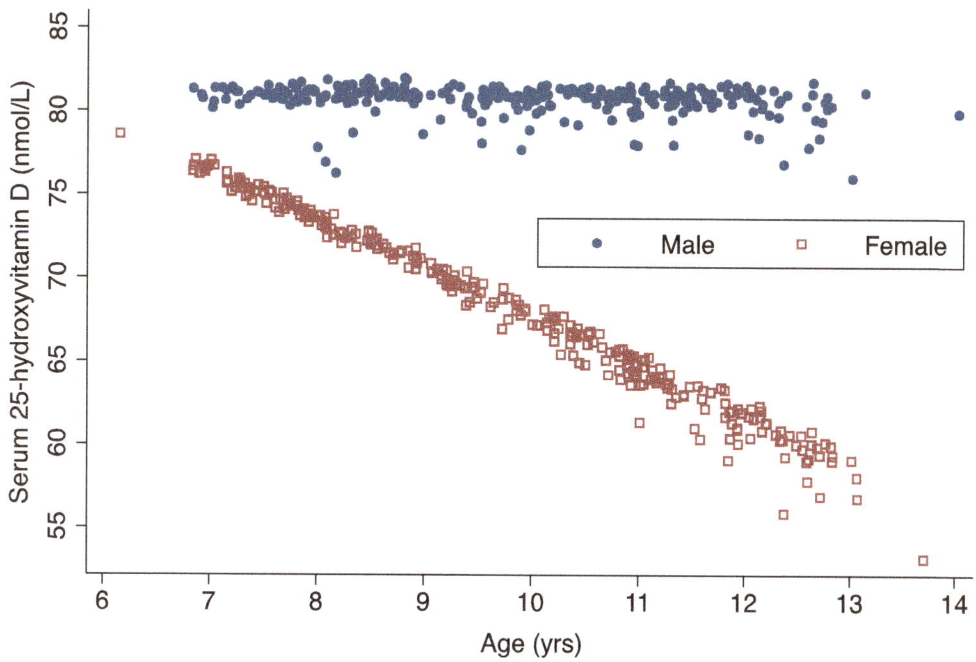

Figure 1. Relation between age in years and serum 25-hydroxyvitamin D (nmol/L) concentrations stratified by gender.

various automated assays [31,32]. However, it is unlikely to be the only reason as geographical location could also contribute to differences in vitamin D status. Data from the Thai National Health Examination Survey demonstrated higher 25(OH)D levels in adults in the northern than in southern regions of the country in addition to lower vitamin D status among those residing in Bangkok, where pollution was higher [22]. Children in the present study were sampled from a single geographical region – the northeast. Consistent with our findings, the prevalence of vitamin D deficiency among Thai adults residing in the northeast region was less than 3% and low serum 25(OH)D levels were associated with being female with mean 25(OH)D levels being approximately 10 nmol/L higher in males [22].

The inverse association of serum 25(OH)D levels with age found only among female participants may reflect reduced sun exposure, however, no measurement of UVB exposure or time spent outdoors was collected in our study. A 2010 survey of sun protection behavior among adolescents in Bangkok demonstrated that females had significantly higher adoption of sun protection behavior compared to males including increase use of sunscreen, staying under the shade and use of umbrellas [33].

Serum concentrations of 1,25(OH)$_2$D in healthy populations have not been well described. In the current study, 1,25(OH)$_2$D concentrations in our sample of Thai children (ranging from an average of 190 and 210 pmol/L among males and females, respectively) were approximately 50 pmol/L higher than those reported in U.S. children [6,34,35]. Serum 1,25(OH)$_2$D concentration is regulated based on its need in calcium homeostasis [36]. A low dietary calcium intake markedly increases serum 1,25(OH)$_2$D [37] and therefore, the differences in 1,25(OH)$_2$D concentrations may be due to the relatively low calcium intakes of our children compared with those of Western counterparts. While dietary intake data were not collected at study endline, baseline median calcium intakes of a randomly selected subsample of our study children (n = 230) were 222 mg/d, as reported previously [20]. Moreover, we found no statistically significant differences in reported calcium intakes between males and females at baseline (regression adjusting for clustering and following log transformation, $P = 0.85$; data not shown).

While there are no data evaluating serum 1,25(OH)$_2$D levels in younger population groups with characteristically low calcium intakes, the higher concentration of 1,25(OH)$_2$D observed in our study was similar to those reported in rural Gambian women with habitually low calcium intakes and sufficient vitamin D status [38]. It has been postulated that the compensatory increased production of 1,25(OH)$_2$D due to low calcium intakes increases the catabolism of 25(OH)D [14–18]. We, however, found no overall relationship between 25(OH)D and 1,25(OH)$_2$D concentrations. This is not unexpected as the circulating levels of 1,25(OH)$_2$D are tightly regulated by gene expression of 1-α-hydroxylase (CYP27B1) and not by the concentration of 25(OH)D. Instead, concentrations of 1,25(OH)$_2$D showed a positive association with serum PTH, which is consistent with the well-known effect of PTH to upregulate CYP27B1 and increase the conversion of 25(OH)D to 1,25(OH)$_2$D in the kidneys [39]. Nonetheless, the existing high serum 25(OH)D status of the study children limits the possibility of indirectly detecting enhanced catabolism of serum 25(OH)D. Additional studies in population groups with lower concentrations of serum 25(OH)D and a direct measurement of 24,25-dihdroxyvitamin D [first metabolic product of 25(OH)D] are needed.

Female children in the current study had significantly higher concentrations of 1,25(OH)$_2$D than male children. Similar findings of a sex difference in 1,25(OH)$_2$D levels are supported by two previous studies [6,34]; however, there is little information available on the influence of gender on vitamin D and calcium homeostasis in this life-cycle group. It has been reported that estrogen replacement therapy increases plasma concentration of 1,25(OH)$_2$D by stimulating renal 1,25(OH)$_2$D production [40]. Although sexual maturation is associated with increasing levels of sex steroids, pubertal staging of participants was not assessed. In Thailand, the onset of puberty in girls has shifted toward a younger age over the last 20 years, with the mean age at menarche

Table 2. Serum 25-hydroxyvitamin D, 1,25-dihyroxyvitamin D and parathyroid hormone concentrations in school-aged children by sex and age group[1].

Variable		Females						Males					
	n	5–8 y	n	8–10 y	n	10+ y	n	5–8 y	n	8–10 y	n	10+ y	n
Serum 25(OH)D, *nmol/L*	529	74.7±1.2	52	70.1±1.2	86	61.9±1.2	130	80.4±1.2	39	78.8±1.2	94	79.4±1.2	128
Serum 1,25(OH)$_2$D, *pmol/L*	523	213.0±1.3	52	203.1±1.3	81	221.7±1.3	129	184.1±1.3	39	182.7±1.3	93	183.4±1.5	129
Serum PTH, *ng/L*	518	36.6±1.4	51	35.8±1.5	81	42.3±1.5	127	31.2±1.5	39	29.4±1.5	93	33.0±1.5	127

[1]Values are geometric mean ± geometric SD. *Note:* Geometric SD is a factor, not a quantity. Powers of the geometric SD can be either multiplied by (or divided into) the geometric mean to determine the set of values that lie n geometric SDs from the mean.

of 12.1 years [41]. In our study, puberty was likely not a significant confounder as menarche had commenced in only 2% (5 of 262) of the female participants studied with 1,25(OH)$_2$D values available.

The significance of the n-shaped association between 1,25(OH)$_2$D and BMI, where participants in the lowest and highest BMI groups displayed lower 1,25(OH)$_2$D concentrations, is unclear and warrants further investigation over a wider range of body mass indices. Very few children in our sample were overweight (n = 17) or obese (n = 13). Several studies have reported an inverse relationship between vitamin D status and childhood body weight [42–45]; however we found no association between 25(OH)D and BMI.

The present data also suggest a positive association between vitamin D metabolites and child height. Few studies have investigated the relationship between vitamin D and linear bone growth in healthy children. An observational study by Lund et al reported a positive association between 1,25(OH)$_2$D and growth velocity in a group of children and adolescents ranging in age from 3 months to 19 years [46]. Currently, there is no simple explanation for this finding; however, there is evidence that suggests a role of the vitamin D endocrine system in regulating growth of the skeleton [47–50]. There is also an interrelation between vitamin D and insulin-like growth factor-1 (IGF-1), an important regulator of skeletal growth and development, albeit the relationship is complex [50,51]. Further studies are required to confirm these findings and establish the mechanisms by which these effects are induced.

Interestingly, while a strong negative association between serum levels of 25(OH)D and PTH was demonstrated, PTH concentrations were within a normal range despite possible low calcium intakes. These results support a similar study in adults where adequate vitamin D status ensured ideal PTH values even when calcium intakes were moderately low [52]. The authors concluded that vitamin D may have a calcium-sparing effect [52]. Although the WHO recommends calcium intakes of 700 mg/d for children 7–9 years of age and 1300 mg/d for children 10–18 years [53], it is increasingly recognized that calcium requirements may be lower for Southeast Asian and East Asian populations [54,55]. A number of dietary factors including phytate, sodium and animal protein, are known to influence the bioavailability of calcium for absorption and/or urinary calcium excretion. In the case of vitamin D, it has been long recognized that vitamin D promotes calcium absorption [56], however, the relation between vitamin D status and intestinal calcium absorption in settings of habitual low calcium intake has not been extensively studied.

This study has several notable strengths including the fairly large sample size of healthy female and male children across a wide age range. Nonetheless, our results are not necessarily generalizable to other geographical regions or population groups. These findings, however, emphasize the need for nationally representative data to appropriately assess the magnitude of vitamin D deficiency, particularly given that our study data are over 10 years old and lifestyle characteristics may have changed including sun exposure protection practices or levels of outdoor activity. Moreover, dietary calcium intakes of participants were not assessed at the time of blood sampling (i.e., study endline; only determined at study baseline). As mentioned above, in order to address the speculation that 25(OH)D concentrations are mediated by the effects of 1,25(OH)$_2$D, additional studies with careful dietary assessment over a wider range of both calcium intakes and vitamin D status are needed. In doing so, careful consideration should also be given to the type of assay employed to measure 1,25(OH)$_2$D as accurate measurement of this vitamin D metabolite is particularly difficult [57].

Table 3. Linear regression model of factors associated with serum 25-hydroxyvitamin D (nmol/L), 1,25-dihydroxyvitamin D (pmol/L) and parathyroid hormone concentrations (ng/L) among Thai schoolchildren aged 6–13 y[1].

	Unadjusted				Adjusted/final[2,3]			
Variable	**n**	**Estimates**	**95% CI**	***P***	**n**	**Estimates**	**95% CI**	***P***
For 25(OH)D					525			
BMI	525	0.99	0.98, 1.00	0.021		0.997	0.987, 1.01	0.515
Sex (male)	526	1.19	1.14, 1.23	<0.001		1.19 [4]	1.14, 1.23	<0.001
Age, y	526	0.98	0.96, 0.99	0.010				
Age, y for boys						1.00	0.98, 1.02	0.895
Age, y for girls						0.96	0.94, 0.97	0.001
Sex × Age interaction								<0.001
Height-for-age Z score	526	0.97	0.94, 0.99	0.017		0.98	0.96, 0.99	0.006
For $1,25(OH)_2D$					510			
BMI	518	1.03	1.00, 1.06	0.028		1.11	1.04, 1.18	0.004
BMI-squared		0.996	0.994, 0.999	0.009		0.997	0.996, 0.999	0.004
Sex (male)	519	0.86	0.83, 0.89	<0.001		0.86	0.82, 0.90	<0.001
Age, y	519	1.02	0.99, 1.05	0.232		1.02	0.99, 1.04	0.17
Height-for-age Z score	519	1.07	1.05, 1.110	<0.001		1.07	1.04, 1.11	0.001
log 25OHD	512	0.91	0.76, 1.08	0.235		1.12	0.95, 1.33	0.153
For PTH					502			
BMI	514	1.02	0.99, 1.04	0.196		0.98	0.96, 1.02	0.365
Sex (male)	515	0.80	0.74, 0.87	<0.001		0.91	0.82, 1.02	0.097
Age, y	515	1.04	1.01, 1.07	0.008		1.03	0.999, 1.07	0.055
Age-squared		1.02	1.00, 1.04	0.037		1.02	1.00, 1.03	0.049
Height-for-age Z score	515	1.10	1.03, 1.18	0.012		1.08	1.02, 1.14	0.016
log 25OHD	509	0.50	0.43, 0.57	<0.001		0.61	0.49, 0.74	<0.001
log $1,25(OH)_2D$	509	1.34	1.09, 1.64	0.012		1.18	0.99, 1.40	0.06

[1]Effect sizes are ratios of geometric means, accompanied by 95% CIs and *P*-values.
[2]Adjusted for variables with $P \leq 0.25$ in univariate analysis.
[3]R^2 of the whole model for 25OHD: 0.24; for $1,25(OH)_2D$: 0.13; for PTH: 0.20.
[4]At the mean age (9.9 y).

In summary, our results suggest that vitamin D status was sufficient in this group of Thai school children, although girls experienced a decline in 25(OH)D levels with increasing age. This association is possibly mediated by reduced sun exposure. Future studies should employ measures to appropriately quantify sun exposure and outdoor activity. In addition, this study is the first to investigate the interrelationship between vitamin D metabolites in a group of healthy children who typically have low calcium intakes. While the increased concentration of 1,25(OH)$_2$D may reflect an adaptive mechanism to maximize calcium absorption, more extensive studies are needed to define the ideal intake of calcium in the presence of an ample supply of vitamin D.

Author Contributions

Conceived and designed the experiments: PW RSG LAH. Performed the experiments: TP SG. Analyzed the data: ARG LAH. Contributed reagents/materials/analysis tools: MJH. Contributed to the writing of the manuscript: LAH.

References

1. Ryan LM, Teach SJ, Singer SA, Wood R, Freishtat R, et al. (2012) Bone mineral density and vitamin D status among African American children with forearm fractures. Pediatrics 130: e553–560.
2. Holick MF (2004) Vitamin D: importance in the prevention of cancers, type 1 diabetes, heart disease, and osteoporosis. Am J Clin Nutr 79: 362–371.
3. Shaw NJ, Mughal MZ (2013) Vitamin D and child health: part 2 (extraskeletal and other aspects). Arch Dis Child 98: 368–372.
4. Al-Ghamdi MA, Lanham-New SA, Kahn JA (2012) Differences in vitamin D status and calcium metabolism in Saudi Arabian boys and girls aged 6 to 18 years: effects of age, gender, extent of veiling and physical activity with concomitant implications for bone health. Public Health Nutr 15: 1845–1853.
5. Razzaghy-Azar M, Shakiba M (2010) Assessment of vitamin D status in healthy children and adolescents living in Tehran and its relation to iPTH, gender, weight and height. Ann Hum Biol 37: 692–701.
6. Carpenter TO, Herreros F, Zhang JH, Ellis BK, Simpson C, et al. (2012) Demographic, dietary, and biochemical determinants of vitamin D status in inner-city children. Am J Clin Nutr 95: 137–146.
7. Weng FL, Shults J, Leonard MB, Stallings VA, Zemel BS (2007) Risk factors for low serum 25-hydroxyvitamin D concentrations in otherwise healthy children and adolescents. Am J Clin Nutr 86: 150–158.
8. Jang HB, Lee HJ, Park JY, Kang JH, Song J (2013) Association between serum vitamin d and metabolic risk factors in korean schoolgirls. Osong Public Health Res Perspect 4: 179–186.
9. Laillou A, Wieringa F, Tran TN, Van PT, Le BM, et al. (2013) Hypovitaminosis D and mild hypocalcaemia are highly prevalent among young Vietnamese children and women and related to low dietary intake. PLoS One 8: e63979.
10. Marwaha RK, Tandon N, Reddy DR, Aggarwal R, Singh R, et al. (2005) Vitamin D and bone mineral density status of healthy schoolchildren in northern India. Am J Clin Nutr 82: 477–482.
11. Khor GL, Chee WS, Shariff ZM, Poh BK, Arumugam M, et al. (2011) High prevalence of vitamin D insufficiency and its association with BMI-for-age among primary school children in Kuala Lumpur, Malaysia. BMC Public Health 11: 95.
12. Neyestani TR, Hajifaraji M, Omidvar N, Eshraghian MR, Shariatzadeh N, et al. (2012) High prevalence of vitamin D deficiency in school-age children in Tehran, 2008: a red alert. Public Health Nutr 15: 324–330.
13. Kumar J, Muntner P, Kaskel FJ, Hailpern SM, Melamed ML (2009) Prevalence and associations of 25-hydroxyvitamin D deficiency in US children: NHANES 2001–2004. Pediatrics 124: e362–70.
14. Clements MR, Johnson L, Fraser DR (1987) A new mechanism for induced vitamin D deficiency in calcium deprivation. Nature 325: 62–65.
15. Halloran BP, Bikle DD, Levens MJ, Castro ME, Globus RK, et al. (1986) Chronic 1,25-dihydroxyvitamin D3 administration in the rat reduces the serum concentration of 25-hydroxyvitamin D by increasing metabolic clearance rate. J Clin Invest 78: 622–628.
16. Davies M, Heys SE, Selby PL, Berry JL, Mawer EB (1997) Increased catabolism of 25-hydroxyvitamin D in patients with partial gastrectomy and elevated 1,25-dihydroxyvitamin D levels. Implications for metabolic bone disease. J Clin Endocrinol Metab 82: 209–212.
17. Batchelor AJ, Compston JE (1983) Reduced plasma half-life of radio-labelled 25-hydroxyvitamin D3 in subjects receiving a high-fibre diet. Br J Nutr 49: 213–216.
18. Clements MR, Davies M, Hayes ME, Hickey CD, Lumb GA, et al. (1992) The role of 1,25-dihydroxyvitamin D in the mechanism of acquired vitamin D deficiency. Clin Endocrinol (Oxf) 37: 17–27.
19. Chusilp K, Somnasang P, Kirdpon W, Wongkham S, Sribonlue P, et al. (1992) Observations on the development of stunting in children of the Khon Kaen region of Thailand. Eur J Clin Nutr 46: 475–487.
20. Gibson RS, Manger MS, Krittaphol W, Pongcharoen T, Gowachirapant S, et al. (2007) Does zinc deficiency play a role in stunting among primary school children in NE Thailand? Br J Nutr 97: 167–175.
21. Heaney RP, Weaver CM, Fitzsimmons ML (1991) Soybean phytate content: effect on calcium absorption. Am J Clin Nutr 53: 745–747.
22. Chailurkit LO, Aekplakorn W, Ongphiphadhanakul B (2011) Regional variation and determinants of vitamin D status in sunshine-abundant Thailand. BMC Public Health 11: 853.
23. Winichagoon P, McKenzie JE, Chavasit V, Pongcharoen T, Gowachirapant S, et al. (2006) A multimicronutrient-fortified seasoning powder enhances the hemoglobin, zinc, and iodine status of primary school children in North East Thailand: a randomized controlled trial of efficacy. J Nutr 136: 1617–1623.
24. Manger MS, McKenzie JE, Winichagoon P, Gray A, Chavasit V, et al. (2008) A micronutrient-fortified seasoning powder reduces morbidity and improves short-term cognitive function, but has no effect on anthropometric measures in primary school children in northeast Thailand: a randomized controlled trial. Am J Clin Nutr 87: 1715–1722.
25. World Health Organization. The WHO Child Growth Standards. Growth reference, 5–19 years Available: http://www.who.int/growthref/en/. Accessed 2014 Jul 21.
26. Maunsell Z, Wright DJ, Rainbow SJ (2005) Routine Isotope-Dilution Liquid Chromatography-Tandem Mass Spectrometry Assay for Simultaneous Measurement of the 25-Hydroxy Metabolites of Vitamins D2 and D3. Clin Chem 51: 1683–1690.
27. Institute of Medicine (2010) Food and Nutrition Board. Dietary reference intakes for calcium and vitamin D.; Ross AC, Taylor CL, Yaktine AL, Del Valle HB, editors. Washington D.C.: National Academy Press.
28. Rojroongwasinkul N, Kijboonchoo K, Wimonpeerapattana W, Purttiponthanee S, Yamborisut U, et al. (2013) SEANUTS: the nutritional status and dietary intakes of 0.5–12-year-old Thai children. Br J Nutr 110 Suppl 3: S36–44.
29. Krobtrakulchai W, Praikanahok J, Visitsunthorn N, Vichyanond P, Manonukul K, et al. (2013) The effect of vitamin d status on pediatric asthma at a university hospital, Thailand. Allergy Asthma Immunol Res 5: 289–294.
30. Nakavachara P, Viprakasit V (2013) Children with hemoglobin E/beta-thalassemia have a high risk of being vitamin D deficient even if they get abundant sun exposure: a study from Thailand. Pediatr Blood Cancer 60: 1683–1688.
31. Schottker B, Jansen EH, Haug U, Schomburg L, Kohrle J, et al. (2012) Standardization of misleading immunoassay based 25-hydroxyvitamin D levels with liquid chromatography tandem-mass spectrometry in a large cohort study. PLoS One 7: e48774.
32. Moon HW, Cho JH, Hur M, Song J, Oh GY, et al. (2012) Comparison of four current 25-hydroxyvitamin D assays. Clin Biochem 45: 326–330.
33. Tempark T, Chatproedprai S, Wananukul S (2012) Attitudes, knowledge, and behaviors of secondary school adolescents regarding protection from sun exposure: a survey in Bangkok, Thailand. Photodermatol Photoimmunol Photomed 28: 200–206.
34. Lewis RD, Laing EM, Hill Gallant KM, Hall DB, McCabe GP, et al. (2013) A Randomized Trial of Vitamin D3 Supplementation in Children: Dose-Response Effects on Vitamin D Metabolites and Calcium Absorption. J Clin Endocrinol Metab.
35. Park CY, Hill KM, Elble AE, Martin BR, DiMeglio LA, et al. (2010) Daily supplementation with 25 mug cholecalciferol does not increase calcium absorption or skeletal retention in adolescent girls with low serum 25-hydroxyvitamin D. J Nutr 140: 2139–2144.
36. Lips P (2006) Vitamin D physiology. Prog Biophys Mol Biol 92: 4–8.
37. Anderson PH, Iida S, Tyson JH, Turner AG, Morris HA (2010) Bone CYP27B1 gene expression is increased with high dietary calcium and in mineralising osteoblasts. J Steroid Biochem Mol Biol 121: 71–75.
38. Aspray TJ, Yan L, Prentice A (2005) Parathyroid hormone and rates of bone formation are raised in perimenopausal rural Gambian women. Bone 36: 710–720.
39. Jones G, Strugnell SA, DeLuca HF (1998) Current understanding of the molecular actions of vitamin D. Physiol Rev 78: 1193–1231.
40. van Hoof HJ, van der Mooren MJ, Swinkels LM, Rolland R, Benraad TJ (1994) Hormone replacement therapy increases serum 1,25-dihydroxyvitamin D: A 2-year prospective study. Calcif Tissue Int 55: 417–419.
41. Mahachoklertwattana P, Suthutvoravut U, Charoenkiatkul S, Chongviriyaphan N, Rojroongwasinkul N, et al. (2002) Earlier onset of pubertal maturation in Thai girls. J Med Assoc Thai 85 Suppl 4: S1127–1134.
42. Gordon CM, Feldman HA, Sinclair L, Williams AL, Kleinman PK, et al. (2008) Prevalence of vitamin D deficiency among healthy infants and toddlers. Arch Pediatr Adolesc Med 162: 505–512.
43. Harkness LS, Cromer BA (2005) Vitamin D deficiency in adolescent females. J Adolesc Health 37: 75.

44. Rockell JE, Green TJ, Skeaff CM, Whiting SJ, Taylor RW, et al. (2005) Season and ethnicity are determinants of serum 25-hydroxyvitamin D concentrations in New Zealand children aged 5–14 y. J Nutr 135: 2602–2608.
45. Saintonge S, Bang H, Gerber LM (2009) Implications of a new definition of vitamin D deficiency in a multiracial US adolescent population: the National Health and Nutrition Examination Survey III. Pediatrics 123: 797–803.
46. Lund B, Clausen N, Lund B, Andersen E, Sorensen OH (1980) Age-dependent variations in serum 1,25-dihydroxyvitamin D in childhood. Acta Endocrinol (Copenh) 94: 426–429.
47. Suarez F, Zeghoud F, Rossignol C, Walrant O, Garabedian M (1997) Association between vitamin D receptor gene polymorphism and sex-dependent growth during the first two years of life. J Clin Endocrinol Metab 82: 2966–2970.
48. Lorentzon M, Lorentzon R, Nordstrom P (2000) Vitamin D receptor gene polymorphism is associated with birth height, growth to adolescence, and adult stature in healthy caucasian men: a cross-sectional and longitudinal study. J Clin Endocrinol Metab 85: 1666–1670.
49. van der Sluis IM, de Muinck Keizer-Schrama SM, Krenning EP, Pols HA, Uitterlinden AG (2003) Vitamin D receptor gene polymorphism predicts height and bone size, rather than bone density in children and young adults. Calcif Tissue Int 73: 332–338.
50. d'Alesio A, Garabedian M, Sabatier JP, Guaydier-Souquieres G, Marcelli C, et al. (2005) Two single-nucleotide polymorphisms in the human vitamin D receptor promoter change protein-DNA complex formation and are associated with height and vitamin D status in adolescent girls. Hum Mol Genet 14: 3539–3548.
51. Ameri P, Giusti A, Boschetti M, Murialdo G, Minuto F, et al. (2013) Interactions between vitamin D and IGF-I: from physiology to clinical practice. Clin Endocrinol (Oxf) 79: 457–463.
52. Steingrimsdottir L, Gunnarsson O, Indridason OS, Franzson L, Sigurdsson G (2005) Relationship between serum parathyroid hormone levels, vitamin D sufficiency, and calcium intake. JAMA 294: 2336–2341.
53. World Health Organization and Food and Agriculture Organization of the United Nations (2004) Calcium. Vitamin and mineral requirements in human nutrition 2nd ed. Geneva, Switzerland: WHO Library.
54. Lee WT, Jiang J (2008) Calcium requirements for Asian children and adolescents. Asia Pac J Clin Nutr 17 Suppl 1: 33–36.
55. Wu L, Martin BR, Braun MM, Wastney ME, McCabe GP, et al. (2010) Calcium requirements and metabolism in Chinese-American boys and girls. J Bone Miner Res 25: 1842–1849.
56. Telfer SV (1926) Studies in calcium and phosphorus metabolism. Quarterly Journal of Medicine 20: 1–6.
57. Farrell CJ, Herrmann M (2013) Determination of vitamin D and its metabolites. Best Pract Res Clin Endocrinol Metab 27: 675–688.

17

Iron Status and Reproduction in US Women: National Health and Nutrition Examination Survey, 1999-2006

Elizabeth M. Miller*

Department of Anthropology, University of South Florida, Tampa, Florida, United States of America

Abstract

Women experience significant changes in iron status throughout their reproductive lifespans. While this is evident in regions with high rates of malnutrition and infectious disease, the extent of reproductive-related changes is less well known in countries with low rates of iron deficiency anemia, such as the United States. The goal of this study is determine the relationship between women's reproductive variables (pregnancy, parity, currently breastfeeding, regular menstruation, hormonal contraceptive use, and age at menarche) and iron status (hemoglobin, ferritin, transferrin receptor, and % transferrin saturation) using an anthropological framework for interpreting the results. Data from women aged 18–49 were taken from the 1999–2006 US NHANES, a nationally representative cross-sectional sample of US women. Using multiple imputation and complex survey statistics, women's reproductive variables were regressed against indicators of iron status. Pregnant women had significantly poorer iron status, by most indicators, than non-pregnant women. All biomarkers demonstrated significantly lower iron levels with increasing parity. Women who were having regular periods had iron indicators that suggested decreased iron levels, while women who used hormonal contraceptives had iron indicators that suggested increased iron levels. Despite relatively good iron status and widespread availability of iron-rich foods in the US, women still exhibit patterns of iron depletion across several reproductive variables of interest. These results contribute to an ecological approach to iron status that seeks to understand variation in iron status, with the hopes that appropriate, population-specific recommendations can be developed to improve women's health.

Editor: James F. Collins, University of Florida, United States of America

Funding: This author has no support or funding to report.

Competing Interests: The author has declared that no competing interests exist.

* Email: emm3@usf.edu

Introduction

Globally, reproductively-active women are at risk of iron-deficiency anemia, which causes significant morbidity and mortality [1,2]. The effects of low iron in women can have broad global effects on their physical and cognitive capabilities as well as specific effects on perinatal outcomes and infant health [3,4]. During pregnancy, iron is allocated to the fetus to a high degree, particularly in the later trimesters [5,6]. This can lead to maternal and fetal iron deficiency anemia, particularly in women with poor iron status pre-pregnancy [4,7–9]. There is also evidence that this can affect women across their reproductive careers: a growing body of literature suggests that increasing parity is associated with decreased indicators of iron status and greater likelihood of iron-deficiency anemia [10–14]. While pregnancy depletes maternal iron stores, after birth women have relatively low iron needs that allows for repletion of iron stores before the next pregnancy [14]. When inter-birth intervals are short or when dietary iron is insufficient, parity-related maternal iron depletion can result [14,15].

Iron status has also been implicated in other aspects of women's reproduction, mainly attributed to the loss of iron via menstrual blood. Menstrual blood loss has been associated with poorer indicators of iron status [16–18], although this perspective is controversial [19]. Fittingly, the use of hormonal contraceptive, which is generally associated with lighter menstrual periods, is associated with better indicators of iron status than in women who do not use hormonal contraceptives [10,17]. Breastfeeding is also associated with lower dietary iron needs [20,21] due to low levels of iron in breast milk and lactational amenorrhea [22–25], particularly in undernourished populations.

The National Health and Nutrition Examination Survey (NHANES) offers a unique opportunity to investigate markers of iron status across a broad cross-section of reproductive-aged US women. Compared to the global population, the United States has low rates of iron-deficiency anemia; however, it does appear that reproduction-related iron depletion can occur, particularly in pregnant women [26] and African American women [12]. This study will investigate the relationship between reproductive variables and markers of iron status using a biological anthropology framework. Specifically, it will explore how pregnancy, parity, breastfeeding, menstruation, hormonal contraceptive use, and menarche are associated with four indicators of iron status:

Table 1. Weighted descriptive statistics for study variables for women aged 18–49 who participated in the NHANES physical examination during 1999–2006, before and after multiple imputation of missing values.

		Pre-imputed weighted descriptive statistics			Imputed weighted descriptive statistics[a]		
		Mean or %	**SE**	*n*	**Mean or %**	**SE**	**95% CI**
Iron Status	Hemoglobin (g/dL)	13.50	0.37	6225	13.50	0.036	13.43, 13.57
	Ferritin (ng/mL)	57.84	1.03	6162	57.72	1.05	55.67, 59.78
	% Transferrin saturation	3.57	0.037	2824	3.70	0.042	3.61, 3.78
	Transferrin receptor (mg/L)[b]	22.60	0.19	6153	22.58	1.18	22.22, 22.94
Reproductive Status	% Pregnant	6.43	0.32	6463	6.52	0.32	5.89, 7.16
	Parity	1.54	0.028	5616	1.53	0.027	1.47, 1.58
	% Currently breastfeeding	2.01	0.34	5107	1.90	0.33	1.26, 2.53
	% Currently using hormonal contraceptive	16.02	0.84	5608	15.86	0.78	14.33, 17.39
	% Ever used hormonal contraceptive	77.46	0.86	5942	77.00	0.87	75.28, 78.70
	% Had regular periods in past year	72.40	0.83	5947	72.58	0.84	70.92, 74.23
	Age at menarche (years)	12.60	0.028	5854	12.60	0.027	12.55, 12.65
Covariates	% Hispanic	15.47	0.13	6603	15.47	0.13	–[c]
	% Non-Hispanic black	13.48	0.11	6603	13.48	0.11	–[c]
	% Non-Hispanic white	65.45	0.10	6603	65.45	0.10	–[c]
	% Other	5.60	0.045	6603	5.60	0.045	–[c]
	BMI (kg/m^2)	27.86	0.16	6468	27.87	0.16	27.56, 28.19
	CRP (g/L)	0.47	0.014	6173	0.47	0.014	0.44, 0.50
	Age (years)	33.99	0.17	6603	33.99	0.17	–[c]
	Dietary iron intake (mg)	13.73	0.14	6252	13.73	0.14	13.46, 14.00

[a]All n = 6603 (except transferrin receptor).
[b]The n for the imputed mean for transferrin receptor is 3295; based on 2003–2006 survey years only.
[c]All variables were available in original data set, so no 95% CI were generated by PROC MIANALYZE.

hemoglobin, ferritin, transferrin receptor, and percent transferrin saturation. This research will test the following hypotheses:

1) Women will show differences in iron status depending on their current and past reproductive history. This hypothesis leads to three predictions: a) Pregnant women will have lower iron status than women who are not pregnant; b) Women who are currently breastfeeding will have iron indicators that indicate post-pregnancy iron recovery; and c) Increasing parity (reproductive history) will be negatively associated with indicators of iron status.
2) Women will experience short- and long-term effects of menstruation on iron status. This hypothesis leads to two predictions: a) Regularly menstruating women will have iron indicators that indicate lower iron status; and b) Earlier age at menarche will be associated with lower iron status.

The US NHANES offers an opportunity to examine several indicators of iron status in reproductive-aged women. Hemoglobin, an iron-containing oxygen carrier protein in red blood cells, is the most common iron indicator used to diagnose anemia. Low hemoglobin is diagnostic of anemia (the lowered ability of the blood to carry oxygen) but cannot necessarily distinguish between iron deficiency anemia and other causes of anemia. Serum ferritin, an iron storage protein, correlates well with global iron stores (except in the presence of inflammation). Low serum ferritin is especially useful in distinguishing between iron deficiency anemia and other forms of anemia [27]. Percent transferrin saturation is the percent iron bound to transferrin (an iron carrier protein), and is also a measure of iron deficiency. Finally, serum transferrin receptor binds to transferrin in order to transfer iron into cells. Transferrin receptor increases during iron deficiency as the body's tissues attempt to increase intercellular iron concentration, and can be used to distinguish iron deficiency anemia from other forms of anemia even when inflammation is present. These four measurements offer similar, but slightly different, perspectives on iron status and can provide insight into the dynamics of iron physiology in reproductive-aged women.

Subjects and Methods

Ethics statement

This study was originally approved by the National Center for Health Statistics Research Ethics Review Board, and participants underwent informed consent before data collection. Because the current study is a secondary analysis of de-identified data, the University of South Florida Institutional Review Board determined that this research is not human subjects research and thus not subject to review.

Sample design

The NHANES is a US-representative survey conducted by the Centers for Disease Control and Prevention (CDC), which has been collecting data on a two-year continuous basis since 1999. The goal of the NHANES is to collect health and nutrition-related data on the general US population. NHANES uses a complex sample design in which participants are weighted according to geographic and census information, and certain groups (such as pregnant women) are oversampled for analytical purposes [28]. Adding to the complexity of the data, not all NHANES participants who took part in the interview decided to take part in the physical examination. There are also considerable missing data, particularly in the reproductive health questionnaire. Although 6603 women between the ages of 18 and 49 participated in the physical examination between 1999 and 2006, rates of missing data were fairly high (see Table 1). Therefore, the current study uses a multiple imputation method to correct for missing responses and increase available sample size.

Variable selection

Iron status. NHANES 1999–2006 has multiple variables relating to iron status. Information relating to laboratory analysis of iron status variables are available in the NHANES documentation on the CDC website. All continuous variables were left as untransformed linear variables for analysis.

Found in red blood cells, hemoglobin is the main oxygen-transporting protein in the body. Each hemoglobin molecule contains one iron ion. Around 70% of the body's iron is located in hemoglobin. Hemoglobin levels are used to diagnose iron-deficiency anemia, with values of <12–12.5 g/dL generally considered anemic in women [29], although can vary by pregnancy status [3]. In the NHANES, hemoglobin was measured as part of the complete blood count using the Coulter HMX Hematology Analyzer [30–33]. Hemoglobin levels (g/dL) are available for all children and adults who completed the physical examination [30–33].

Ferritin is an iron-storage protein that is indirectly used as a measure of iron levels in the body. Ferritin levels of <12 ng/mL are considered indicative of iron deficiency [29]. Ferritin levels (ng/mL) are available for all adults and children from survey years 1999–2002 and in reproductive aged-women (12–49 years) in survey years 2003–2006 [30–33]. Two different assays were used to measure ferritin across data years: in years 1999–2003 BioRad Laboratories' two-site immunoradiometric assay kit was used, while in 2004 and later years the Roche/Hitachi immunoturbidity assay was used. The Roche/Hitachi method gives a higher ferritin estimate than the BioRad assay, and must be normalized using a derived piecewise linear equation [34]. While the 2003 data were normalized to the 2004 data prior to release, investigators that use the 1999–2002 data with later releases, including the current study, must adjust the earlier values using provided equations [34]. Ferritin levels are increased during acute-phase inflammation [35], so C-reactive protein (CRP) should be included in multivariate models as a control variable.

Transferrin receptor is a carrier protein for transferrin, providing transportation for iron into cells and helping maintain iron homeostasis in the body. Transferrin receptor is upregulated in the case of low body iron in order to help maintain intracellular iron levels, and is frequently elevated in pregnancy [36–38]. Previous research has indicated that the cutoff for iron deficiency for transferrin receptor in reproductive-aged women is > 5.33 mg/L [39]. In the NHANES, serum transferrin receptor was measured via immunoturbidity assay using Roche kits on the Hitachi Mod P clinical analyzer [32,33]. Serum transferrin receptor (mg/L) was available for all women aged 12–49 years in survey years 2003–2006, but was only available for pregnant women in survey years 1999–2002 [30–33]. While multiple imputation would theoretically replace the missing data in the earlier survey years, in practice multiple imputation of all 8 years lead to biased data and models that would not converge. Therefore, the decision was made to perform analyses on transferrin receptor for 2003–2006 only, and impute the missing data only in those years.

Percent transferrin saturation is a measure of the total body iron that is bound to transferrin, which is a blood protein that binds to and controls the release of the body's iron. Percent transferrin saturation was calculated using the formula: serum iron/total iron-binding capacity x 100%. Serum iron and total iron-binding capacity were measured using automated AAII-25 colorimetric method modified to be performed on the Alpkem Flow Solutions 3000 system [30–33]. Percent transferrin saturation was available in 1999–2000 for men and women of all ages and in 2001–2006 for women between the ages of 12 and 59 years [30–33]. Percent transferrin saturation is considered deficient when values fall below 16% [29].

Reproductive history variables. Reproduction-related variables are available for all women above the age of 12 in the reproductive health questionnaire. Some reproductive variables were constructed using more than one variable in order to accurately represent the survey methods and the population's response. For all constructed reproductive variables, respondents with missing values for both questions were left missing.

Pregnancy status was determined by the results of the urine pregnancy test. A continuous parity variable was constructed based on a combined variable, first by using a variable that asks if women had ever been pregnant and for those that said yes, using the number of reported live births. Women who had no pregnancies were reported to have a parity of 0; for all others, the reported live births were used as their parity value.

A dichotomous variable for currently breastfeeding women was created using three variables: First, women who reported never being pregnant were coded as not currently breastfeeding. Second, women who had given birth within the past two years were asked if they were currently breastfeeding; those that said yes were coded as currently breastfeeding and those that said no were coded as not currently breastfeeding. Finally, women who had reported giving birth 2 or more years ago were coded as not currently breastfeeding (the NHANES survey made the assumption during data collection that women 2 or more years post birth were not currently breastfeeding).

Two dichotomous variables for hormonal contraceptive use were created: one, for current use of hormonal contraception, and two, for using hormonal contraception at any point during the life span.

Reported having regular menstrual periods over the previous 12 months was included as a dichotomous variable. To assess the long-term effects of menstrual history, recalled age at menarche was included as a continuous variable.

Control variables. Regression analyses were controlled for the following variables: Age, CRP level, body mass index (BMI), survey year, ethnicity, dietary iron intake from 24-hour recall, and household income. Age, BMI, CRP, and dietary iron intake were included as continuous variables. Yearly household income was coded as dummy variables in \$5000 increments, up to \$75,000+. Ethnicity was coded as dummy variables for Hispanic (including Mexican Americans), non-Hispanic black and other, with non-Hispanic white as the reference category. Survey year for each two-year data-release period was included as dummy variables.

Eight-year examination sample weights were calculated using the 4-year weight for survey years 1999–2002 and two-year weights for 2003-2004 and 2005–2006. The 4-year weights were multiplied by ½ and the 2-year weights were multiplied by ¼ to create the 8-year weight variable. To create the 4-year weights for the transferrin receptor models for 2003–2004 and 2005–2006, the 2-year examination sample weights were multiplied by ½ [28].

Statistical methods

Excluding individuals who have missing values from analysis can lead to biased results [40,41]. Multiple imputation (MI) is a statistical method for replacing missing variables in a data set. Imputation models use a probability model on both complete and missing data in a set to generate likely variables for missing values. In multiple imputation, several imputed data sets are generated, and the desired statistical analysis is performed on each one. After analysis, the results from each imputed set are averaged across variables to help control for the variance introduced by the imputation process [40,41].

Multiple imputation proceeds through three steps: 1) the generation of the MI data sets, which generates likely values for missing variables based on available data; 2) complex survey regression analyses based on the MI data sets; and 3) the synthesis of the imputed data sets and regression analyses, which combines the imputed results and reports the variability introduced by the imputation process [41,42]. The MI process was performed in SAS 9.3 (SAS Institute, Inc., Cary, North Carolina). Statistical significance was assessed at $\alpha = 0.05$ (two-sided).

The multiple imputation of data sets was performed using PROC MI in SAS. In SAS, PROC MI uses a Markov chain Monte Carlo method that assumes arbitrary missing data and multivariate normality. Standard usage of MI data sets suggests that at least 5 imputed data sets should be used, although this number may be higher for data sets with more missing data [43]. Due to the high levels of missing values for some variables in the data set, $n = 50$ imputations were performed in this analysis. For 50 imputations, reliability estimates for each variable were above 95%. All variables mentioned above were included in the imputation analysis, but income variables were dropped from regression analysis because they were not statistically significant and had no biological rationale for being included as a control variable.

A special mention should be made of dichotomous variables in MI procedures. Imputed dichotomous variables are not dichotomous themselves, but instead range as a proportion between 0 and 1. Some practitioners round the imputed fractions to the nearest 0 or 1; however, this practice leads to biased estimates of these variables [44]. Analysis of a variety of methods for handling dichotomous variables suggests that for the majority of cases, imputed fractions should be left alone for regression analysis [45]. Therefore, imputed dichotomous variables in this study were left as-is for analysis.

Analysis of imputed data sets was performed using PROC SURVEYMEANS for descriptive statistics and PROC SURVEYREG for linear regression. All survey analyses (descriptive and regression) were adjusted using NHANES-provided variables for strata and cluster, and the adjusted 8-year sample weight described above (or the 4-year sample weight for the transferrin receptor model). The imputed data sets were added to the model as part of the domain statement. This allows the analyses to be performed on each imputed data set.

For the PROC SURVEYREG analyses, four models were run with each iron biomarker (hemoglobin, ferritin, transferrin receptor, and % transferring saturation) as dependent variables. Independent variables for each model were as follows: current pregnancy, parity, currently breastfeeding, currently using contraceptive pills, ever used contraceptive pills, having regular periods in the past 12 months, and age at menarche. All models were adjusted for ethnicity (with white ethnicity as the reference variable), survey release years (with 1999–2000 as the reference variable except the transferrin receptor model, which used 2003–2004 as the reference variable), BMI, CRP, age, and 24-hour recall of dietary iron intake.

To complement MI analysis, it is recommended that an analysis of all complete cases (cases with no missing data) be performed in order to assess potential areas of bias, either in the complete case or in the multiple imputation [46]. In this study, complete case analyses were performed for each model using PROC SUR-

VEYREG and was adjusted for examination weight, strata, and cluster as described above. The subdomain for this analysis was female exam participants ages 18–49. Descriptive statistics for the non-imputed, original data were performed using PROC SURVEYMEANS and the parameters described above.

The final step was performed using PROC MIANALYSIS. This procedure synthesizes the results of the 50 imputed data sets, providing summary means and adjusted variances for PROC SURVEYMEANS, and summary parameter estimates and adjusted variances for the results of PROCSURVEYREG. This method also provides 95% confidence intervals for means and parameter estimates. Using these three steps, results are adjusted for both the multiple imputation process and the complex survey design of NHANES.

Results

Descriptive statistics were performed on both the original data sets and the imputed data sets using PROC SURVEYMEANS, to adjust for the complex survey design (Table 1). The percent missing data, derived from the total number of eligible women ($n = 6603$), ranged from 0% to 32.7% depending on the variable of interest. Graphs of the weighted association between iron biomarkers and pregnancy are found in Figure 1 and iron biomarkers and parity in Figure 2. Hemoglobin, ferritin, and % transferrin saturation declined with increasing parity and was also reduced in pregnant women. Transferrin receptor increased with increasing parity, and was higher in non-pregnant women compared to pregnant women. Table 2 shows the percentage of women who fall below the cutoff value for each iron biomarker, as well as the percentage of women considered iron deficient, as defined by having two out of three values of hemoglobin, ferritin, and % transferrin saturation below their respective cutoff values [47].

Complete case results (estimates and p-values) for survey regression for the four models is found in Table 3. In general, there were between 60–65% complete cases for each model out of the eligible women in the study population. Results do not appear to differ significantly between the complete case results and the imputed results, reported in Table 4.

Imputed estimates, 95% confidence intervals, and p-values for each of the four models (analyzed using imputed values and PROC SURVEYREG) can be found in Table 4. In the hemoglobin model, there was a significant negative association between pregnancy and hemoglobin, parity and hemoglobin, and having regular periods and hemoglobin. In addition, white American women had significantly higher hemoglobin than all other ethnicities.

In the ferritin model, ferritin was significantly negatively associated with pregnancy, parity, and having regular periods. Ferritin was significantly positively associated with taking hormonal contraceptive. Several covariates were also statistically significant. Hispanic women had significantly lower ferritin levels while women whose ethnicity was given as "other" had significantly higher ferritin levels. Ferritin was also significantly positively associated with current age and CRP level.

Transferrin receptor levels were significantly positively associated with having regular menstrual periods and parity. Transferrin receptor was negatively associated with pregnancy and taking hormonal contraceptive pills. Transferrin receptor levels were also significantly higher in non-Hispanic black women and in women with higher BMIs.

Percent transferrin saturation was significantly negatively associated with parity and having regular menstrual periods. Hispanic and non-Hispanic black women had significantly lower % transferrin saturation than white women. Finally, % transferrin saturation was significantly negatively associated with BMI and CRP.

Discussion

Pregnancy had a clear effect on some, but not all, of the iron status measures. Pregnancy was associated with lower levels of hemoglobin and ferritin, indicating that iron availability to red blood cells and iron storage is compromised during pregnancy. This is a typical finding for pregnant women, as the fetus's high iron needs depletes mothers' iron stores, particularly as pregnancy progresses. Similarly, % transferrin saturation was lower in pregnant women than non-pregnant women, but not significantly so. Curiously, transferrin receptor levels were significantly lower in pregnant women compared to non-pregnant women. As transferrin receptor is usually higher under conditions of low body iron, this result is opposite of what would be predicted by previous literature [36,37]. However, it may be an expected result in the context of maternal-fetal iron transfer. Maternal physiology is hypothesized to negotiate the allocation of resources between maternal and fetal somatic needs, which may sometimes conflict with fetal interests [48,49]. In the case of maternal-fetal iron transfer, previous research suggests that fetal iron transfer has priority over maintaining maternal iron stores [50], and that fetal iron deficiency only occurs after maternal iron stores have been severely compromised [51,52]. The current results suggest that transferrin receptor may be downregulated during pregnancy in an attempt to allocate iron away from the mother's tissues and toward the fetus. These results hint at a pregnancy iron transfer system that depletes bodily iron during pregnancy in favor of fetal iron stores, supporting previous findings. However, more research is necessary to confirm the physiological mechanisms that may underlie such a mechanism.

There were no significant effects of breastfeeding on any iron status values. Unfortunately, analysis of this variable was hampered by the low rate of breastfeeding in US women: only 2% of women reported that they were currently breastfeeding. Replicating these findings in a population of women with higher breastfeeding rates would better test the hypothesis that the postpartum period is a time of iron repletion in reproducing women.

These results provide evidence that postpartum iron repletion is incomplete in US women, and has an additive negative effect with each child. Increasing parity was found to have a small but statistically significant impact on all indicators of iron status. These results replicate parity-related maternal iron depletion findings in developing countries with high rates of iron-deficiency anemia, albeit with smaller statistical estimates [14]. Despite the relatively good overall iron status of the US population, high-parity women are vulnerable to poor iron status. This effect may be particularly worrisome in high parity women who become pregnant [26].

The results show that having regular periods across the past 12 months is associated with lower iron stores than not having regular periods, and that taking hormonal contraceptive pills is associated with higher iron status. This seemingly points to the traditional view that menstrual blood loss directly affects iron status, and that contraception's protective effect is due to lighter menstrual periods while on the pill [16,17]. More recently, however, mouse models have demonstrated a direct relationship between estrogen and iron homeostasis [53,54]. Work on this relationship shows that that estrogen directly inhibits the expression of hepcidin, a liver-produced peptide hormone that inhibits iron intake across the gut

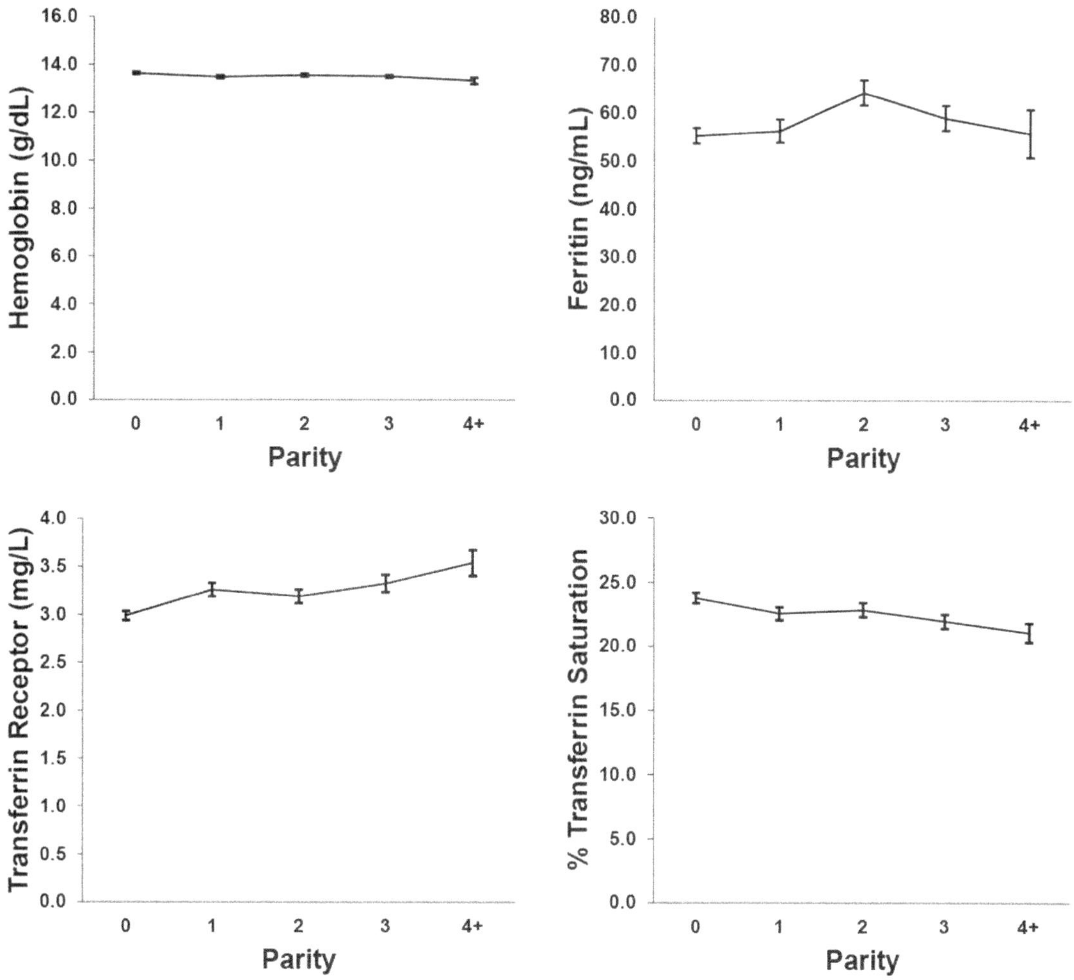

Figure 1. Weighted (unimputed) means and ±1 standard error of the mean for measures of iron status by pregnancy status.

and is a regulator of iron homeostasis in the body [55]. When estrogen is high, hepcidin is low and iron uptake into the body is increased. The authors proposed that this is a mechanism to regulate iron uptake across the menstrual cycle, and can explain the higher level of iron in women who take hormonal contraceptives [55].

Despite the immediate impact of having regular periods and using contraceptive pills on iron status, there appears to be no long-term effects: history of contraceptive pill use and age at menarche were not significantly associated with iron stores in this population. It could be hypothesized that menstruation-related iron loss should accumulate, particularly in a population who spends a high proportion of their reproductive careers menstruating [56]. However, these results call into question the idea that blood loss is the sole cause of altered iron stores in menstruating women. This perspective has also been advanced by Clancy et al. [19], who note that a thicker endometrium (and greater potential menstrual blood loss) is actually associated with higher hemoglobin in reproductive-aged Polish women. Contrary to established wisdom, their work shows menstruation is associated with better, not worse, iron status, and suggests that iron is a sensitive indicator of reproductive condition. Rather than assume that menstrual blood loss leads to anemia, a closer examination of the co-relationship between hepcidin, iron absorption, estrogen, and reproduction in women is warranted. It is more likely that menstruation-related iron homeostasis is tightly regulated, even in women who continually menstruate throughout their reproductive career.

The results showed significantly different measures of iron status between ethnic groups in the US. Non-Hispanic white women had higher hemoglobin compared to other groups, Hispanic women had lower ferritin and % transferrin saturation compared to the reference group (non-Hispanic white women), and non-Hispanic black women had higher levels of transferrin receptor and lower % transferrin saturation compared to the reference group. These differences raise several questions. First, what is the normal range of variation in US women? Why does it vary between groups, and what are the factors that contribute to this reaction norm? Some researchers suggest a lower threshold for iron-deficiency anemia for African-American women [3], for example, but what drives this difference? Second, it also demonstrates that there may be no one picture of low iron status in women, and that each iron indicator may offer a slightly different interpretation of the physiological processes involved in the body's response to low iron. Further research would untangle the meaning of these different pathways, particularly in the context of women's reproduction. Finally, it is worth investigating population-specific reproductive outcomes due to poor iron status. There are well-known consequences of maternal iron-deficiency anemia, including preterm birth, low birth weight, increased maternal morbidity,

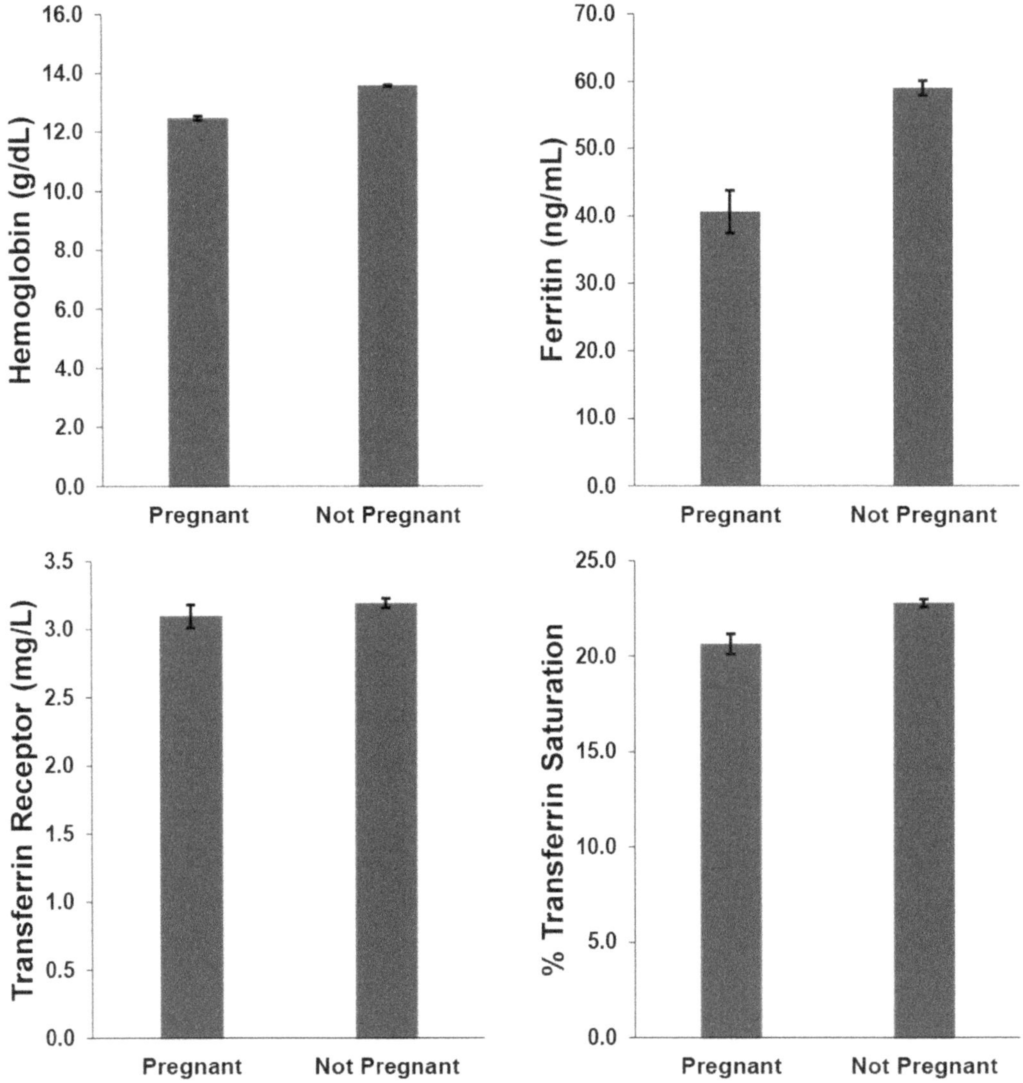

Figure 2. Weighted (unimputed) means and ±1 standard error of the mean for measures of iron status by parity.

increased risk of infant iron-deficiency, poor neurocognitive development in infants, and others [4,7]. However, meta-analyses indicate that most of these adverse outcomes (with the exception of pre-term birth) are not consistent across studies [57]. Rather than doubt the possibility of these adverse outcomes, an anthropological approach would instead posit that there may be ecological variation in the appearance of these outcomes. Instead, the question becomes: who do these adverse outcomes happen to, and why? Further work from an anthropological perspective may

Table 2. Non-imputed, weighted percentages of NHANES women who are below iron indicator cutoffs by pregnancy status (See Table 1 for number of non-missing values in each category).

	Non-pregnant women	Pregnant women
Hemoglobin (<12 g/dL)	6.9%	29.1%
Ferritin (<12 ng/mL)	10.9%	18.5%
Transferrin receptor (>5.33 mg/L)[a]	5.4%	5.7%
% Transferrin saturation (<16%)	29.7%	39.1%
% Iron deficient[b]	9.8%	25.4%

[a]Percentages based on 2003–2006 survey years only.
[b]Calculated based on percentage of women who had two of three values (hemoglobin, ferritin, and % transferrin saturation) below cutoff.

Table 3. Weighted estimates and p-values for complete case survey regression models of hemoglobin, ferritin, % transferrin saturation, and transferrin receptor as dependent variables, reproductive variables as independent variables, and ethnicity, survey release year, and other covariates as control variables.

		Hemoglobin		Ferritin		% Transferrin Saturation		Transferrin Receptor[a]	
		n=4255		*n*=4252		*n*=4245		*n*=2019	
		$R^2=0.15$		$R^2=0.071$		$R^2=0.095$		$R^2=0.099$	
		Estimate	*p*	Estimate	*p*	Estimate	*p*	Estimate	*p*
Reproductive Status	Currently pregnant	−1.02	<0.0001	−19.94	<0.0001	−0.58	0.48	−0.033	0.74
	Parity	−0.081	0.0003	−2.27	0.0026	−0.66	0.0002	0.047	0.17
	Currently breastfeeding	0.037	0.78	3.41	0.5687	−0.98	0.35	0.37	0.14
	Current birth control use	−0.034	0.59	9.97	0.0108	1.44	0.042	−0.33	0.0001
	Ever use birth control	0.026	0.69	−0.062	0.98	−0.042	0.95	−0.00070	0.99
	Having regular periods	−0.20	0.0032	−16.62	<0.0001	−1.22	0.067	0.013	0.93
	Age at menarche	−0.024	0.076	−0.65	0.3056	−0.070	0.59	−0.0051	0.74
Ethnicity[b]	Hispanic	−0.29	<0.0001	−4.09	0.0355	−1.49	0.016	−0.053	0.60
	Non-Hispanic black	−1.06	<0.0001	−0.022	0.9935	−2.84	<0.0001	0.54	<0.0001
	Other	−0.47	0.0004	7.73	0.0711	−1.85	0.034	0.29	0.12
Survey Release[c,d]	2001–2002	−0.033	0.70	−10.39	0.0011	−0.22	0.75	–	–
	2003–2004	0.14	0.11	2.61	0.4303	0.41	0.60	–	–
	2005–2006	0.094	0.28	0.14	0.9627	0.025	0.97	−0.25	0.0023
Other Covariates	BMI (kg/m^2)	0.0018	0.55	0.11	0.5819	−0.27	<0.0001	0.029	0.0002
	CRP (g/L)	−0.087	0.0017	10.54	<0.0001	−2.34	<0.0001	0.053	0.18
	Age (years)	−0.00020	0.96	0.73	<0.0001	0.040	0.16	−0.00060	0.90
	Dietary iron intake (mg)	−0.00010	0.95	0.044	0.7448	−0.013	0.63	0.0043	0.32

[a]Transferrin receptor model is based on survey years 2003–2006 only.
[b]Reference category is white ethnicity.
[c]Reference category is survey release year 1999–2000 (hemoglobin, ferritin, and % transferrin saturation models).
[d]Reference category is survey release year 2003–2004 (transferrin receptor model only).

Table 4. Weighted estimates, 95% confidence intervals, and p-values for imputed survey regression models of hemoglobin, ferritin, % transferrin saturation, and transferrin receptor as dependent variables, reproductive variables as independent variables, and ethnicity, survey release year, and other covariates as control variables.

		Hemoglobin[a]			Ferritin[a]			% Transferrin Saturation[a]			Transferrin Receptor[b]		
		$R^2 = 0.17$[c]			$R^2 = 0.12$[c]			$R^2 = 0.093$[c]			$R^2 = 0.10$[c]		
		Estimate	95% CI	*p*	Estimate	95% CI	*p*	Estimate	95% CI	*p*	Estimate	95% CI	*p*
Reproductive Status	Currently pregnant	−1.12	−1.24, −0.99	<0.0001	−19.60	−27.03, −12.16	<0.0001	−0.58	−1.84, 0.67	0.36	−0.29	−0.51, −0.057	0.014
	Parity	−0.066	−0.10, −0.030	0.0003	−2.94	−4.55, −1.34	0.0003	−0.62	−0.90, −0.34	<0.0001	0.10	0.052, 0.15	<0.0001
	Currently breastfeeding	−0.076	−0.34, 0.19	0.57	−7.40	−21.12, 6.32	0.29	−0.95	−3.38, 1.48	0.44	0.37	−0.14, 0.88	0.15
	Current birth control use	−0.077	−0.20, 0.043	0.21	14.74	6.24, 23.23	0.0007	1.18	−0.084, 2.45	0.067	−0.40	−0.57, −0.23	<0.0001
	Ever use birth control	0.057	−0.056, 0.17	0.32	0.56	−4.36, 5.47	0.82	−0.0058	−1.08, 1.06	0.99	−0.059	−0.25, 0.13	0.55
	Having regular periods	−0.28	−0.37, −0.19	<0.0001	−32.25	−38.43, −26.08	<0.0001	−1.42	−2.34, −0.50	0.0025	0.29	0.068, 0.52	0.011
	Age at menarche	−0.012	−0.035, 0.011	0.29	−0.70	−1.91, 0.51	0.26	0.022	−0.20, 0.25	0.84	0.015	−0.024, 0.053	0.45
Ethnicity[d]	Hispanic	−0.25	−0.35, −0.14	<0.0001	−4.09	−7.92, −0.26	0.036	−1.59	−2.55, −0.63	0.0012	0.042	−0.13, 0.21	0.62
	Non-Hispanic black	−1.08	−1.17, −0.98	<0.0001	6.57	−0.27, 13.41	0.060	−2.53	−3.34, −1.73	<0.0001	0.91	0.68, 1.14	<0.0001
	Other	−0.31	−0.49, −0.13	0.0008	11.76	2.37, 21.16	0.014	−1.45	−2.89, −0.0058	0.049	0.086	−0.15, 0.33	0.48
Survey Release[e,f]	2001–2002	−0.0031	−0.18, 0.18	0.97	−6.80	−12.06, −1.53	0.012	−0.10	−1.17, 0.96	0.85	—	—	—
	2003–2004	0.21	0.057, 0.37	0.0077	9.38	4.95, 13.81	<0.0001	0.94	−0.20, 2.08	0.11	-	-	-
	2005–2006	0.11	−0.05, 0.28	0.17	3.11	−2.18, 8.40	0.25	0.054	−1.00, 1.11	0.92	−0.052	−0.21, 0.10	0.51
Other Covariates	BMI (kg/m^2)	0.00064	−0.0043, 0.0056	0.80	0.23	−0.17, 0.62	0.26	−0.27	−0.31, −0.22	<0.0001	0.033	0.025, 0.042	<0.0001
	CRP (g/L)	−0.032	−0.082, 0.017	0.20	12.61	7.49, 17.73	<0.0001	−1.96	−2.43, −1.48	<0.0001	−0.016	−0.090, 0.057	0.66
	Age (years)	0.000067	−0.0050, 0.0052	0.98	1.16	0.90, 1.41	<0.0001	0.067	0.021, 0.11	0.0046	−0.0026	−0.012, 0.0065	0.58
	Dietary iron intake (mg)	−0.0017	−0.0062, 0.0028	0.45	−0.12	−0.37, 0.14	0.37	−0.024	−0.067, 0.019	0.27	0.0024	−0.0063, 0.011	0.59

[a]The *n* for the hemoglobin, ferritin, and % transferrin saturation model is 6603 (all years).
[b]The *n* for the transferrin receptor model is 3295 (survey years 2003–2006 only).
[c]Mean R^2 of 50 imputations.
[d]Reference category is white ethnicity.
[e]Reference category is survey release year 1999–2000 (hemoglobin, ferritin, and % transferrin saturation models).
[f]Reference category is survey release year 2003–2004 (transferrin receptor model only).

provide better insight into the ecology of iron use in women's reproduction.

One interesting finding in this study is that reported levels of dietary iron intake in the current study were not significantly associated with indicators of iron status in statistical analyses. Interestingly, the reported dietary intake of iron in this sample of women (13.73 mg/day) was lower than the recommended daily intake of 18 mg/day for reproductive-aged women; however, rates of iron deficiency were 9.8% in non-pregnant women and 25.4% in pregnant women (Table 2). These results show that while women in the US have clear reproductive-related changes in iron status, low iron is considerably less prevalent in non-pregnant women, despite their lower-than-recommended dietary intake.

When viewed through an anthropological framework, these results challenge current interpretations of the variation in women's reproduction in several ways. First, rather than use cut-off levels that determine iron deficiency, this study instead examined iron status as continuous variables, as is typical in biological anthropology. Therefore, these results do not make recommendations relating to supplementation or the avoidance of reproductive-related low iron in the US. Rather, they are intended to show associated patterns and to help identify potential future research areas of interest to both anthropologists and nutritional scientists. Second, although many of these results are statistically significant, they may not all be biologically significant. For example, the parity results, although significant, would require a large number of children in most cases to find a biologically meaningful effect. While this is uncommon among US women, populations with higher fertility rates should be advised of parity-related effects. Third, the results from this study challenge what is considered a "normal" iron status in US women. These results show evidence of reproduction-related changes in iron status in US women despite the widespread availability of iron-rich foods and supplements. Perhaps rather than viewing every case of low iron during pregnancy as a problem in need of correction, low iron should be viewed as a normal function of women's pregnancy, provided these women and their infants do not experience adverse outcomes [58,59]. This falls in line with other research that suggests that pregnant women should have lower cutoff thresholds for anemia, and that these cutoffs may vary by ethnicity [3]. Finally, these results highlight the contradictory nature of recommending supplementation while stating that some degree of low iron is normal in reproducing women. To reconcile the contradiction, it may be true that US women need iron supplementation during their pregnancy, but might not need the daily high doses of iron recommended by health officials. For example, a meta-analysis of the literature has found that intermittent iron supplementation prevents iron deficiency in pregnant women as well as daily supplementation, with fewer adverse effects [60]. The current results do suggest that certain situations may require more attention to risk factors that might require iron supplementation, such as very high parity women and non-white women. By incorporating some tolerance of low iron as "normal," and by understanding the ecological variation in iron status between populations, supplementation recommendations can help avoid under- and over-treating low iron in reproductive-aged women. These results can help point researchers to more specific iron supplementation recommendations for pregnant and non-pregnant women, both in the US and on the global stage.

There are several limitations to this study. First, these results are limited by the data collection. The NHANES was not specifically designed for a study of this nature, so data are limited and missing in many cases. This was partially corrected by means of multiple imputation, but the limitations on data between survey releases could not be statistically overcome, particularly in the case of transferrin receptor data. Similarly, there are limited types of questions available in the survey, and not all questions of interest could be asked using this data. For example, women's interbirth interval is a very important data point when considering the pregnancy-depletion/postpartum-repletion cycle and parity-related iron depletion. Despite these limitations, these results offer insight into the mechanisms of reproductive-related iron status in US women and suggest future research into the mechanisms of reproductive iron homeostasis.

Acknowledgments

The author would like to thank Kate Clancy and an anonymous reviewer for greatly improving this manuscript.

Author Contributions

Conceived and designed the experiments: EMM. Analyzed the data: EMM. Wrote the paper: EMM.

References

1. Balarajan Y, Ramakrishnan U, Özaltin E, Shankar AH, Subramanian SV (2011) Anaemia in low-income and middle-income countries. Lancet 378: 2123–2135.
2. Kassebaum NJ, Jasrasaria R, Johns N, Wulf S, Chou D, et al. (2013) A systematic analysis of global anaemia burden between 1990 and 2010. Lancet 381: S72.
3. Cao C, O'Brien KO (2013) Pregnancy and iron homeostasis: an update. Nutr Rev 71: 35–51.
4. Allen LH (2000) Anemia and iron deficiency: effects on pregnancy outcome. Am J Clin Nutr 71: 1280s–1284s.
5. Milman N (2006) Iron and pregnancy: A delicate balance. Ann Hematol 85: 559–565.
6. Bothwell TH (2000) Iron requirements in pregnancy and strategies to meet them. Am J Clin Nutr 72: 257S–264S.
7. Scholl TO (2005) Iron status during pregnancy: setting the stage for mother and infant. Am J Clin Nutr 81: 1218S–1222S.
8. Scholl TO, Reilly T (2000) Anemia, iron and pregnancy outcome. J Nutr 130: 443.
9. Allen LH (1997) Pregnancy and iron deficiency: Unresolved issues. Nutr Rev 55: 91–101.
10. Milman N, Kirchhoff M, JØrgensen T (1992) Iron status markers, serum ferritin and hemoglobin in 1359 Danish women in relation to menstruation, hormonal contraception, parity, and postmenopausal hormone treatment. Ann Hematol 65: 96–102.
11. Kessel E, Sastrawinata S, Mumford SD (1985) Correlates of fetal growth and survival. Acta Pædiatr 74: 120–127.
12. Chang S-C, O'Brien KO, Nathanson MS, Mancini J, Witter FR (2003) Hemoglobin concentrations influence birth outcomes in pregnant African-American adolescents. J Nutr 133: 2348–2355.
13. Desalegn S (1993) Prevalence of anaemia in pregnancy in Jima town, southwestern Ethiopia. Ethiop Med J 31: 251–258.
14. Miller EM (2010) Maternal hemoglobin depletion in a settled northern Kenyan pastoral population. Am J Hum Biol 22: 768–774.
15. Winkvist A, Rasmussen KM, Habicht JP (1992) A new definition of maternal depletion syndrome. Am J Public Health 82: 691–694.
16. Milman N, Clausen J, Byg KE (1998) Iron status in 268 Danish women aged 18–30 years: influence of menstruation, contraceptive method, and iron supplementation. Ann Hematol 77: 13–19.
17. Milman N, Rosdahl N, Lyhne N, Jørgensen T, Graudal N (1993) Iron status in Danish women aged 35–65 years: Relation to menstruation and method of contraception. Acta Obstetr et Gynecol Scand 72: 601–605.
18. Beard JL (2000) Iron requirements in adolescent females. J Nutr 130: 440.
19. Clancy KB, Nenko I, Jasienska G (2006) Menstruation does not cause anemia: endometrial thickness correlates positively with erythrocyte count and hemoglobin concentration in premenopausal women. Am J Hum Biol 18: 710–713.
20. Dewey KG (2004) Impact of breastfeeding on maternal nutritional status. Adv Exp Med Biol 554: 91–100.

21. Dewey KG, Cohen RJ (2007) Does birth spacing affect maternal or child nutritional status? A systematic literature review. Matern Child Nutr 3: 151–173.
22. Labbok MH (2001) Effects of breastfeeding on the mother. Ped Clin N Am 48: 143–158.
23. Fransson G-B, Lönnerdal B (1980) Iron in human milk. J Pediatr 96: 380–384.
24. Lonnerdal B (1984) Iron and breast milk. In: Stekel A, editor. Iron Nutrition in Infancy and Childhood. New York: Vevy/Raven Press. pp. 95–118.
25. Quinn EA (2014) Too much of a good thing: Evolutionary perspectives on infant formula fortification in the United States and its effects on infant health. Am J Hum Biol 26: 10–17.
26. Mei Z, Cogswell ME, Looker AC, Pfeiffer CM, Cusick SE, et al. (2011) Assessment of iron status in US pregnant women from the National Health and Nutrition Examination Survey (NHANES), 1999–2006. Am J Clin Nutr 93: 1312–1320.
27. Jacobs A, Miller F, Worwood M, Beamish M, Wardrop C (1972) Ferritin in the serum of normal subjects and patients with iron deficiency and iron overload. BMJ 4: 206.
28. CDC (2006) Analytic and reporting guidelines. The National Health and Nutrition Examination Survey (NHANES) Atlanta, GA: Center for Disease Control and Prevention.
29. Cook JD, Baynes RD, Skikne BS (1992) Iron deficiency and the measurement of iron status. Nutr Res Rev 5: 198–202.
30. National Center for Health Statistics. 1999–2000 National Health and Nutrition Examination Survey (NHANES). Available: http://wwwn.cdc.gov/nchs/nhanes/search/nhanes99_00.aspx. Accessed 2014 May 26.
31. National Center for Health Statistics. 2001–2002 National Health and Nutrition Examination Survey (NHANES). Available: http://www.cdc.gov/nchs/nhanes/nhanes01_02.htm. Accessed 2014 May 26.
32. National Center for Health Statistics. 2003–2004 National Health and Nutrition Examination Survey (NHANES). Available: http://www.cdc.gov/nchs/nhanes/nhanes03_04.htm. Accessed 2014 May 26.
33. National Center for Health Statistics. 2005–2006 National Health and Nutrition Examination Survey (NHANES). Available: http://www.cdc.gov/nchs/nhanes/nhanes05_06.htm. Accessed 2014 May 26.
34. CDC (2006) National Health and Nutrition Examination Survey. 2003–2004 Data documentation, codebook, and frequencies. Ferritin and transferrin receptor. Atlanta, GA: Center for Disease Control.
35. Thurnham DI, McCabe LD, Haldar S, Wieringa FT, Northrop-Clewes CA, et al. (2010) Adjusting plasma ferritin concentrations to remove the effects of subclinical inflammation in the assessment of iron deficiency: a meta-analysis. Am J Clin Nutr 92: 546–555.
36. Akesson A, Bjellerup P, Berglund M, Bremme K, Vahter M (1998) Serum transferrin receptor: a specific marker of iron deficiency in pregnancy. The American journal of clinical nutrition 68: 1241–1246.
37. Carriaga MT, Skikne BS, Finley B, Cutler B, Cook JD (1991) Serum transferrin receptor for the detection of iron deficiency in pregnancy. Am J Clin Nutr 54: 1077–1081.
38. Choi JW, Im MW, Pai SH (2000) Serum transferrin receptor concentrations during normal pregnancy. Clin Chem 46: 725–727.
39. Mei Z, Pfeiffer CM, Looker AC, Flores-Ayala RC, Lacher DA, et al. (2012) Serum soluble transferrin receptor concentrations in US preschool children and non-pregnant women of childbearing age from the National Health and Nutrition Examination Survey 2003–2010. Clin Chim Acta 413: 1479–1484.
40. Little RJ, Rubin DB (2002) Statistical analysis with missing data. New York, NY: Wiley.
41. Royston P (2004) Multiple imputation of missing values. Stata Journal 4: 227–241.
42. Berglund PA (2010) An introduction to multiple imputation of complex sample data using SAS v9.2. SAS Global Forum Proceedings Cary, NC: SAS Institute Inc.
43. Graham JW, Olchowski AE, Gilreath TD (2007) How many imputations are really needed? Some practical clarifications of multiple imputation theory. Prev Sci 8: 206–213.
44. Horton NJ, Lipsitz SR, Parzen M (2003) A potential for bias when rounding in multiple imputation. Am Stat 57: 229–232.
45. Allison PD (2005) Imputation of categorical variables with PROC MI. SAS Users Group International, 30th Meeting (SUGI 30): Citeseer.
46. Sterne JA, White IR, Carlin JB, Spratt M, Royston P, et al. (2009) Multiple imputation for missing data in epidemiological and clinical research: Potential and pitfalls. BMJ 338.
47. Looker AC, Dallman PR, Carroll MD, Gunter EW, Johnson CL (1997) Prevalence of iron deficiency in the United States. JAMA 277: 973–976.
48. Abrams ET, Meshnick SR (2009) Malaria during pregnancy in endemic areas: a lens for examining maternal-fetal conflict. Am J Hum Biol 21: 643–650.
49. Haig D (1993) Genetic conflicts in human pregnancy. Q Rev Biol 68: 495–532.
50. Van Santen S, de Mast Q, Luty AJF, Wiegerinck ET, Van der Ven AJAM, et al. (2011) Iron homeostasis in mother and child during placental malaria infection. Am J Trop Med Hygiene 84: 148–151.
51. McArdle HJ, Gambling L, Kennedy C (2014) Iron deficiency during pregnancy: the consequences for placental function and fetal outcome. Proc Nutr Soc 73: 9–15.
52. Gambling L, Lang C, McArdle HJ (2011) Fetal regulation of iron transport during pregnancy. Am J Clin Nutr: 1903S–1907S.
53. Ikeda Y, Tajima S, Izawa-Ishizawa Y, Kihira Y, Ishizawa K, et al. (2012) Estrogen regulates hepcidin expression via GPR30-BMP6-dependent signaling in hepatocytes. PLOS ONE 7: e40465.
54. Hou Y, Zhang S, Wang L, Li J, Qu G, et al. (2012) Estrogen regulates iron homeostasis through governing hepatic hepcidin expression via an estrogen response element. Gene 511: 398–403.
55. Yang Q, J J, Katz S, Abramson SB, Huang X (2012) 17β-Estradiol Inhibits Iron Hormone Hepcidin Through an Estrogen Responsive Element Half-Site. Endocrinology 153: 3170–3178.
56. Strassmann BI (1997) The biology of menstruation in Homo sapiens: Total lifetime menses, fecundity, and nonsynchrony in a natural-fertility population. Curr Anthropol 38: 123–129.
57. Xiong X, Buekens P, Alexander S, Demianczuk N, Wollast E (2000) Anemia during pregnancy and birth outcome: a meta-analysis. Am J Perinatol 17: 137–146.
58. Beaton GH (2000) Iron needs during pregnancy: do we need to rethink our targets? Am J Clin Nutr 72: 265S–271S.
59. Yip R (2000) Significance of an abnormally low or high hemoglobin concentration during pregnancy: special consideration of iron nutrition. Am J Clin Nutr 72: 272S–279S.
60. Pena-Rosas JP, De-Regil LM, Dowswell T, Viteri FE (2012) Intermittent oral iron supplementation during pregnancy. Cochrane Database Syst Rev 7: Cd009997.

18

Iodine Deficiency and Excess Coexist in China and Induce Thyroid Dysfunction and Disease

Yang Du[¶], Yanhui Gao[¶], Fangang Meng, Shoujun Liu, Zhipeng Fan, Junhua Wu, Dianjun Sun*

Center for Endemic Disease Control, Chinese Center for Disease Control and Prevention, Harbin Medical University; Key Lab of Etiology and Epidemiology, Education Bureau of Heilongjiang Province & Ministry of Health (23618504), Harbin, China

Abstract

Background: In spite of the salt iodization, iodine deficiency disorders (IDD) have not been sustainably eliminated in China. There are coastal areas with low iodized salt coverage rates (iodine nutrition is inadequate) and other areas with excessive amounts of iodine in the drinking water.

Objective: This study aimed to clarify the association of iodine deficiencies resulting from a low coverage rate of iodized salt, excess iodine intake from drinking water with thyroid function and disease in adults.

Design: A cross-sectional study was conducted in adults in different iodine nutrition areas in three provinces in China.

Results: The prevalence of thyroid nodules was 15.52%, 8.66% and 22.17% in the iodine excess, sufficient and deficient groups, respectively. The prevalence of subclinical hypothyroidism was 20.09%, 10.41%, and 2.25% in the excess, sufficient and deficient iodine groups, respectively. The prevalence of subclinical hyperthyroidism and overt hyperthyroidism in the iodine deficient group was higher than that in the iodine excess group ($\chi^2 = 9.302$, $p = 0.002$) and iodine sufficient group ($\chi^2 = 7.553$, $p = 0.006$). Thyroid-stimulating hormone (TSH) was significantly correlated with excess iodine intake ($\beta = 1.764, P = 0.001$) and deficient iodine intake ($\beta = -1.219$, $P = 0.028$).

Conclusions: Thyroid nodules are more likely to be present in the iodine excess and deficient areas than in the iodine sufficient areas. Subclinical hyperthyroidism and overt hyperthyroidism are more likely to be prevalent in the iodine deficient areas than in the iodine excess or sufficient areas. Subclinical hypothyroidism is more likely to be prevalent in the high iodine intake areas than in the iodine deficient or sufficient areas. Median TSH may be deemed as an alternative indicator for monitoring the iodine nutrition status of the adult population in iodine excess and deficient areas.

Editor: Eliseo A. Eugenin, Rutgers University, United States of America

Funding: This study was supported by the Special Fund for National Health Scientific Research in the Public Interest by the Ministry of Health of China (No. 201202012). The funders had no role in study design, data collection and analysis, decision to publish, or preparation of the manuscript.

Competing Interests: The authors have declared that no competing interests exist.

* Email: hrbmusdj@163.com

¶ These authors contributed equally to this work.

Introduction

Iodine is an essential trace element required for the synthesis of thyroid hormones (including thyroxine and triiodothyronine), and it is indispensable for normal growth and fetal brain development in human beings [1,2]. Both iodine deficiency and excess intake may lead to thyroid dysfunction or disease. Iodine deficiency has widespread implications, which include cretinism, endemic goiter, intellectual impairments, increased pregnancy loss and infant mortality [3,4,5,6,7]. Excess iodine intake may lead to endemic goiter and thyroid dysfunction [8,9]. It is reported that thirty countries remain iodine deficient and ten countries have excessive iodine intake across the world [10]. The best strategy to prevent iodine deficiency disorders (IDD) is the addition of iodine to dietary salt in most countries [11]. To date, IDD has been primarily controlled in China. A common reason for iodine excess intake in many countries is the over iodization of salt and/or poor monitoring of salt iodization [12]. However, unlike other iodine excess countries, China has excess iodine areas resulting from high iodine concentrations in water [13]. Moreover, there are iodine deficient areas due to the low coverage rate of iodized table salt along the coast. Previous studies of iodine excess or deficiency have primarily focused on the vulnerable populations such as children, pregnant women and lactating women [14,15,16,17,18]. The last study in China was performed in Henan, Hebei, Shanxi and Shandong province (four main excess iodine areas by historical

Yellow River flushing, and are representative of Chinese iodine excess area) and published in 2014, this study focused on the iodine excess in the vulnerable population, and suggested that excessive iodine intake was associated with impaired thyroid function of children, pregnant women and lactating women [19]. Studies on the impact of iodine deficiency or excess on the adults are scarce. Therefore, the main objective of this study is to clarify the relationship between adult iodine malnutrition (including iodine deficiency due to low coverage rate of iodized salt and excess iodine intake from drinking water) and thyroid abnormalities (dysfunction and disease).

Subjects and Methods

Subjects

According to the recent national IDD surveillance data and water iodine surveillance data, three populations with different iodine nutrition levels were selected in three provinces. Fengrun and Yangfang village in Qingxu County, Dongwenzhuang village in Xiaodian District of Shanxi Province, and Caizhuang village in Cao County of Shandong Province were selected as areas where residents consume high iodine water. Shuangzhai, Houhuangtai, Lizhuang, Anrong and Hutong villages in Shanyin County and Xicuan village in Xiaodian District of Shanxi Province were selected as areas where residents have sufficient iodine nutrition. Tieshangang District in Beihai City, Guangxi Autonomous Region, was selected as a coastal area with low coverage rates of iodized salt and regarded as an area with iodine deficiency. The income of most participants in these areas is similar (4000–5000 RMB yuan/person/year, equivalent to USD 640–800/person/year). A cluster random sampling method was adopted in these areas. All participants who had lived in the region for more than 10 years and were older than 18 years were eligible for recruitment. Subjects taking anti-thyroid drugs during the time of this study were excluded.

Methods

Questionnaire. A standard questionnaire was designed to obtain demographic information, including name, gender, age, personal or family history of thyroid disease, smoking and drinking habits, economic income and source of drinking water and drinking duration. For the smoking habit, participants were divided into four grades: non smoker, mild smokers (1–10 cigarettes/day), moderate smokers (11–20 cigarettes/day) and heavy smokers (>20 cigarettes/day). For the alcohol consumption habit, participants were divided into three categories: non-drinking, occasional light consumption (<1 time/week) and heavy consumption (≥1 times/week). The investigation was performed face to face in dialect by well-trained staff.

Drinking Water Collection and Analysis. In the preselected high iodine water and iodine sufficient villages, at least four water samples were collected from the east, west, south, north and central directions of each village with scattered water supplies; one water sample was collected from each village with centralized water supplies. In the preselected iodine deficient area (Tieshangang District), each participant provided a water sample. Each water sample was more than 15 ml and kept at 4°C until analysis. The iodine concentration of the drinking-water was determined by arsenic–cerium catalytic spectrophotometry [20].

Urine Sample Collection and Analysis. Morning spot urine samples were collected in clean plastic tubes for each participant. Urinary iodine concentration was determined by the acid digestion method ($As^{3+}-Ce^{4+}$catalytic spectrophotometry [21]). The internal quality control samples for urine iodine and water iodine were provided by the China National Iodine Deficiency Disorders Reference Laboratory.

Coverage Rate of Iodized Salt. In the preselected iodine excess or sufficient areas, the iodized salt coverage rates were calculated by the Information Management System of National Iodized Salt Surveillance, which is managed by our organization. In the preselected iodine deficient area (Tieshangang District), each participant provided a table salt sample of at least 100 g. The salt iodine levels were determined using the General Test Method of the salt industry for the determination of iodine [22]. The standard for salt iodine level in Shandong, Shanxi province and Guangxi Autonomous Region is 25 mg/kg. The salt type was defined as follows: non-iodized salt, salt iodine less than 5 mg/kg, qualified iodized salt, salt iodine more than 18 mg/kg and less than 50 mg/kg, others, unqualified iodized salt.

Blood Sample and Analysis. Blood samples were collected from the cubital vein and stored in a glass tube. The serum samples were prepared by centrifugation (3000 r/m, 10 mins) after standing for an hour and were frozen at −70°C until determination. Serum thyroid-stimulating hormone (TSH), free triiodothyronine (FT3), free tetraiodothyronine (FT4), thyroid peroxidase antibody (TPOAb) and thyroglobulin antibody (TGAb) were tested. These indexes were tested by chemiluminescent immunoassay (Fluorometric magnetic beads enzyme immunoassay, TOSOH Corporation, Japan). The thyrotropin receptor antibody (TRAb) was tested by chemiluminescent immunoassay (Snibe Co., Ltd, China).

Thyroid Ultrasound. Thyroid ultrasonography was performed using a 7.5-MHz transducer by one experienced examiner (mainly measure the thyroid volume, nodule diameter and echo). The thyroid lobe volume was calculated by measuring the depth (d), the width (w) and the length (l) of each lobe by the following formula: V (ml) $= 0.479 \times d \times w \times l$ (mm)/1000. The thyroid volume was recorded as the sum of both lobes. The normal volume for adult males and females is less than 25 ml or 18 ml, respectively [23].

Diagnostic Criteria for Thyroid Diseases. The diagnostic criteria for thyroid diseases were listed in Table 1 [24,25].

Statistical Analysis. All data were recorded with EpiData3.1, the data processing and statistical analyses were performed using IBM SPSS statistics version 19 and SigmaPlot 12.5 software. Comparison of the proportions among the three groups was performed by the chi-square test ($\alpha = 0.05$); if the null hypothesis was rejected, pairwise comparisons were performed ($\alpha = 0.0125$). Normally distributed data were expressed as the mean ±SD; abnormally distributed data were described as the median with the 25th and 75th percentiles. Binary logistic regression analysis was used to calculate the odds ratio (OR) and 95% Confidence Intervals (CIs) for thyroid diseases by iodine nutrition status and other risk factors. The dependent variables entered into the logistic regression models were goiter, autoimmune thyroiditis, subclinical hyperthyroidism and overt hyperthyroidism, nodules and subclinical hypothyroidism. Gender, age, smoking status, alcohol consumption, goiter, nodules, iodine status, TPOAb positive and TGAb positive were entered as explanatory variables. First, univariate logistic regression was performed to select the potentially significant variables for the multivariate model. Then, based on the results of univariate logistic analysis, the significant variables, gender and age were put into the multivariate logistic model. The pairwise comparisons of the TSH values among the three groups were compared by the Kruskal-Wallis test. The relativity between TSH and urinary iodine concentration was tested using the Spearman rank correlation.

Table 1. Diagnostic criteria for the thyroid diseases included in this study.

Thyroid disease	Diagnostic criteria*
Goiter	Thyroid volume >25 ml (male) or >18 ml (female)
Diffuse	Goiter without nodules
Nodular	Goiter with nodules >10 mm in diameter
Single nodule	Normal thyroid volume with a single nodule >3 mm in diameter
Multiple nodules	Normal thyroid volume with >2 nodules >3 mm in diameter
Overt hypothyroidism	TSH>5.57 mIU/L, FT4<10.06 pmol/L
Subclinical hypothyroidism	TSH>5.57 mIU/L, FT4 within the normal range
Over hyperthyroidism	TSH<0.38 mIU/L; FT4>23.99 pmol/L, FT3>5.85 pmol/L, or both
Subclinical hyperthyroidism	TSH<0.38 mIU/L, FT3 and FT4 within the normal ranges
Graves' disease	Hyperthyroidism. Diffuse goiter on ultrasound. TPOAb>2.6 IU/ml or TRAb>30 IU/ml
Autoimmune thyroiditis	Hypothyroidism or subclinical hypothyroidism. TPOAb>2.6 IU/ml or TgAb>14.58 IU/ml
Hashimoto's thyroiditis	With goiter
Atrophic thyroiditis	Without goiter

*Reference ranges: FT3, 2.77–5.85 pmol/L; FT4, 10.06–23.99 pmol/L; TSH, 0.38–5.57 mIU/L; TPOAb, 0–2.6 IU/ml; TgAb, 0–14.58 IU/ml; TRAb, 0.11–30 IU/ml. Reference ranges were provided by the second affiliated hospital of Harbin Medical University.

Ethical Statement. The study was approved by the Ethical Review Board of Harbin Medical University (HMUIRB 20120021). Written informed consent was obtained from all participants ahead of the survey. No specific permits were required for the locations or activities associated with the drinking water sample collection in this field study. The locations were not privately owned or protected in any way and this field study did not involve endangered or protected species.

Results

A total of 2147 adults were recruited for this survey, the sample sizes were presented in Table 2. The demographic characteristics of the participants were presented in Table 3.

Iodine Concentration in Urine Sample

Each village was a unit, the villages were divided into excess, sufficient and deficient groups according to the median urinary iodine (MUI) of each village. The grouping criteria was as follows: iodine excess group, MUI>400 μg/L; iodine sufficient group, 100 μg/L<MUI<300 μg/L; and iodine deficient group, MUI< 100 μg/L. The MUI of the participants was 750.18 μg/L, 228.70 μg/L and 62.03 μg/L for iodine excess, sufficient and deficient groups, respectively, as shown in Table 2.

Iodine Concentration in Drinking Water

The detailed iodine concentrations in the drinking water of each survey site were presented in Table 2. The median iodine concentration of the drinking water ranged from 272.98 μg/L to 629.90 μg/L in the iodine excess group and 7.69 μg/L to 77.77 μg/L in the iodine sufficient group. The median in the iodine deficient group was 2.84 μg/L.

Coverage Rate of Iodized Table Salt

In Shanyin County, the coverage rates of iodized salt and qualified iodized salt were 99.67% and 98%, respectively. In high iodine water areas of Xiaodian District and Cao County, the coverage rates of iodized table salt were 0% and 1.67%, respectively. In the iodine deficient areas of Tieshangang, the coverage rates of iodized salt and qualified iodized salt were 24.29% and 17.14%, respectively.

The Prevalence of Thyroid Diseases

Nodule. The prevalence of thyroid nodules in the different iodine nutrition groups was presented in Table 4. For single and multiple nodules, the prevalence of thyroid nodules differed significantly among the three groups ($\chi^2 = 39.779$, $p = 0$), between the iodine deficient group and iodine sufficient group ($\chi^2 = 39.234$, $p = 0$), between the iodine excess group and iodine sufficient group ($\chi^2 = 13.964$, $p = 0$), and between the iodine excess group and iodine deficient group ($\chi^2 = 11.125$, $p = 0.001$). The prevalence of thyroid nodules for males and females was shown in Figure 1. In males, a significant difference in the prevalence of thyroid nodules was found among the three groups ($\chi^2 = 18.401$, $p = 0$), between the iodine deficient group and iodine sufficient group ($\chi^2 = 13.67$, $p = 0$), and between the iodine deficient group and iodine excess group ($\chi^2 = 11.916$, $p = 0.001$), but not between the iodine excess group and iodine sufficient group ($\chi^2 = 0.389$, $p = 0.533$). In females, the prevalence of thyroid nodules differed significantly among the three groups ($\chi^2 = 21.463$, $p = 0$), between the iodine excess group and iodine sufficient group ($\chi^2 = 11.775$, $p = 0.001$), and between the iodine deficient group and iodine sufficient group ($\chi^2 = 21.629$, $p = 0$), but not between iodine excess group and iodine deficient group ($\chi^2 = 2.998$, $p = 0.083$). The prevalence of single nodule differed significantly among the three groups ($\chi^2 = 20.624$, $p = 0$), between the iodine excess group and iodine sufficient group ($\chi^2 = 10.999$, $p = 0.001$), and between the iodine deficient group and iodine sufficient group ($\chi^2 = 20.809$, $p = 0$), but not between the iodine excess group and iodine deficient group ($\chi^2 = 2.96$, $p = 0.085$). For multiple nodules, the prevalence of nodules in the iodine deficient group was higher than that in other groups (Iodine sufficient group vs. Iodine deficient group, $\chi^2 = 17.918$, $p = 0$; Iodine excess group vs. Iodine deficient group, $\chi^2 = 12.933$, $p = 0$), as shown in Table 4. Logistic-regression analysis indicated that female or elder age, excess iodine intake or iodine deficiency, smoking 11–20 cigarettes per day and goiter were risk factors for developing thyroid nodules (Table 5).

Table 2. A summary of the samples collected and the iodine nutrition status of the survey sites.

Survey sites		Participant numbers	Water samples		Urine samples		Blood samples	Ultrasound samples	Table salt samples
			n	Median (Interquartile range) (μg/L)	n	Median (Interquartile range) (μg/L)			
Iodine excess group	Caizhuang	285	246	272.98 (171.95,393.33)	281	473.38 (270.51,758.51)	282	285	—
	Dongwenzhuang	156	1	629.90	145	1183.96 (793.26,1557.11)	156	156	—
	Fengrun	145	1	571.20	108	896.55 (525.03,1264.95)	137	139	—
	Yangfang	344	1	460.20	254	823.90 (573.05, 1219.88)	286	335	—
	Sum	930	249	—	788	750.18 (451.84, 1188.55)	861	915	—
Iodine sufficient group	Xicuan	122	2	77.77	116	264.72 (195.85, 380.04)	122	121	—
	Shuangzhai	68	20	23.15 (9.94, 32.96)	56	272.41 (175.95, 328.72)	56	66	—
	Houhuangtai	163	20	10.90 (1.62, 19.52)	111	188.45 (112.48, 258.75)	146	158	—
	Lizhuang	65	20	13.13 (1.0, 30.92)	53	229.50 (108.39, 288.78)	61	63	—
	Anrong	86	25	7.69 (1.46, 11.37)	71	239.50 (124.10, 324.50)	80	78	—
	Hutong	46	20	15.29 (10.51, 28.02)	43	209.99 (126.94, 293.20)	44	45	—
	Sum	550	107	—	450	228.70 (134.13, 322.73)	509	531	—
Iodine deficient group	Tieshangang	667	336	2.84 (1.93,5.87)	642	62.03 (36.24, 99.10)	667	636	280

Table 3. Demographic characteristics of the participants in the three different iodine nutrition groups.

Characteristics		Iodine excess group	Iodine sufficient group	Iodine deficient group
Participants number		930	550	667
Gender				
	Male	281	212	157
	Female	649	338	510
Age				
	Mean ±SD	55.46±12.44	57.71±12.11	51.89±15.10
	≤40	181	91	247
	41–60	432	254	214
	61-	317	205	206
Education level※				
	Illiteracy	238	91	61
	Primary school	396	282	197
	Junior high school	227	140	217
	Senior high school	55	16	120
	College	14	5	72
Marital status▲				
	Single	4	2	27
	Married	914	533	614
	Divorced/widowed	12	2	26
Smoking★				
	None	789	432	628
	1–10	29	33	21
	11–20	29	3	12
	>20	66	77	6
Alcohol consumption△				
	None	809	490	592
	Light	65	28	51
	Heavy	37	22	24

※16 missing.
▲13 missing.
★22 missing.
△29 missing.

Goiter. No significant difference was found in the prevalence of goiter among the three groups ($\chi^2 = 1.871$, $p = 0.392$). Logistic-regression analysis indicated that female, TPOAb positive, TGAb positive and having nodules were risk factors for developing goiter (Table 5).

Hypothyroidism. The prevalence of overt hypothyroidism was 2.56%, 1.18% and 1.05% for the iodine excess, sufficient and deficient groups, respectively. A significant difference was found among the three groups ($\chi^2 = 6.215$, $p = 0.045$). However, there were no significant differences in the pairwise comparisons (Iodine excess group vs. Iodine sufficient group, $\chi^2 = 3.027$, $p = 0.082$; Iodine excess group vs. Iodine deficient group, $\chi^2 = 4.576$, $p = 0.032 > 0.0125$; Iodine sufficient group vs. Iodine deficient group, $\chi^2 = 0.044$, $p = 0.834$). No significant difference was found among the three groups in males or females (males, $p = 0.253$; females, $p = 0.183$) as shown in Table 6.

The prevalence of subclinical hypothyroidism was 20.09%, 10.41%, and 2.25% for the iodine excess, sufficient and deficient iodine groups, respectively. There were significant differences in the prevalence of subclinical hypothyroidism among the comparisons in males or females. In males, the prevalence of subclinical hypothyroidism differed significantly among all three groups ($\chi^2 = 24.159$, $p = 0$), between the iodine excess group and iodine sufficient group ($\chi^2 = 9.315$, $p = 0.002$), and between the iodine excess group and iodine deficient group ($\chi^2 = 18.911$, $p = 0$), but not between the iodine sufficient group and iodine deficient group ($\chi^2 = 3.763$, $p = 0.052$). In females, there were significant differences among the three groups ($\chi^2 = 95.232$, $p = 0$), between the iodine excess group and iodine sufficient group ($\chi^2 = 10.816$, $p = 0.001$), and between the iodine sufficient group and iodine deficient group ($\chi^2 = 37.349$, $p = 0$), and between the iodine excess group and iodine deficient group ($\chi^2 = 95.295$, $p = 0$). Logistic-regression results indicated that females were more susceptible to subclinical hypothyroidism than males, and people living in the excess and sufficient areas were more susceptible to subclinical hypothyroidism than those in the deficient areas. Thyroid nodules and TPOAb positive were risk factors for subclinical hypothyroidism (Table 5).

Table 4. Prevalence of thyroid nodules and goiter within the different iodine nutrition groups.

Thyroid diseases	Iodine excess group number of cases (percent)	Iodine sufficient group number of cases (percent)	Iodine deficient group number of cases (percent)
Nodules	142 (15.52)	46 (8.66)	141 (22.17)
Single nodule	121 (13.22)	40 (7.53)	104 (16.35)
Multiple nodules	21 (2.30)	6 (1.13)	37 (5.82)
Goiter	23 (2.51)	12 (2.26)	22 (3.46)
Diffuse	21 (2.30)	9 (1.69)	15 (2.36)
Nodular	2 (0.22)	3 (0.56)	7 (1.10)

Hyperthyroidism. There were no significant differences in the prevalence of overt hyperthyroidism ($\chi^2 = 3.590$, $p = 0.166$) and Graves' disease ($p = 0.593$, Fisher's exact test) among the three groups. The prevalence of subclinical hyperthyroidism differed significantly among the three groups ($\chi^2 = 11.596$, $p = 0.003$); significant differences were found between the iodine sufficient group and deficient group ($\chi^2 = 7.538$, $p = 0.006$), but not between the iodine excess group and deficient group ($\chi^2 = 6.045$, $p = 0.014 > 0.0125$).

The prevalence of subclinical hyperthyroidism and overt hyperthyroidism was 1.16%, 0.98% and 3.44% for the iodine excess, sufficient and deficient groups, respectively. The prevalence of subclinical hyperthyroidism and overt hyperthyroidism differed significantly among the three groups ($\chi^2 = 13.628$, $p = 0.001$), between the iodine deficient group and iodine excess group ($\chi^2 = 9.302$, $p = 0.002$), and between the iodine deficient group and iodine sufficient group ($\chi^2 = 7.553$, $p = 0.006$). Logistic-regression results indicated that female, living in an iodine deficient area, and young or middle aged were risk factors for developing overt hyperthyroidism or subclinical hyperthyroidism.

Autoimmune Thyroiditis. The prevalence of autoimmune thyroiditis differed significantly among the three groups ($\chi^2 = 21.564$, $p = 0$), between the iodine excess group and iodine deficient group ($\chi^2 = 21.805$, $p = 0$), and between the iodine sufficient group and iodine deficient group ($\chi^2 = 9.249$, $p = 0.002$). The prevalence of atrophic thyroiditis differed among the three groups ($\chi^2 = 15.808$, $p = 0$), between the iodine sufficient group and iodine deficient group ($\chi^2 = 7.615$, $p = 0.006$), and between the iodine excess group and iodine deficient group ($\chi^2 = 15.964$, $p = 0$), but not between the iodine excess group and iodine sufficient group ($\chi^2 = 1.003$, $p = 0.317$) (Table 6).

TSH Level

The results of the Kruskal-Wallis test indicated that the TSH levels differed significantly among the three groups (among all the three groups, $p = 0$; Iodine excess group vs. Iodine sufficient group, $p = 0$; Iodine excess group vs. Iodine deficient group, $p = 0$; Iodine sufficient group vs. Iodine deficient group, $p = 0$). Figure 2 showed the correlation between the MUI and median TSH, with the increasing MUI correlating with the increasing median TSH. By spearman correlation analysis, the urinary iodine concentration was positively related with the TSH value ($r = 0.414$, $p = 0$). By multiple linear regression analysis, after adjusting for gender and age, the TSH value was significantly correlated with excess iodine

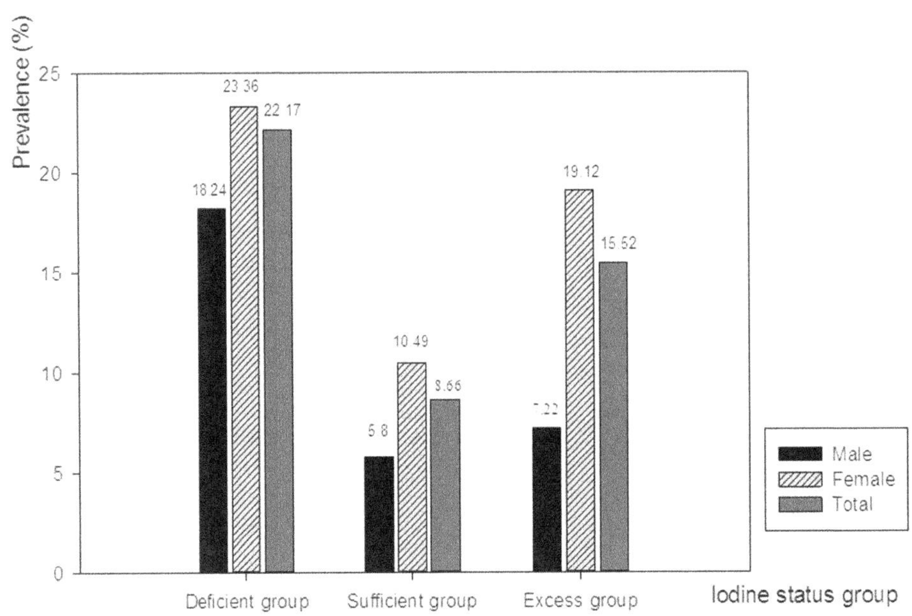

Figure 1. The prevalence of thyroid nodules among different iodine nutrition groups.

Table 5. Associations between thyroid diseases and different iodine nutrition status and other potential risk factors.

Factors		Sub-group Number	Goiter	Autoimmune thyroiditis	Subclinical hyperthyroidism and overt hyperthyroidism	Nodules	Subclinical hypothyroidism
			OR (95% CI)	OR (95% CI)	OR (95% CI)	OR (95% CI)	OR (95% CI)
Gender	Female	1497	1	1	1	1	1
	Male	650	0.251 (0.097, 0.647)**	0.849 (0.558, 1.292)	0.214 (0.050, 0.909)*	0.478 (0.332, 0.689)**	0.666 (0.473, 0.940)*
Age	≤40	519	1	1	1	1	1
	41–60	900	0.687 (0.319, 1.478)	1.472 (0.856, 2.531)	0.575 (0.280, 1.180)	1.602 (1.146, 2.240)**	1.363 (0.907, 2.046)
	61–	728	1.583 (0.775, 3.233)	1.465 (0.830, 2.588)	0.216 (0.071, 0.653)**	1.913 (1.354, 2.702)**	1.186 (0.768, 1.832)
Iodine status	Sufficient	550				1	
	Excess	930				1.865 (1.299, 2.678)**	
	Deficient	667				2.973 (2.046, 4.321)**	
Iodine status	Deficient	667	1	1	1		1
	Sufficient	550	0.979 (0.448, 2.143)	2.162 (1.168, 4.001)*	0.401 (0.146, 1.102)		5.791 (3.161, 10.611)**
	Excess	930	0.981 (0.524, 1.836)	3.012 (1.742, 5.209)**	0.404 (0.186, 0.880)*		11.717 (6.742, 20.362)**
Smoking	Never	1849				1	
	1–10	83				1.502 (0.708, 3.186)	
	11–20	44				2.530 (1.054, 6.071)*	
	>20	149				0.940 (0.455, 1.940)	
Alcohol consumption	None	1891				1	
	Light	144				0.709 (0.364, 1.383)	
	Heavy	83				0.717 (0.298, 1.725)	
TPOAb	Negative	1686	1		1		1
	Positive	351	2.582 (1.274, 5.233)**		2.124 (0.879, 5.130)		2.20 (1.454, 3.327)**
TGAb	Negative	1640	1		1		1
	Positive	397	2.373 (1.171, 4.812)*		2.289 (0.952, 5.501)		1.398 (0.935, 2.091)
Thyroid nodules	No	1753	1	1			1
	Yes	329	4.383 (2.455, 7.826)**	0.492 (0.252, 0.960)*			1.769 (1.222, 2.561)**
Goiter	No	2025				1	1
	Yes	57				3.477 (1.997, 6.055)**	1.918 (0.963, 3.818)

*$p<0.05$.
**$p<0.01$.

Table 6. Prevalence of thyroid disease within the different iodine nutrition groups.

Thyroid disease	Iodine excess group number of cases (percent)			Iodine sufficient group number of cases (percent)			Iodine deficient group number of cases (percent)		
	Total (n = 861)	Male (n = 256)	Female (n = 605)	Total (n = 509)	Male (n = 197)	Female (n = 312)	Total (n = 667)	Male (n = 157)	Female (n = 510)
Subclinical hypothyroidism	173 (20.09)	39 (15.23)	134 (22.15)	53 (10.41)	12 (6.09)	41 (13.14)	15 (2.25)	3 (1.91)	12 (2.35)
Overt hypothyroidism	22 (2.56)	6 (2.34)	16 (2.64)	6 (1.18)	1 (0.51)	5 (1.60)	7 (1.05)	1 (0.64)	6 (1.18)
Subclinical hyperthyroidism and overt hyperthyroidism	10 (1.16)	1 (0.39)	9 (1.49)	5 (0.98)	0	5 (1.60)	23 (3.44)	1 (0.64)	22 (4.31)
Subclinical hyperthyroidism	5 (0.58)	1 (0.39)	4 (0.66)	1 (0.20)	0	1 (0.32)	13 (1.95)	0	13 (2.55)
Overt hyperthyroidism	5 (0.58)	0	5 (0.83)	4 (0.79)	0	4 (1.28)	10 (1.50)	1 (0.64)	9 (1.76)
Graves' disease	3 (0.35)	0	3 (0.50)	3 (0.59)	0	3 (0.96)	5 (0.75)	1 (0.64)	4 (0.78)
Autoimmune thyroiditis	70 (8.13)	23 (8.98)	47 (7.77)	31 (6.09)	8 (4.06)	23 (7.37)	17 (2.55)	4 (2.55)	13 (2.55)
Hashimoto's thyroiditis	9 (1.05)	2 (0.78)	7 (1.16)	2 (0.39)	0	2 (0.64)	0	0	0
Atrophic thyroiditis	61 (7.08)	21 (8.20)	40 (6.61)	29 (5.70)	8 (4.06)	21 (6.73)	17 (2.55)	4 (2.55)	13 (2.55)

intake ($\beta = 1.764, P = 0.001$), iodine deficient intake ($\beta = -1.219$, $P = 0.028$) and TGAb positivity ($\beta = 3.038$, $P = 0$) (Table 7).

Discussion

Interestingly, our findings indicated that thyroid nodules were likely to be prevalent when the population has excess or deficient iodine intake. The correlation between iodine deficiency and thyroid nodules has been reported in many countries [26,27,28,29]. Takahashi et al. found that moderate iodine deficiency might be responsible for the increase of thyroid nodules in the Marshallese population [27]. The study performed by Gutekunst et al. concluded that moderate dietary iodine deficiency might cause both goiters and thyroid nodules [28]. However, research on the relationship between excess iodine intake and thyroid nodules is scarce. Recently, a cross-sectional study on the relationship between non-iodized salt and thyroid nodules conducted in Hangzhou (a foreland city in China) found a significant correlation between low urine iodine concentration and high thyroid nodules prevalence. However, in contrast to our findings, the Hangzhou study did not find a significant relationship between high and excess iodine intake and thyroid nodules [30]. In that study, the excessive iodine intake population selection didn't depend on the MUI of the population, but depended on the individual urine iodine concentration [30]. In fact, Hangzhou is another environmental iodine deficient area [31]. Future study is needed to investigate the relationship between excess iodine intake and the prevalence of thyroid nodules. Our study demonstrated that smoking 11–20 cigarettes per day was significantly related with the presence of thyroid nodules. The main reason for this might be the sample size of the 11–20 cigarettes per day group, which was much smaller than the other groups.

The results indicated that subclinical hypothyroidism was more likely to be prevalent in high iodine intake areas than in deficient or sufficient areas, while overt hyperthyroidism and subclinical hyperthyroidism were more likely to be prevalent in iodine deficient areas than in excess or sufficient areas. Likewise, our study results are similar to Andersen's study [32], in which they found more hypothyroidism and less hyperthyroidism in elderly people (aged 75–80) with sufficient iodine nutrition compared to those with mild iodine deficiency. A study conducted in China found that children had a higher concentration of TSH and a higher prevalence of thyroid diseases in the excess iodine area than in the iodine adequate area, especially for subclinical hypothyroidism [16].

It's well documented in previous studies that the prevalence of goiter in school children is higher in iodine excess or deficient areas than in iodine sufficient areas [4,33,34,35,36]; the prevalence of goiter in school-age children is usually used as a major indicator of IDD surveillance [37]. The results of this study, which included both diffuse and nodular goiter, indicated that goiter prevalence was low (<5%) in all three groups, regardless of iodine excess or deficiency. In addition, females were more susceptible to goiter. In Teng's study, the prevalence of goiter in adults in the more than adequate iodine area was higher than that in the excess iodine areas [25]. The goiter prevalence was different between adults and school children. Based on the above evidence, it could be concluded that thyroid goiter might not be an accurate indicator for assessing the iodine status in adults.

The results of this study indicated that iodine nutrition status play an important role in the TSH level, and iodine excess or deficiency influenced the TSH level. It is reported that neonatal blood TSH concentrations are an indicator for monitoring iodine deficiency in many countries [38,39,40]. Based on our survey,

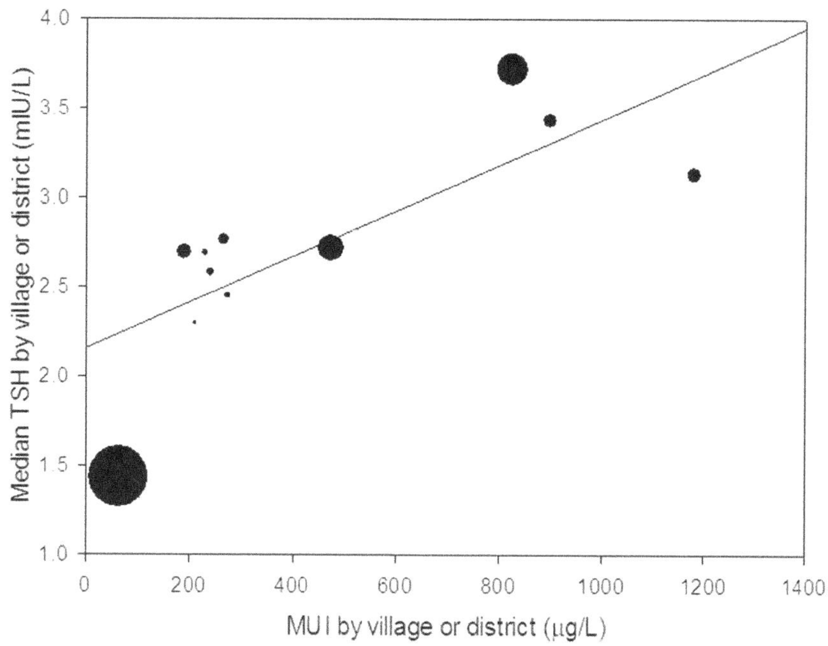

Figure 2. Bubble plot (clustered by village or district) of median TSH vs. MUI with a linear trend line. The size of the bubbles reflects the sample size for each village or district.

except for MUI, median TSH could be deemed as an alternative indicator for monitoring the iodine nutrition status of the adult population in iodine excess or deficient areas. Our results suggested that autoimmune thyroiditis might be prevalent in iodine excess or sufficient areas, which was in line with the previous study [25].

IDD was widespread in China until 1994 when universal salt iodization (USI) was carried out as a mandatory effective strategy to prevent IDD. Afterward, according to the IDD Surveillance Report of China, the government adjusted the iodine concentration in iodized salt three times to maintain the iodine nutrition at an appropriate level. However, at present, there are extra environmental iodine deficient areas with low iodized salt coverage in China and iodine deficiency remains a public health problem. The results of the present study indicate that Tieshangang District of Beihai City is a mild iodine deficient area with a high prevalence of thyroid nodules, overt hyperthyroidism and subclinical hyperthyroidism. The coverage rates of iodized salt and qualified iodized salt are low in Tieshangang District, and the extra environmental iodine nutrition is deficient, such as drinking

Table 7. Simple and multivariate linear regression analyses of TSH on determinants.

Variables	β	95% CI	P
Simple linear regression			
Age	0.038	0.007–0.068	0.016
Gender	0.371	−0.526–1.268	0.471
Smoking	0.353	−0.027–0.733	0.069
Drinking	−0.394	−1.308–0.52	0.398
Iodine status	1.574	1.101–2.047	0
TPOAb positive	3.041	1.96–4.121	0
TGAb positive	3.815	2.791–4.839	0
Multivariate linear regression			
Age	0.023	−0.008–0.054	0.14
Gender	0.484	−0.415–1.384	0.291
TGAb positive	3.038	1.787–4.288	0
TPOAb positive	1.307	−0.001–2.616	0.050
Excess group*	1.764	0.746–2.781	0.001
Deficient group*	−1.219	−2.307– −0.131	0.028

*Dump variable: the reference is the sufficient group.

water. In the coastal areas, there are illegal private salt plants that produce coarse salt (non-iodized salt), the price of course salt is lower than that of iodized salt, and thus it is easier to obtain for the households living in the coastal areas. This situation in the coastal areas highlights the necessity of consolidating the USI and ensuring a high coverage rate of qualified iodized salt, which are indispensable for preventing IDD, especially in coastal areas in China. Adequate iodine nutrition protects the health of the thyroid and prevents a high prevalence of thyroid disease. There are 30 million people living in the high iodine water areas distributed in 734 towns in China [13]. One of the effective measures to prevent excess iodine intake is to sell non-iodized salt in the market in high iodine water areas; the water authorities seldom pay attention to the iodine concentration in the water improvement program. This study demonstrated that the current intervention of supplying non-iodized salt was not enough to prevent excess iodine intake in high iodine water areas; therefore, changing to a safe water source may be the most effective measure for the prevention of the harm resulted from excess iodine intake.

Currently, the subjects of regular iodine nutrition surveillance are children, pregnant women and lactating women. However, our study suggested that both excess and deficient iodine intake could cause thyroid dysfunction or disease in adults; therefore, the adult population should also be under surveillance.

The present study has some limitations. First, the proportion of gender among the three different iodine nutrition groups was different, which might result in a bias for the prevalence of the thyroid disease; however, we applied the multivariable regression analysis to exclude the potential influence of confounders. Second, our survey sites were selected from three provinces in China, the dietary habits may be different in these sites, and we did not conduct a dietary survey, which may affect the results of this study.

In conclusion, iodine deficiency and iodine excess coexist in China. We have demonstrated that both iodine excess and deficiency induce thyroid dysfunction or diseases. The high iodine water areas should decrease iodine intake by changing to a safe water source without providing non-iodized salt, whereas in coastal areas, the non-iodized salt should be forbidden and we should encourage the household to buy iodized salt. These measures should be adopted to make sure that the MUI is maintained at an optimal level (100–199 μg/L) as suggested by the WHO [37]. Our study has provided important baseline data for monitoring the iodine nutrition and thyroid function in iodine excess or deficient areas. In view of our findings, it is recommended that, in the future, except for children, pregnant women and lactating women, an increased emphasis should be placed on monitoring the iodine status of the adult population, especially in the endemic regions.

Acknowledgments

We thank all the organizations that participated in this survey: the provincial (municipality) Centers for Disease Control (CDC) and the Centers for Endemic Disease Control in Shandong, Shanxi and Guangxi, and the residents of Cao County, Shanyin County, Qingxu County, Xiaodian District and Tieshangang District who participated in this survey.

Author Contributions

Conceived and designed the experiments: DS. Performed the experiments: FM SL ZF JW. Analyzed the data: YG. Wrote the paper: YD.

References

1. Zimmermann MB (2009) Iodine deficiency. Endocrine reviews 30: 376–408.
2. Zimmermann MB, Jooste PL, Pandav CS (2008) Iodine-deficiency disorders. Lancet 372: 1251–1262.
3. Mitka M (2013) Even mild iodine deficiency during gestation may impair brain function in children. JAMA 309: 2428–2428.
4. District C (2013) Prevalence of Goitre in School Children of Chamarajanagar District, Karnataka, India. Journal of Clinical and Diagnostic Research 7: 2807–2809.
5. Matthys B, Davlatmamadova M, Karimova G, Jean-Richard V, Zimmermann MB, et al. (2013) Iodine nutritional status and risk factors for goitre among schoolchildren in South Tajikistan. BMC endocrine disorders 13: 50.
6. Zimmermann MB (2012) The effects of iodine deficiency in pregnancy and infancy. Paediatric and perinatal epidemiology 26: 108–117.
7. Pearce EN (2012) Effects of iodine deficiency in pregnancy. Journal of Trace Elements in Medicine and Biology 26: 131–133.
8. Roti E, Uberti ED (2001) Iodine excess and hyperthyroidism. Thyroid 11: 493–500.
9. Li M, Liu DR, Qu CY, Zhang PY, Qian QD, et al. (1987) Endemic goitre in central China caused by excessive iodine intake. Lancet 2: 257–259.
10. Pearce EN, Andersson M, Zimmermann MB (2013) Global iodine nutrition: where do we stand in 2013? Thyroid 23: 523–528.
11. Andersson M, de Benoist B, Rogers L (2010) Epidemiology of iodine deficiency: salt iodisation and iodine status. Best Practice & Research Clinical Endocrinology & Metabolism 24: 1–11.
12. Zimmermann MB (2013) Iodine deficiency and excess in children: worldwide status in 2013. Endocrine Practice 19: 839–846.
13. Shen H, Liu S, Sun D, Zhang S, Su X, et al. (2011) Geographical distribution of drinking-water with high iodine level and association between high iodine level in drinking-water and goitre: a Chinese national investigation. British Journal of Nutrition 106: 243–247.
14. Lv S, Xu D, Wang Y, Chong Z, Du Y, et al. (2014) Goitre prevalence and epidemiological features in children living in areas with mildly excessive iodine in drinking-water. British Journal of Nutrition 111: 86–92.
15. Kapil U, Prakash S, Sareen N, Bhadoria A, Khenduja P, et al. (2014) Status of iodine deficiency among pregnant mothers in Himachal Pradesh, India. Public health nutrition 17: 1971–1974.
16. Sang Z, Chen W, Shen J, Tan L, Zhao N, et al. (2013) Long-Term Exposure to Excessive Iodine from Water Is Associated with Thyroid Dysfunction in Children. The Journal of nutrition 143: 2038–2043.
17. Sang Z, Wei W, Zhao N, Zhang G, Chen W, et al. (2012) Thyroid dysfunction during late gestation is associated with excessive iodine intake in pregnant women. The Journal of Clinical Endocrinology & Metabolism 97: E1363–E1369.
18. Lv S, Zhao J, Xu D, Chong Z, Jia L, et al. (2012) An epidemiological survey of children's iodine nutrition and goitre status in regions with mildly excessive iodine in drinking water in Hebei Province, China. Public health nutrition 15: 1168–1173.
19. Liu P, Liu L, Shen H, Jia Q, Wang J, et al. (2014) The Standard, Intervention Measures and Health Risk for High Water Iodine Areas. PLoS One 9: e89608.
20. Jin Y, E X, Chen Y, Zhang L, Chen C, et al. (2006) Standard exanination methods for drinking water-Nonmetal parameters(GB/T5750.5–2006). Beijing, China: China Criteria Publishing House.
21. Yan Y, Zhang Y, Liu L, Liu J, Li W, et al. (2006) Method for determination of iodine in urine by As $^{3+}$-Ce^{4+} catalytic spectrophotometry (WS/T 107–2006). Beijing, China: People's Medical Publishing House.
22. Tong Y, Huo J (2012) General test method in salt industry: Determination of iodine (GB/T 13025.7–2012). Beijing, China: China Criteria Publishing House.
23. Liu S, Chen Z, Jia Q, Su X, Zhang S (2007) Diagnostic criterion of endemic goiter(WS 276–2007). Beijing, China: People's Medical Publishing House.
24. Zou S, Wu F, Guo C, Song J, Huang C, et al. (2012) Iodine nutrition and the prevalence of thyroid disease after salt iodization: a cross-sectional survey in Shanghai, a coastal area in China. PLoS One 7: e40718.
25. Teng W, Shan Z, Teng X, Guan H, Li Y, et al. (2006) Effect of iodine intake on thyroid diseases in China. N Engl J Med 354: 2783–2793.
26. Yu X, Fan C, Shan Z, Teng X, Guan H, et al. (2008) A five-year follow-up study of goiter and thyroid nodules in three regions with different iodine intakes in China. J Endocrinol Invest 31: 243–250.
27. Takahashi T, Fujimori K, Simon SL, Bechtner G, Edwards R, et al. (1999) Thyroid nodules, thyroid function and dietary iodine in the Marshall islands. International journal of epidemiology 28: 742–749.
28. Gutekunst R, Smolarek H, Hasenpusch U, Stubbe P, Friedrich H-J, et al. (1986) Goitre epidemiology: thyroid volume, iodine excretion, thyroglobulin and thyrotropin in Germany and Sweden. Acta Endocrinologica 112: 494–501.
29. Szabolcs I, Podoba J, Feldkamp J, Dohan O, Farkas I, et al. (1997) Comparative screening for thyroid disorders in old age in areas of iodine deficiency, long-term iodine prophylaxis and abundant iodine intake. Clin Endocrinol (Oxf) 47: 87–92.
30. Chen Z, Xu W, Huang Y, Jin X, Deng J, et al. (2013) Associations of noniodized salt and thyroid nodule among the Chinese population: a large cross-sectional study. The American journal of clinical nutrition 98: 684–692.

31. Lu Y-l, Wang N-j, Zhu L, Wang G-x, Wu H, et al. (2005) Investigation of iodine concentration in salt, water and soil along the coast of Zhejiang, China. Journal of Zhejiang University SCIENCE B 6: 1200–1205.
32. Andersen S, Iversen F, Terpling S, Pedersen KM, Gustenhoff P, et al. (2009) More hypothyroidism and less hyperthyroidism with sufficient iodine nutrition compared to mild iodine deficiency—A comparative population-based study of older people. Maturitas 64: 126–131.
33. Mesele M, Degu G, Gebrehiwot H (2014) Prevalence and associated factors of goiter among rural children aged 6-12 years old in Northwest Ethiopia, cross-sectional study. BMC public health 14: 130.
34. Ahmed M, Zama SY, Nagarajarao V, Khan MA (2014) Iodine deficiency in children: A comparative study in two districts of south-interior Karnataka, India. Journal of family & community medicine 21: 48–52.
35. Medani AMM, Elnour AA, Saeed AM (2013) Excessive iodine intake, water chemicals and endemic goitre in a Sudanese coastal area. Public health nutrition 16: 1586–1592.
36. Henjum S, Barikmo I, Gjerlaug AK, Mohamed-Lehabib A, Oshaug A, et al. (2010) Endemic goitre and excessive iodine in urine and drinking water among Saharawi refugee children. Public health nutrition 13: 1472–1477.
37. WHO UNICEF, ICCIDD (2007) Assessment of iodine deficiency disorders and monitoring their elimination: a guide for programme managers.
38. Evans C, Nix AB, Hillier S, Moat SJ (2014) Neonatal blood TSH concentration in Wales (UK): an indicator of iodine sufficiency. Clinical Endocrinology 81: 606–609.
39. Eltom A, Eltom M, Idris M, Gebre-Medhin M (2001) Thyroid function in the newborn in relation to maternal thyroid status during labour in a mild iodine deficiency endemic area in Sudan. Clinical endocrinology 55: 485–490.
40. Sukkhojaiwaratkul D, Mahachoklertwattana P, Poomthavorn P, Panburana P, Chailurkit L-o, et al. (2014) Effects of maternal iodine supplementation during pregnancy and lactation on iodine status and neonatal thyroid-stimulating hormone. Journal of Perinatology 34: 594–598.

Stunting, Poor Iron Status and Parasite Infection Are Significant Risk Factors for Lower Cognitive Performance in Cambodian School-Aged Children

Marlene Perignon[1]*, Marion Fiorentino[1], Khov Kuong[2], Kurt Burja[3], Megan Parker[4], Sek Sisokhom[5], Chhoun Chamnan[2], Jacques Berger[1], Frank T. Wieringa[1]

1 Institut de Recherche pour le Développement, Montpellier, France, **2** Department of Fisheries Post-Harvest Technologies and Quality Control, Ministry of Agriculture, Forestry and Fisheries, Phnom Penh, Cambodia, **3** United Nations World Food Programme, Phnom Penh, Cambodia, **4** PATH, Seattle, Washington, United States of America, **5** Department of Psychology, Royal University of Phnom Penh, Phnom Penh, Cambodia

Abstract

Background: Nutrition is one of many factors affecting the cognitive development of children. In Cambodia, 55% of children <5 y were anemic and 40% stunted in 2010. Currently, no data exists on the nutritional status of Cambodian school-aged children, or on how malnutrition potentially affects their cognitive development.

Objective: To assess the anthropometric and micronutrient status (iron, vitamin A, zinc, iodine) of Cambodian schoolchildren and their associations with cognitive performance.

Methods: School children aged 6–16 y (n = 2443) from 20 primary schools in Cambodia were recruited. Anthropometry, hemoglobin, serum ferritin, transferrin receptors, retinol-binding protein and zinc concentrations, inflammation status, urinary iodine concentration and parasite infection were measured. Socio-economic data were collected in a sub-group of children (n = 616). Cognitive performance was assessed using Raven's Colored Progressive Matrices (RCPM) and block design and picture completion, two standardized tests from the Wechsler Intelligence Scale for Children (WISC-III).

Results: The prevalence of anemia, iron, zinc, iodine and vitamin A deficiency were 15.7%; 51.2%, 92.8%, 17.3% and 0.7% respectively. The prevalence of stunting was 40.0%, including 10.9% of severe stunting. Stunted children scored significantly lower than non-stunted children on all tests. In RCPM test, boys with iron-deficiency anemia had lower scores than boys with normal iron status (−1.46, $p<0.05$). In picture completion test, children with normal iron status tended to score higher than iron-deficient children with anemia (−0.81; $p = 0.067$) or without anemia (−0.49; $p = 0.064$). Parasite infection was associated with an increase in risk of scoring below the median value in block design test (OR = 1.62; $p<0.05$), and with lower scores in other tests, for girls only (both $p<0.05$).

Conclusion: Poor cognitive performance of Cambodian school-children was multifactorial and significantly associated with long-term (stunting) and current nutritional status indicators (iron status), as well as parasite infection. A life-cycle approach with programs to improve nutrition in early life and at school-age could contribute to optimal cognitive performance.

Editor: Shantanu Sengupta, CSIR-Institute of Genomics and Integrative Biology, India

Funding: This work has been funded by the United Nations World Food Programme (WFP)- DSM consortium, the United States Department of Agriculture/Foreign Agricultural Service (USDA/FAS), and the Institut de Recherche pour le Développement (IRD). The WFP had a role in study design. The IRD had a role in study design, data collection and analysis, decision to publish, and preparation of the manuscript. The USDA/FAS had no role in study design, data collection and analysis, decision to publish, or preparation of the manuscript.

Competing Interests: The authors have declared that no competing interests exist.

* Email: perignonmarlene@gmail.com

Introduction

Worldwide, undernutrition and micronutrient deficiencies substantially impair human health and socio-economic development. Both developed and developing countries are concerned by the burden of micronutrient deficiencies disorders, although the highest prevalence exist in Sub-Saharan Africa and South Asia [1]. In Cambodia, despite a considerable reduction in national poverty since the mid-1990s, undernutrition remains a major problem, and approximately one fifth of the population was still living on less than $1.25 per day in 2009. According to the most recent Cambodia Demographic and Health Survey (CDHS 2010), 40% of children are stunted, 11% are wasted, and 55% of children of 6–59 months are anemic [2].

Nutrition is one of many key factors affecting mental development of children. Deficiencies of critical micronutrients such as iron, folate or iodine can lead to impaired cognitive functions due to their decisive role in brain development. For example, iron deficiency (ID) has been estimated to impair the optimal mental development of 40% to 60% of the developing world's infants [3]. Indirectly, deficiencies of other micronutrients like vitamin A or zinc can increase the risk of morbidity thereby increasing school absenteeism and reducing learning abilities and school performance.

Iron deficiency anemia (IDA), the most severe degree of ID, has been associated with poorer cognitive performance but it is still unclear if malnutrition has detrimental effects on cognitive performance independent of anemia in school-aged children [4]. Some recent systematic reviews based on randomized controlled trials provided evidence for a positive effect of iron supplementation on different measures of cognition in anemic and non-anemic children >5 y [5], on attention and concentration in adolescents and women [6], and beneficial effect of micronutrient interventions (food-based or supplementation) on short term memory [7]. In addition to IDA, stunting is a known risk factor for impaired child development [8]. Despite a general decrease of the global prevalence, stunting still affects one third of the children under 5 y in the developing world [9]. Several studies have documented the relationship between cognitive ability and stunting in young children [10,11] but few have explored it within school-aged children [12–14].

School-aged children are often omitted from public health research. Early child development programs typically focus on the nutritional status and milestones of children under 5 y. Thus, our knowledge regarding the prevalence and impact of micronutrient deficiencies on children >5 y remains scarce. Yet, some areas of the brain and higher cognitive functions continue to develop throughout childhood and adolescence [15]. The myelination of frontal lobes which are thought to be responsible for executive, "higher-order" cognitive activities, starts around 6 mo and continues until adulthood. Changes in the volumes of cortical gray and white matters, significantly correlated to children's performance on a verbal learning task, occur during childhood and adolescence [16]. As during infancy, this ongoing brain development throughout childhood is likely to be affected by detrimental effect of poor nutritional status, hence warranting further research on the impact of nutritional status on cognitive performance of school-aged children. In Cambodia, there is currently no data available concerning the nutritional status of children >5 y, nor how malnutrition potentially affects their mental development.

The present study aimed to evaluate the anthropometric and micronutrient status (iron, vitamin A, zinc and iodine) of Cambodian children aged 6–16 y and to determine if these outcomes are associated with cognitive performance.

Subjects and Methods

Study population and design

Data were collected as part of a randomized placebo-controlled trial investigating the impact of multi-micronutrient fortified rices on health and development of Cambodian schoolchildren (FORISCA UltraRice+NutriRice study, FOrtified RIce for School meals in CAmbodia). Baseline data collection was conducted in November 2012 in 20 primary schools from 5 districts of Kampong Speu province in Cambodia. Kampong Speu is one of the 23 provinces of Cambodia, situated 60 km west of the capital Phnom Penh. Agriculture is predominant, with rice farming as the main occupation and income source. The schools were randomly selected from primary schools participating in school meal or take-home ration programs of the UN World Food Program (WFP). Children attending the selected schools were eligible to be part of the study if they were between 6 16 y of age, had written informed consent from parents/caregivers and did not have any mental or severe physical handicap. In each school, 132 children were randomly selected after stratification by sex and grade, hence 2640 children. 197 children were not recruited because they were absent on the day of data collection or refused to participate. Hence, a total of 2443 schoolchildren aged 6–16 y participated in the study. The study was approved by the National Ethic Committee for Health Research (NECHR) of the Ministry of Health, Phnom Penh, Cambodia, the Ministry of Education, Youth and Sports, Phnom Penh, Cambodia, and the Research Ethics Committee of PATH, Seattle, USA.

Anthropometric measurements

Height and weight were measured using standardized procedures [17,18]. Children wore minimum clothing and no shoes. Height was measured in duplicate to the nearest 0.1 cm with a wooden stadiometer. Weight was measured once, to the nearest 0.1 kilogram using an electronic scale (Seca, 881 U, Germany). Z-scores for height-for-age (HAZ) were calculated with AnthroPlus software version 1.0.4 using the WHO 2007 standards. Moderate and severe stunting were respectively defined as $-3<HAZ<-2$ and $HAZ<-3$ respectively.

Cognitive performance tests

The cognitive performance evaluation included three tests: the Raven's Colored Progressive Matrices test (RCPM), and two standardized tests from the Wechsler Intelligence Scale for Children (WISC III): block design and picture completion. RCPM, the coloured form of Raven's Progressive Matrices test for use with children, is a widely used nonverbal test of intelligence which was designed as a measure of overall intellectual ability [19,20]. The WISC III, designed for children aged 6–16 y, is one of the most widely used tests of the intelligence of children [21]. Block design is a measure of problem solving to assess executive functions [21]. Picture completion evaluates alertness to detail and visual discrimination. The cognitive tests were conducted by 25 students from Psychology department of Royal University of Phnom Penh. The interviewers were trained in a 1 week workshop to ensure standardization in the assessment and scoring procedures. Each child was tested individually using standardized test protocols translated into Khmer language. Since norms are not available for Cambodia, interpretations of the scores of cognitive test were used as raw scores. For all cognitive tests, higher scores indicate better performance.

Blood and urine samples collection

Blood samples (5 ml) were collected by venipuncture and aliquoted in a trace-element free vacutainers with no anticoagulant (Vacuette, Greiner Bio One, Austria). Urine samples were collected from the children in a sterile plastic container. Blood and urine samples were then stored in cool-boxes containing ice-packs and transported to Phnom Penh within 5 h of collection. The blood samples were centrifuged at 2700 rpm (1300 g) for 10 min at room temperature. Serum and urine were then aliquoted in capped Eppendorf tubes and stored at −30°C until transfer for analysis.

Hemoglobin concentration

Hemoglobin concentrations were determined immediately after blood taking using the HemoCue (301+ system, HemoCue Angholm, Sweden). Anemia was defined as hemoglobin concentration <115 g/L for children between the ages 6 and 11 y,

Table 1. Characteristics of school-children participating in the study.

	BOYS	GIRLS	ALL	p-value
n	1223	1220	2443	
Age	9.75±2.34	9.54±2.17	9.65±2.26	p<0.05
% inflammation	41.6 (n = 491)	37.5 (n = 446)	39.5 (n = 937)	p<0.05
% parasite infection	20.0 (n = 177)	16.1 (n = 148)	18.0 (n = 325)	p<0.05
ANTHROPOMETRY				
HAZ	−1.80±1.00 (n = 1219)	−1.71±1.06 (n = 1216)	−1.75±1.03 (n = 2435)	p<0.05
% HAZ<−2SD	41.6 (n = 507)	38.5 (n = 468)	40.0 (n = 965)	NS
% HAZ<−3SD	11.1 (n = 135)	10.8 (n = 131)	10.9 (n = 266)	NS
IRON STATUS				
Hb (g/L)	123.8±9.9 (n = 1203)	124.5±9.5 (n = 1206)	124.2±9.7 (n = 2409)	NS
% anemia	16.8 (n = 202)	14.7 (n = 177)	15.7 (n = 379)	NS
% severe anemia	0.1 (n = 1)	0.2 (n = 2)	0.1 (n = 3)	
FER[1,2] (μg/L)	66.28±1.68 (n = 1181)	68.63±1.68 (n = 1190)	67.45±1.68 (n = 2371)	NS
% FER[1] <15 μg/L	1.9 (n = 22)	1.2 (n = 14)	1.5 (n = 36)	NS
TfR[2] (mg/L)	8.56±1.32 (n = 1181)	8.41±1.30 (n = 1190)	8.48±1.31 (n = 2371)	NS
% TfR >8.3 mg/L	51.8 (n = 612)	50.3 (n = 598)	51.0 (n = 1210)	NS
% ID[3] total	52.2 (n = 616)	50.3 (n = 599)	51.2 (n = 1215)	NS
% ID[3] with anemia	10.8 (n = 127)	9.3 (n = 111)	10.0 (n = 238)	NS
Body iron (mg/kg)	5.90±2.27 (n = 1181)	6.09±2.21 (n = 1190)	5.99±2.24 (n = 2371)	p<0.05
% body iron <0	2.5 (n = 29)	1.6 (n = 19)	2.0 (n = 48)	NS
% body iron <2	5.0 (n = 59)	5.0 (n = 59)	5.0 (n = 118)	NS
% body iron <4	14.5 (n = 171)	13.3 (n = 158)	13.9 (n = 329)	NS
VITAMIN A STATUS				
RBP[1] (μmol/L)	1.54±0.41 (n = 1181)	1.62±0.45 (n = 1190)	1.58±0.43 (n = 2371)	p<0.01
% marginal VA status[4]	9.2 (n = 109)	6.6 (n = 79)	7.9 (n = 188)	p<0.05
% VAD[5]	0.8 (n = 10)	0.6 (n = 7)	0.7 (n = 17)	NS
IODINE STATUS				
% iodine deficiency[6]	14.8 (n = 175)	19.8 (n = 233)	17.3 (n = 408)	p<0.05
% above requirements[7]	52.5 (n = 620)	47.9 (n = 564)	50.2 (n = 1184)	p<0.05
ZINC STATUS				
% zinc deficiency[8]	93.7 (n = 931)	91.9 (n = 907)	92.8 (n = 1838)	NS
SOCIO-ECONOMIC STATUS (on a sub-group n = 616)				
Income[9] ($/year)	1995 (495; 4291)	1825 (500; 4050)	1935 (500; 4150)	
Caretaker's level of education:				
% no or informal schooling	11.9 (n = 35)	14.8 (n = 42)	13.3 (n = 77)	NS
% primary school	65.3 (n = 192)	59.0 (n = 167)	62.2 (n = 359)	NS
% secondary school	22.8 (n = 67)	26.1 (n = 74)	24.4 (n = 141)	NS

Results are mean ± SD unless stated, [1]corrected for inflammation, [2]geometric mean ± SD, [3]based on FER[1] <15 μg/L and/or TfR >8.3 mg/L, [4] 0.7≤ RBP[1] <1.05 μmol/L, [5]RBP[1] <0.7 μmol/L, [6]UIC <100 μg/L, [7]UIC ≥200 μg/L, [8]zinc <0.66 mg/L for girls ≥10 y, <0.70 mg/L for boys ≥10 y, and <0.65 mg/L for boys and girls <10 y, [9]median (10th; 90th), HAZ: height-for-age z-scores, Hb: hemoglobin, FER: ferritin, TfR: transferrin receptors, ID: iron-deficiency, NS: not significant, RBP: retinol binding protein, VA: vitamin A, VAD: vitamin A deficiency.

<120 g/L for children between the ages 12 and 14 y and girls aged 15 y and older and <130 g/L for boys aged 15 y and older according to WHO guidelines [22].

Laboratory analysis

Ferritin (FER), soluble transferrin Receptor (TfR), retinol-binding protein (RBP), C-reactive protein (CRP), α1-acid-glycoprotein (AGP) and zinc serum concentrations. Serum samples were sent on dry ice to the VitMin laboratory (Willstaett, Germany) for determination of retinol-binding protein (RBP), C-reactive protein (CRP), ferritin (FER), soluble transferrin receptor (TfR) and α1-acid-glycoprotein (AGP), and to National Institute of Nutrition (Hanoi, Vietnam) for zinc analysis. RBP, FER, TfR, CRP, AGP were measured by a sandwich enzyme-linked immunosorbent assay (ELISA) technique [23]. Zinc concentration was measured using a flame atomic absorption spectrophotometer (GBC, Avanta+) using trace element-free procedures. Inflammation was defined as high CRP

Table 2. Factors associated with cognitive performance in RCPM test among participating school children.

Variable	n	Estimated mean[1] ± SE	Estimated mean difference[1] (95% CI)	p-value		Estimated mean difference (95% CI) adjusted for all variables[9]	p-value
Gender							
male	1201	16.88±0.14					
female	1224	16.44±0.14	−0.44 (−0.77; −0.12)	0.008		−0.72 (−1.12; −0.33)	p<0.001
Stunting							
normal status	1500	17.03±0.13					
−3< HAZ <−2	677	16.41±0.26	−0.62 (−1.32; 0.08)	0.10		−0.56 (−1.12; 0.006)	0.053
HAZ <−3	244	15.12±0.29	−1.91 (−2.70; −1.12)	p<0.001		−1.97 (−2.81; −1.12)	p<0.001
Parasite infection							
not infected	1471	17.49±0.11					
infected	324	17.00±0.28	−0.49 (−1.09; 0.11)	0.11	M	0.29 (−0.49; 1.08)	0.47
					F	−1.43 (−2.18; −0.68)	0.016
Iron deficiency[2]							
no ID	1148	17.21±0.13					
ID without anemia	968	16.93±0.14	−0.28 (−0.73; 0.18)	0.43	M	−0.31 (−1.10; 0.48)	1.00
					F	−0.31 (−1.01; 0.38)	0.84
ID with anemia	236	16.41±0.35	−0.81 (−1.70; 0.086)	0.092	M	−1.46 (−2.73; −0.18)	0.019
					F	−0.36 (−1.56; 0.84)	1.00
FER[3] (mg/L)							
≥50	1811	17.19±0.10					
15–50	507	16.69±0.20	−0.50 (−1.03; 0.02)	0.068			
<15	34	16.50±1.07	−0.69 (−3.26; 1.87)	1.00			
TfR (mg/L)							
≤8.3	1152	17.21±0.13					
>8.3	1200	16.86±0.12	−0.348 (−0.698; 0.01)	0.052			
Body iron (mg/kg)							
>4	2028	17.16±0.09					
0–4	278	16.42±0.28	−0.75 (−1.44; −0.06)	0.029			
<0	46	15.85±0.82	−1.32 (−3.29; 0.65)	0.33			
VA status							
normal VA status	2170	16.69±0.12					
marginal VA status[4]	173	16.48±0.42	−0.21 (−1.06; 0.65)	0.63			
VAD[5]	15	16.15±1.26	−0.54 (−3.02; 1.95)	0.67			
Iodine status							

Table 2. Cont.

Variable	n	Estimated mean[1] ± SE	Estimated mean difference[1] (95% CI)	p-value	Estimated mean difference (95% CI) adjusted for all variables[9]	p-value
adequate	763	17.21±0.18				
iodine deficiency[6]	406	16.72±0.33	−0.49 (−1.39; 0.41)	0.57		
above requirements[7]	1171	17.33±0.14	1.12 (−0.42; 0.65)	1.00		
Zinc status						
normal status	140	17.62±0.51				
zinc deficiency[8]	1827	17.08±0.11	−0.54 (−1.57; 0.49)	0.30		

[1]adjusted for age, [2]defined by FER[3]<15 µg/L and/or TFR >8.3 mg/L, [3]corrected for inflammation, [4]0.7≤ RBP[3] <1.05 µmol/L, [5]RBP[3] <0.7 µmol/L, [6]UIC <100 mg/L, [7]UIC ≥200 mg/L, [8]zinc <0.66 mg/L for girls ≥10 y, <0.70 mg/L for boys ≥10 y, and <0.65 mg/L for boys and girls <10 y, [9]significant interactions between gender and parasite, and gender and iron deficiency, ID: iron deficiency, FER: ferritin, TfR: transferrin receptors, VA: vitamin A, VAD: VA deficiency, M: male, F: female, RCPM: Raven's colored progressive matrices.

(>5 mg/L) and/or high AGP concentrations (>1 g/L). Inflammation status was then categorized in four groups based on CRP and AGP levels: no inflammation (normal CRP and AGP), incubation (high CRP and normal AGP), early convalescence (high CRP and AGP), and late convalescence (normal CRP and high AGP) [24]. FER is affected by presence of infection or inflammation, therefore FER concentrations were adjusted using correction factors published by Thurnham et al., namely 0.77, 0.53 and 0.75 for children respectively in incubation, early convalescence, and late convalescence phases. Low FER (corrected value <15 µg/L) was used as indicator of depleted iron stores [22], and high TfR (>8.3 mg/L) as indicator of tissue iron deficiency [25,26]. Iron deficiency was defined using both FER and TfR indicators, i.e. by depleted iron stores or tissue iron deficiency. Total body iron (BI) was calculated from FER corrected for inflammation and TfR as described by Cook *et al.* [27]. Serum retinol is bound to RBP in a 1-to-1 complex, hence RBP concentrations were used to evaluate vitamin A status [28]. RBP concentrations were adjusted for the presence of inflammation using correction factors of 1.15, 1.32 and 1.12 for incubation, early convalescence and late convalescence phases respectively [29]. Corrected RBP cut-offs were used to define marginal vitamin A status (0.70 µmol/L ≤ corrected RBP<1.05 µmol/L), vitamin A deficiency (<0.70 µmol/L) and severe vitamin A deficiency (< 0.35 µmol/L) respectively [28,30]. Zinc deficiency was defined using the following cut-offs: serum zinc concentration <0.66 mg/L for girls ≥10 y, <0.70 mg/L for boys ≥10 y, and <0.65 mg/L for boys and girls <10 y [31].

Urinary iodine concentration. Urine samples were sent on dry ice to the Provincial Preventive Medicine Center (Thai Nguyen, Vietnam) for determination of urinary iodine concentration (UIC) using spectrophotometric methods [32]. Iodine deficiency (IDD) was defined by a median UIC below 100 µg/L and/or a proportion of participants below 50 µg/L higher than 20%, and iodine nutrition above requirements by a median UIC above 200 µg/L [33].

Parasite infestation

Plastic containers and instructions for fecal sample collection were distributed to the children on the day of data collection and requested to be returned with fecal sample to the school the following day. Samples were then stored in a cool box, transported to the National Malaria Center (CNM, Phnom Penh, Cambodia) and stored at 4°C until analysis. Quantitative parasite egg counts were performed by CNM using the Kato-Katz method [34]. The egg output was expressed as eggs per gram feces (epg).

Socio-economic survey

Socio-economic information was collected on a sub-sample (n = 616 children, FORISCA-NutriRice study) by trained interviewers during household visits. Questionnaires were answered by parents or caretaker and included information about household characteristics, caretaker's level of education and amount and source of household income.

Data management and statistical analysis

Data entry, including quality checks and validation by double entry of questionnaires, was performed with EpiData version 3.1 (EpiData Association, Odense, Denmark). Data management and analyses were performed using SPSS version 20.0 software (SPSS, Inc., Chicago, IL). Normality of distributions was evaluated using Kolmogorov-Smirnoff test. Not normally distributed data were considered to be reasonably close to normality to allow parametric tests when skewness and kurtosis values ranged between −1.0 and

Table 3. Factors associated with cognitive performance in Picture completion test among participating school children.

Variable	n	Estimated mean[1] ± SE	Estimated mean difference[1] (95% CI)	p-value	Estimated mean difference (95% CI) adjusted for all variables[9]	p-value
Gender						
male	1201	7.38±0.13				
female	1224	7.29±0.14	−0.09 (−0.41; 0.23)	0.60		
Stunting						
normal status	1500	7.80±0.13				
−3< HAZ <−2	677	6.69±0.25	−1.11 (−1.79; −0.43)	p<0.001	−1.07 (−1.62; −0.52)	p<0.001
HAZ <−3	244	5.99±0.29	−1.81 (−2.58; −1.04)	p<0.001	−1.68 (−2.50; −0.86)	p<0.001
Parasite infection						
not infected	1485	7.69±0.18				
infected	304	7.09±0.31	−0.60 (−1.30; 0.10)	0.095	M 0.02 (−0.73; 0.77)	0.96
					F −0.85 (−1.61; −0.09)	0.028
Iron deficiency[2]						
no ID	1148	7.43±0.17				
ID without anemia	968	7.24±0.18	−0.19 (−0.78; 0.40)	1.00	−0.49 (−1.01; 0.02)	0.064
ID with anemia	236	7.00±0.36	−0.43 (−1.39; 0.52)	0.82	−0.81 (−1.66; 0.04)	0.067
FER[3] (mg/L)						
≥50	1811	7.89±0.10				
15–50	507	7.53±0.19	−0.36 (−0.88; 0.15)	0.27		
<15	34	8.11±1.05	0.22 (−2.31; 2.74)	1.00		
TfR (mg/L)						
≤8.3	1152	7.98±0.12				
>8.3	1200	7.64±0.12	−0.35 (−0.69; −0.01)	0.048		
Body iron (mg/kg)						
>4	2028	7.90±0.09				
0–4	278	7.13±0.27	−0.77 (−1.45; −0.10)	0.019		
<0	46	7.33±0.80	−0.57 (−2.51; 1.36)	1.00		
VA status						
normal VA status	2170	7.36±0.11				
marginal VA status[4]	173	7.56±0.41	0.19 (−0.82; 1.21)	1.00	0.08 (−0.84; 0.99)	1.00
VAD[5]	15	4.79±1.22	−2.57 (−5.52; 0.37)	0.11	−0.86 (−3.43; 1.71)	1.00
Iodine status						
adequate	763	7.73±0.17				
iodine deficiency[6]	406	7.72±0.33	−0.01 (−0.90; 0.88)	1.00		

Table 3. Cont.

Variable	n	Estimated mean[1] ± SE	Estimated mean difference[1] (95% CI)	p-value	Estimated mean difference (95% CI) adjusted for all variables[9]	p-value
above requirements[7]	1171	8.03±0.14	0.30 (−0.23; 0.83)	0.51		
Zinc status						
normal status	140	8.21±0.50				
zinc deficiency[8]	1827	7.83±0.10	−0.38 (−1.38; 0.62)	0.45		

[1]adjusted for age, [2]defined by FER[3] <15 μg/L and/or TFR >8.3 mg/L, [3]corrected for inflammation, [4]0.7≤ RBP[3] <1.05 μmol/L, [5]RBP[3] <0.7 μmol/L, [6]UIC <100 mg/L, [7]UIC ≥200 mg/L, [8]zinc <0.66 mg/L for girls ≥10 y, <0.70 mg/L for boys ≥10 y, and <0.65 mg/L for boys and girls <10 y, [9]significant interactions between gender and parasite, ID: iron deficiency, FER: ferritin, TfR: transferrin receptors, VA: vitamin A, VAD: vitamin A deficiency, M: male, F: female.

+1.0. Continuous variables that were not normally distributed were log-transformed. Block design score was categorized as score below and above median value. All analyses took into account characteristics of the cluster sampling design (school clusters). The main effects of explanatory variables on cognitive tests scores were first assessed in univariate analysis using ANCOVA for RCPM and Picture completion tests, and logistic regression for Block design test, with all analysis including age as covariate. Multivariate analyses were then performed to evaluate the associations between cognitive tests scores and variables assessing nutritional status (stunting, anemia and micronutrient status) while taking into account the effect modification or confounding of other variables (age, gender, parasite infection, socio-economic status). Any variable having a p-value <0.25 in the univariate test was considered for the multivariate analysis. Interactions were tested and if significant at the 0.05 level, analyses were run separately at each level of the variable modifying the effect. Multiple comparisons were conducted by using the Bonferroni post-hoc test.

Results

Characteristics of the studied sample

A total of 2443 children from grades 1–6 participated in the study. Characteristics of the participants are presented in **Table 1**. The mean ± SD age of children was 9.6±2.3 y and half (49.9%) were girls. The prevalence of anemia was 15.7% including 0.1% severe anemia. There was no significant difference in anemia prevalence between boys and girls, or age groups; however, prevalence varied between 4.8% and 30.0% across the schools. The overall prevalence of stunting (HAZ<−2SD) was 40.0%, including 10.9% severe stunting (HAZ<−3SD). Children ≥10 y were significantly more affected by stunting (54.0% and 29.6% respectively) or severe stunting (18.5% and 5.3% respectively) than children <10 y, but no difference was found between gender. Inflammation (CRP>5 mg/L and/or AGP>1 g/L) was found in more than one third of the children (39.5%), with boys being more affected than girls. Parasite infection was found in 18% of the children, boys being more affected than girls (p<0.05). Only 1.5% of the children had depleted iron stores (FER<15 μg/L) whereas 50.1% had tissue iron deficiency (TfR>8.3 mg/L). There was no significant difference between age groups or genders for both indicators. Prevalence of iron deficiency, as defined by low FER and/or high TfR, was 51.2% without any difference between age groups or gender. Only 2% of the children had negative body iron stores but marginal body iron stores (total body iron <4 mg/kg body weight) were prevalent (13.9%). Prevalence of iron-deficiency anemia was 10.0% with no difference between boys and girls. Prevalence of vitamin A deficiency (VAD) was 0.7%, with no severe VAD. However, 7.9% of the children had marginal VA status (0.7≤ corrected RBP<1.05 μmol/L). Children <10 y were significantly more affected by marginal VA status (9.4% and 6% respectively) than children >10 y (p<0.05). Prevalence of marginal VA status was also higher in boys than in girls (9.2% and 6.6% respectively, p<0.05). Most children (93%) exhibited low serum zinc concentrations, indicative of zinc deficiency. Approximately one fifth (17%) of the children were iodine deficient while half (50.2%) had iodine intake above requirements.

Factors associated with cognitive performance

Cognitive scores were associated with stunting and micronutrient status (**Table 2** (RCPM test), **Table 3** (Picture completion test) and **Table 4** (Block design test)). Children with severe stunting scored significantly lower than non stunted children in all

Table 4. Univariate and multivariate analysis of factors associated with poor performance in Block design test among participating schoolchildren.

Variable	n	odds-ratio[1] (95% CI)	p-value	odds-ratio adjusted for all variables (95% CI)	p-value
Gender					
male	1208	1		1	
female	1213	1.28 (1.06; 1.55)	0.009	1.27 (0.99; 1.63)	0.058
Stunting					
normal status	1446	1		1	
−3< HAZ <−2	706	1.88 (1.50; 2.37)	p<0.001	1.73 (1.29; 2.33)	p<0.001
HAZ <−3	263	3.67 (2.56; 5.26)	p<0.001	2.35 (1.47; 3.75)	p<0.001
Parasite infection					
not infected	1471	1		1	
infected	324	1.64 (1.21; 2.24)	0.002	1.73 (1.24; 2.42)	0.001
Iron deficiency[2]					
no ID	1148	1		1	
ID without anemia	968	0.95 (0.77; 1.17)	0.62	1.09 (0.83; 1.43)	0.52
ID with anemia	236	1.32 (0.95; 1.85)	0.10	1.17 (0.74; 1.85)	0.26
FER[3] (mg/L)					
≥50	1811	1			
15–50	507	1.11 (0.88; 1.40)	0.39		
<15	34	1.31 (0.60; 2.90)	0.50		
TfR (mg/L)					
≤8.3	1152	1			
>8.3	1200	1.01 (0.83; 1.23)	0.93		
Body iron (mg/kg)					
>4	2028	1			
0–4	278	1.23 (0.92; 1.66)	0.17		
<0	46	1.24 (0.62; 2.49)	0.54		
VA status					
normal VA status	2149	1			
marginal VA status[4]	186	0.91 (0.64; 1.30)	0.60		
VAD[5]	17	1.67 (0.48; 5.89)	0.42		
Iodine status					
adequate	763	1			
iodine deficiency[6]	406	0.91 (0.68; 1.21)	0.52		
above requirements[7]	1171	0.94 (0.74; 1.19)	0.60		
Zinc status					
normal status	140	1		1	
zinc deficiency[8]	1827	1.43 (0.95; 2.15)	0.091	1.32 (0.82; 2.13)	0.26

[1]adjusted for age, [2]defined by FER[3] <15 µg/L and/or TFR >8.3 mg/L, [3]corrected for inflammation, [4]0.7≤ RBP[3] <1.05 µmol/L, [5]RBP[3] <0.7 µmol/L, [6]UIC <100 mg/L, [7]UIC ≥200 mg/L, [8]zinc <0.66 mg/L for girls ≥10 y, <0.70 mg/L for boys ≥10 y, and <0.65 mg/L for boys and girls <10 y, ID: iron deficiency, FER: ferritin, TfR: transferrin receptors, VA: vitamin A, VAD: vitamin A deficiency, M: male, F: female.

tests ($p<0.001$ for all), with reduction of score reaching up to −2 points in RCPM test (12% of mean score), or −1.7 points in picture completion test (22% of mean score) after adjustment on all variables. Children with moderate stunting scored significantly lower (Picture completion and Block design tests, both $p<0.001$) or tend to score lower (RCPM test, $p=0.053$) when compared with non-stunted children. For the block design test, severely stunted children were 2.5 times more likely to score below the median value than children with normal height status (OR = 2.53, $p<0.001$).

Univariate analysis showed that positive but marginal body iron stores (0<body iron ≤4 mg/kg) were associated with significantly lower scores in RCPM and picture completion tests (both $p<0.05$). After adjustment on all variables, boys with iron-deficiency anemia (IDA) scored significantly lower than children with normal iron status in RCPM test (−1.46; $p<0.05$). Score difference was not significant for girls with IDA. For the picture completion test, children with normal iron status tended to score higher than iron-deficient children with anemia (−0.81; $p=0.067$) or without anemia (−0.49; $p=0.064$), for both genders. Vitamin A deficien-

Table 5. Factors associated with cognitive performance in RCPM test before and after adjustment on socio-economic status in a sub-sample of school children (n = 616).

Variable	n		mean difference[1] (95% CI)	p-value		mean difference[2, 3] (95% CI) after adjustment for SES	p-value
Gender							
male	311						
female	305		−0.29 (−1.06; 0.48)	0.47		−0.47 (−1.27; 0.33)	0.25
Stunting							
normal status	367						
−3< HAZ <−2	176		−0.33 (−1.42; 0.75)	1.00		−0.55 (−1.67; 0.57)	0.71
HAZ <−3	67		−1.68 (−3.33; −0.04)	0.044		−1.60 (−3.29; 0.08)	0.067
Parasite infection							
not infected	387						
infected	48	M	−0.09 (−1.85; 1.66)	0.92	M	0.20 (−1.63; 2.03)	0.83
		F	−2.32 (−4.24; −0.40)	0.018	F	−2.27 (−4.25; −0.29)	0.025
Iron deficiency[4]							
no ID	261						
ID without anemia	262	M	0.13 (−1.49; 1.74)	1.00	M	−0.01 (−1.63; 1.65)	1.00
		F	−0.25 (−1.75; 1.24)	1.00	F	−0.26 (−1.77; 1.25)	1.00
ID with anemia	65	M	−2.09 (−4.60; 0.42)	0.14	M	−2.23 (−4.78; 0.32)	0.11
		F	−1.05 (−3.25; 1.15)	0.76	F	−0.95 (−3.31; 1.41)	1.00
Socio-economic status							
Household income[5]	616					0.03 (0.00; 0.05)	0.048
Caretaker's education[6]	616					0.18 (0.02; 0.34)	0.024

[1]variables in the model: age, gender, stunting, parasite infection, iron deficiency, [2]variables in the model: age, gender, stunting, parasite infection, iron deficiency, caretaker's level of education, income, [3]interaction between gender and parasite infection, and gender and iron-deficiency, [4]defined by FER (corrected for inflammation) <15 µg/L and/or TFR >8.3 mg/L, [5]x100 US$/year, [6]years of schooling, ID: iron deficiency, SES: socio-economic status, M: male, F: female.

cy, iodine disorders (deficiency or excessive intake) and zinc deficiency were not significantly associated with cognitive performance.

Girls scored significantly lower than boys in the RCPM test (-0.72; $p<0.01$) and were more likely ($OR = 1.27$; $p<0.05$) to score below the median value in the block design test. Parasite infection was associated with an increased risk of scoring below median value for the block design test ($OR = 1.62$; $p<0.05$), and with lower scores in RCPM and picture completion tests, but only for girls (both $p<0.05$).

In the sub-sample of school children for which data were available ($n = 616$), socio-economic status (caretaker's level of education and household's income) was significantly associated with scores in RCPM test, but not in Picture completion and Block design tests. In RCPM test, higher household's income and caretaker's level of education were both associated with higher test score (both $p<0.05$, **Table 5**). Results of multivariate analysis of association between RCPM scores and explanatory variables before and after adjustment on socio-economic status are given in **Table 5**. The results obtained for this sub-group were similar to those obtained on all children, with lower statistical significance as a consequence of smaller number of subjects. Adjustment on socio-economic status did not change the results: severe stunting and parasite infection were associated with lower scores in RCPM test, as well as IDA for boys.

Discussion

Within this large cross-sectional survey of Cambodian school children, both long-term nutritional deficits as reflected by stunting and current micronutrient status, especially iron status, significantly affected cognitive performance. According to the WHO classification system, the observed prevalence of anemia (15.7%) indicated a mild public health problem in Cambodia, with only 3 cases of severe anemia. The prevalence of depleted iron stores (1.5%) or negative body iron (2%) were both very low. In contrast, more than half of the children had high TFR concentrations. TFR reflects tissue iron needs but may have also been increased by factors like hemoglobinopathy or inflammation [35,36]. TFR levels were actually higher in children showing abnormal Hb type (HbE) or inflammation, but prevalence of high TFR was still important in the sub-sample of children with normal Hb profile (48.5%) or without inflammation (42.1%). Iron stores being adequate for most of the children (as indicated by the high ferritin concentrations), high TfR concentration suggests a functional tissue iron deficiency due to either an impaired release of iron from stores or impaired systems for transporting iron to target tissues.

The prevalence of iron-deficiency anemia (10%) represented about two-thirds of the overall anemia prevalence. Also, approximately one tenth (9%) of the children exhibited low VA status, with 0.7% being deficient, and >90% had low serum zinc concentrations, indicating a very high prevalence of zinc deficiency in this population. Hence, this population of school children exhibited concurrent deficiencies of micronutrients, as reported previously for younger children in SE Asia [37,38].

Poor iron status was associated with lower cognitive ability, however the effect was modified by gender: children with IDA, especially boys, scored lower than iron-replete children. Interestingly, ID was associated with lower scores in the picture completion test even without anemia. Also, lower scores in two of the three tests were found for children with positive but marginal total body iron stores (0–4 mg/kg) as compared to children with replete stores. Thus, the findings from this study indicate that marginal iron status may have impaired cognitive performance before the onset of anemia. This evidence suggests that interventions are needed to improve iron status in school children even in the absence of IDA.

Stunting is an indicator of early-life chronic malnutrition, with most of the growth deficit occurring in the first 2 y of life [39]. In the present study, stunting was a high risk factor for lower scores in all tests after controlling for age, gender and micronutrient status (iron, vitamin A, zinc, iodine), and also for socio-economic status in the sub-sample of children. Furthermore, this study showed that the prevalence of stunting, both moderate and severe, was higher in children ≥10 y than in children <10 y. One possible explanation could be that nutritional status of young children has improved considerably over the last decade in this area, but the national data reported a consistent 40% of stunting among children <5 y in 2005 and 2010 [2,40]. Another explanation could be that growth faltering continues after 5 y of age. Thus, considering also the extremely high prevalence of zinc deficiency found in the studied 6–16 y children (93%), interventions like zinc fortification could possibly help to limit worsening of stunting and, as a consequence, of cognitive performance impairment.

Children infected by parasites, especially girls, exhibited poorer cognitive performance than non infested children. Possible links between parasite infection and cognitive outcomes are reduced school attendance due to illness, loss of concentration, or through nutrition by affecting absorption of micronutrients such as iron and iodine [41,42]. In the present study, parasite infections remained a highly significant factor in the multivariate analysis which included anthropometry and micronutrient status indicators, suggesting an effect of parasite infection on cognition independent from nutrition. Therefore, the negative effect of parasite infection on cognition might be associated to higher absenteeism from school due to illness. Regardless of the underlying mechanisms, deworming programs could benefit school performance in Cambodian school children.

Although not available for all studied children, socio-economic status was included in analysis for a sub-sample of children ($n = 616$). The results obtained from this sub-group were similar to the whole sample and remained unchanged after correcting for confounding effect of caretaker's level of education and household' s income. Thus, we can reasonably assume that associations between cognitive outcomes and variables reflecting nutritional status found for the 2443 children are not due to confounding effects of socio-economic status.

Thus, the present study showed that poor cognitive performance was multi-factorial, with nutritional factors as stunting and iron deficiency and non-nutritional factors such as parasite infection being implicated. These results are consistent with recent studies showing a relationship between cognitive abilities below average and low HAZ in school children in South East Asia [13], and a beneficial effect or iron supplementation on attention, concentration and different measures of cognition [5,6]. Hence, as stunting and iron deficiency in school-aged children reflect long-term and current nutritional status respectively, interventions at different periods of age could have a beneficial effect on cognitive abilities. Nutritional programs in early life to ensure good nutrition and prevent stunting before start of schooling are crucial. In addition, strategies at school-age like deworming, surveys for early recognition and prevention of iron deficiency before the onset of anemia, or interventions to prevent worsening of growth faltering should be considered to contribute to optimal cognitive development. Combining nutrition specific interventions, such as food fortification, with nutrition sensitive interventions, such as deworming, might have synergistic benefits.

Acknowledgments

We would like to thank all school children and their parents in Kampong Speu province for their participation in the study.

Author Contributions

Conceived and designed the experiments: FTW JB KB CC SS M. Parker. Performed the experiments: M. Perignon MF KK FTW. Analyzed the data: M. Perignon. Contributed to the writing of the manuscript: M. Perignon FTW.

References

1. Black RE, Victora CG, Walker SP, Bhutta ZA, Christian P, et al. (2013) Maternal and child undernutrition and overweight in low-income and middle-income countries. The Lancet 382: 427–451.
2. National Institute of Statistics, Directorate General for Health, Macro I (2011) Cambodia demographic and health survey in 2010.
3. UNICEF MI (2004) Vitamin and Mineral Deficiency - A Global Progress Report.
4. McCann JC, Ames BN (2007) An overview of evidence for a causal relation between iron deficiency during development and deficits in cognitive or behavioral function. Am J Clin Nutr 85: 931–945.
5. Hermoso M, Vucic V, Vollhardt C, Arsic A, Roman-Vinas B, et al. (2011) The Effect of Iron on Cognitive Development and Function in Infants, Children and Adolescents: A Systematic Review. Annals of Nutrition and Metabolism 59: 154–165.
6. Falkingham M, Abdelhamid A, Curtis P, Fairweather-Tait S, Dye L, et al. (2010) The effects of oral iron supplementation on cognition in older children and adults: a systematic review and meta-analysis. Nutr J 9: 4.
7. Khor GL, Misra S (2012) Micronutrient interventions on cognitive performance of children aged 5–15 years in developing countries. Asia Pacific Journal of Clinical Nutrition 21: 476–486.
8. Walker SP, Wachs TD, Gardner JM, Lozoff B, Wasserman GA, et al. (2007) Child development: risk factors for adverse outcomes in developing countries. Lancet 369: 145–157.
9. Black RE, Allen LH, Bhutta ZA, Caulfield LE, de Onis M, et al. (2008) Maternal and child undernutrition 1 - Maternal and child undernutrition: global and regional exposures and health consequences. Lancet 371: 243–260.
10. Crookston BT, Dearden KA, Alder SC, Porucznik CA, Stanford JB, et al. (2011) Impact of early and concurrent stunting on cognition. Matern Child Nutr 7: 397–409.
11. Grantham-McGregor S (2002) Linear growth retardation and cognition. The Lancet 359: 542.
12. Sokolovic N, Selvam S, Srinivasan K, Thankachan P, Kurpad AV, et al. (2014) Catch-up growth does not associate with cognitive development in Indian school-age children. European Journal of Clinical Nutrition 68: 14–18.
13. Sandjaja, Poh BK, Rojroonwasinkul N, Nyugen BKL, Budiman B, et al. (2013) Relationship between anthropometric indicators and cognitive performance in Southeast Asian school-aged children. British Journal of Nutrition 110: S57–S64.
14. Best C, Neufingerl N, van Geel L, van den Briel T, Osendarp S (2010) The nutritional status of school-aged children: why should we care? Food Nutr Bull 31: 400–417.
15. Bryan J, Osendarp S, Hughes D, Calvaresi E, Baghurst K, et al. (2004) Nutrients for cognitive development in school-aged children. Nutr Rev 62: 295–306.
16. Sowell ER, Thompson PM, Toga AW (2004) Mapping changes in the human cortex throughout the span of life. Neuroscientist 10: 372–392.
17. Cogill B, Food, Project NTA (2003) Anthropometric Indicators Measurement Guide: Food and Nutrition Technical Assistance Project, Academy for Educational Development.
18. WHO (1995) Physical status: the use and interpretation of anthropometry: report of a WHO Expert Committee. WHO Technical Report Series: World Health Organization.
19. Kaplan RM, Saccuzzo DP (2009) Psychological Testing: Principles, Applications, and Issues: Principles, Applications, and Issues: Wadsworth Cengage Learning.
20. Isaacs E, Oates J (2008) Nutrition and cognition: assessing cognitive abilities in children and young people. Eur J Nutr 47 Suppl 3: 4–24.
21. Hughes D, Bryan J (2003) The assessment of cognitive performance in children: considerations for detecting nutritional influences. Nutr Rev 61: 413–422.
22. WHO (2001) Iron Deficiency Anaemia Assessment, Prevention and Control. A guide for programme managers. Geneva: World Health Organization.
23. Erhardt JG, Estes JE, Pfeiffer CM, Biesalski HK, Craft NE (2004) Combined measurement of ferritin, soluble transferrin receptor, retinol binding protein, and C-reactive protein by an inexpensive, sensitive, and simple sandwich enzyme-linked immunosorbent assay technique. Journal of Nutrition 134: 3127–3132.
24. Thurnham DI, McCabe LD, Haldar S, Wieringa FT, Northrop-Clewes CA, et al. (2010) Adjusting plasma ferritin concentrations to remove the effects of subclinical. Am J Clin Nutr 92: 546–555.
25. Zimmermann MB, Molinari L, Staubli-Asobayire F, Hess SY, Chaouki N, et al. (2005) Serum transferrin receptor and zinc protoporphyrin as indicators of iron status. Am J Clin Nutr 81: 615–623.
26. Skikne BS, Flowers CH, Cook JD (1990) Serum transferrin receptor: a quantitative measure of tissue iron deficiency. Blood 75: 1870–1876.
27. Cook JD, Flowers CH, Skikne BS (2003) The quantitative assessment of body iron. Blood 101: 3359–3364.
28. de Pee S, Dary O (2002) Biochemical indicators of vitamin A deficiency: Serum retinol and serum retinol binding protein. Journal of Nutrition 132: 2895S–2901S.
29. Thurnham DI, McCabe GP, Northrop-Clewes CA, Nestel P (2003) Effects of subclinical infection on plasma retinol concentrations and assessment of prevalence of vitamin A deficiency: meta-analysis. Lancet 362: 2052–2058.
30. Gibson RS (2005) Principles of Nutritional Assessment: Oxford University Press.
31. Gibson RS, Hess SY, Hotz C, Brown KH (2008) Indicators of zinc status at the population level: a review of the evidence. British Journal of Nutrition 99: S14–S23.
32. Dunn JT, Crutchfield HE, Gutekunst R, Dunn AD (1993) Methods for measuring iodine in urine: ICCIDD, UNICEF, WHO.
33. WHO (2007) Assessment of iodine deficiency disorders and monitoring their elimination. A guide for programme managers. 3rd ed. World Health Organization. pp. 32–33.
34. Ash LR, Savioli L, Orihel TC, World Health Organization (1994) Bench aids for the diagnosis of intestinal parasites. Geneva: World Health Organization.
35. Zimmermann MB (2008) Methods to assess iron and iodine status. British Journal of Nutrition 99: S2–S9.
36. Knowles J, Thurnham DI, Phengdy B, Houamboun K, Philavong K, et al. (2013) Impact of inflammation on the biomarkers of iron status in a cross-sectional survey of Lao women and children. Br J Nutr 110: 2285–2297.
37. Dijkhuizen MA, Wieringa FT, West CE, Muherdiyantiningsih Muhilal (2001) Concurrent micronutrient deficiencies in lactating mothers and their infants in Indonesia. Am J Clin Nutr 73: 786–791.
38. Thurlow RA, Winichagoon P, Pongcharoen T, Gowachirapant S, Boonpraderm A, et al. (2006) Risk of zinc, iodine and other micronutrient deficiencies among school children. Eur J Clin Nutr 60: 623–632.
39. Victora CG, de Onis M, Hallal PC, Blossner M, Shrimpton R (2010) Worldwide timing of growth faltering: revisiting implications for interventions. Pediatrics 125: e473–480.
40. National Institute of Public Health, National Institute of Statistics Macro O (2006) Cambodia Demographic and Health Survey 2005.
41. Hall A (2007) Micronutrient supplements for children after deworming. The Lancet Infectious Diseases 7: 297–302.
42. Hall A, Hewitt G, Tuffrey V, de Silva N (2008) A review and meta-analysis of the impact of intestinal worms on child growth and nutrition. Matern Child Nutr 4 Suppl 1: 118–236.

20

Intra-Individual Double Burden of Overweight and Micronutrient Deficiencies among Vietnamese Women

Arnaud Laillou[1]*, Elizabeth Yakes[2], Thi Hop Le[3], Frank Tammo Wieringa[4], Bach Mai Le[3], Regina Moench-Pfanner[5], Jacques Berger[4]

1 UNICEF, Maternal Child Health and Nutrition section, Phnom Penh, Cambodia, **2** University of New Mexico, Department of Individual, Family and Community Education and Department of Family and Community Medicine, Albuquerque, New Mexico, United States of America, **3** National Institute of Nutrition (NIN), Nutrition section, Hanoi, Vietnam, **4** Institut de Recherche pour le Développement (IRD), Unité Mixte de Recherche 204 "Prévention des malnutritions et des pathologies associées", Montpellier, France, **5** Global Alliance for Improved Nutrition (GAIN), Singapore Office, Singapore, Singapore

Abstract

Background: Vietnamese Living Standard Surveys showed that the rate of overweight and obese in Vietnamese adults doubled between 1992 and 2002, from 2% to 5.5%, respectively with no significant difference in the proportions of overweight/obesity between men and women.

Objectives: Considering the increasing public health concern over the double burden of malnutrition in Vietnam, we investigated micronutrient deficiencies among women of reproductive age according to their Body Mass Index.

Methods: A transversal study was conducted in 2010 among 1530 women of reproductive age from 19 provinces. Participating women were asked to give a non-fasting blood sample for plasma iron, vitamin A, folate, vitamin B_{12} and zinc assessment.

Results: Although % body fat was associated with haemoglobin, ferritin, retinol and zinc concentrations, BMI category was only associated with marginal vitamin A status (19% among underweight vs 7% among overweight/obese; $p<0.0001$) and not with iron deficiency anemia, zinc deficiency, vitamin B_{12} deficiency or folate status. The prevalence of iron, and vitamin B_{12} deficiencies was respectively 11.4% and 15% among the 20% overweight/obese women; prevalence of zinc deficiency and marginal/deficient folate status was much higher, affecting respectively 61.1% and 25.8%. Intra-individual double burden of malnutrition (overweight/obesity (OW) and micronutrient deficiency) was observed among 2.0% for OW-anemia, 2.3% OW-iron deficient, 3.0% for OW-Vitamin B_{12} deficiency, 12.2% for OW-Zinc deficiency and 5.2% for OW-marginal/deficient folate status.

Conclusions: This large, cross-sectional survey demonstrated that micronutrient deficiencies are an issue across the weight spectrum among women in Vietnam, with only vitamin A status being better among overweight than underweight women. It is therefore essential for Vietnam to actively prevent women of reproductive age from overweight/obesity and at same time to control micronutrient deficiencies in this population to limit their economic and health consequences.

Editor: Marià Alemany, Faculty of Biology, Spain

Funding: Global Alliance for Improved Nutrition (GAIN) has funded this research as they were interested to understand the micronutrient deficiencies in Vietnam. The funders had no role in study design, data collection and analysis, decision to publish, or preparation of the manuscript.

Competing Interests: The authors have declared that no competing interests exist.

* Email: alaillou@unicef.org.org

Background

Obesity is a major health concern worldwide. According to the World Health Organization (WHO), there were approximately 1.5 billion overweight adults and 300 million obese women worldwide in 2008 [1]. Rapid social change, urbanisation and changes in the food supply and dietary patterns, along with demographic and other behaviour changes has caused a "nutrition transition" in many lower- and middle income countries. This transition has been characterized by an increase in overweight/obesity and related chronic diseases [2]. For example, economic growth, ageing of populations and urbanization with the associated lifestyle changes is likely to lead to a 54% increase in worldwide diabetes prevalence by 2030 [3].

Cardiovascular diseases and their risk factors, such as hypertension and obesity, are emerging as the leading causes of morbidity and mortality in many developing countries, including Vietnam [4]. As with many countries experiencing rapid economic growth, Vietnam is facing the so-called "double burden of malnutrition," defined as the presence of both under-nutrition and over-nutrition in the population[5]. The Vietnamese Living Standard Surveys showed that the prevalence of overweight(BMI≥25 kg/m^2) in Vietnamese adults doubled between 1992 and 2002, from 2% to 5.5%, respectively [6]. The National Adult Obesity study, using the Asian BMI cut-off of 23 kg/m^2, showed an even higher prevalence of overweight in 2005 (16.3%), a sharp increase compared to 11.7% in 2000 [5]. This situation is likely to worsen, as a recent survey in Ho Chi Minh showed that the prevalence of combined overweight/obesity increased from 13.8% to 21.0% in a 6-year period among adolescents [7].

Individuals experiencing over-nutrition (overweight/obesity) due to excess energy intake may also suffer from micronutrient deficiencies. This has been particularly showed in relation to iron deficiency [8]. In addition, some recent studies showed that inadequate vitamin D and/or zinc status have been associated overweight and obesity and other metabolic syndromes [9–11]. Given the health risks associated with both excess adiposity and micronutrient deficiencies, their co-occurrence may have particularly dire consequences for the health of a population. The recent 2010 Vietnamese nationwide micronutrient deficiencies study showed high prevalence of zinc deficiency (~67%) and vitamin B_{12} deficiency (~12%) among women of reproductive age [12]. Prevalence of folate deficiency and vitamin A deficiency were considered negligible, but approximately 25% of women had marginal folate status and low iron stores, while 14% had marginal vitamin A status [12]. This survey also found an overweight/obesity (BMI≥23 kg/m^2) prevalence of 20%. Considering the increasing public health concern over the double burden of malnutrition in Vietnam, the objective of the present paper is to examine predictors of overweight/obesity among Vietnamese women of reproductive age and to quantify micronutrient deficiencies among Vietnamese women by weight status (underweight, healthy weight, overweight/obese) from the recent 2010 nationwide micronutrient data.

Methods

Study design and sampling

The sample size for this study was estimated to evaluate the prevalence of micronutrient deficiency among women of reproductive age with a hypothesis of 50% prevalence, a precision of 5.0% and an expected design effect of 2.0. Anticipating an estimated 17% refusal or absence of women in the selected households, 840 women per stratum (urban/rural) were required [12]. Consequently, a total of 56 urban and 56 rural clusters of 15 households were selected and 1526 women of reproductive age were surveyed.Non-pregnant women of reproductive age (15–49 years) with no severe or chronic illness or current acute infection (e.g. fever, diarrhea, acute respiratory infection) were included in the survey after obtaining informed consent.

Anthropometry and body composition

The women were invited to come to the Commune Health Center in the early morning. Women were weighed without shoes or sandals and wearing light clothes using a balance with a precision of 0.1 kg (Body Composition Monitor Scale Tanita BC-543, Tokyo, Japan). Height was measured using a wooden height board with a precision of 0.1 cm (UNICEF supply). The percentage of body fat and water and the bone mineral mass were measured with the same balance using Bioelectric Impedance Analysis taking gender, age, height and weight into account.

Anthropometric data were entered into EpiData (version 6.0). Body mass index (BMI) was calculated and women were classified using the BMI cut-off points for Asian populations: underweight (BMI<18.5 kg/m^2), healthy weight (BMI 18.5–22.9 kg/m^2), overweight (BMI 23.0–27.49 kg/m^2), and obese (BMI≥27.5 kg/m^2) [13].

Blood sampling and analysis

After anthropometry data collection (between 0700 and 0900 hours), a non-fasting venous blood sample (6 ml)was withdrawn by venipuncture into trace-element free heparinized sampling tubes (Vacuette, Greiner Bio One, Austria) by licensed medical technicians. Blood samples were stored in the dark in a cool box and transported within 4 hours of collection to the Provincial Medical Center (PMC) laboratory for hemoglobin determination. Hemoglobin concentration (Hb) was then measured immediately according to the manufacturer's instructions using a HemoCue device (Hemocue 301, Ängelholm, Sweden) and control material provided by Hemocue (HemoCue - HemoTrol, Keplerlaan, Netherland). Thereafter, plasma was obtained by centrifugation at 3000 g for 10 min at 4°C. Plasma was aliquoted into 200 µL pre-labelled Eppendorf tubes and kept frozen at −20°C at the Provincial Medical Center before being sent, within two weeks, on dry ice to the National Institute of Nutrition (NIN) in Hanoi, where samples were stored at −70°C until analysis.

Plasma concentrations of ferritin, retinol, zinc, and C-reactive protein (CRP) were determined at the NIN Micronutrient Laboratory. Plasma ferritin was measured by ELISA using commercial kits that included reference samples (Ramco Laboratories Inc, Houston, Texas). The accuracy was tested with Bio-Rad liquicheck control (Bio-Rad Laboratories, USA). Plasma retinol concentration was determined by reverse-phase HPLC (LC-10 ADVP, Shimadzu, Japan) according to the method of the International Vitamin A Consultative Group in a dimly lighted room [14]. Zinc was analysed using a flame atomic absorption spectrophotometer (GBC, Avanta+) using trace element-free procedures and powder free gloves (Latex Surgical Glove), and results were verified using reference materials (Liquicheck, Bio-Rad Laboratories, USA). A control for potential contamination of material used for blood sampling and blood processing by external zinc was carried out by analysing zinc content of at least 20 sets of materials (needle, syringe, vacutainers and eppendorf tubes) where blood was replaced by bi-distilled water. CRP, an acute phase protein, was used to quantify the acute phase response as a marker of inflammation and infection. Plasma CRP was measured by ELISA using a commercial kit from GenWay (Biotech, Inc., San Diego, California), with reference materials included in each assay (Liquicheck, Bio-Rad Laboratories, USA).

Aliquots of plasma were sent to the Swiss Vitamin Institute (Epalinges, Switzerland) for analysis of folate and vitamin B_{12} using a microbiological assay. Extracted folates were diluted with basal medium containing all required growth nutrients except folate[15]. The growth response of *Lactobacillus casei*, subspecies rhamnosus (ATCC 7469) to extracted folates was compared to the growth response to calibration solutions with known concentrations. Vitamin B_{12} was measured for a randomly selected subsample of 505 women. Vitamin B_{12} was analyzed turbidimetrically using *Lactobacillus plantarum* (ATCC 8014) as the test organism [16–18]. The growth response of *Lactobacillus plantarum* is proportional to the quantity of vitamin B_{12} in the sample[19]. The within-assay variability for plasma ferritin, retinol, folate, zinc, vitamin B_{12}, and CRP was <6%.

Anemia was defined according to WHO standards as hemoglobin below 120 g/l for women of reproductive age [20]. Iron deficiency was defined as plasma ferritin <15 µg/L for women [20] using a correction factor of 0.65 for ferritin concentration from subjects with sub-clinical inflammation as indicated by increased concentrations of CRP (>5 mg/l) [21]. Sub-clinical

Table 1. Prevalence of underweight, healthy weight, overweight and obesity among Vietnamese women.

Maternal BMI (kg/m^2) Category	n*	Prevalence (%)	Standard Error of Prevalence (SEP)	95% CI for prevalence**
Severe underweight (BMI<16)	30	2.0	0.4	1.3–2.7
Moderate underweight (BMI 16–16.9)	58	3.9	0.5	2.9–4.8
Mild underweight (BMI 17–18.49)	220	14.7	1.1	12.5–16.8
Healthy weight (BMI 18.5–22.9)	893	59.5	1.4	56.7–62.3
Overweight (BMI 23.0–27.4)	264	17.6	1.1	15.5–19.7
Obese (BMI≥27.5)	36	2.4	0.4	1.5–3.2

*24 of 1526 women did not have any anthropometric measurements.
**: CI: confidence interval.

vitamin A deficiency was defined using WHO cut-offs of plasma retinol <0.7 µmol/l [20], while marginal status was defined as plasma retinol between 0.7 and 1.05 µmol/l [22]. Plasma retinol concentrations were corrected where sub-clinical infection existed [23]. Zinc deficiency was defined using the International Zinc Nutrition Consultative Group (IZiNCG) cut off of zinc < 10.1 µmol/l for women [24]. Vitamin B_{12} deficiency was defined as plasma vitamin B_{12} values below 148 pmol/l; vitamin B_{12} status was considered marginal when the plasma concentration was between 148–220 pmol/l [25]. Folate deficiency and marginal status was defined as plasma folate concentrations <13.4 nmol/l [25].

Socioeconomic status

The Demographic and Health Survey (DHS) Wealth Index was used to divide the surveyed households into five socio-economic quintiles: the "extreme poor" (category 1), the "poor" (category 2), the "intermediate" (categories 3 and 4), and the "wealthy" (category 5). The Wealth Index was constructed from recorded data on household assets such as tables, chairs, refrigerator, air conditioners and beds and also from housing conditions (materials of house floor, house roof, main wall) and facilities (energy for cooking, electricity and latrines) [26].

Ethical approval

The Scientific Committees of the National Institute of Nutrition (NIN) (Hanoi, Vietnam) and the Ministry of Health (Hanoi, Vietnam) reviewed and approved the study protocol. All women were informed verbally and in writing about the aims and procedures of the study, and written informed consent was obtained from all women before enrolment.

Statistical analysis

Data entry, including quality checks was performed with Excel 2007. Data management and analysis were performed with SAS software version 9.3 (SAS, V9.3; SAS institute, Cary, NC). All analyses accounted for the cluster sampling design using appropriate SAS survey procedures. Categorical variables are expressed as percentages and standard error percentages (surveyfreq procedure). Bivariate relationships between categorical variables were assessed using the Rao-Scott Chi-Square Test. Bivariate and multivariate relationships between age category, socioeconomic category, ethnic group, urban/rural location, region, education level, and micronutrient status and BMI category (dependent variable) were assessed using ordinal logistic regression or multinomial logistic regression in cases where the proportional odds assumption was not met (surveylogistic procedure). Continuous variables are expressed as means and standard error of the mean (surveymeans procedure). Associations between maternal BMI category, age, and socio economic status and continuous dependent variables (plasma micronutrient concentrations, percent body fat, bone mass) were assessed using linear regression models (surveyreg procedure). Plasma micronutrient concentrations were transformed to natural logarithms as necessary to meet the assumptions of normality of residuals and homogeneity of variance.

Results

Using the BMI cut-offs for Asian populations, 20.5% of the Vietnamese women were underweight (UW, **Table 1**), while 20.0% were overweight including only 2.4% of obese women. For the remainder of this paper, overweight and obese women (OW) are combined into one category (overweight/obese; BMI≥23 kg/m^2) with an average BMI in this category of 25±2 kg/m^2. BMI was highly correlated to maternal body fat ($\beta = 0.91$; $P<0.001$), but less strong to Wealth Index (beta = −0.07 $p<0.001$) and age (beta = 0.03; $p = 0.012$).

Average maternal body fat significantly increased with BMI category ($p<0.001$), with percent body fat averages (mean±SEM) of 21.0%±0.2% for UW (95% CI: 20.6–21.4), 27.7%±0.1% for healthy weight women (HW, 95% CI: 27.5–28.0) and 35.3%±0.2% for OW (95% CI: 34.8–35.8). Maternal bone density also significantly ($p<0.001$) increased with BMI category, with bone density averages of 1.66 g/cm^2±0.02 for UW (95% CI: 1.63–1.70), 1.88 g/cm^2±0.01 for HW (95% CI: 1.86–1.90) and 2.13g/cm^2±0.02 for OW (95% CI: 2.09–2.16).

In bivariate analyses, weight status was significantly associated (**Table 2**) with age, daily energy intake, socioeconomic category, ethnicity, urban/rural location, and region. The prevalence of overweight/obesity steadily increased with older age category with 64% of the 300 OW being 36.0 year old or older. OW had significantly higher energy intakes with half of them consuming more than 1900 kcal/day (7955 kJ/day) while ~60% of UW consumed less than 1660 kcal/day (6950 kJ/day). There was a 55% to 89% reduction in the unadjusted odds of overweight/obesity among women in younger age groups compared to women ≥36 years old (**Figure 1**). Women from the highest socioeconomic group (group 5) clearly had the lowest prevalence of underweight (13.3%) and the highest prevalence of OW. There was a 54% to 79% decrease in the unadjusted odds of overweight/obesity among women in the lowest three socioeconomic groups compared to women in group 5 (**Figure 1**). The prevalence of overweight/obesity was significantly higher among the Kinh ethnic group compared to minority groups and among urban dwellers compared to rural dwellers (22.2% vs. 17.9%), with an 35% increase in the unadjusted odds of overweight/obesity among Kinh vs. minority and urban vs. rural populations (**Figure 1**). The prevalence of overweight/obesity differed significantly by region of the country, ranging from 11.4% in the Central North to an alarming 56.4% in the Central south (**Table 2**). Higher educated women tended to have a lower prevalence of overweight/obesity than less educated women, with an 45 to 59% increased unadjusted odds of overweight/obesity among women with a primary school or high school level education compared to the higher educated women (**Figure 1**). Controlling only for age, % body fat was significantly associated to concentrations of hemoglobin (beta = 0.12; $p<0.001$), ferritin (beta = 0.05; $p = 0.049$), retinol (beta = 0.12; $p<0.001$) and zinc (beta = 0.08; $p = 0.02$) Given the high correlation between % body fat and BMI, it was not surprising there were significant bivariate relationships between BMI category and hemoglobin, ferritin and retinol concentrations (Table 3), which were significantly lower for UW and HW compared to OW. These relationships persisted after controlling for maternal age and socio economic status, with the exception of ferritin that was no longer significant ($p>0.05$). A significant association was also observed between BMI category and marginal vitamin A status ($p<0.0001$). There was, a 66% decrease in the odds of marginal vitamin A status among OW compared to UW (**Figure 2**). Among OW, one of ten women had anemia and iron deficiency whereas 15% had vitamin B_{12} deficiency, 25% marginal/deficient folate status and more than 60% zinc deficiency (Table 3). Consequently, among the women surveyed nation-wide, the intra-individual double burden of malnutrition (overweight/obesity and micronutrient deficiency) was observed among 2.0% (95% CI: 1.3–2.7) for OW-anemia, 2.3% (95% CI: 1.4–3.1) OW-Iron deficiency, 3.0% (95% CI: 1.7–4.3) for OW-Vitamin B_{12} deficiency, 12.2% (95% CI: 10.7–13.7) for OW-Zinc deficiency and 5.2% (95% CI: 4.0–6.3) for OW-marginal/deficient folate status.

Discussion

Earlier, we reported a double burden of malnutrition at the country level among Vietnamese women of reproductive age, with an overall prevalence of both underweight and overweight/obesity

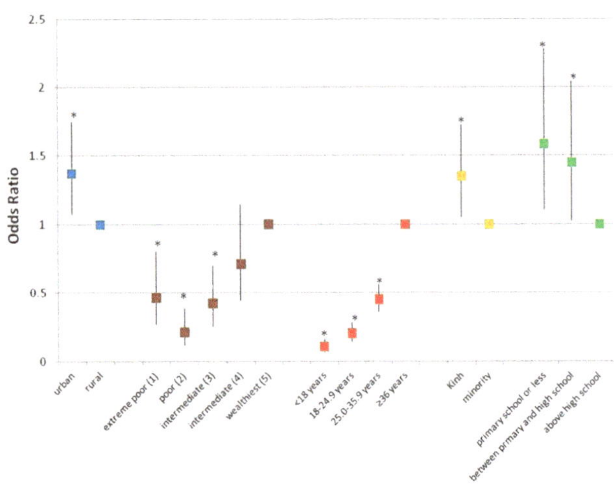

Figure 1. Unadjusted odds ratios for overweight/obesity for Vietnamese women of reproductive age.

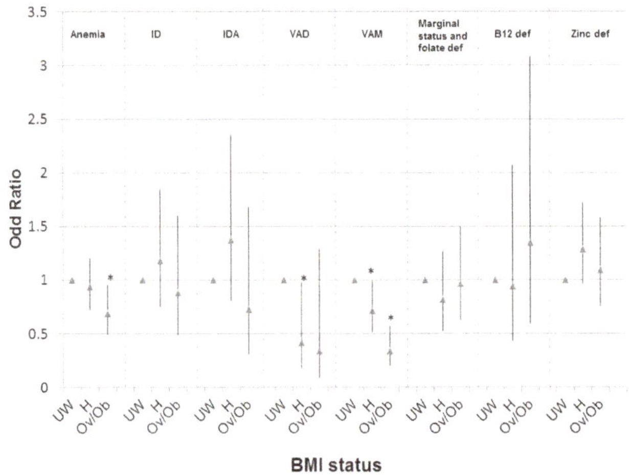

Figure 2. Unadjusted odds ratios for overweight/obesity for Vietnamese women of reproductive age. Note: UW: underweight women; H: healthy women; Ov/Ob: overweight or obese women; ID: iron deficiency; IDA: Iron deficiency anemia; VAD: vitamin A deficiency; VAM: vitamin A marginal status; def: deficiency.

of approximately 20% [12]. The present study demonstrates that a significant proportion of Vietnamese women of reproductive age experience the double burden of malnutrition at intra-individual level, with overweight/obesity and micronutrient deficiency being present in the same individual. Especially zinc deficiency was prevalent, both in overweight/obese and normal weight women, with >60% of the women affected. Only the prevalence of vitamin A deficiency was lower in OW women, as compared to UW women, whereas the prevalence of deficiency or marginal status of iron, folate or vitamin B_{12} did not differ between underweight, normal weight and overweight/obese women.

The poor status of vitamin B_{12} (15%) and folic acid (26%) in these overweight/obese Vietnamese women, even though not different in prevalence to normal weight women, is reason for concern as deficiency of either vitamin B_{12} or folic acid can lead to an increase in plasma homocysteine levels [27,28], which is a powerful risk factor for cardiovascular disease [29]. Combined with the elevated BMI, these women are even at a higher risk for cardiovascular disease. Therefore national strategies to improve vitamin B_{12} and folic acid status in the general population are needed.

Ferritin concentrations (corrected for inflammation [21]), increased significantly with BMI as reported earlier from finding in the USA [30]. There is some controversy around iron status in obese subjects. Some authors have suggested that higher hepcidin levels in obesity may contribute to lower iron absorption and hence to iron deficiency in obesity [31]. Also, obesity is characterized by higher rates of inflammation, which will lead to higher concentrations of plasma ferritin, thereby causing under-estimation of iron deficiency in subjects with obesity [32]. In the present study, we corrected ferritin concentrations for inflammation, using the factors derived by Thurnham et al [21] that have been confirmed relevant for obesity recently [32]. Even after correction for inflammation, higher % body fat (and hence higher BMI) is still associated with higher ferritin concentrations, showing that in this population, overweight/obesity is not a risk factor for iron deficiency, and even associated with better iron status. This is in accordance with another study showing that overweight Mexican women had similar anemia and iron status (measured with transferrin saturation) compared to normal weight women

Table 2. Bivariate relationships betweenage, socioeconomic status, ethnicity, location (rural/urban), region and the prevalence of underweight, normal weight, overweight and obesity among Vietnamese women.

	BMI Category (kg/m²)												p*
	Underweight (BMI<18.5)				Healthy Weight (BMI 18.5–22.9)				Overweight/Obese (BMI≥23.0)				
Category	n	Prevalence (%)	SEP	95% CI	n	Prevalence (%)	SEP	95% CI	n	Prevalence (%)	SEP	95% CI	
Maternal Age (years)**													<0.0001
<18	64	49.6	4.7	40.3–58.9	60	46.5	4.4	37.8–55.2	5	3.8	1.7	0.5–7.2	
18–24.9	77	32.1	3	26.1–38.1	150	62.5	3.2	56.2–68.8	13	5.4	1.4	2.7–8.1	
25.0–34.9	102	18.9	1.8	15.2–22.5	348	64.3	2.2	60.0–68.6	91	16.8	1.4	14.1–19.6	
≥36.0	65	11	1.5	8.1–13.9	335	56.7	2.1	52.5–60.9	191	32.3	2.2	28.0–36.6	
Maternal daily Energy intake (kcal)**													<0.0001
<1600 kcal/day	46	59.7	6.7	46.3–73.1	29	37.7	7.1	23.5–51.8	2	2.6	1.7	0.0–6.1	
1600–1899 kcal/day	93	19.8	1.9	15.9–23.7	328	69.8	2.1	65.6–73.9	49	10.4	1.4	7.6–13.2	
≥1900 kcal/day	12	4.1	1.1	2.0–6.2	136	46.6	2.9	40.8–52.3	144	49.3	3	43.4–55.3	
Socioeconomic category**													<0.0001
1	58	23.5	3.5	16.6–30.3	142	57.3	3.8	50.0–65.0	47	19	2.7	13.7–24.3	
2	62	27.3	3.2	20.9–33.7	142	62.6	3.5	55.7–69.5	23	10.1	2	6.1–14.2	
3	64	23.4	3.1	17.4–29.5	162	59.3	3.6	52.2–66.5	47	17.2	2.4	12.5–21.9	
4	66	21	2.1	16.8–25.2	166	52.9	2.7	47.5–58.3	82	26.1	2.5	21.2–31.0	
5	58	13.3	1.7	10.16.6	277	63.5	1.9	59.8–67.2	101	23.2	1.8	19.5–26.8	
Ethnicity**													0.05
Kinh	220	19.1	1.4	16.2–22.0	693	60.2	1.6	57.0–63.3	239	20.7	1.3	18.1–23.3	
Minority groups	82	25.9	2.5	20.9–30.9	178	56.2	3.2	49.8–62.5	57	18	2.3	13.5–22.4	
Education level**													0.09
1	103	18.7	1.7	15.2–22.1	330	59.9	1.9	56.0–63.8	118	21.4	1.9	17.6–25.2	
2	153	20.4	1.7	17.0–23.8	446	59.5	1.8	55.9–63.0	151	20.1	1.5	17.2–23.1	
3	47	28.3	3.4	21.5–35.1	92	55.4	3.7	48.0–62.8	27	16.3	3	10.3–22.3	
Location**													0.02
Rural	180	23.3	2	19.3–27.3	454	58.8	2.2	54.5–63.1	138	17.9	1.6	14.8–21.0	
Urban	128	17.6	1.5	14.6–20.5	439	60.2	1.7	56.8–63.6	162	22.2	1.6	19.0–25.5	
Region**													<0.0001
Central Highland	19	13.2	2.5	8.2–18.1	101	70.1	3.6	63.1–77.2	24	16.7	2.6	11.6–21.7	
Central North	30	38	7.3	23.5–52.4	40	50.6	6.1	38.5–62.8	9	11.4	3.4	4.7–18.1	
Central South	40	18.7	3.3	12.1–25.3	118	55.1	2.5	50.1–60.1	56	56.4	3.5	49.5–63.2	
Mekong River Delta	27	16.4	3.1	10.2–22.6	93	56.4	3.5	49.5–63.2	45	27.3	2.8	21.7–32.8	
North East	60	25.5	2.8	20.1–31.0	145	61.7	4	53.8–69.6	30	12.8	2.2	8.4–17.1	
North West	13	13.5	3.5	6.6–20.5	61	63.5	7.1	49.5–77.6	22	22.9	3.9	15.1–30.7	

Table 2. Cont.

Category	BMI Category (kg/m²)												p*
	Underweight (BMI<18.5)				Healthy Weight (BMI 18.5–22.9)				Overweight/Obese (BMI≥23.0)				
	n	Prevalence (%)	SEP	95% CI	n	Prevalence (%)	SEP	95% CI	n	Prevalence (%)	SEP	95% CI	
Red River Delta	20	16.5	2.9	10.7–22.3	78	64.5	3.1	58.2–70.7	23	19	2.6	13.9–24.1	
South East	99	22.1	2.3	17.5–26.8	257	57.5	2.5	52.6–62.4	91	20.4	2.3	15.7–25.0	

Note: *Based on bivariate analysis; Rao-Scott Chi-Square Test.
**Number of women with missing data varies by variable: age (n = 25), region (n = 25),location (n = 25), socioeconomic data (n = 29), ethnicity (n = 57), education level (n = 59).
Education level. 1: primary school degree or less; 2 more than primary school but not over high school degree; 3: over high school degree.

[33]. In the same study however, obese women had lower iron status. In the present study, most of the women were overweight (average BMI: 25±2 kg/m2), based on cut-offs adapted for Asian population [13], with only 0.6% having a BMI over 30 kg/m2 [12], the obesity cut-off used in studies in Western populations, perhaps explaining this difference with the study from Mexico.

In contrast to the water-soluble vitamins, there were clear differences for vitamin A status between underweight, normal weight and overweight Vietnamese women, with vitamin A status being highest in overweight/obese women, with significant higher plasma retinol concentrations and an Odd Ratio of 0.38 for marginal vitamin A status among overweight/obese women compared to underweight women. Another study from Mexico [34] among 580 women of reproductive age did not find any difference in serum vitamin A concentration among BMI categories. However, the authors did not correct retinol concentrations for inflammation. Retinol concentrations are known to decrease with inflammation [23]. Hence, vitamin A status in these obese Mexican women might have been underestimated.

The higher iron and especially retinol status among Vietnamese overweight/obese population could be explained by a higher dietary diversity. We showed that overweight/obese participants had much higher energy intake than underweight women and higher socio-economic level. This energy increase might have consequently induced higher micronutrient intakes as a previous study in Vietnam shows that non-poor Vietnamese households experienced an significant increases in calorie intake and dietary diversity during the period 1997/1998–2004 [35] while poor households did not experience such an increase. Furthermore, in Vietnam, the consumption of vitamin A has been positively correlated to the household expenditure [36]. As both iron and vitamin A deficiency are associated with anemia [37,38], the better iron and retinol status in overweight women may also explain the higher haemoglobin concentration observed in overweight/obese Vietnamese women.

In conclusion, in the present study there was a positive association between % body fat on one side, and hemoglobin and plasma retinol, zinc and ferritin concentrations on the other side, even after correcting retinol and ferritin concentrations for inflammation. The apparent discrepancy between studies on iron and vitamin A status in overweight/obese subjects is likely due to the effect of inflammation on indicators of iron and vitamin A status [39]. No correction for inflammation seems to lead to an overestimation of iron status, and an underestimation of vitamin A status in overweight/obese subjects. Another factor which could explain the discrepancies is the prevalence of overweight and obese subjects in the study population, with different effects being reported between overweight and obese subjects. When using global cut-offs for obesity, in contrast to Asian cut-offs, the prevalence of obesity was very low in the present study (0.6% of the women [12]). The higher iron and vitamin A status in our population is most likely due to a higher food intake which has not lead to a better status of water-soluble vitamins (folate and B_{12}). Knowing the close link of folate and B_{12} deficiency and the risk for cardiovascular disease, it is essential for Vietnam to actively monitor the progress of overweight and obesity to limit health consequences for the population as well as the economic burden for the country [40]. It may also be worthwhile to monitor waist circumference, as excess of central adiposity is strongly associated with the increase of non-communicable disease prevalence [41]. But BMI should be also kept as an indicator as other research says that no strong evidence supports replacing BMI in clinical or public health practice with other adiposity measures [42].

Table 3. Bivariate relationships between micronutrient status and the prevalence of underweight, normal weight, and overweight/obesity among Vietnamese women.

	Maternal BMI Category (kg/m²)												p*
	Underweight (BMI<18.5)				Healthy Weight (BMI 18.5–22.9) Increasing but acceptable risk				Overweight/Obese (BMI≥23.0) Increased/High Risk				
Category	n	Prevalence (%)/mean	SEP/SEM***	95% CI	n	Prevalence (%)/mean	SEP/SEM***	95% CI	n	Prevalence (%)/mean	SEP/SEM***	95% CI	
Plasma concentration													
Hemoglobin in g/l	308	130.8	0.07	129.9–132.1	892	131.2	0.05	130.3–132.1	300	132.9	0.07	131.6–134.2	0.04
Ferritin in µg/l	307	70.48	6.89	56.81–84.15	892	73.98	3.18	67.58–80.20	298	91.01	6.56	80–104.03	0.03
serum retinol in µmol/l	298	1.32	0.03	1.27–1.37	861	1.47	0.03	1.42–1.52	290	1.61	0.05	1.51–1.70	<0.0001
Folate in nmol/l	286	18.4	0.6	17.3–19.6	809	18.5	0.4	17.6–19.3	266	18.0	0.5	16.9–19.1	0.543
Vitamin B_{12} in pmol/l	95	580.1	40.4	499.1–661.1	300	660.2	27.1	606.4–713.9	100	577.3	46.5	484.3–670.2	0.106
Zinc in µmol/l	307	9.6	0.2	9.2–9.9	891	9.4	0.1	9.2–9.7	298	9.7	0.2	9.3–10.0	0.097
*Anemia***													0.62
No	273	88.6	1.8	85.0–92.3	785	88.0	1.3	85.4–90.6	270	90.0	1.7	86.5–93.5	
Yes	35	11.4	1.8	7.7–15.0	107	12.0	1.3	9.4–14.6	30	10.0	1.7	6.5–13.5	
Iron deficiency													
No	268	87.3	2.2	83.0–91.6	761	85.3	1.4	82.5–88.1	264	88.6	2.2	84.3–92.9	0.39
Yes	39	12.7	2.2	8.4–17.0	131	14.7	1.4	11.9–17.5	34	11.4	2.2	7.1–15.7	
Iron deficiency anemia													0.09
No	293	95.4	1.1	93.3–97.6	836	93.8	0.9	92.1–95.6	288	96.6	1.0	94.6–98.7	
Yes	14	4.6	1.1	2.4–6.7	55	6.2	0.9	4.4–7.9	10	3.4	1.0	1.3–5.4	
*Vitamin A deficiency***													0.08
No	289	97.0	1	94.9–99.1	850	98.7	0.4	98.0–99.4	287	99.0	0.6	97.8–100.0	
Yes	9	3.0	1	1.0–5.1	11	1.3	0.4	0.6–2.0	3	1.0	0.6	0.0–2.2	
*Marginal vitamin A status***													<0.0001
No	242	81.2	2.2	76.8–85.6	739	85.8	1.3	83.3–88.4	269	92.8	1.5	89.7–95.8	
Yes	56	18.8	2.2	14.4–23.2	122	14.2	1.3	11.6–16.7	21	7.2	1.5	4.2–10.3	
*Zinc deficiency***													0.18

Table 3. Cont.

Category	Maternal BMI Category (kg/m^2)												p*
	Underweight (BMI<18.5)				Healthy Weight (BMI 18.5–22.9) Increasing but acceptable risk				Overweight/Obese (BMI≥23.0) Increased/High Risk				
	n	Prevalence (%)/mean	SEP/SEM***	95% CI	n	Prevalence (%)/mean	SEP/SEM***	95% CI	n	Prevalence (%)/mean	SEP/SEM***	95% CI	
No	126	41.0	4	33.2–48.9	313	35.1	2.9	29.4–40.9	116	38.9	3.8	31.4–46.4	
Yes	181	59.0	4	51.1–66.8	578	64.9	2.9	59.1–70.6	182	61.1	3.8	53.6–68.6	
*Vitamin B_{12} deficiency***													0.58
No	84	88.4	3.6	81.2–95.6	267	89.0	2.2	84.7–93.3	85	85.0	3.3	78.5–91.5	
Yes	11	11.6	3.6	4.4–18.8	33	11.0	2.2	6.7–15.3	15	15.0	3.3	8.5–21.5	
*Folate deficiency and marginal status***													0.71
No	211	71.5	2.9	65.9–77.2	623	72.1	2.0	68.2–76.1	213	74.2	2.9	68.5–80.0	
Yes	84	28.5	2.9	22.8–34.1	241	27.9	2.0	23.9–31.8	74	25.8	2.9	20.0–31.5	

Note: *: Based on linear regression (with variables log transformed as needed to meet the assumptions of normality of residuals and homogeneity of variance) for mean and the Rao-Scott Chi-Square Test for prevalence.
**Number of women with missing data differ by micronutrient: folate (n = 80), vitamin B_{12} (n = 1031), zinc (n = 30), vitamin A (n = 77), and anemia (n = 28).
***SEP/SEM: Standard Error of the Mean/Standard Error of the Prevalence.

Conclusions

This large, cross-sectional survey demonstrates that micronutrient deficiencies were an issue across the weight spectrum among women in Vietnam. Thus it is important to not only focus on underweight women but also on overweight/obese women for micronutrient deficiency prevention programs, even in higher socioeconomic strata. Improving micronutrient status of overweight/obese women is particularly important because micronutrient deficiencies may increase chronic disease risk. The findings of this study highlight the importance of targeting interventions to improve micronutrient status for whole populations, and not restrict those to populations selected on basis of specific nutritional status only (such as low BMI).

Given the demonstrated health and economic costs of micronutrient deficiencies and obesity, heart disease and diabetes, it is urgent that national interventions and policies address both the trend towards increasing overweight/obesity and the on-going problem of micronutrient deficiencies in Vietnam.

Acknowledgments

We would like to thank NIN for their support during the study. All authors read and approved the final manuscript.

Author Contributions

Conceived and designed the experiments: JB AL THL FTW BML RMP. Performed the experiments: THL BML FTW JB AL. Analyzed the data: EY AL FTW JB. Contributed reagents/materials/analysis tools: THL BML FTW. Contributed to the writing of the manuscript: AL FTW JB EY.

References

1. World Health Organisation (2011) Obesity and overweight. Fact Sheet N° 311.
2. Popkin BM Jr. (2002) The shift in stages of the nutrition transition in the developing world differs from past experiences! Malays J Nutr 8: 109–124.
3. Shaw JE, Sicree RA, Zimmet PZ (2010) Global estimates of the prevalence of diabetes for 2010 and 2030. Diabetes Res Clin Pract 87: 4–14.
4. Mackay J, Mensah G (2004) The atlas of heart diseases and stroke. Geneva, Switzerland: World Health Organization.
5. Ha do TP, Feskens EJ, Deurenberg P, Mai le B, Khan NC, et al. (2011) Nationwide shifts in the double burden of overweight and underweight in Vietnamese adults in 2000 and 2005: two national nutrition surveys. BMC Public Health 11: 62.
6. Nguyen MD, Beresford SA, Drewnowski A (2007) Trends in overweight by socio-economic status in Vietnam: 1992 to 2002. Public Health Nutr 10: 115–121.
7. Nguyen PVN, Hong TK, Hoang T, Nguyen DT, Robert A (2013) High prevalence of overweight among adolescents in Ho Chi Minh City, Vietnam. BMC Public Health 13: 141.
8. Zimmermann MB, Zeder C, Muthayya S, Winichagoon P, Chaouki N, et al. (2008) Adiposity in women and children from transition countries predicts decreased iron absorption, iron deficiency and a reduced response to iron fortification. International Journal of Obesity 32: 1098–1104.
9. Reis JP, von Muhlen D, Miller ER 3rd, Michos ED, Appel LJ (2009) Vitamin D status and cardiometabolic risk factors in the United States adolescent population. Pediatrics 124: e371–379.
10. García OP, Long KZ, Rosado JL (2009) Impact of micronutrient deficiencies on obesity. Nutrition Reviews 67: 559–572.
11. Via M (2012) The Malnutrition of Obesity: Micronutrient Deficiencies that Promote Diabetes. ISRN Endocrin doi:10.5402/2012/103472.
12. Laillou A, Pham TV, Tran NT, Le HT, Wieringa F, et al. (2012) Micronutrient Deficits Are Still Public Health Issues among Women and Young Children in Vietnam. PLoS One 7: e34906.
13. WHO expert consultation(2004) Appropriate body-mass index for Asian populations and its implications for policy and intervention strategies. Lancet 363: 157–163.
14. IVACG (1982) Biochemical methodology for assessement of vitamin A status. Washington DC, USA: Nutrition Foundation.
15. European Committee for Standardization (2003) Foodstuffs- Determination of folate by microbiological assay. Brussel: Management Centre.
16. Barton-Wright EC (1952) Practical Methods for Microbiological Assay of the Vitamin B Complex and Essential Amino Acids. Ashe Laboratories, Ltd, London.
17. Wiss O (1950) Mikrobiologische Vitamin- and Aminosaurebestimmungen. Hyg: 225–258.
18. AOAC International(1995) Official Methods and Analysis of AOAC international. 95–96 p.
19. Bui MH (1999) Internat. J Vit Nutr Res 69: 362.
20. Allen L, de Benoist B, Dray O, Hurrell R (2006) Guidelines on food fortification with micronutrients. WHO/FAO.
21. Thurnham DI, McCabe LD, Haldar S, Wieringa FT, Northrop-Clewes CA, et al. (2010) Adjusting plasma ferritin concentrations to remove the effects of subclinical inflammation in the assessment of iron deficiency: a meta-analysis. Am J Clin Nutr 92: 546–555.
22. de Pee S, Dary O (2002) Biochemical indicators of vitamin A deficiency: serum retinol and serum retinol binding protein. J Nutr 132: 2895S–2901S.
23. Thurnham DI, McCabe GP, Northrop-Clewes CA, Nestel P (2003) Effects of subclinical infection on plasma retinol concentrations and assessment of prevalence of vitamin A deficiency: meta-analysis. The Lancet 362: 2052–2058.
24. Gibson RS, Hess SY, Hotz C, Brown KH (2008) Indicators of zinc status at the population level: a review of the evidence. Br J Nutr 99 Suppl 3: S14–23.
25. Jones KM, Ramirez-Zea M, Zuleta C, Allen LH (2007) Prevalent vitamin B-12 deficiency in twelve-month-old Guatemalan infants is predicted by maternal B-12 deficiency and infant diet. J Nutr 137: 1307–1313.
26. Rutstein S The DHS Wealth Index: Approaches for rural and urban areas. USAID.
27. Stabler SP (1995) Screening the older population for cobalamin (vitamin B_{12}) deficiency. J Am Geriatr Soc. 43(11): p. 1290–7.
28. Kang S, Wonga P, Norusis M (1987) Homocysteinemia due to folate deficiency Metabolism. 36(5): p. 458–462.
29. Allen LH (2005) Multiple micronutrients in pregnancy and lactation: an overview. Am J Clin Nutr. 81(5): p. 1206S–1212S.
30. Ausk KJ, Ioannou GN (2008) Is obesity associated with anemia of chronic disease? A population-based study. Obesity (Silver Spring). 16(10): p. 2356–61.
31. Aeberli I, Hurrell RF, Zimmermann MB (2009) Overweight children have higher circulating hepcidin concentrations and lower iron status but have dietary iron intakes and bioavailability comparable with normal weight children. Int J Obes. 33(10): p.1111–7.
32. Gartner A, Berger J, Bour A, Ati AE, Traissac P, et al. (2013) Assessment of iron deficiency in the context of the obesity epidemic: importance of correcting serum ferritin concentrations for inflammation Am J Clin Nutr 98: 3 821–826.
33. Cepeda-Lopez AC, Aeberli I, Zimmermann MB (2010) Does obesity increase risk for iron deficiency? A review of the literature and the potential mechanisms. Int J Vitam Nutr Res 80: 263–270.
34. Garcia O, Ronquillo D, Caamano Md, Camacho M, Long K, et al. (2012) Zinc, vitamin A, and vitamin C status are associated with leptin concentrations and obesity in Mexican women: results from a cross-sectional study. Nutrition & Metabolism 9: 59.
35. Dien le, Thang NM, Bentley ME (2004) Food consumption patterns in the economic transition in Vietnam. Asia Pac J Clin Nutr. 13(1): p. 40–7.
36. Khan NC, Mai LB, Minh ND, Do TT, Khoi HH, et al. (2008) Intakes of retinol and carotenoids and its determining factors in the Red River Delta population of northern Vietnam. Eur J Clin Nutr 62: 810–816.
37. Suharno D, Muhilal, Karyadi D, West CE, Hautvast JG (1993) Supplementation with vitamin A and iron for nutritional anaemia in pregnant women in West Java, Indonesia. The Lancet Volume 342, 8883: 1325–1328.
38. Nguyen TH, Sandalinas F, de Sesmaisons A, Laillou A, Nguyen PT, et al. (2012). Multi-micronutrient-fortified biscuits decreased the prevalence of anaemia and improved iron status, whereas weekly iron supplementation only improved iron status in Vietnamese school children. Brit. J. Nutr., 108: 1419–1427.
39. Wieringa FT, Dijkhuizen MA, West CE, Northrop-Clewes C, Muhilal (2002). Estimation of the Effect of the Acute Phase Response on Indicators of Micronutrient Status in Indonesian Infants J. Nutr. 132: 10 3061–3066.
40. Withrow D, Alter DA (2011) The economic burden of obesity worldwide: a systematic review of the direct costs of obesity. Obesity Reviews 12: 131–141.
41. The Decoda Study G, Nyamdorj R (2008) BMI Compared With Central Obesity Indicators in Relation to Diabetes and Hypertension in Asians. Obesity 16: 1622–1635.
42. Taylor AE, Ebrahim S, Ben-Shlomo Y, Martin RM, Whincup PH, et al. (2010) Comparison of the associations of body mass index and measures of central adiposity and fat mass with coronary heart disease, diabetes, and all-cause mortality: a study using data from 4 UK cohorts. The American Journal of Clinical Nutrition 91: 547–556.

Effects of a High-Fat Diet on Spontaneous Metastasis of Lewis Lung Carcinoma in Plasminogen Activator Inhibitor-1 Deficient and Wild-Type Mice

Lin Yan*, Lana C. DeMars

Grand Forks Human Nutrition Research Center, United States Department of Agriculture, Agricultural Research Service, Grand Forks, North Dakota, United States of America

Abstract

This study investigated the effects of a high-fat diet on spontaneous metastasis of Lewis lung carcinoma (LLC) in plasminogen activator inhibitor-1 deficient (PAI-$1^{-/-}$) and wild-type mice. The high-fat diet increased the number of pulmonary metastases by 60% ($p<0.01$), tumor cross-sectional area by 82% ($p<0.05$) and tumor volume by 130% ($p<0.05$) compared to the AIN93G diet. Deficiency in PAI-1 reduced the number of metastases by 35% ($p<0.01$) compared to wild-type mice. In mice fed the high-fat diet, PAI-1 deficiency reduced tumor cross-sectional area by 52% ($p<0.05$) and tumor volume by 61% ($p<0.05$) compared to their wild-type counterparts; however, PAI-1 deficiency affected neither area nor volume in mice fed the AIN93G diet. Adipose and plasma concentrations of PAI-1 were significantly higher in high-fat fed wild-type mice than in their AIN93G-fed counterparts. Adipose and plasma PAI-1 were not detectable in PAI-$1^{-/-}$ mice regardless of the diet. Mice deficient in PAI-1 showed significantly greater plasma concentrations of monocyte chemotactic protein-1, tumor necrosis factor-α, leptin, vascular endothelial growth factor, tissue inhibitor of metalloproteinase-1 and insulin compared to wild-type mice, indicating a compensatory overproduction of inflammatory cytokines, angiogenic factors and insulin in the absence of PAI-1. We conclude that PAI-1 produced by the host, including that by adipose tissue, promotes high-fat enhanced metastasis of LLC.

Editor: Adriano Angelucci, University of L'Aquila, Italy

Funding: Funding for this work was provided by the U.S. Department of Agriculture, ARS, Research project 5450-51000-045-00D. The funders had no role in study design, data collection and analysis, decision to publish, or preparation of the manuscript.

Competing Interests: The authors have declared that no competing interests exist.

* Email: lin.yan@ars.usda.gov

Introduction

Plasminogen activator inhibitor-1 (PAI-1), a serine protease inhibitor, is a major component of the urokinase plasminogen activation system. It is the principal inhibitor of urokinase-type plasminogen activator (uPA) that catalyzes the conversion of latent plasminogen to plasmin, which is responsible for proteolysis of extracellular matrix during cancer invasion and metastasis. Paradoxically, PAI-1 may participate in the pathophysiology of cancer progression, because elevated PAI-1 expression in primary tumors is associated with poor prognosis and substantially increased risk of recurrence [1,2]. Laboratory studies have found that PAI-1 promotes tumor growth [3] and experimental metastasis [4] and that depletion of PAI-1 inhibits tumor growth [5], invasion and vascularization [6] and metastasis [7]. However, others have reported that PAI-1 did not affect tumor growth [8] and metastasis [8,9].

Recurrent or metastatic cancer, the spread of malignant cells from a primary tumor to different sites of the same organ or to distant organs, remains the most devastating aspect of cancer. Its occurrence directly affects the prognosis and survival of cancer patients, presenting a great challenge not only for cancer patients but also for physicians and researchers. Metastasis is a multistep process, from dissemination of malignant cells from a primary tumor, to intravasation into blood circulatory system, arrest in a distant vascular bed, extravasation into the interstitium of a target organ and proliferation to form metastases in the target organ. Stimulation of any of these steps can be expected to enhance malignant spread, whereas inhibition of any can be expected to reduce metastasis.

Obesity is a leading risk factor for cancer, second only to smoking. Being obese at the time of diagnosis of primary cancer can be predictive of poor prognosis. For example, breast cancer patients who are obese are at a greater risk of recurrence [10] with a shorter disease-free interval than those with normal body weight [11], and obese or overweight prostate cancer patients are more likely to have recurrence after radical prostatectomy than those of normal weight [12,13].

Adipose tissue has been considered an endocrine organ that produces adipokines contributing to obesity. The expression of the adipokine PAI-1 is elevated in obese subjects [14,15], and plasma levels of PAI-1 are elevated in mice fed obesigenic, high-fat diets [16,17]. We reported that a high-fat diet enhances the malignant spread of Lewis lung carcinoma (LLC) in mice and this enhancement is accompanied by increases in plasma concentrations of PAI-1 [18,19]. We hypothesized that PAI-1 participates in the spread of LLC and that the pro-metastatic effect of a high-fat feeding involves the up-regulation of PAI-1. The present experiments were conducted to test that hypothesis in PAI-1 deficient mice using a spontaneous metastasis model.

Materials and Methods

This study was approved by the Animal Care and Use Committee of the U.S. Department of Agriculture, Agricultural Research Service, Grand Forks Human Nutrition Research Center. The procedures followed the National Institute of Health guidelines for the care and use of laboratory animals [20].

Animals and diets

Four to five-week-old male PAI-1 deficient mice (PAI-1$^{-/-}$, B6.129S2-*Serpine1*^{tm1Mlg}/J) with a C57BL/6J background and C57BL/6J wild-type mice were purchased from The Jackson Laboratory (Bar Harbor, ME). The AIN93G diet [21] and AIN93G diet modified to include 45% of energy from dietary fat (hereafter referred to as the high-fat diet) were used in this study (Table 1). Gross energy of each diet (Table 1) was analyzed by oxygen bomb calorimetry (Model 6200, Oxygen Bomb Calorimeter, Parr Instrument, Moline, IL). Mice were shipped in two separate cohorts within 2 weeks. In each cohort, mice were randomized to 4 treatment groups (n = 11 per group for PAI-1$^{-/-}$ mice fed the AIN93G or the high-fat diet, n = 14 per group for wild-type mice fed the AIN93G or the high-fat diet). Mice were maintained in a pathogen-free room on a 12:12-hour light-dark cycle with a temperature of 22±1°C. Mice were weighed weekly, and they had free access to their diets and deionized water. Food intake was recorded for 3 weeks before cancer cell inoculation. All diets were powdered diets, and they were stored at −20°C until being provided to mice. Body composition was assessed in conscious, immobilized mice 1 week before cancer cell injection using quantitative magnetic resonance (Echo whole-body composition analyzer, Model 100, Echo Medical System, Houston, TX).

Lewis lung carcinoma cells

Lewis lung carcinoma cell line, a variant that metastasizes specifically to lungs [22], was obtained from Dr. Pnina Brodt, McGill University, Montreal, Quebec, Canada. The cells were cultured with RPMI-1640 medium containing 10% heat-inactivated fetal bovine serum and maintained in a humidified atmosphere of 5% CO_2 in air at 37°C. Cells used for animal studies were *in vivo*-selected once [19]. The cells were monitored for phenotype (by microscopic examination of cell morphology), proliferation properties (by growth curve analysis) and metastatic capability (by injecting cells subcutaneously into mice and examining metastatic formation in lungs). Cells were free of mycoplasma based on Hoechst DNA staining and direct culture tests performed by American Type Cell Collection (Manassas, VA). These assessments showed that cell identity and metastatic behavior were similar to those of original stocks from the institution providing the cell line.

Experimental design

Mice (n = 22 per group for PAI-1$^{-/-}$ mice, n = 28 per group for wild-type mice) were fed their respective AIN93G or high-fat diet for 7 weeks before they were subcutaneously injected with 2.5×10^5 viable LLC cells per mouse into the lower dorsal region. The resulting primary tumor was removed surgically 12 days later when it was approximately 1 cm in diameter. Following removal, the mice were maintained on their respective diets for an additional 10 days. An additional 13 wild-type mice were fed the AIN93G diet but not injected with LLC cells. At the end of the study, plasma was collected from these mice to use as a control in comparison with AIN93G-fed LLC-bearing wild-type mice to assess the effect of metastasis on changes in plasma concentrations of adipokines, angiogenic factors and related biomarkers. Mice

Table 1. Composition of experimental diets.

Ingredient	AIN93G g	AIN93G kcal	High-Fat g	High-Fat kcal
Corn starch	397.5	1590	33.5	134
Casein	200	800	200	800
Sucrose	100	400	100	400
Dextrin	132	528	200	800
Corn oil	70	630	201.5	1813.5
Cellulose	50	0	50	0
AIN93 mineral mix[a]	35	30	35	30
AIN93 vitamin mix[a]	10	39	10	39
L-cystine	3	12	3	12
Choline bitartrate	2.5	0	2.5	0
tert-butylhydroquinone	0.014	0	0.014	0
Total	1000	4029	835.5	4029
Calculated composition fat, % kCal	16		45	
Analyzed composition				
gross energy, kCal/g[b]	4.37±0.01		5.27±0.05	

[a]Reference 21.
[b]n = 3 for each diet.

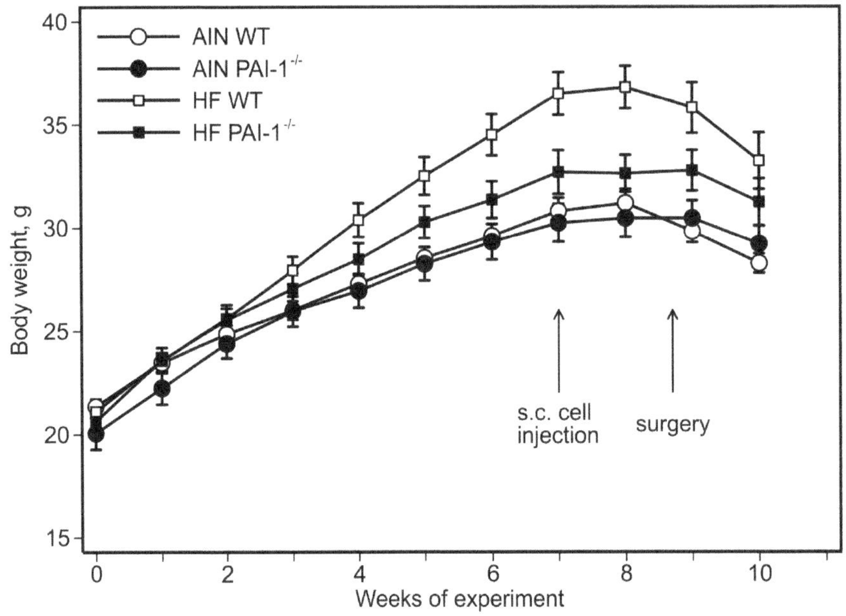

Figure 1. Body weight. Two-way ANOVA and Tukey contrasts were performed to test for differences among the groups. The high-fat diet, compared to the AIN93G diet, increased body weights; the difference was significant starting 4 weeks after the initiation of experimental feeding ($p<0.01$), and the significant increase continued throughout the experiment. Compared to wild-type mice, PAI-1 deficiency lowered body weights, and the difference was significant starting at week 6 of the experiment ($p\leq0.05$). Values are means ± SEM (n = 11 per group for PAI-1$^{-/-}$ mice, n = 14 per group for wild-type mice; second cohort). AIN WT: AIN93G-fed wild-type mice, AIN PAI-1$^{-/-}$: AIN93G-fed PAI-1$^{-/-}$ mice, HF WT: high-fat fed wild-type mice, HF PAI-1$^{-/-}$: high-fat fed PAI-1$^{-/-}$ mice.

were terminated by intraperitoneal injection of a mixture of ketamine and xylazine. Lungs were removed and fixed with Bouin's solution. The number of pulmonary metastases was counted [23] and the cross-sectional area and the volume of each metastasis were analyzed [24] using an ImagePro-Plus software (Media Cybernetics, Silver Spring, MD) and a camera-equipped stereomicroscope. Tumor cross-sectional area was defined as the surface area of each lung metastasis. Tumor volume was estimated by assuming that tumors were spherical and using their average diameter [24]. The average diameter was the average measured at two degree intervals joining two outline points and passing through the centroid. Epididymal adipose tissue and plasma were collected and stored at −80°C for further analyses.

Quantification of adipokines, angiogenic factors and related biomarkers

Concentrations of PAI-1 in epididymal adipose tissue, plasma and 24-hours-old conditioned medium from LLC cells were quantified using a sandwich enzyme-linked immunosorbent assay kit (Molecular Innovation, Novi, MI). An extract of adipose tissue was obtained by the protocol of Ortega et al [25]. Concentrations of PAI-1 in adipose extract and conditioned medium were normalized to protein content. Total protein concentration in each adipose extract and LLC cell lysate was estimated by BCA protein assay (Thermo Scientific, Waltham, MA). Plasma concentrations of uPA (Cell Sciences, Canton, MA), monocyte chemotactic protein-1 (MCP-1), tumor necrosis factor-α (TNF-α), leptin, vascular endothelial growth factor (VEGF), tissue inhibitor of metalloproteinase-1 (TIMP-1), insulin (all were from R&D Systems, Minneapolis, MN) and glucose (Cayman Chemical, Ann Arbor, MI) were quantified using sandwich enzyme-linked immunosorbent assay kits following manufacturers' protocols. Samples were read within the linear range of the assay, and the accuracy of the analysis was confirmed by the controls provided in each kit.

Statistical Analyses

The effects of diet (AIN93G or high-fat), genotype (PAI-1$^{-/-}$ or wild-type) and their interaction were tested using two-way analysis of variance (ANOVA). If a significant interaction between diet and genotype occured, Tukey contrasts were performed to compare the 4 treatment groups. To examine the effect of metastasis on changes of plasma concentrations of adipokines, angiogenic factors and related biomarkers, *a priori* contrasts were used to test for differences in wild-type mice fed the AIN93G diet with or without LLC. A mixed model ANOVA with mouse as the random blocking factor and with diet, genotype and their interaction as fixed effects was used to test for differences in cross-sectional area and volume of metastases among the groups. All data are presented as means ± standard error of the mean (SEM). Differences with a p-value of 0.05 or less were considered statistically significant. All analyses were performed using SAS software (version 9.3, SAS Institute, Cary, NC).

Results

Consumption of the high-fat diet increased body weights compared to the AIN93G diet. The difference was statistically significant 4 weeks after the initiation of experimental feeding (high-fat vs. AIN93G: $p<0.01$), and the significant increase continued throughout the experiment (Fig. 1). Starting at week 6, PAI-1$^{-/-}$ mice weighed significantly less than wild-type mice (PAI-1$^{-/-}$ vs. wild-type: $p<0.05$, Fig. 1), a difference more marked in the high-fat fed mice. Compared to the AIN93G diet, high-fat diet consumption increased body fat mass by 43% (high-fat vs. AIN93G: $p<0.01$) with a concomitant reduction in body lean mass by 9% ($p<0.01$) (Table 2). Compared to wild-type mice,

Table 2. Body fat mass ratio, lean mass ratio, absolute lean mass weight and caloric intake of mice[1].

	Treatment				*p* value		
	AIN WT	AIN PAI-1$^{-/-}$	HF WT	HF PAI-1$^{-/-}$	Diet	Gene	Diet × Gene
Fat mass ratio, %	19.0±0.8	16.8±1.3	27.9±1.5	23.1±1.3	<0.01	<0.01	0.29
Lean mass ratio, %	72.0±0.8	73.9±1.1	64.1±1.4	68.3±1.1	<0.01	<0.01	0.32
Lean mass weight, g	21.1±0.3	21.9±0.4	21.8±0.3	22.2±0.4	0.12	0.07	0.45
Caloric intake, kCal/day	16.1±0.3	14.6±0.5	17.3±0.6	15.9±0.7	<0.05	<0.05	0.92

[1]Two-way ANOVA was performed to test for differences among the groups. Values are means ± SEM (n = 22 per group for PAI-1$^{-/-}$ mice, n = 28 per group for wild-type mice or n = 6 per group for caloric intake). AIN WT: AIN93G-fed wild-type mice, AIN PAI-1$^{-/-}$: AIN93G-fed PAI-1$^{-/-}$ mice, HF WT: high-fat fed wild-type mice, HF PAI-1$^{-/-}$: high-fat fed PAI-1$^{-/-}$ mice.

PAI-1$^{-/-}$ mice had a 15% reduction in fat mass (PAI-1$^{-/-}$ vs. wild-type: $p<0.01$) and a 5% increase in lean mass ($p<0.01$) (Table 2). Neither the high-fat diet nor PAI-1 deficiency affected absolute lean mass weight (Table 2). Consumption of the high-fat diet increased caloric intake by 8% (high-fat vs. AIN93G: $p<0.05$) and PAI-1 deficiency lowered caloric intake by 9% (PAI-1$^{-/-}$ vs. wild-type: $p<0.05$) compared to their respective controls (Table 2).

Subcutaneous injection of LLC cells resulted in primary tumor and pulmonary metastasis. Compared to the AIN93G diet, high-fat diet consumption increased the number of lung metastases by 60% (high-fat vs. AIN93G: $p<0.01$; Fig. 2a). Mice deficient in PAI-1 had 35% less metastases than wild-type mice (PAI-1$^{-/-}$ vs. wild-type: $p<0.01$; Fig. 2a). The high-fat diet increased tumor cross-sectional area by 82% ($p<0.05$, Fig. 2b) and tumor volume by 130% ($p<0.05$, Fig. 2c) in wild-type mice compared to AIN93G-fed controls. Deficiency in PAI-1 reduced tumor cross-sectional area by 52% ($p<0.05$, Fig. 2b) and tumor volume by 61% ($p<0.05$, Fig. 2c) in high-fat fed mice, but the deficiency did not affect either cross-sectional area or volume in mice fed the AIN93G diet (Fig. 2b, 2c), compared to their respective wild-type controls. Necropsy at the end of the study found no metastatic growth in other organs.

There was no significant difference in adipose PAI-1 between LLC-bearing and non-tumor-bearing mice fed the AIN93G diet (Table 3). Compared to the AIN93G diet, the high-fat diet increased adipose PAI-1 by 147% ($p<0.05$, Table 3). Lewis lung carcinoma increased plasma PAI-1 by 407% in wild-type mice compared to non-tumor-bearing controls ($p<0.01$, Table 3). The high-fat diet further increased plasma PAI-1 by 102% compared to the AIN93G diet ($p<0.05$, Table 3). Plasminogen activator inhibitor-1 in adipose tissue and plasma was not detectable in PAI-1$^{-/-}$ mice regardless of the diet (Table 3). The conditioned medium from LLC cells contained 32.7±7.7 ng PAI-1/mg protein (n = 6).

Plasma levels of uPA were increased in tumor-bearing mice by 115% compared to non-tumor-bearing controls ($p<0.01$, Table 3). Compared to the AIN93G diet, the high-fat diet increased plasma uPA by 112% (high-fat vs. AIN93G: $p<0.01$, Table 3). There was no significant difference in plasma uPA between PAI-1$^{-/-}$ and wild-type mice (Table 3).

Compared to non-tumor-bearing controls, mice with LLC had a 443% increase in plasma MCP-1 ($p<0.01$) and a 397% increase in TNF-α ($p<0.01$) (Table 3). The high-fat diet, compared to the AIN93G diet, increased MCP-1 by 144% (high-fat vs. AIN93G: $p<0.01$) and TNF-α by 69% (high-fat vs. AIN93G: $p<0.01$) (Table 3). Compared to wild-type mice, PAI-1$^{-/-}$ mice had a 24% increase in plasma MCP-1 (PAI-1$^{-/-}$ vs. wildtype: $p<0.01$) and 7% increase in TNF-α (PAI-1$^{-/-}$ vs. wildtype: $p<0.05$) (Table 3). Lewis lung carcinoma did not affect plasma levels of leptin (Table 3). The high-fat diet, compared to the AIN93G diet, increased plasma leptin by 106% (high-fat vs. AIN93G: $p<0.01$, Table 3). Plasminogen activator inhibitor-1 deficiency increased leptin by 29% (PAI-1$^{-/-}$ vs. wild-type: $p = 0.01$, Table 3).

Mice with LLC exhibited an 11% increase in plasma concentrations of VEGF ($p<0.01$) and a 47% increase in TIMP-1 ($p<0.01$) compared to non-tumor-bearing controls (Table 4). The high-fat, compared to the AIN93G diet, increased plasma VEGF by 12% (high-fat vs. AIN93G: $p = 0.01$) and TIMP-1 by 71% (high-fat vs. AIN93G: $p<0.01$) (Table 4). Deficiency in PAI-1 increased plasma VEGF by 11% (PAI-1$^{-/-}$ vs. wild-type: $p<0.05$) and TIMP-1 by 27% (PAI-1$^{-/-}$ vs. wild-type: $p<0.01$) (Table 4).

There were no differences in plasma concentrations of insulin and glucose between LLC-bearing and non-tumor-bearing mice

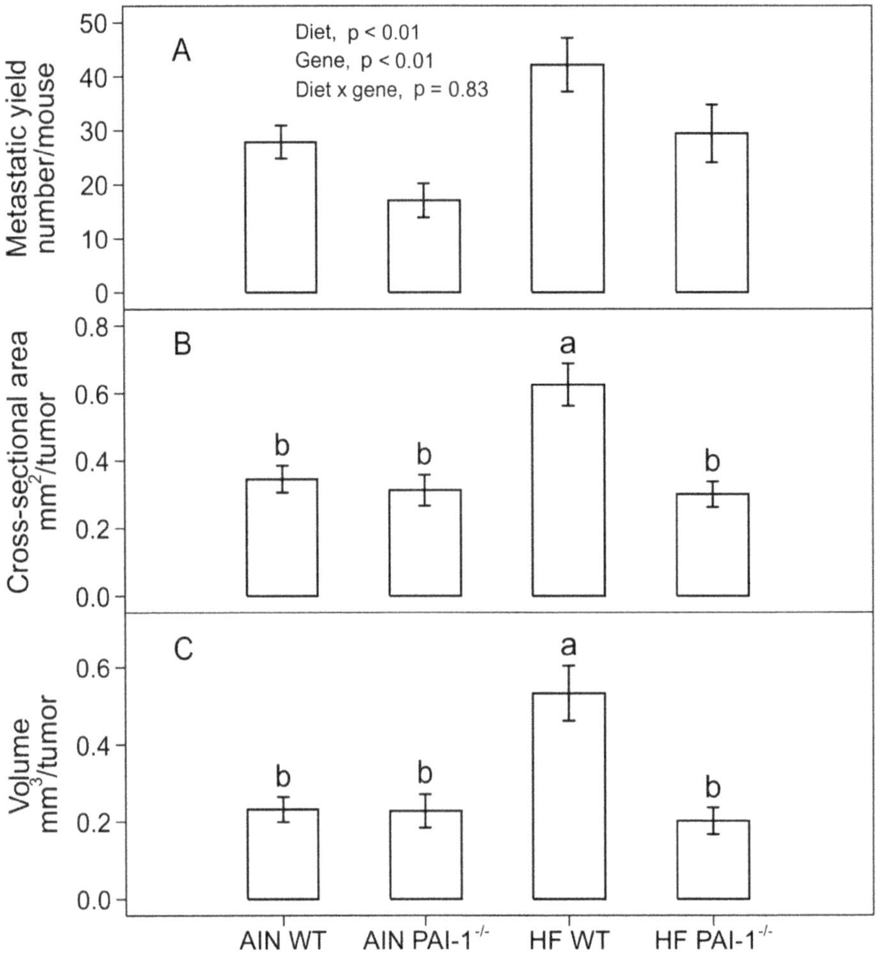

Figure 2. The number (*a*), cross-sectional area (*b*) and volume (*c*) of pulmonary metastases in PAI-1$^{-/-}$ and wild-type mice fed the AIN93G or the high-fat diet. Two-way ANOVA and Tukey contrasts were performed to test for differences among the groups. Values (means ± SEM) with different superscripts are significantly different at $p \leq 0.05$ (n = 22 per group for PAI-1$^{-/-}$ mice, n = 28 per group for wild-type mice). AIN WT: AIN93G-fed wild-type mice, AIN PAI-1$^{-/-}$: AIN93G-fed PAI-1$^{-/-}$ mice, HF WT: high-fat fed wild-type mice, HF PAI-1$^{-/-}$: high-fat fed PAI-1$^{-/-}$ mice.

(Table 4). The high-fat diet, compared to the AIN93G diet, increased plasma insulin by 111% (high-fat vs. AIN93G: $p<0.01$) and glucose by 23% (high-fat vs. AIN93G: $p<0.01$) (Table 4). Deficiency in PAI-1 increased plasma insulin by 15% (PAI-1$^{-/-}$ vs. wild-type: $p=0.01$, Table 4). There was no significant difference in plasma glucose between PAI-1$^{-/-}$ and wild-type mice (Table 4).

Discussion

The present study demonstrates that PAI-1 participates in spontaneous metastasis of LLC and that PAI-1 deficiency reduces metastasis enhanced by the high-fat diet.

Malignant spread is an important and critical step of metastatic development. The finding of a significant reduction in pulmonary metastases in PAI-1$^{-/-}$ mice indicates that host-produced PAI-1 may play an active role in metastasis. This is supported by previous reports that the absence of host PAI-1 prevents invasion of transplanted malignant keratinocytes *in vivo* [6]. Plasma concentrations of uPA in PAI-1$^{-/-}$ mice were similar to those of their wild-type counterparts, indicating that the action of PAI-1 on cancer spread may be independent on uPA. However, there is evidence suggesting that both PAI-1 and uPA are necessary for maximal metastatic progression. Lung cancer cells expressing only uPA and its receptor display no invasive capability [26].

When fed the high-fat diet, PAI-1$^{-/-}$ mice had a significant smaller metastasis size compared to the wild-type mice. This finding indicates that PAI-1 expression is needed for high-fat feeding enhancement of growth of metastases.

Adipose PAI-1 was depleted in PAI-1$^{-/-}$ mice, regardless of the diet. This finding indicates that it is the PAI-1 derived from adipose tissues that participates in LLC progression and contributes to enhanced malignant spread and growth by the high-fat diet. Although LLC produces PAI-1, the present results suggest that the amount of PAI-1 contributed by LLC in this model is insufficient to overcome the host deficiency of this adipokine. It indicates the importance of exogenous PAI-1 in metastasis of PAI-1 dependent malignancies.

The present study demonstrates that plasma concentrations of inflammatory cytokines (MCP-1, TNF-α, leptin), angiogenic factors (VEGF, TIMP-1) and insulin are elevated in PAI-1$^{-/-}$ mice. These elevations apparently compromise a compensation for the absence of PAI-1. Monocyte chemotactic protein-1 [27] and TNF-α [28,29] are tumorigenic and angiogenic. Leptin is known

Table 3. Adipose concentration of PAI-1 and plasma concentrations of adipokines (PAI-1, MCP-1, TNF-α, leptin) and uPA[1].

	Treatment					p value		
	Control	AIN WT	AIN PAI-1$^{-/-}$	HF WT	HF PAI-1$^{-/-}$	Diet	Gene	D × G
PAI-1,[2] ng/mg protein	0.22±0.03	0.17±0.04^{b}	N.D.	0.42±0.07^{a}	N.D.	<0.01	<0.01	<0.01
PAI-1, ng/mL	0.44±0.10*	2.23±0.30^{b}	N.D.	4.50±0.48^{a}	N.D.	<0.01	<0.01	<0.01
uPA, ng/mL	0.82±0.06*	1.76±0.20	1.51±0.23	3.77±0.35	3.15±0.33	<0.01	0.14	0.51
MCP-1, pg/mL	7.32±1.97*	39.77±4.85^{b}	43.21±2.27^{b}	87.77±3.65^{a}	114.88±8.37^{a}	<0.01	<0.01	<0.05
TNF-α, pg/mL	1.93±0.64*	9.60±0.30	10.53±0.32	16.51±0.39	17.49±0.47	<0.01	<0.05	0.94
Leptin, ng/mL	4.53±0.42	4.57±0.35	6.48±0.60	10.18±0.75	12.53±1.14	<0.01	0.01	0.77

[1]Two-way ANOVA and Tukey contrasts were performed to compare differences among the groups of LLC-bearing mice; *a priori* contrasts were performed to compare differences in AIN93G-fed wild-type mice with or without LLC (control vs. AIN WT). Values (means ± SEM) in a row with different superscripts are significantly different at $p \leq 0.05$ for LLC-bearing groups (n = 10 per group).
*$p<0.01$ compared to AIN WT. Control: AIN93G-fed non-tumor-bearing wild-type mice, AIN WT: AIN93G-fed wild-type mice, AIN PAI-1$^{-/-}$: AIN93G-fed PAI-1$^{-/-}$ mice, HF WT: high-fat fed wild-type mice, HF PAI-1$^{-/-}$: high-fat fed PAI-1$^{-/-}$ mice, D × G: diet × gene interaction, N.D.: not detectable.
[2]Adipose PAI-1.

Table 4. Plasma concentrations of angiogenic factors (VEGF, TIMP-1), insulin and glucose[1].

	Treatment					p value		
	Control	AIN WT	AIN PAI-1$^{-/-}$	HF WT	HF PAI-1$^{-/-}$	Diet	Gene	D × G
VEGF, pg/mL	69.41±1.23*	77.1±2.86	84.34±5.98	85.00±1.76	96.16±2.97	0.01	<0.05	0.60
TIMP-1, ng/mL	0.81±0.04*	1.19±0.09	1.49±0.08	2.01±0.10	2.57±0.11	<0.01	<0.01	0.18
Insulin, ng/mL	0.32±0.01	0.32±0.01^{b}	0.31±0.01^{b}	0.59±0.01^{a}	0.74±0.05^{a}	<0.01	0.01	<0.01
Glucose, mg/mL	0.84±0.04	0.82±0.04	0.87±0.03	1.08±0.03	1.00±0.03	<0.01	0.64	0.07

[1]Two-way ANOVA and Tukey contrasts were performed to compare differences among the groups of LLC-bearing mice; *a priori* contrasts were performed to compare differences in AIN93G-fed wild-type mice with or without LLC (control vs. AIN WT). Values (means ± SEM) in a row with different superscripts are significantly different at $p \leq 0.05$ for LLC-bearing groups (n = 10 per group). *$p<0.01$ compared to AIN WT. Control: AIN93G-fed non-tumor-bearing wild-type mice, AIN WT: AIN93G-fed wild-type mice, AIN PAI-1$^{-/-}$: AIN93G-fed PAI-1$^{-/-}$ mice, HF WT: high-fat fed wild-type mice, HF PAI-1$^{-/-}$: high-fat fed PAI-1$^{-/-}$ mice, D × G: diet × gene interaction.

to be angiogenic [30] and to modulate tumor growth by increasing VEGF expression [31]. Vascular endothelial growth factor [32] and TIMP-1 [33] contribute to metastatic development. Hyperinsulinemia enhances growth and progression of mammary tumors [34,35]. Thus, observed elevations of these factors suggest that they may contribute to the less aggressive development and growth of LLC in the absence of PAI-1 in PAI-1$^{-/-}$ mice.

Plasminogen activator inhibitor-1 together with uPA has been recommended as prognostic biomarkers in breast cancer [36]. RNA aptamers specific to PAI-1 were generated for preclinical testing for potential clinical applications [37]. PAI-039, a small molecule inhibitor of PAI-1 that was investigated clinically for treatments of acute and arterial thrombosis [38], has been tested for its efficacy in preclinical tumor angiogenesis mouse models [39]. The present results suggest that treatments targeting PAI-1 may be counteracted by the compensatory overproduction of inflammatory cytokines and angiogenic factors. This warrants further investigation, particularly in those studies aimed at long-term PAI-1 inhibition.

That PAI-1 was not detectable in plasma from LLC-bearing PAI-1$^{-/-}$ mice suggests that LLC-produced PAI-1 is not responsible for the significant elevated plasma PAI-1 in AIN93G-fed wild-type mice with LLC. Plasminogen activator inhibitor-1 is an acute phase reactant [40]. The concentration of PAI-1 in mouse liver is relatively low [41]; however, PAI-1 gene expression in the liver is up-regulated markedly by endotoxin and inflammatory mediators [41,42]. Because cancer has an inflammatory component, the presence of LLC in wild-type mice may be up-regulating PAI-1 production from liver and other organs, resulting in significantly higher plasma PAI-1 than in the non-tumor-bearing wild-type mice.

Reductions in caloric intake and body fat mass in PAI-1$^{-/-}$ mice fed the high-fat diet may have contributed to the inhibition of malignant progression, particularly metastatic growth, in those mice. Dietary energy restriction reduces primary tumorigenesis and metastasis [43]. Caloric restriction, which lowers adiposity and production of inflammatory cytokines, may be a useful adjuvant in the prevention and treatment of obesity-related cancer. The present results suggest that better outcomes in studies aimed at PAI-1 inhibition may come from subjects with healthy body weights, whereas overweight/obesity or excessive caloric intake may be additive to PAI-1 deficiency-related compensatory increases in inflammatory cytokines and angiogenic factors.

Significant reduction in body fat mass and increases in plasma concentrations of leptin and insulin in PAI-1$^{-/-}$ mice were not expected considering the existing understanding that blood levels of leptin and insulin are positively associated with adiposity [44,45]. However, it has been reported that plasma insulin was increased in PAI-1$^{-/-}$ mice compared to wild-type mice, even though there was no difference in gonadal fat pad weight between the groups [46]. Considering the significant increases in adipokines and angiogenic factors in PAI-1$^{-/-}$ mice in the present study, the increase in leptin, as well as insulin, is likely through an overproduction compensatory mechanism in the absence of PAI-1, which may be independent of body fat mass or body weight.

That LLC-associated increases in plasma concentrations of inflammatory cytokines PAI-1, MCP-1, TNF-α, protease uPA and angiogenic factors VEGF, TIMP-1 indicate the aggressiveness of this carcinoma model. High expressions of PAI-1 [2,47], MCP-1 [48,49], TNF-α [50], uPA [2], VEGF [51] and TIMP-1 [52] have been associated with regional or distant metastasis and poor prognosis in cancer patients. Elevations of these cytokines [3,53,54], uPA [55,56] and angiogenic markers [19,33] have been reported in animal models of various malignancies. The present results are consistent with the existing knowledge and confirm the usefulness of the LLC model to study spontaneous metastasis.

The present study used corn oil as the source of dietary fat, which is comprised of 57% linoleic acid [57] and provided 25% of total energy in the high-fat diet. This diet was low in α-linolenic acid (0.5% of dietary energy), which comprises 1% of fatty acids in corn oil [57]. It is possible that this low α-linolenic acid/linoleic acid ratio [58] may have contributed to the effects observed for the high-fat diet because of its low content of α-linolenic acid, which has been suggested to be anticarcinogenic [59,60]. This possibility warrants further investigation.

In summary, results from the present study indicate that PAI-1 contributes to the metastasis of LLC and that PAI-1 deficiency ameliorates metastasis enhanced by the high-fat diet. These findings are consistent with others showing that PAI-1 participates in cancer progression [3,4]. Furthermore, the present study demonstrates that host-produced PAI-1 including that from adipose tissues was a significant determinant of malignant progression. Adipose tissue is a modifiable source of PAI-1, particularly in obesity. Weight loss through caloric restriction alone or in combination with exercise reduces blood levels of PAI-1 [61,62]; thus, these practices can be useful adjuvants to achieving the best outcomes of chemoprevention. The compensatory increases in production of inflammatory cytokines, angiogenic factors and insulin in PAI-1$^{-/-}$ mice suggest that these compensatory responses may counteract treatments aimed at PAI-1 inhibition.

Acknowledgments

The authors greatly acknowledge the assistance of the following staff of Grand Forks Human Nutrition Research Center: Kay Keehr for technical support, James Linlauf for preparing experimental diets, LuAnn Johnson for advice in statistical analysis and vivarium staff for providing high quality animal care. Notes: The U.S. Department of Agriculture, Agricultural Research Service, Northern Plains Area, is an equal opportunity/affirmative action employer and all agency services are available without discrimination. Mention of trade names or commercial products in this article is solely for providing specific information and does not imply recommendation or endorsement by the U.S. Department of Agriculture.

Author Contributions

Conceived and designed the experiments: LY. Performed the experiments: LY LD. Analyzed the data: LY. Contributed reagents/materials/analysis tools: LY LD. Contributed to the writing of the manuscript: LY.

References

1. Janicke F, Schmitt M, Pache L, Ulm K, Harbeck N, et al. (1993) Urokinase (uPA) and its inhibitor PAI-1 are strong and independent prognostic factors in node-negative breast cancer. Breast Cancer Res Treat 24: 195–208.
2. Seetoo DQ, Crowe PJ, Russell PJ, Yang JL (2003) Quantitative expression of protein markers of plasminogen activation system in prognosis of colorectal cancer. J Surg Oncol 82: 184–193.
3. McMahon GA, Petitclerc E, Stefansson S, Smith E, Wong MK, et al. (2001) Plasminogen activator inhibitor-1 regulates tumor growth and angiogenesis. J Biol Chem 276: 33964–33968.
4. Tsuchiya H, Sunayama C, Okada G, Matsuda E, Tomita K, et al. (1997) Plasminogen activator inhibitor-1 accelerates lung metastasis formation of human fibrosarcoma cells. Anticancer Res 17: 313–316.
5. Gutierrez LS, Schulman A, Brito-Robinson T, Noria F, Ploplis VA, et al. (2000) Tumor development is retarded in mice lacking the gene for urokinase-type

plasminogen activator or its inhibitor, plasminogen activator inhibitor-1. Cancer Res 60: 5839–5847.
6. Bajou K, Noel A, Gerard RD, Masson V, Brunner N, et al. (1998) Absence of host plasminogen activator inhibitor 1 prevents cancer invasion and vascularization. Nat Med 4: 923–928.
7. Maillard CM, Bouquet C, Petitjean MM, Mestdagt M, Frau E, et al. (2008) Reduction of brain metastases in plasminogen activator inhibitor-1-deficient mice with transgenic ocular tumors. Carcinogenesis 29: 2236–2242.
8. Almholt K, Nielsen BS, Frandsen TL, Brunner N, Dano K, et al. (2003) Metastasis of transgenic breast cancer in plasminogen activator inhibitor-1 gene-deficient mice. Oncogene 22: 4389–4397.
9. Eitzman DT, Krauss JC, Shen T, Cui J, Ginsburg (1996) Lack of plasminogen activator inhibitor-1 effect in a transgenic mouse model of metastatic melanoma. Blood 87: 4718–4722.
10. Daniell HW (1988) Increased lymph node metastases at mastectomy for breast cancer associated with host obesity, cigarette smoking, age, and large tumor size. Cancer 62: 429–435.
11. Loi S, Milne RL, Friedlander ML, McCredie MR, Giles GG, et al. (2005) Obesity and outcomes in premenopausal and postmenopausal breast cancer. Cancer Epidemiol Biomarkers Prev 14: 1686–1691.
12. Bassett WW, Cooperberg MR, Sadetsky N, Silva S, DuChane J, et al. (2005) Impact of obesity on prostate cancer recurrence after radical prostatectomy: data from CaPSURE. Urology 66: 1060–1065.
13. Amling CL, Riffenburgh RH, Sun L, Moul JW, Lance RS, et al. (2004) Pathologic variables and recurrence rates as related to obesity and race in men with prostate cancer undergoing radical prostatectomy. J Clin Oncol 22: 439–445.
14. McGill JB, Schneider DJ, Arfken CL, Lucore CL, Sobel BE (1994) Factors responsible for impaired fibrinolysis in obese subjects and NIDDM patients. Diabetes 43: 104–109.
15. Alessi MC, Bastelica D, Morange P, Berthet B, Leduc I, et al. (2000) Plasminogen activator inhibitor 1, transforming growth factor-beta1, and BMI are closely associated in human adipose tissue during morbid obesity. Diabetes 49: 1374–1380.
16. Yan L, DeMars LC, Johnson LK (2012) Long-term voluntary running improves diet-induced adiposity in young adult mice. Nutr Res 32: 458–465.
17. Yan L, Graef GL, Claycombe KJ, Johnson LK (2013) Effects of voluntary running and soy supplementation on diet-induced metabolic disturbances and inflammation in mice. J Agric Food Chem 61: 9373–9379.
18. Yan L, Combs GF Jr (2014) Consumption of a high-fat diet abrogates inhibitory effects of methylseleninic acid on spontaneous metastasis of Lewis lung carcinoma in mice. Carcinogenesis 35: 2308–2313.
19. Yan L, Demars LC (2010) Effects of dietary fat on spontaneous metastasis of Lewis lung carcinoma in mice. Clin Exp Metastasis 27: 581–590.
20. Institute for Laboratory Animal Research (2011) Guide for the Care and Use of Laboratory Animals; National Research Council DoEaLS, Institute for Laboratory Animal Research, editor. Washington, D.C.: National Academies Press.
21. Reeves PG, Nielsen FH, Fahey GCJ (1993) AIN-93 purified diets for laboratory rodents: final report of the American Institute of Nutrition ad hoc writing committee on the reformulation of the AIN-76A rodent diet. J Nutr 123: 1939–1951.
22. Brodt P (1986) Characterization of two highly metastatic variants of Lewis lung carcinoma with different organ specificities. Cancer Res 46: 2442–2448.
23. Fidler IJ (1978) General considerations for studies of experimental cancer metastasis. In: Busch H, editor. Methods in Cancer Research. New York: Academic Press. 399–439.
24. Welch DR, Neri A, Nicolson GL (1983) Comparison of 'spontaneous' and 'experimental' metastasis using rat 13726 mammary adenocarcinoma metastatic cell clones. Invasion Metastasis 3: 65–80.
25. Ortega FJ, Moreno-Navarrete JM, Mayas D, Garcia-Santos E, Gomez-Serrano M, et al. (2012) Breast cancer 1 (BrCa1) may be behind decreased lipogenesis in adipose tissue from obese subjects. PLoS One 7: e33233.
26. Liu G, Shuman MA, Cohen RL (1995) Co-expression of urokinase, urokinase receptor and PAI-1 is necessary for optimum invasiveness of cultured lung cancer cells. Int J Cancer 60: 501–506.
27. Salcedo R, Ponce ML, Young HA, Wasserman K, Ward JM, et al. (2000) Human endothelial cells express CCR2 and respond to MCP-1: direct role of MCP-1 in angiogenesis and tumor progression. Blood 96: 34–40.
28. Kulbe H, Thompson R, Wilson JL, Robinson S, Hagemann T, et al. (2007) The inflammatory cytokine tumor necrosis factor-alpha generates an autocrine tumor-promoting network in epithelial ovarian cancer cells. Cancer Res 67: 585–592.
29. Waters JP, Pober JS, Bradley JR (2013) Tumour necrosis factor and cancer. J Pathol 230: 241–248.
30. Sierra-Honigmann MR, Nath AK, Murakami C, Garcia-Cardena G, Papapetropoulos A, et al. (1998) Biological action of leptin as an angiogenic factor. Science 281: 1683–1686.
31. Rene Gonzalez R, Watters A, Xu Y, Singh UP, Mann DR, et al. (2009) Leptin-signaling inhibition results in efficient anti-tumor activity in estrogen receptor positive or negative breast cancer. Breast Cancer Res 11: R36.
32. Yan L, Demars LC (2012) Dietary supplementation with methylseleninic acid, but not selenomethionine, reduces spontaneous metastasis of Lewis lung carcinoma in mice. Int J Cancer 131: 1260–1266.
33. Kopitz C, Gerg M, Bandapalli OR, Ister D, Pennington CJ, et al. (2007) Tissue inhibitor of metalloproteinases-1 promotes liver metastasis by induction of hepatocyte growth factor signaling. Cancer Res 67: 8615–8623.
34. Dool CJ, Mashhedi H, Zakikhani M, David S, Zhao Y, et al. (2011) IGF1/insulin receptor kinase inhibition by BMS-536924 is better tolerated than alloxan-induced hypoinsulinemia and more effective than metformin in the treatment of experimental insulin-responsive breast cancer. Endocr Relat Cancer 18: 699–709.
35. Fierz Y, Novosyadlyy R, Vijayakumar A, Yakar S, LeRoith D (2010) Insulin-sensitizing therapy attenuates type 2 diabetes-mediated mammary tumor progression. Diabetes 59: 686–693.
36. Harris L, Fritsche H, Mennel R, Norton L, Ravdin P, et al. (2007) American Society of Clinical Oncology 2007 update of recommendations for the use of tumor markers in breast cancer. J Clin Oncol 25: 5287–5312.
37. Blake CM, Sullenger BA, Lawrence DA, Fortenberry YM (2009) Antimetastatic potential of PAI-1-specific RNA aptamers. Oligonucleotides 19: 117–128.
38. Hennan JK, Elokdah H, Leal M, Ji A, Friedrichs GS, et al. (2005) Evaluation of PAI-039 [{1-benzyl-5-[4-(trifluoromethoxy)phenyl]-1H-indol-3-yl}(oxo)acetic acid], a novel plasminogen activator inhibitor-1 inhibitor, in a canine model of coronary artery thrombosis. J Pharmacol Exp Ther 314: 710–716.
39. Leik CE, Su EJ, Nambi P, Crandall DL, Lawrence DA (2006) Effect of pharmacologic plasminogen activator inhibitor-1 inhibition on cell motility and tumor angiogenesis. J Thromb Haemost 4: 2710–2715.
40. Kruithof EK, Gudinchet A, Bachmann F (1988) Plasminogen activator inhibitor 1 and plasminogen activator inhibitor 2 in various disease states. Thromb Haemost 59: 7–12.
41. Sawdey MS, Loskutoff DJ (1991) Regulation of murine type 1 plasminogen activator inhibitor gene expression in vivo. Tissue specificity and induction by lipopolysaccharide, tumor necrosis factor-alpha, and transforming growth factor-beta. J Clin Invest 88: 1346–1353.
42. Quax PH, van den Hoogen CM, Verheijen JH, Padro T, Zeheb R, et al. (1990) Endotoxin induction of plasminogen activator and plasminogen activator inhibitor type 1 mRNA in rat tissues in vivo. J Biol Chem 265: 15560–15563.
43. Phoenix KN, Vumbaca F, Fox MM, Evans R, Claffey KP (2010) Dietary energy availability affects primary and metastatic breast cancer and metformin efficacy. Breast Cancer Res Treat 123: 333–344.
44. Staiger H, Tschritter O, Machann J, Thamer C, Fritsche A, et al. (2003) Relationship of serum adiponectin and leptin concentrations with body fat distribution in humans. Obes Res 11: 368–372.
45. Schwartz MW, Woods SC, Porte D, Jr., Seeley RJ, Baskin DG (2000) Central nervous system control of food intake. Nature 404: 661–671.
46. Morange PE, Lijnen HR, Alessi MC, Kopp F, Collen D, et al. (2000) Influence of PAI-1 on adipose tissue growth and metabolic parameters in a murine model of diet-induced obesity. Arterioscler Thromb Vasc Biol 20: 1150–1154.
47. Czekay RP, Loskutoff DJ (2004) Unexpected role of plasminogen activator inhibitor 1 in cell adhesion and detachment. Exp Biol Med (Maywood) 229: 1090–1096.
48. Ueno T, Toi M, Saji H, Muta M, Bando H, et al. (2000) Significance of macrophage chemoattractant protein-1 in macrophage recruitment, angiogenesis, and survival in human breast cancer. Clin Cancer Res 6: 3282–3289.
49. Chavey C, Bibeau F, Gourgou-Bourgade S, Burlinchon S, Boissiere F, et al. (2007) Oestrogen receptor negative breast cancers exhibit high cytokine content. Breast Cancer Res 9: R15.
50. Ferrajoli A, Keating MJ, Manshouri T, Giles FJ, Dey A, et al. (2002) The clinical significance of tumor necrosis factor-alpha plasma level in patients having chronic lymphocytic leukemia. Blood 100: 1215–1219.
51. Guo RP, Zhong C, Shi M, Zhang CQ, Wei W, et al. (2006) Clinical value of apoptosis and angiogenesis factors in estimating the prognosis of hepatocellular carcinoma. J Cancer Res Clin Oncol 132: 547–555.
52. Ree AH, Florenes VA, Berg JP, Maelandsmo GM, Nesland JM, et al. (1997) High levels of messenger RNAs for tissue inhibitors of metalloproteinases (TIMP-1 and TIMP-2) in primary breast carcinomas are associated with development of distant metastases. Clin Cancer Res 3: 1623–1628.
53. Kimura Y, Sumiyoshi M (2007) High-fat, high-sucrose, and high-cholesterol diets accelerate tumor growth and metastasis in tumor-bearing mice. Nutr Cancer 59: 207–216.
54. Okahara H, Yagita H, Miyake K, Okumura K (1994) Involvement of very late activation antigen 4 (VLA-4) and vascular cell adhesion molecule 1 (VCAM-1) in tumor necrosis factor alpha enhancement of experimental metastasis. Cancer Res 54: 3233–3236.
55. Achbarou A, Kaiser S, Tremblay G, Ste-Marie LG, Brodt P, et al. (1994) Urokinase overproduction results in increased skeletal metastasis by prostate cancer cells in vivo. Cancer Res 54: 2372–2377.
56. Kido A, Tsutsumi M, Iki K, Takahama M, Tsujiuchi T, et al. (1999) Overexpression of matrix metalloproteinase (MMP)-9 correlates with metastatic potency of spontaneous and 4-hydroxyaminoquinoline 1-oxide (4-HAQO)-induced transplantable osteosarcomas in rats. Cancer Lett 137: 209–216.
57. Corn Refiners Association. Corn Oil (5th Edition, 2006). Corn Refiners Association website. Available: http://www.corn.org/wp-content/uploads/2009/12/CornOil.pdf. 1–22. Accessed 2014 Oct 7.
58. Barcelo-Coblijn G, Murphy EJ (2009) Alpha-linolenic acid and its conversion to longer chain n-3 fatty acids: benefits for human health and a role in maintaining tissue n-3 fatty acid levels. Prog Lipid Res 48: 355–374.

59. Gerber M (2012) Omega-3 fatty acids and cancers: a systematic update review of epidemiological studies. Br J Nutr 107 Suppl 2: S228–239.
60. Algamas-Dimantov A, Davidovsky D, Ben-Ari J, Kang JX, Peri I, et al. (2012) Amelioration of diabesity-induced colorectal ontogenesis by omega-3 fatty acids in mice. J Lipid Res 53: 1056–1070.
61. Kockx M, Leenen R, Seidell J, Princen HM, Kooistra T (1999) Relationship between visceral fat and PAI-1 in overweight men and women before and after weight loss. Thromb Haemost 82: 1490–1496.
62. Mavri A, Stegnar M, Krebs M, Sentocnik JT, Geiger M, et al. (1999) Impact of adipose tissue on plasma plasminogen activator inhibitor-1 in dieting obese women. Arterioscler Thromb Vasc Biol 19: 1582–1587.

PERMISSIONS

All chapters in this book were first published in PLOS ONE, by The Public Library of Science; hereby published with permission under the Creative Commons Attribution License or equivalent. Every chapter published in this book has been scrutinized by our experts. Their significance has been extensively debated. The topics covered herein carry significant findings which will fuel the growth of the discipline. They may even be implemented as practical applications or may be referred to as a beginning point for another development.

The contributors of this book come from diverse backgrounds, making this book a truly international effort. This book will bring forth new frontiers with its revolutionizing research information and detailed analysis of the nascent developments around the world.

We would like to thank all the contributing authors for lending their expertise to make the book truly unique. They have played a crucial role in the development of this book. Without their invaluable contributions this book wouldn't have been possible. They have made vital efforts to compile up to date information on the varied aspects of this subject to make this book a valuable addition to the collection of many professionals and students.

This book was conceptualized with the vision of imparting up-to-date information and advanced data in this field. To ensure the same, a matchless editorial board was set up. Every individual on the board went through rigorous rounds of assessment to prove their worth. After which they invested a large part of their time researching and compiling the most relevant data for our readers.

The editorial board has been involved in producing this book since its inception. They have spent rigorous hours researching and exploring the diverse topics which have resulted in the successful publishing of this book. They have passed on their knowledge of decades through this book. To expedite this challenging task, the publisher supported the team at every step. A small team of assistant editors was also appointed to further simplify the editing procedure and attain best results for the readers.

Apart from the editorial board, the designing team has also invested a significant amount of their time in understanding the subject and creating the most relevant covers. They scrutinized every image to scout for the most suitable representation of the subject and create an appropriate cover for the book.

The publishing team has been an ardent support to the editorial, designing and production team. Their endless efforts to recruit the best for this project, has resulted in the accomplishment of this book. They are a veteran in the field of academics and their pool of knowledge is as vast as their experience in printing. Their expertise and guidance has proved useful at every step. Their uncompromising quality standards have made this book an exceptional effort. Their encouragement from time to time has been an inspiration for everyone.

The publisher and the editorial board hope that this book will prove to be a valuable piece of knowledge for researchers, students, practitioners and scholars across the globe.

LIST OF CONTRIBUTORS

Hamid Jan Jan Mohamed and See-Ling Loy
Nutrition Program, School of Health Sciences, Universiti Sains Malaysia, Kubang Kerian, Kelantan, Malaysia

Angela Rowan
Fonterra Co-operative Group Ltd, Palmerston North, NewZealand

Bertram Fong
Fonterra Research and Development Centre, Palmerston North, New Zealand

Francis Biville, Christophe Brézillon, Dario Giorgini and Muhamed-Kheir Taha
Unitédes Infections Bactériennes invasives, Département Infectionet Epidémiologie, Institut Pasteur, Paris, France

Justyna Czech-Kowalska, Julita Latka-Grot, Dorota Bulsiewicz and Anna Dobrzanska
Department of Neonatology and Neonatal Intensive Care, The Children's Memorial Health Institute, Warsaw, Poland

Maciej Jaworski, Pawel Pludowski, Elzbieta Karczmarewicz and Edyta Czekuc-Kryskiewicz
Department of Biochemistry, Radioimmunology, and Experimental Medicine, The Children's Memorial Health Institute, Warsaw, Poland

Grazyna Wygledowska
Department of Neonatology, Miedzyleski Specialist Hospital, Warsaw, Poland

Bogdan Chazan and Beata Pawlus
Department of Neonatology, Holy Family Hospital, Warsaw, Poland

Anna Zochowska
Department of Neonatology, Public Hospital, Otwock, Poland

Maria K. Borszewska-Kornacka
Department of Neonatology, Warsaw Medical University Hospital, Warsaw, Poland

Carolin Lechtermann, Berthold P. Hauffa and Corinna Grasemann
Department of Pediatric Endocrinology and Diabetology, Kinderklinik II, Universitätsklinikum-Essen and the University of Duisburg-Essen, Essen, Germany

Ralf Herrmann
Department of Pediatric Endocrinology and Diabetology, Kinderklinik II, Universitätsklinikum-Essen and the University of Duisburg-Essen, Essen, Germany
Department of Neonatology, Kinderklinik I, Universitätsklinikum -Essen and the University of Duisburg-Essen, Essen, Germany

Michael M. Schündeln
Department of Pediatric Oncology and Hematology, Kinderklinik III, Universitätsklinikum -Essen and the University of Duisburg-Essen, Essen, Germany

Alexandra Gellhaus
Institute of Molecular Biology, Universitätsklinikum -Essen and the
University of Duisburg-Essen, Essen, Germany

Markus Schmidt
Department of Gynecology and Obstetrics, Klinikum Duisburg and the University of Duisburg-Essen, Duisburg, Germany

Ayalew Mentewab and Shanice Robinson
Biology Department, Spelman College, Atlanta, Georgia, United States of America

Kinnari Matheson
Biology Department, Spelman College, Atlanta, Georgia, United States of America
Molecular Biology Department, Princeton University, Princeton, New Jersey, United States of America

Morayo Adebiyi
Biology Department, Spelman College, Atlanta, Georgia, United States of America
The Graduate School of Biomedical Sciences, University of Texas Health Science Center at Houston, Houston, Texas, United States of America

Brianna Elston
Biology Department, Spelman College, Atlanta, Georgia, United States of America
College of Health Care Sciences, Nova Southeastern University, Davie, Florida, United States of America

Sangita Choudhury, Soochan Bae, Qingen Ke, Ji Yoo Lee, Sylvia S. Singh, Federica del Monte and Peter M. Kang
Cardiovascular Institute, Beth Israel Deaconess Medical Center and Harvard Medical School, Boston, Massachusetts, United States of America

René St-Arnaud
Shriners Hospital and Departments of Surgery and Human Genetics, McGill University, Montreal, Canada

Amy Woods and Kevin G. Thompson
University of Canberra, Research Institute for Sport and Exercise, Canberra, Australia

Laura A. Garvican-Lewis
University of Canberra, Research Institute for Sport and Exercise, Canberra, Australia
Australian Institute of Sport, Canberra, Australia

Philo U. Saunders, Greg Lovell, David Hughes, Ruth Fazakerley, Bev Anderson and Christopher J. Gore
Australian Institute of Sport, Canberra, Australia

Sarah E. Montgomery and John D. Wangsgaard
Department of Applied Human Nutrition, Mount Saint Vincent University, Halifax, Nova Scotia, Canada

Amir A. Sepehry
College for Interdisciplinary Studies, Graduate program in Neuroscience, University of British Columbia (UBC), Vancouver, BC, Canada
UBC Division of Neurology, Department of Medicine, University of British Columbia (UBC), Vancouver, BC, Canada

Jeremy E. Koenig
Faculty of Computer Science, Dalhousie University, Halifax, NS, Canada

Wei Zhao, Cheng Han, Xiaoguang Shi, Chuhui Xiong, Jie Sun, Zhongyan Shan and Weiping Teng
Department of Endocrinology and Metabolism, Institute of Endocrinology, Liaoning Provincial Key Laboratory of Endocrine Diseases, the First Affiliated Hospital of China Medical University, Shenyang, Liaoning Province, People's Republic of China

Benjamin J. Ryan and William C. Byrnes
Department of Integrative Physiology, University of Colorado Boulder, Boulder, Colorado, United States of America

Nadine B. Wachsmuth and Walter F. Schmidt
Department of Sports Medicine/Sports Physiology, University of Bayreuth, Bayreuth, Germany

Colleen G. Julian and Robert C. Roach
Altitude Research Center, Department of Emergency Medicine, University of Colorado Anschutz Medical Campus, Aurora, Colorado, United States of America

Andrew T. Lovering
Department of Human Physiology, University of Oregon, Eugene, Oregon, United States of America

Andrew W. Subudhi
Altitude Research Center, Department of Emergency Medicine, University of Colorado Anschutz Medical Campus, Aurora, Colorado, United States of America
Department of Biology, University of Colorado Colorado Springs, Colorado Springs, Colorado, United States of America

Małgorzata Lenartowicz, Paweł Grzmil, Aleksandra Bednarz, Mateusz Ogórek and Olga Pierzchała
Department of Genetics and Evolution, Institute of Zoology, Jagiellonian University, Kraków, Poland

Rafał R. Starzyński, Robert Staroń, Anna Gajowiak and Paweł Lipiński
Department of Molecular Biology, Institute of Genetics and Animal Breeding, Polish Academy of Sciences, Magdalenka, Poland

Wojciech Krzeptowski
Department of Cell Biology and Imaging, Institute of Zoology, Jagiellonian University, Kraków, Poland

Mazliza Ramly, Karuthan Chinna and Suhaili Suboh
Department of Social and Preventive Medicine, Faculty of Medicine, University of Malaya, Kuala Lumpur, Malaysia

Moy Foong Ming
Julius Centre University of Malaya, Department of Social and Preventive Medicine, Faculty of Medicine, University of Malaya, Kuala Lumpur, Malaysia

Rokiah Pendek
Department of Medicine, Faculty of Medicine, University of Malaya, Kuala Lumpur, Malaysia

Lily Li, Marvin Lin, Maria Krassilnikova, Katya Ostrow, Amanda Bader, Brian Radbill, Anita Mehrotra, Jaime Uribarri, Joji Tokita, Staci Leisman and Vijay Lapsia
Division of Nephrology, Icahn School of Medicine at Mount Sinai, New York, New York, United States of America
Department of Medicine, Icahn School of Medicine at Mount Sinai, New York, New York, United States of America

Randy A. Albrecht
Department of Microbiology, Icahn School of Medicine at Mount Sinai, New York, New York, United States of America
Global Health and Emerging Pathogens Institute, Icahn School of Medicine at Mount Sinai, New York, New York, United States of America

Adolfo García-Sastre
Department of Medicine, Icahn School of Medicine at Mount Sinai, New York, New York, United States of America
Department of Microbiology, Icahn School of Medicine at Mount Sinai, New York, New York, United States of America
Global Health and Emerging Pathogens Institute, Icahn School of Medicine at Mount Sinai, New York, New York, United States of America

Andrea D. Branch
Department of Medicine, Icahn School of Medicine at Mount Sinai, New York, New York, United States of America
Division of Liver Diseases, Icahn School of Medicine at Mount Sinai, New York, New York, United States of America

Peter S. Heeger
Division of Nephrology, Icahn School of Medicine at Mount Sinai, New York, New York, United States of America
Department of Medicine, Icahn School of Medicine at Mount Sinai, New York, New York, United States of America
Recanati Miller Transplantation Institute, Icahn School of Medicine at Mount Sinai, New York, New York, United States of America
Immunology Institute, Icahn School of Medicine at Mount Sinai, New York, New York, United States of America

Vincent Billard, Alain Ourry, Anne Maillard and Philippe Etienne
Normandie Université, Caen, France
UNICAEN, UMR 950 Ecophysiologie Végétale, Agronomie et nutritions N, C, S, Caen, France
INRA, UMR 950 Ecophysiologie Végétale, Agronomie et nutritions N, C, S, Caen, France

Maria Garnica and José Maria Garcia-Mina
Timac Agro Spain, Poligono de Arazuri-Orcoyen, Orcoyen, Spain

Laurent Coquet and Thierry Jouenne
Plateforme de protéomique PISSARO, UMR6270 CNRS Facultédes Sciences de Rouen, Mont-Saint-Aignan, France

Florence Cruz and Jean-Claude Yvin
Centre de Recherche International en Agroscience, CRIAS-TAI, Groupe Roullier, Dinard, France

Julia Gollhofer, Roman Timofeev and Thomas J. Buckhout
Institute of Biology, Humboldt University Berlin, Berlin, Germany

Ping Lan
State Key Laboratory of Soil and Sustainable Agriculture, Institute of Soil Science, Chinese Academy Sciences, Nanjing, PR China

Wolfgang Schmidt
Academia Sinica, Institute of Plant and Microbial Biology, Taipei, Taiwan
Graduate Institute of Biotechnology, National Chung Hsing University, Taichung, Taiwan

Genome and Systems Biology Degree Program, College of Life Science, National Taiwan University, Taipei, Taiwan

Lisa A. Houghton, Michelle J. Harper and Rosalind S. Gibson
Department of Human Nutrition, University of Otago, Dunedin, New Zealand

Andrew R. Gray
Department of Preventive and Social Medicine, University of Otago, Dunedin, New Zealand

Pattanee Winichagoon,Tippawan Pongcharoen and Sueppong Gowachirapant
Institute of Nutrition, Mahidol University, Salaya, Thailand

Elizabeth M. Miller
Department of Anthropology, University of South Florida, Tampa, Florida, United States of America

Yang Du., Yanhui Gao., Fangang Meng, Shoujun Liu, Zhipeng Fan, Junhua Wu and Dianjun Sun
Center for Endemic Disease Control, Chinese Center for Disease Control and Prevention, Harbin Medical University; Key Lab of Etiology and Epidemiology, Education Bureau of Heilongjiang Province & Ministry of Health (23618504), Harbin, China

Marlene Perignon, Marion Fiorentino, Jacques Berger and Frank T. Wieringa
Institut de Recherche pour le Développement, Montpellier, France

Khov Kuong and Chhoun Chamnan
Department of Fisheries Post-Harvest Technologies and Quality Control, Ministry of Agriculture, Forestry and Fisheries, Phnom Penh, Cambodia

Kurt Burja
United Nations World Food Programme, Phnom Penh, Cambodia

Megan Parker
PATH, Seattle, Washington, United States of America

Sek Sisokhom
Department of Psychology, Royal University of Phnom Penh, Phnom Penh, Cambodia

Arnaud Laillou
UNICEF, Maternal Child Health and Nutrition section, Phnom Penh, Cambodia

Elizabeth Yakes
University of New Mexico, Department of Individual, Family and Community Education and Department of Family and Community Medicine, Albuquerque, New Mexico, United States of America

Thi Hop Le and Bach Mai Le
National Institute of Nutrition (NIN), Nutrition section, Hanoi, Vietnam

Frank Tammo Wieringa and Jacques Berger
Institut de Recherche pour le Développement (IRD), Unité Mixte de Recherche 204 "Prévention des malnutritions et des pathologies associé es", Montpellier, France

Regina Moench-Pfanner
Global Alliance for Improved Nutrition (GAIN), Singapore Office, Singapore, Singapore

Lin Yan and Lana C. DeMars
Grand Forks Human Nutrition Research Center, United States Department of Agriculture, Agricultural Research Service, Grand Forks, North Dakota, United States of America

Index